AF699350

WITHDRAWN

The Chemistry and Physiology of the Human Plasma Proteins

Pergamon Titles of Related Interest

Abraham Microscopic Innervation of the Heart and Blood Vessels in Vertebrates Including Man

Birke et al Physiology and Pathophysiology of Plasma Protein Metabolism

Fareed et al Perspectives in Hemostasis

Kelemen Physiopathology and Therapy of Human Blood Disease

Maupin Blood Platelets in Man and Animals

Peeters/Wright Plasma Protein Pathology

Rosenoer et al Albumin Structure, Function and Uses

The Chemistry and Physiology of the Human Plasma Proteins

Proceedings of a Conference
Held 19-21 November 1978 in
Boston, Massachusetts
Sponsored by the
Center for Blood Research

Edited by

David H. Bing

Pergamon Press
NEW YORK • OXFORD • TORONTO • SYDNEY • FRANKFURT • PARIS

Pergamon Press Offices:

U.S.A.	Pergamon Press Inc., Maxwell House, Fairview Park, Elmsford, New York 10523, U.S.A.
U.K.	Pergamon Press Ltd., Headington Hill Hall, Oxford OX3 0BW, England
CANADA	Pergamon of Canada, Ltd., 150 Consumers Road, Willowdale, Ontario M2J, 1P9, Canada
AUSTRALIA	Pergamon Press (Aust) Pty. Ltd., P O Box 544, Potts Point, NSW 2011, Australia
FRANCE	Pergamon Press SARL, 24 rue des Ecoles, 75240 Paris, Cedex 05, France
FEDERAL REPUBLIC OF GERMANY	Pergamon Press GmbH, 6242 Kronberg/Taunus, Pferdstrasse 1, Federal Republic of Germany

Copyright © 1979 Pergamon Press Inc.

QP
99.3
.P7
C43
1979

Library of Congress Cataloging in Publication Data
Main entry under title:

The chemistry and physiology of the human plasma proteins.

Proceedings of a meeting held November 19-21, 1978 in Boston and sponsored by the Center for Blood Research.
Includes index.
1. Blood proteins—Congresses. I. Bing, David H.
II. Center for Blood Research. [DNLM: 1. Blood proteins—Congresses. 2. Chemistry, Physical—Congresses.
WH400 C517 1978]
QP99.3.P7C43 612′.12 79-10742
ISBN 0-08-023860-2

All Rights reserved. No part of this publication may be reproduced, stored in a retrieval system or transmitted in any form or by any means: electronic, electrostatic, magnetic tape, mechanical, photocopying, recording or otherwise, without permission in writing from the publishers.

Printed in the United States of America

CONTENTS

PREFACE

On November 19-21, 1978, the Center for Blood Research held a meeting in Boston, Massachusetts to commemorate fifty years of research on the proteins of human plasma carried out by the Harvard Medical School Group working under the leadership of Dr. E.J. Cohn, and by their successors in laboratories all over the world. The meeting coincided with the 25th anniversary of the founding of the Protein Foundation, the parent organization of the Center for Blood Research. This book contains the proceedings of that conference.

I would like to thank a number of people for their assistance in organizing this meeting and the subsequent publication of this book. First, I would like to express by gratitude to all the participants for their excellent presentations and contributions to this book. The Center for Blood Research is indebted to The Commonwealth Fund for its support in the publication of this book. Without the unfailing efforts of Mr. Francis G. Shaw and Mrs. Jean S. Gregory, the meeting would never have taken place. I would like to recognize the dedicated help of Mrs. Rachelle Rosenbaum, not only with the meeting, but in the typing, editing and indexing of this book. Finally, I would like to express gratitude to the individuals at Pergamon Press, and Mr. Laszlo Straka in particular, for their help in preparation of this book.

David H. Bing, Ph.D.
Center for Blood Research
Boston, Massachusetts

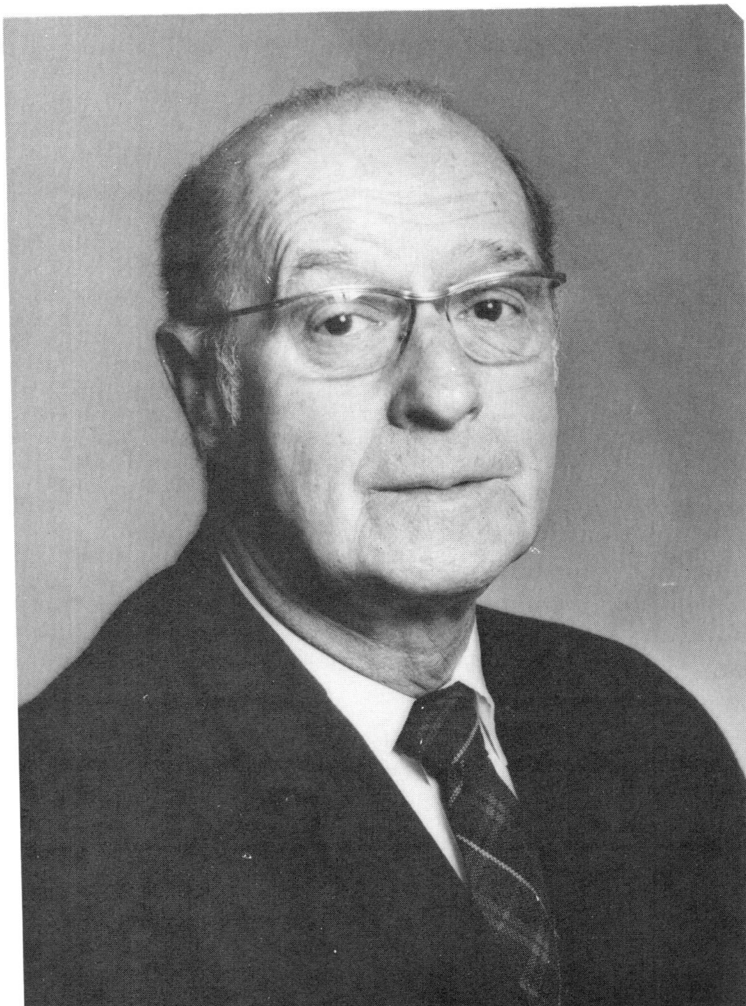

Robert B. Pennell
Director of Laboratories
Center for Blood Research
Boston, Massachusetts

INTRODUCTION

It is appropriate to dedicate this volume to Robert B. Pennell. In the last twenty-five years of the fifty years of research being commemorated by this congress, his energies, scholarship and administrative skills were applied totally and undividedly to the pursuit of goals and the execution of initiatives made by Doctor Edwin Cohn. His long and distinguished career has encompassed translocations, from Harvard Medical School to the Bussey Laboratories to the Center for Blood Research, and the several reorganizations, from the University Laboratory of Physical Chemistry related to Medicine and Public Health to the Protein Foundation, the Blood Research Institute and now the Center for Blood Research.

All of Doctor Pennell's formal education was taken at Michigan State University where he earned a B.S. in 1930, the M.S. in 1932 and the Ph.D. in immunology in 1937 under Doctor I.F. Huddleson. In 1939 he joined Sharp and Dohme Co. in Philadelphia as Research Associate, where, in 1950, he became Assistant Director of Immunochemical Research in the Sharpe and Dohme Division of Merck and Company. While here, he became acquainted with Doctor Cohn when sent to Boston to learn Cohn fractionation methods 6 and 9. After three years of long range collaboration with Doctor Cohn and associates, he was recruited in 1953 to join the newly created Protein Foundation. He was its first employee, assuming the title of Chief of the Chemical Division. In 1956, he became Lecturer in Immunology at Harvard School of Public Health. When the reorganization to form Blood Research Institute occurred in 1966, he was named Acting Scientific Director, a post he held for the ensuing five years.

We first met Bob Pennell by telephone from Boston to Philadelphia, having been referred to him by Doctor Cohn for help in obtaining leukocytes for the study of blood lysozyme. In his usual gracious and cooperative way, he promised buffy coat white cells from the days collection of blood. That night, when we met the plane, we were astonished to receive a gallon jug with buffy coat "cream" skimmed from two thousand donors! It was a supply which took years to consume. Bigness was a characteristic of Doctor Cohn's group, from brains and concepts, to engineering, technology and accomplishments. Bob Pennell was an integral member.

In the historical reminiscences made by the eminent speakers at the opening session of these meetings, one can discern many and varied ways that Bob Pennell quietly, modestly, but always competently, carried out the functions of investigator, administrator, and good friend to his colleagues. Reference was made by Doctor Surgenor of the size of the plasma fractionation industry at the present day, a descendant of the pioneering days; and Doctor Janeway traced its early trials. The World War II caused acute needs for blood and attempts to make and use bovine albumin were modestly successful, but troublesome immunologically. The military, pressured and reluctant, was persuaded artfully by Cohn to support the fractionation of human plasma, and the group was on its way. The complete reversal in attitude of the military to the acceptance of Cohn methods and the extent to which they were developed and applied is exemplified in 1970 by the gift by the

Defense Department to Blood Research Institute of 2,000 pounds (that's right, one ton!) of surplus, outdated, human albumin, condemned because of pyrogens. It was Bob Pennell's frustrating duty to collect it from laboratories and industries around the country and try to find a way to salvage the material. The Navy, too, invested heavily in a program of cryogenic red cell preservation at the Chelsea Naval Hospital under Doctors Tullis, Pyle and Pennell at a time when red cell freezing was a laboratory curiosity. Today, blood freezing has spawned a new industry and the Navy Blood Preservation Laboratory, now independent, is the foremost in the world.

Bob Pennell participated in the pioneering research on fractionation and the methods of blood collection now in standard use. The use of ion-exchange resins as anticoagulants to remove calcium ion was explored and eventually abandoned. Nevertheless, these efforts launched the career of Doctor Harry Antoniades, Senior Investigator at the Center for Blood Research, who observed that insulin activity, and later Hageman factor and serum growth factor, were removed from plasma by the resins. During this developmental period of the refinement of fractionation methodology and new applications, Doctor Pennell served for fifteen years on the Subcommittee on Plasma of the Division of Medical Sciences of the National Research Council, the last nine years of which he chaired the Committee. It was the function of this Committee to advise government agencies related to health and defense on all research relative to use of blood and its components. The many forums and symposia it sponsored were the most stimulating any young investigator could be privileged to attend. Indeed, they were in many respects like the sessions of the meeting published in this volume.

In the opening session of these symposia, Doctor Alper began his remarks by exhibiting a bottle containing 100 gms of properdin found among the old stock of chemicals moved from the Bussey Laboratories into the new building of the Center for Blood Research, --- obviously impressed with the grand style and scope of Doctor Cohn's program. All but a few were unaware that the isolation and properties of properdin was the subject of the Ph.D. thesis many years earlier by Fred Rothstein, present in the audience, but then a graduate student in biochemistry at Harvard under Doctors Oncley and Pennell.

In the transition from the glorious times of Doctor Cohn through the hard economic period which followed after his death, Bob Pennell devoted most of his energies to keeping the Protein Foundation and later the Blood Research Institute solvent and functioning. Operating from a tiny cubicle office in the multi-partitioned and overcrowded Bussey Laboratory, his responsibilities were compounded many-fold when the happy dream, a new building on the present site, became a reality. He coordinated moves of the senior staff from various scattered laboratories, coped with architects, builders, staff, the city, and neighbors. Only a few of us fully appreciated his unstinting, tireless, and unselfish dedication to the truly Herculean task. We all tried to continue to function, with the minimum of interruption while he sacrificed his own scientific work to make us comfortable and productive. In this most difficult period (1970-1973) he was also responsible for renewing annually the Institute Program Project Grant, the main source of operational funds. Single-handedly (almost) he wrote voluminous progress reports and renewal proposals, often just from data or rough copy supplied by busy investigators. From 1961-1971, as principal investigator, he was responsible for and successfully raised these funds. With what time he could generate, he and his close friend and colleague, Jack Bergen of the Worcester Foundation, conducted research on the identification of chemical factors in plasma related to schizophrenia. After the merger with Blood Grouping Laboratory made time available to him to concentrate on research, one of his biggest frustrations ever was his inability to raise funds through grant channels to continue the project.

To dedicate a volume to Bob Pennell without commenting on his extraordinary character would be an injustice. The adjectives, kind, gentle, self-effacing, courteous, considerate, unassuming, and the cliche, gentleman's gentleman, do not exaggerate. In the opening session, remarks by Doctor Tullis, bedridden with flu and unable to attend, were read by Pennell. Doctor Tullis cited the difficult times of 1952 when he and Pennell met weekly to struggle with financial problems and decide how to meet the payroll. The tenure of the Protein Foundation "hung by a gossamer thread". For these years and many to follow Bob Pennell was the thread.

Fabian J. Lionetti
Senior Investigator
Center for Blood Research
November 27, 1978

PHYSICAL CHEMISTRY AT HARVARD MEDICAL SCHOOL: THE FIRST TWENTY YEARS

John T. Edsall
Harvard University, Biological Laboratories, Cambridge, Massachusetts 02138

THE FOUNDING OF THE DEPARTMENT OF PHYSICAL CHEMISTRY

The Department of Physical Chemistry at Harvard Medical School was unique, both in name and in character, among medical school departments. To explain its origins I must note that my father, David Linn Edsall, had become Dean of Harvard Medical School in 1918. One of the early problems that faced him was that of holding Lawrence J. Henderson at Harvard. Henderson was the discoverer of buffer action, and the author of a series of papers on the physical chemistry of blood -- studies that were to culminate ten years later in his great monograph "Blood". He was also the author of an influential monograph on the biological significance of the properties of matter: "The Fitness of Environment" and of a sequel entitled "The Order of Nature". He had been teaching a pioneer course on the history of science in Harvard College for some years. Yet, in spite of his brilliance and his versatility --- partly indeed perhaps because his range of interests was so broad --- he had not yet received adequate recognition from the Harvard Administration. Johns Hopkins University was trying to lure him away with a very attractive offer, and David Edsall was determined to keep him at Harvard if possible. Suitable action became possible because the Medical School had just received a gift of two million dollars, later increased to four million, through the will of an enterprising industrialist, Captain Joseph R. DeLamar. This was the largest single gift that the Medical School had ever received up to that time, and it went to support research in several departments. David Edsall used a fraction of it to set up a new Department of Physical Chemistry with Henderson in charge. Its responsibility was to pursue research fundamental to medicine, with no specific obligations for teaching medical students. Henderson happily accepted the proposal, and decided to stay at Harvard.

Henderson had long ceased to be a laboratory worker, and he needed someone to take charge of the laboratory in the new Department. For this he turned to his former student, Edwin Joseph Cohn, who had done his Ph.D. thesis partly with Henderson, and partly with Frank Lillie at Chicago and Woods Hole. After completing his Ph.D. thesis, Cohn made the decision to devote his scientific life to the study of proteins. He began by going to the laboratory of the foremost protein chemist in the country --- Thomas Burr Osborne in New Haven. Our involvement in World War I soon brought him back to Harvard, to take part with Henderson in a project for making bread from potatoes and other sources; what flour was in short supply, during the war, and making bread from other sources was an important practical problem.

With the war over, Cohn received one of the first of the National Research Council Fellowships, and went in 1919 to Copenhagen to work with the great Danish protein chemist S.P.L. Sørensen. Although he spent only about six months there, this experience was crucial for Cohn's subsequent career, and greatly influenced his choice of research problems in the next few years. He returned to Harvard Medical School in 1920, to take up the work of the Department of Physical Chemistry. From the beginning Henderson gave him a very free hand, and within a relatively short time he was for practical purposes the head of the laboratory. Henderson turned his main energies to research on blood and his associates at the Massachusetts General Hospital, and later at the Fatigue Laboratory in the Harvard Business School.

In those early years the Department occupied only part of the fourth floor of Building C1 at the Medical School; later it gradually expanded. On the floor below were the Laboratories of Physiology, under the direction of Walter B. Cannon. Professor Cannon had an operating room for this animal experiments on the fourth floor, adjoining Cohn's Department. At the farther end of the hall, in what later became Edwin Cohn's office, was Professor William T. Porter, another physiologist. When Porter retired in 1928, Cohn took over that section of the fourth floor also. With Cohn in the laboratory were Ronald M. Ferry, later to become Master of John Winthrop House at Harvard, and Selig Hecht, who was in the early stages of his distinguished career in the physiology of vision, before he moved permanently to Columbia. Jessie L. Hendry was the first expert laboratory assistant, followed not long after by Ruth E.L. Berggren and Adela M. Prentiss.

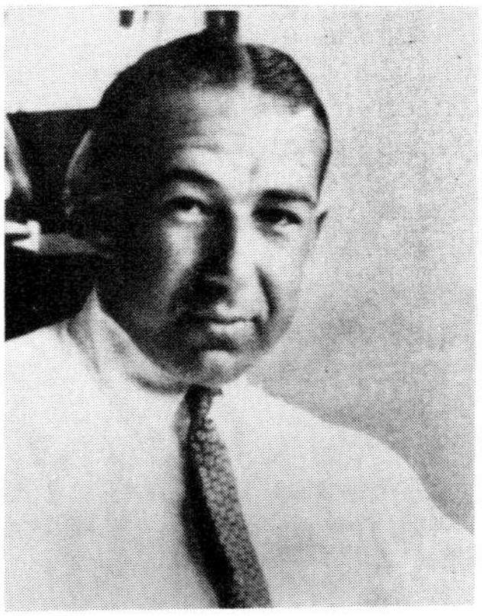

Fig. 1 Edwin J. Cohn as a young man. From M. Florkin "History of Biochemistry" in M. Florkin and E.H. Stotz (editors) Comprehensive Biochemistry, Vol. 30. Elsevier Publishing Co., Amsterdam and New York 1972.

EARLY RESEARCH ON PROTEINS

From the beginning, Cohn (of whom an early photograph is shown in Fig. 1) concentrated on the factors determining the solubility of proteins, and on their behavior as acids and bases --- problems that had already been intensively studied in Sørensen's laboratory. From the beginning Cohn assumed, like his mentors Osborne and Sørensen, that the general laws of physical chemistry applied to proteins, provided that one made due allowance for their large sizes and multiple electric charges. In his titration studies he did his best to correlate the capacity of proteins to take up or release protons with their content of acidic and basic amino acid residues. The correlation was often imperfect, owing largely to the great difficulties that existed in those days in doing amino acid analyses.

Cohn did not do such analyses himself, but relied on the best available data in the literature, and sought advice from his friend H.B. Vickery in New Haven. The titration curves were done on the hydrogen electrode; glass electrodes did not come into use in the laboratory until the middle 1930s. From the start Cohn rejected the notion, then still fashionable among many of the colloid chemists, that proteins might bind hydrogen or hydroxyl ions by some rather vaguely defined process of adsorption. He held strictly to the view that combination occurred by chemical binding to acid or basic amino acid side chains. At that time he tacitly assumed that all the acid and basic side chains were freely titratable in the native protein. The idea that proteins could unfold reversibly, in acid or alkaline solution, so as to make groups titratable which had been inaccessible in the native protein, was not to emerge until much later, and Cohn was by no means the first to perceive it.

The studies on solubility involved both the "salting in" of euglobulins by dilute salt solutions, and their salting out in concentrated salt. Both phenomena, of course, had long been known; and Hofmeister in Strassburg, about 1890, had described the series of salts (or rather of anions and cations) that bears his name, in terms of their capacity to precipitate proteins at high salt concentration. Cohn's first notable contribution to the interpretation of salting out was his plot of the logarithm of the protein solubility (S) against the salt concentration (C_S) or the ionic strength, which have a straight line at high salt concentrations, according to the equation:

$$\text{Log } S = \beta - K_S C_S \qquad (1)$$

Here K_S is the salting out coefficient, and β is a constant.

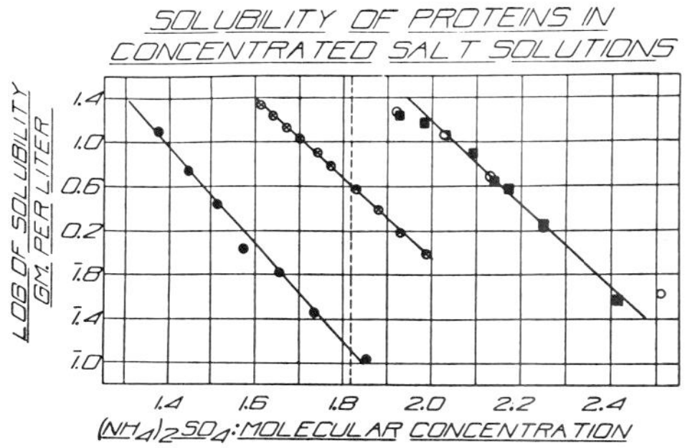

Investigators	*Protein*	*Symbol*
Chick and Martin (45, Table 1)	Egg albumin	○
Chick and Martin (45, Table 2)	Egg albumin	■
Sørensen and Høyrup (323, Table 40)	Egg albumin	⊗
Sørensen (319)	Pseudoglobulin	●

Fig. 2 The linear logarithmic relation for the salting out of proteins. From E.J. Cohn (1925) Physiol. Reviews 5, 349.

The equation is illustrated in Fig. 2, taken from Cohn's original plot in his comprehensive review of 1925. The data are not his; he took them from the published papers of Chick and Martin and of Sørensen, who certainly had had no thought of such a logarithmic relation. The fit to the linear relation is impressive, and it is interesting to note that it is just as good for Sørensen's pseudoglobulin, which was certainly a heterogeneous mixture of components, as for the highly purified ovalbumin.

Cohn's thinking about salting out, and many other matters, was certainly greatly influenced by his friend George Scatchard of M.I.T. Cohn and Scatchard had known each other as undergraduates at Amherst, and they were not then particularly congenial; but, as Scatchard was later to write in his Cohn Memorial Lecture: "Soon after I came to M.I.T. in 1923, Cohn and I attended a reception of the Science Club of Amherst College for Niels Bohr. We stayed with a mutual friend and drive back to Cambridge together. I was surprised to find that he thought more like me than anybody I had ever met. His thoughts were more developed and polished than mine, but there was little other difference. From that day we became close friends and frequent collaborators although we never published a paper together." Scatchard was much more deeply grounded than Cohn in fundamental physical chemistry and mathematics. Cohn was the more dynamic of the two, eith driving force as an organizer, and a remarkable capacity for bringing diverse people together in cooperative research. Their abilities were in many ways complementary. I well remember the important part that George Scatchard played in the departmental seminars, from the very beginning of my work in the laboratory in 1926. It was very rare, indeed almost unheard of, in those days for a "pure" physical chemist like Scatchard to come and listen to biochemists, and even to clinical investigators, and discuss their problems with them, patiently and at length. His scientific publications were generally hard reading, with rigorous thinking and highly condensed presentation. Students in his undergraduate course were reported to have a hard time understanding him. Some indeed referred to the time of his lectures as "the mystery hour". Nevertheless in personal discussion he could be almost endlessly patient in going over difficult points, with others less deeply versed in physical chemistry, until his interlocuter gradually began to take it all in. I am glad to express my own enduring gratitude to him for generout help and advice over many years. There are others in this gathering who can say the same.

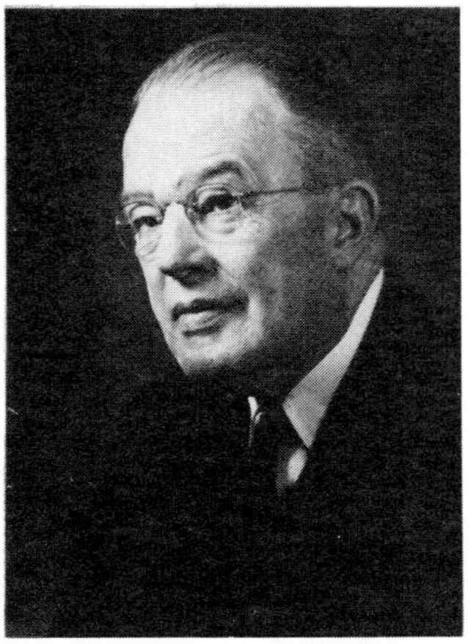

Fig. 3 George Scatchard in 1954.

A masterly experimenter in the solubility work was Dr. Arda Alden Green, who did an outstanding series of studies on horse carboxyhemoglobin. She determined both salting in and salting out curves, for a variety of salts, as well as studying the influence of pH on solubility. The solubility of course was at a minimum, at or near the isoelectric point of the protein, and it increased on going either to lower or to higher pH. She found the salting out coefficient, K_s, for any given salt, to be independent of temperature and pH; change of either of these variables displaced the linear portion of the salting out curve up or down, parallel to itself, but did not change the slope. Figure 4 gives an example of her solubility data for several salts over a wide range of ionic strength.

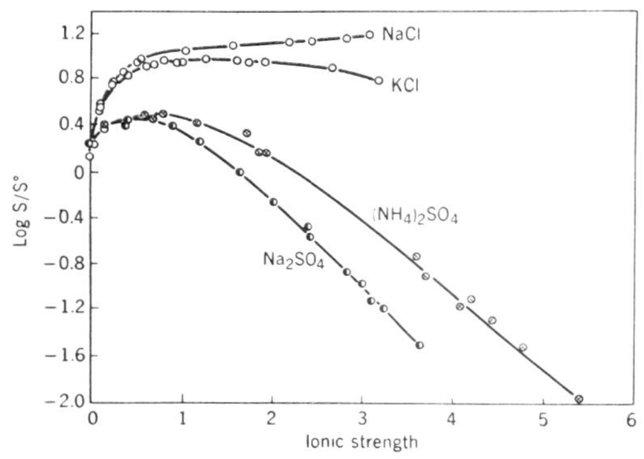

Fig. 4 The salting-in and salting-out of horse carboxy-hemoglobin by various salts. From the work of Arda A. Green [J. Biol. Chem. 93, 495-516, 517-542 (1931); 95, 47-66 (1932)] as plotted by E.J. Cohn and J.T. Edsall (1943, p. 608).

Beginning about 1926 Cohn, while actively continuing his protein studies, devoted much effort to an attempt to purify the anti-pernicious anemia factor in liver. George R. Minot's work had demonstrated the curative properties of liver in this disease, and a search for the active principle was obviously called for. The work of Cohn and his associates was a practical triumph, for they prepared a concentrated liver extract that saved patients from the previous necessity of eating about 200 g of liver a day in order to stay well. Yet for Cohn the outcome was a bitter disappointment, for he never got the active principle in pure form; indeed his extracts never even approached purity. Attempts to find an assay for the active component in animals proved fruitless. It was not until much later, in 1948, that a successful bacterial assay was developed, and pure vitamin B-12 was at last obtained, but not in Cohn's laboratory.

When I joined the laboratory in 1926, working in my limited free time while I was a third year medical student, Cohn set me to work on a globulin from muscle which had already been studied before me by W.T. Salter. It was messy stuff to handle, and gave extremely viscous solutions. I sometimes came close to despair in working on it. The arrival of Alexander von Muralt from Switzerland in 1928 opened entirely new vistas, when he showed us that a flowing solution of the globulin showed strong double refraction, which disappeared when the flow stopped. This indicated that the protein particles were long and asymmetrical. That simple observation led us to two years of joint research, in which Alex's superb experimental resourcefulness, and his knowledge of physics in relation to biology, enabled us to learn much about what was evidently an important component of the structural basis of muscular contraction. Following earlier workers, we called the protein myosin. Today it is clear, from the work of Albert Szent-Gyorgyi and others, that it was a form of what would now be termed actomyosin.

THE SECOND DECADE: THE STUDY OF AMINO ACIDS AND PEPTIDES AS PROTEIN MODELS

Beginning about 1930, and continuing for almost exactly a decade, the Laboratory undertook a far-reaching study of the physical chemistry of amino acids and peptides. It had become apparent that proteins were such complex molecules, with still unknown structures, that even the beautiful solubility studies of Arda Green were largely uninterpretable in theoretical terms. It was necessary to turn back to studies on simpler compounds of known structure, the amino acids, peptides, and related molecules, which contained the characteristic groups present in proteins, to provide models for interpreting the protein studies.

The initial emphasis was on the electrostatic interactions arising from the charged groups present in amino acids, peptides, and proteins. E.Q. Adams in a pioneer study in 1915, and Niels Bjerrum in a more comprehensive analysis eight years later had pointed out clearly that a simple amino acid, like glycine, at its isoelectric point, must exist in aqueous solution predominantly as the zwitterion, or dipolar ion, with a positively charged ammonium and a negatively charged carboxylate group. Comparison of the ionization constants of the amino acids with those of closely related compounds made this plain; in retrospect it seemed astonishing that no one had perceived it before. Thus isoelectric amino acids should be involved in strong electrostatic interactions with other molecules and ions in the solution. At pH values well above or below their isoelectric points they would of course be ions carrying a net charge, which would also be involved in electrostatic interactions of longer range.

The effects of the electrostatic forces between ions on the thermodynamic properties of salts, especially in media of high dielectric constant, had been elucidated by Debye and Hückel in 1923. Their treatment was strictly accurate only at low ionic strength, but it brought order and clarity into a field of research that had been highly confused. From the time their work had appeared, Cohn and Scatchard had been well aware of its important implications for protein studies. However, Debye and Hückel had developed their theory only for ions carrying a net charge. Similar forces must be important between the dipolar ions, such as amino acids, and their surroundings; but the quantitative relations must be quite different. In an α-amino acid, the centers of positive and negative charge are only about 3 Å apart. The electrostatic forces around such a dipole must fall off much more rapidly with distance than in the case of an ion carrying a net charge. In 1930 there was no adequate theory for such systems. At a series of informal discussions and seminars in the Department, in which George Scatchard was heavily involved, the matter was debated. Fortunately a younger colleague of Scatchard at M.I.T., John G. Kirkwood, was drawn into the discussion. Scatchard and Kirkwood developed a theory for a so-called dumbbell model of an amino acid --- two charged spheres, one positive, one negative, connected by a rigid rod. This proved useful for some calculations, but the model was clearly inadequate. Kirkwood then carried the analysis much further by calculating the behavior of spherical and ellipsoidal models, with charges located inside them at suitable positions. These models proved to be readily applicable to the actual solubility data on amino acids and peptides that were being obtained by Cohn and by T.L. McMeekin, who had joined the Department in 1930.

The experiments showed, in accord with Kirkwood's calculations, that simple amino acids like glycine were salted in by neutral salts. However, as predicted, the logarithm of the solubility of the amino acid, at low ionic strength, was a linear function of the first power of the ionic strength, not of its square root as in the case of interaction between two salts. If one decreased the dielectric constant of the solvent, for instance by working in an ethanol-water mixture instead of water as solvent, the solubility of a dipolar ion at zero ionic strength was greatly diminished; but the effect of added ions in increasing the solubility was greater than in water, because the electrostatic forces were stronger in medium of low dielectric constant.

Isoelectric cystine, which is a quadrupole with two positive and two negative charges, gave solubility curves that showed salting in at low, and salting out at high, ionic strength. The form of the curves, and the relative effects of different salts, as shown in Fig. 5, are strikingly similar qualitatively to Arda Green's data for hemoglobin; but the magnitude of the effects in cystine is very much smaller. It is a sort of miniature model for the behavior of hemoglobin.

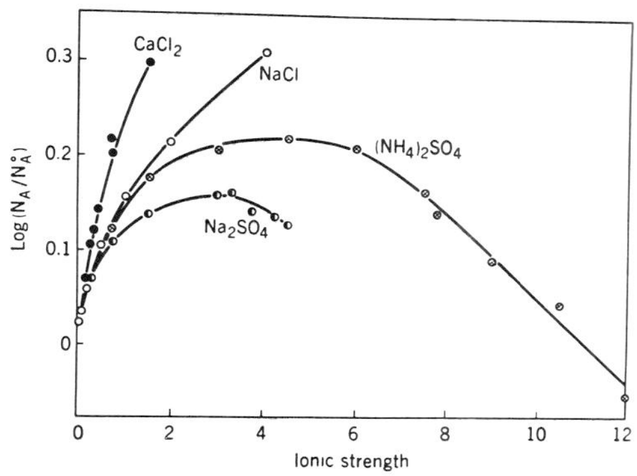

Fig. 5 The salting-in and salting-out of cystine. Data of T.L. McMeekin, E.J. Cohn and M.H. Blanchard, J. Amer. Chem. Soc. (1937) 59, 2717-2723. Compare with the data of Fig. 4 on hemoglobin; note the difference in scale of both abscissa and ordinate on the two figures.

The solubility studies revealed also the great importance of non-polar groups in determining relative solubility in different media. For this work I think we are much indebted to Dr. McMeekin, who studied the solubilities of a wide range of shrewdly chosen organic compounds. There was so much discussion, and interchange of ideas within the group, that it is impossible to say just who suggested what, but I would certainly assign much of the credit to McMeekin.

One specific example will illustrate the relations involved. Glycine at 25°C is about 7400 times as soluble in water as in ethanol, expressing the solubility in moles per liter. Alanine, with one more CH_2 group, is about 2200 times as soluble in water as in ethanol. In other words, the added CH_2 group reduces the value of this solubility ratio by a factor slightly greater than three; and such a ratio is characteristic of methylene groups generally, making allowance for a few special conditions that I need not discuss here. Similar rules were found to apply for other non-polar groups. These effects, which we certainly recognized as of major importance, are due to what would today be called hydrophobic interactions. Yasuhiko Nozaki and Charles Tanford have explored them in greater depth and refinement in recent years, and have formulated rules for calculating the free energy of transfer between various media in their relation to the nature of the polar and non-polar groups involved. Let me add that we certainly make no claim to having discovered hydrophobic interactions in the 1930s. That had happened long before, and the man who deserves the initial credit is probably Isidor Traube, who had observed such effects of non-polar groups when studying surface tensions of aqueous solutions, near the end of the nineteenth century.

Even an α-amino acid should have a very high dipole moment in water, of the order of 15 Debye units. Peptides, or β, γ, δ, and ε amino acids, with a greater separation between the charged groups, should have still higher moments. One would thus expect their aqueous solutions to have higher dielectric constants than that of pure water, for which the value is very high to begin with (78.5 at 25°C). Jeffries Wyman, who had spent a year in Cohn's laboratory in 1927-28, and then moved to the Harvard Biology Department in Cambridge, undertook the study of dielectric constants, and developed an instrument that was a great improvement on anything previously available. The results, obtained in collaboration with McMeekin, were striking. A one molar solution of glycine had a dielectric constant 22.5 units higher than pure water; a one molar solution of glycylglycine had an increment of 70 units. Indeed these increments turned out to be a simple linear function of the number of atoms in the chain, between the positively charged amino and the negatively charged carboxyl group. This was probably the most direct evidence of all for the dipolar ion structure of these compounds. It also led Wyman to propose relations governing dielectric properties of polar liquids, which stimulated Onsager at Yale, and Kirkwood at Cornell, to develop theories of major importance for such systems.

The dipolar ion structure had other implications that we had never suspected when the research started. For example, the partial molal volume of an amino acid dissolved in water --- that is, the increment in volume when one mole of amino acid is dissolved in a very large amount of water --- was substantially smaller than the corresponding value for an isomeric compound that was not a dipolar ion. Thus the value for glycine was some 13 cm^3/mole less than for the isomeric compound glycolamide. The difference was due, not to any shrinkage of the amino acid molecule itself, but to the interactions of its charged groups with the surrounding water which cause the water molecules to pack more tightly around the charged groups in the amino acid; a phenomenon known as electrostriction. These volume effects were first reported in a paper by Cohn, McMeekin, Muriel Blanchard and myself in 1934; and I would pay tribute here to Mrs. Blanchard, whose superb technical skill made an essential contribution, not only to this research, but to a number of the others I have mentioned.

Electrostriction effects also showed up dramatically in the study of heat capacities. At 5°C the addition of a small amount of glycine to water actually lowers the heat capacity of the system, due to the relative immobilization of water molecules around the charged groups of the amino acid. On the other hand, the added CH_2 group in alanine, compared to glycine, induces an extraordinary increase in the heat capacity increment when the amino acid dissolves in water; the increment per CH_2 in aqueous solution, for a homologous series of compounds, is of the order of 20-23 cal deg^{-1} mol^{-1}, whereas it is only 6-8, in the same units, in a homologous series of pure organic liquids. This is another manifestation of hydrophobic interactions, which was not at all understood at the time, and is still something of a puzzle, but all subsequent work has confirmed it. Nobody in the Harvard laboratory was competent to do such heat capacity measurements; fortunately we were able to enlist Professor Frank T. Gucker, then at Northwestern University, who did very beautiful and convincing measurements.

In studies of Raman spectra of amino acids and related compounds in water, I was able to observe the characteristic vibrational frequencies of various ionizable groups, both in the charged and in the uncharged state. This also proved to give decisive evidence for the dipolar ion character of amino acids and peptides.

Dr. Jesse P. Greenstein, later to become a leader in cancer biochemistry at the National Cancer Institute in Bethesda, was through all of this period an extraordinary resourceful investigator in the synthesis of peptides, and in studying their ionization constants and other properties. Later, while still in the

Harvard Laboratory, he undertook important studies on protein denaturation, and on the reactivity of sulfhydryl groups in native and denatured proteins.

Although the main emphasis of the laboratory in the 1930s was on amino acids and peptides, there was still an active concern with proteins. When Larry Oncley moved over from M.I.T. to the Medical School in 1935, he launched the Department into a nre realm of research, with his studies on the dielectric properties of protein solutions. These gave not only the dielectric increments and dipole moments of the proteins, from measurements at low frequencies, but also permitted him to study their rotary diffusion coefficients and relaxation times, by work at higher frequencies. From this, some inferences could be drawn, concerning both the size and shape of a protein molecule. Moreover in 1938 the Laboratory acquired its first ultracentrifuge --- an air-driven model of the type developed by Beams and Pickels, the forerunner of the Spinco instrument; and Dr. Oncley was in charge of the ultracentrifuge also. John D. Ferry arrived in 1936, working with Oncley on the dielectric properties of proteins, and beginning those studies on the mechanical properties of substances of high molecular weight, which he has later pursued with outstanding results. John W. Mehl came to us from Berkeley, also in 1936, and continued very effectively the studies of flow birefringence that von Muralt and I had begun earlier on myosin.

By 1938 Edwin Cohn was eager to return to the study of proteins. The work on amino acids and peptides had provided a theoretical background for a more rational attack on the problems of fractionating individual proteins from the complex mixtures found in nature. With Ronald Ferry he was measuring the solubility of carboxyhemoglobin in ethanol-water mixtures at -5°C, and was turning his attention also to the proteins of blood plasma.

With the outbreak of war in Europe in 1939, and the evidence that the United States might soon be involved, the pace of work in the laboratory accelerated, and its character changed. The work of the 1930s had involved absorbing problems of basic research; the work seemed highly abstract to many of our colleagues at Harvard Medical School, some of whom doubted whether it would ever have any relevance to medicine. Within two years, from 1939 to 1941, the situation had become transformed by the insistent demand of the Armed Forces for blood, blood plasma, and plasma fractions, for those who were in service in the field, at sea, and in the air. The Department of Physical Chemistry, guided by the vision of Edwin Cohn entered a new era, very unlike anything it had known before, which was to make it famous in many research centers and clinics throughout the world --- but that takes us far beyond my story of this afternoon.

REFERENCES

Since this article deals with events long past, I have not tried to cite individual references in the text, but offer instead here a list of references that provide further detail concerning the people and events I have discussed.

Concerning Harvard Medical School, Including the Department of Physical Chemistry

H. K. Beecher and M. D. Altschule, in Medicine at Harvard: the First Three Hundred Years, University Press of New England, Hanover, N.H., p. xiv + 587 (1977).

On Research in the Department of Physical Chemistry, to 1940:

E. J. Cohn, The physical chemistry of the proteins, Physiol. Rev. 5, 349-437 (1925).

E. J. Cohn and J. T. Edsall, in *Proteins, Amino Acids and Peptides as Ions and Dipolar Ions*, Reinhold, New York, p. xviii + 700 (1943); reprint by Hafner, New York (1965).

On the History of the Department, 1920-1950:

J. T. Edsall, A historical sketch of the Department of Physical Chemistry, Harvard Medical School, 1920-1950, *Am. Scientist* 38, 580-593 (1950). In slightly extended form, this formed part of a booklet "University Laboratory of Physical Chemistry related to Medicine and Public Health, 1950", published by the University Laboratory (copies are now very scarce).

Biographical Articles and Personal Recollections:

J. T. Edsall, Edwin J. Cohn, *Ergebnisse der Physiol.* 48, 23-48 (1955). This contains an extensive bibliography of the work of Cohn's associates, as well as his own papers.

J. T. Edsall, Edwin Joseph Cohn 1892-1953, *Biog. Mem. Nat. Acad. Sci.* 35, 47-84 (1961).

G. Scatchard, in *Equilibrium in Solutions* and *Surface and Colloid Chemistry*, Harvard University Press, p. xxxv + 306 (1976). The introduction, by I. H. Scheinberg, contains personal recollections by several associates of Scatchard and Cohn, and a short autobiography by Scatchard.

G. Scathard, Edwin J. Cohn and protein chemistry, *Vox Sanguinis* 17, 37-44 (1969).

J. T. Edsall and W. H. Stockmayer, George Scatchard, 1892-1973, *Biog. Mem. Nat. Acad. Sci.* in press (1979).

CELLULAR PRESERVATION AND INTERACTION OF CELLS AND COAGULATION PROTEINS

James L. Tullis
New England Deaconess Hospital and Center for Blood Research, Boston, Massachusetts

This paper is intended to be both historical and current in content. It was my privilege to join Dr. Cohn's distinguished group in early 1949 on the suggestion of Dr. Louis K. Diamond. The plasma fractionation work of the prior decade which resulted from the fundamental studies, as reviewed so well by Dr. Edsall, had led to a vast storehouse of protein fractions for potential therapeutic work. However, Dr. Cohn was aware that half of the content of each unit of blood was discarded before the plasma fractionation process began as the logistics of red cell use did not permit simplified distribution. He foresaw the economic and sociologic need to salvage this precious commodity. "Would you be interested," he asked, "in starting a cytology section in the laboratory to work on the separation, stabilization and preservation of red cells, white cells and platelets and when that is completed to devote time to a study of the interaction of such cells with coagulation proteins?" Does a rat like cheese? It may have taken me a day to begin work, but it was more like four hours, three of which were spent in saying yes I would work in his lab, provided I need not give up clinical medicine and one hour of which was spent by Dr. Cohn explaining that he would tolerate such abberant behavior if I confined clinical medicine to the hours between 3:00 A.M. and breakfast when he occasionally rested.

What were some of the sequelae of this brief companionate marriage, which only lasted the few years from then until his untimely death; but which influenced my personal research and that of the subsequent students to whom I have been privileged to pass the baton over the subsequent three decades?

The first was the completion and development of biomechanical equipment for the collection and processing of blood. Dr. Cohn made the oft-repeated statement that one would never know the true state in nature of blood cells and plasma proteins unless each part could be isolated promptly and atraumatically from the other substances with which it normally interacted. And certainly, the then common practice of collecting blood through rubber tubing, into naked (uncoated) glass bottles containing a sea of warm citrate at a pH of about 5, was not physiologic. Because of this, Dr. Cohn conceived the scheme of a centrifuge connected directly to a donor in which a film of blood flowed through the centrifugal field with the lighter plasma rising to the central core and overflowing as an effluent stream while the red cells, white cells and platelets aligned themselves in layers according to density following which they too were displaced into separate containers (1)(2)(3). In 1951, Dr. Cohn asked me to accompany him to Portugal to demonstrate a model of this apparatus which had been assembled in the Harvard Medical School shops. Two events stand out clearly from that memorable week. Directly before we appeared on the program of the Blood Congress, Henry Sloviter who had been working in Aubrey Smith's laboratory in England, demonstrated the freezing of a test tube containing glycerolized blood and its subsequent thawing without red cell lysis. I was so impressed with the absence of broken cells I could talk of little else. But Dr. Cohn's thoughts raced ahead. "Freezing will not be practical for blood preservation unless you get the glycerol back out," he blurted. It's alright for the preservation of bull sperm" - which incidentally had prompted the experiments - "but stored blood is transfused back into an 0.3 osmolar aqueous solution." Turning, he said, "When we get home, I want you to adapt this machine to glycerolizing and deglycerolizing red cells in a simple, bacteriologically sterile system." I don't recall that he even said, "please." Protestations that my interests were in platelets and clotting proteins would have been useless. I heard myself reply, "Yes" (4)(5)(6).

With the constant collaboration and support of Mr. Robert Tinch, with whom I have been privileged to labor during the subsequent 30 years, and with the vision and encouragement of Dr. Surgenor and others, it was possible after Cohn's death to adapt this awkward apparatus into a centrifuge which not only would glycerolize and wash red cells, but which was able to be adapted for such widespread uses as plateletpheresis, leucophoresis, plasmapheresis, and diverse other clinical applications. Those of us who were in on the beginning of such developments occasionally look with petulance at the manifold plastic copies which have sprung up on every side. However, it is fitting that reproductions should appear. If Cohn were here, he would say piracy is flattery.

The other event I recall from that remote congress in Lisbon was the actual demonstration of that early model of the blood separator. While Cohn lectured on the principles of continuous flow centrifugation, it was my duty to stick a needle into the vein of a volunteer donor on an examining table down on the floor of the amphitheater. The event began faultlessly. Blood coursed through the tubing and entered the centrifuge bowl which in those days was made of glass. A spotlight was trained on the bowl. The audience leaned forward in their seats to see the whirling container of blood layer itself neatly into red cells, yellow plasma and white buffy coat. If all went well, the first effluent plasma would overflow in 4½ minutes. As I held the phlebotomy needle with one hand on the donor's arm and Dr. Cohn talked on, I held an old-fashioned pocket watch in my other hand. Four minutes 10 seconds, 4 minutes 20 seconds, 4 minutes 30 seconds. Suddenly, there was a cacophony of sound as congress members in the lower four rows of the amphitheater scrambled over the backs of their seats to reach higher ground. Little did Dr. Cohn or I know that the night before we had sailed to Portugal, an enthusiast in the Harvard shops had siliconed the whole apparatus, to please us with non-wettable surfaces (7). The silicone had of course plugged up the effluent hole, causing the revolving seal to break down when the pressure of the entering blood reached a critical full-bowl level - thus sending a sunburst shower of good Portuguese Rosé blood over the lower tier of the auditorium.

I should like to jump over the next 26 years with only a precis, as that period included the tenuous era when the survival of Protein Foundation hung by a gossamer thread. Dr. Pennell and I would meet for lunch once a month with George Batchelder and Charles Janeway, not to dream of grandiose experiments in the field of blood, but to face such mundane matters as how to meet the next month's payroll for that small hard core of loyal employees that remained with us. During that period, the work with which it was possible to move forward was heavily weighted toward studies on the interaction of platelets and clotting proteins. The by-line of first the Protein Foundation, then the Blood Research Institute and finally, the Center for Blood Research also accompanied the development of such clotting fractions for human use as factor-VIII-rich fibrinogen (8), factor V or Ac globulin (9) as it was then known - truly a protein in search of a disease, factor II - VII - IX - X concentrate for the treatment of Christmas disease (10) and of course platelet concentrates for treatment of thrombocytopenia and as an in-vitro reagent for platelet antibody tests (11).

That moves us to recent years. To illustrate the present state of the art, I would like to make brief reference to the current work of two former students and present colleagues of mine - Drs. Murray Bern and Francis Chao. There are numerous others whom I don't want to demean by omission. I mention these two only because they epitomize the traditions which have passed down from the original group in the University Laboratory of Physical Chemistry at Harvard Medical School of which I was only transiently a part. Dr. Bern has shown well the manner in which human platelets play an innocent bystander role in diverse immune events. This had been hypothesized by many workers especially in the field of renal allograft transplants due to the profound thrombocytopenia and organ specific D.I.C. which heralds rejection. The unique feature is, that he dared to cross disciplinary lines - a difficult task when it comes time to get results accepted for publication. By immunizing rabbits with tuberculin, he was able to demonstrate selective adhesion of arterial platelets to beads which were coated with appropriate antigen (12). Dr. Chao, on the other hand, has made his greatest contribution by exemplifying the adage to work with simple mixtures when studying cell-protein interactions in-vitro. By observing the effects of physical variables such as concentration, on a simple 3-phase system of platelets, fibrinogen and thrombin, he uncovered the startling fact that platelets are stimulative to the action of thrombin on fibrinogen in high concentrations of thrombin and inhibitory when the concentration of thrombin is reduced to a few thousand molecules per platelet (13). This is illustrated in Figure 1 which shows a standardized thrombin time in which the effect of platelet concentration is evident.

Figure 1. Effect of Platelet Concentration on Thrombin Time.

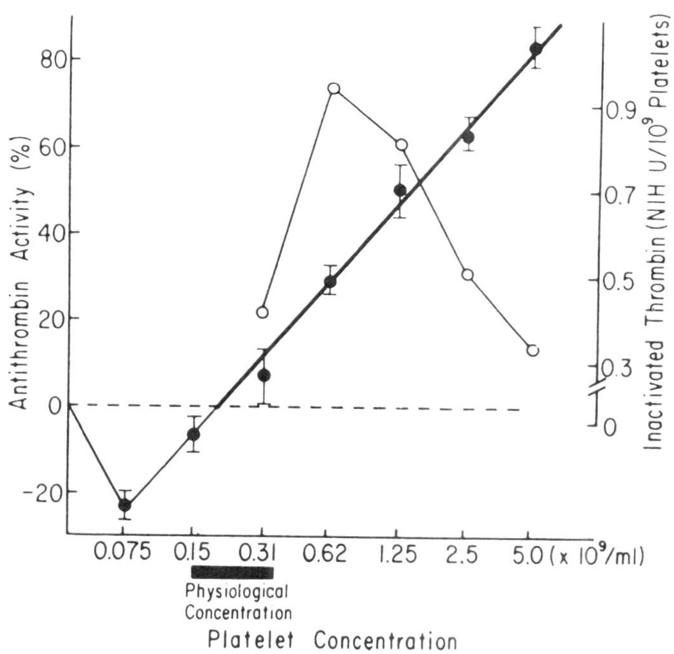

In low platelet numbers there is a negative antithrombin activity. Once the platelet numbers exceed .15 x 10^9, there is a stepwise increase in antithrombin activity as plotted on the solid circles or decrease in amount of thrombin inactivated as plotted on the open circles. I remember the excitement with which Dr. Chao showed me this data one evening about 8:00 P.M. when we both should have been home eating supper with our weary wives. Our first concerns were that this represented only an artifact of washing the platelets before placing them in the system. However, we subsequently were able to show by a simple sequential concentration of platelets in their native plasma (Table 1) that unwashed platelets also inhibit the action of thrombin on fibrinogen when one works at very low thrombin concentrations.

TABLE 1

PLATELET ANTITHROMBIN
Effect Count on Thrombin Time

Platelet Concentration/mm^3	Percent Thrombin Inactivated Thrombin Concentration	
	2U	1U
10,000,000	38	79
4,000,000	33	57
2,000,000	13	47
1,000,000	13	21
500,000	3	10
200,000	3	13
P.P.P.	0	0

Final test = 0.2 ml platelet suspension + 0.2 ml Thrombin mixture

As can be seen in the left hand column where 2 units of thrombin/ml were employed, there is a stepwise increase in thrombin inhibition as the platelet numbers are increased from standard concentrations of normal blood up to a maximum of 10 million/mm^3 which can be reached in-vivo under extreme conditions of excess marrow activity. In this instance there was a maximum inactivation of 38% of the added thrombin. In a similar system shown on the right hand column of Table 1, the thrombin concentration is further reduced to 1 unit/ml. The percent inactivated by platelets then rises to 79% at the highest platelet concentration.

Thus, our knowledge of platelet antithrombin began. Time prevents a detailed discussion of its nature. However, subsequent studies in the past two years have shown that it is comprised of two separate interactions (14)(15). Approximately 75% of the activity represents membrane binding of thrombin at specific binding sites on platelets demonstrated elsewhere by Ganguly et al. Twenty-five percent is due to binding of thrombin to extruded intracellular fibrinogen at the time of platelet activation. Platelet antithrombin is totally distinct from the well known plasma antithrombins, and it is not inactivated by antithrombin III antibody. Having thus found evidence of a new role for platelets in the physiology of hemostasis in the microcirculation, the next step was to develop a routine assay that could quantitate this observation and make possible a delineation of the role, if any, of platelet antithrombin under physiologic and pathologic conditions. The two-stage test, as devised by Dr. Watanabe, a hematology fellow who worked with us, is simple and consists of a 10-minute incubation of 1 x 10^9 washed platelets and 2 units of thrombin following which the residual unbound thrombin is measured in a standard fibrinogen clotting time. In assays on several hundred controls and patients with non-thrombotic or hemorrhagic disorders, it was found that the thrombin inactivation ranged from 34 to 71% with a median of almost exactly 50%. In an equally broad study of thrombotic disorders, we have identified platelet antithrombin deficiencies in myeloproliferative diseases such as polycythemia vera, and primary thrombocythemia in which there is a close correlation between the thrombotic phase of the disease, and evidence of decreased thrombin binding by this assay. Figure 2 shows such a relationship.

Figure 2

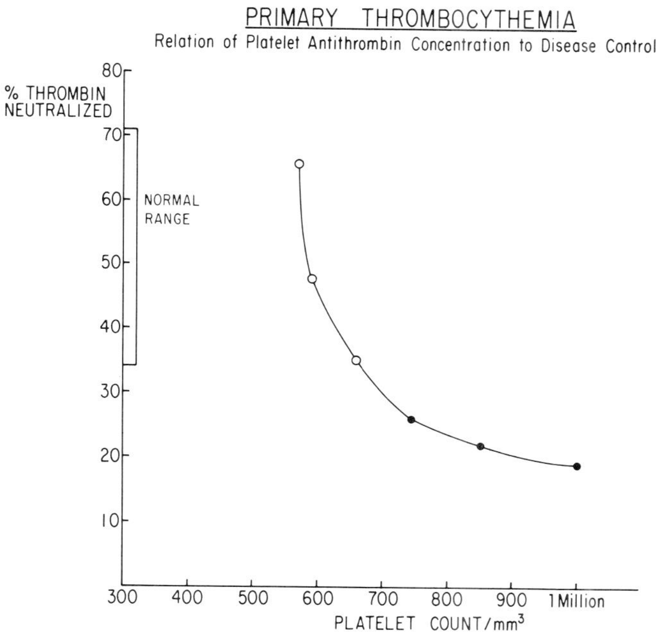

This patient with a typical thrombocythemia accompanied by clotting rather than bleeding has been repeatedly followed during uncontrolled phases of her disease and subsequent remissions induced by chemotherapy, or radiation. It can be seen that when her disease is uncontrolled as evidenced by high concentrations of circulating platelets in the range of 1 million, platelet samples removed from her circulation and tested in standard normal concentrations in the antithrombin test show a striking reduction in thrombin binding to 18%. With stepwise improvement in her platelet numbers as a reflection of improvement in her disease after radiation theraphy, there is proportional increase in thrombin binding per individual platelet until one sees normal values at the time the population of abnormal platelets is essentially suppressed.

In separate studies it also has been possible to identify a large family in whom a congenial deficiency of this activity is present (16). In recently published data we have advanced the thesis that the families who have been identified elsewhere with congenial antithrombin III plasma deficiency may actually represent a deficiency of platelet antithrombin activity, with their plasma antithrombin deficiency being only a secondary phenomenon.

This vignette of current work is presented as an illustration of which traditions are passed on through succeeding generations of laboratory workers. It is only the people who change, not ideas. The standards of excellence promulgated by the members of that original group of Dr. Cohn's have endured and will keep reappearing like dominant genes.

REFERENCES

(1) J.L. Tullis, D.M. Surgenor, R.J. Tinch, M. D'Hont, F. Gilchrist, S. Driscoll, W.H. Batchelor, New principle of closed system centrifugation, Science 124, 792 (1956).

(2) J.L. Tullis, R.J. Tinch, J.G. Gibson, P. Baudanza, A simplified centrifuge for the separation and processing of blood cells, Transf. 7, 232 (1967).

(3) J.L. Tullis, R.J. Tinch, P. Baudanza, J.G. Gibson, S. Diforte, G. Conneely, K. Murthy, Platelet-pheresis in a disposable system, Transf. 11, 386 (1971).

(4) J.L. Tullis, M.M. Ketchel, H.M. Pyle, R.B. Pennell, J.G. Gibson, R.J. Tinch, S. Driscoll, Studies on the in-vivo survival of glycerolized and frozen human red blood cells, J.A.M.A. 168, 399 (1958).

(5) M.M. Ketchel, J.L. Tullis, R.J. Tinch, S. Driscoll, D.M. Surgenor, Use of biomechanical equipment for the long-term preservation of erythrocytes, J.A.M.A. 168, 404 (1958).

(6) J.L. Tullis, J.G. Gibson, R.J. Tinch, J. Hinman, P. Baudanza, S. DiForte, T. Smith, A.T. Breed, Disposable plastic centrifuge bowls for separation of red blood cells and plasma in the processing of frozen blood, Transf. 11, 358 (1971).

(7) J.L. Tullis and E.G. Rochow, Non-wettable surfaces, Blood 7, 850 (1952).

(8) D.M. Surgenor, C.W. McMillan, L.K. Diamond, B.B. Steele, Studies with AHF-rich fibrinogen in classical hemophilia, Vox Sang. 5, 80 (1960).

(9) D.M. Surgenor, M. Melin, A.S. Henry, L.P. Wheaton, N.A. Wilson, J.L. Tullis, Preparation of Factor V for clinical use, Vox Sang. 5, 77 (1960).

(10) J.L. Tullis, M. Melin, P. Jurigian, Clinical use of human prothrombin complexes, New Engl. J. Med. 273, 667 (1965).

(11) J.L. Tullis, D.M. Surgenor, P. Baudanza, Preserved platelets: their preparation, storage and clinical use, Blood 14, 456 (1969).

(12) M.M. Bern, Platelet immune adhesion to glass beads coated with purified protein derivatives of tuberculosis, Fed. Am. Soc. Exp. Biol. (Abstract) p.217 (1975).

(13) F.C. Chao, J.L. Tullis, D.M. Kenney, Concentration effects of platelets, fibrinogen and thrombin on platelet aggregation and fibrin clotting, Thromb. Diath. Haemorrh. 32, 216, (1974).

(14) K. Watanabe, F.C. Chao, J.L. Tullis, Antithrombin activity of intact human platelets, Thromb. Diath. Haemorrh. 34, 115 (1975).

(15) K. Watanabe, F.C. Chao, J.L. Tullis, Platelet antithrombins: roles of thrombin binding and the release of platelet fibrinogen, Br. J. Haematol. 35, 119 (1977).

(16) J.L. Tullis and K. Watanabe, Platelet antithrombin deficiency, Am. J. Med. 65, 472 (1978).

PROPERDIN, PAST AND PRESENT*

Chester A. Alper
Center for Blood Research, Boston, Massachusetts

In rummaging through the storage areas of the Center for Blood Research, two things emerged. One was a large brown bottle labeled "Human Properdin, Lot 1734, 300 gm," the other was the fact that nothing was ever thrown out at the Protein Foundation. The properdin was purified in the mid 1950's from plasma by the alcohol fractionation methods developed by Dr. E. J. Cohn and his colleagues. It provides me with the opportunity to bridge the historical aspects of this Symposium with the more recent interests of some of us at the descendent organization of the Protein Foundation, the Center for Blood Research.

The history of the properdin or alternative pathway of complement activation is intricately enmeshed in the history of complement research itself and perhaps began with the observation in 1884 that cell-free blood plasma was capable of killing bacteria and other microorganisms (1). This capacity was soon found to be destroyed by heating to 55° for 1 hr (2). Over the next few years, it became apparent from the work of Buchner (3, 4), Pfeiffer and Issaeff (5), Metchnikoff (6), and particularly Bordet (7) and Ehrlich and Morgenroth (8) that "classical" complement activity required antibody for its generation and that the specificity of complement-mediated hemolysis of antibody-sensitized bacteria or red cells resided in the specificity of the antibodies involved. Classical complement activity could be separated into first component (euglobulin) and second component (pseudoglobulin) (9, 10) which interacted with antibody in that order.

More specific information about the alternative pathway probably began with the report in 1894 (11) that serum from rabbits injected with lethal doses of snake venom lost its bactericidal activity. The interaction of cobra venom with mammalian complement was further explored by Stephens and Myers (12, 13) at the

*Supported in part by grants AI 14157, AI 13626, AM 16392 and AI 15033 from the National Institutes of Health, and in part by grant 6-183 from The National Foundation-March of Dimes, and The Charles E. Merrill Trust.

very end of the last century. These authors showed that cobra venom incubated with whole human or animal blood produced hemolysis. At higher doses of venom, no hemolysis occurred, but at lower, effective doses, the hemolytic activity was enhanced by mammalian serum. The ability of serum to mediate the hemolytic action of cobra venom was abolished by heating to 58° for 10 min. These phenomena were pursued further by Flexner and Noguchi (14) who related them to complement as it was then understood. They showed that when mammalian serum was incubated with snake venom, it lost complement activity manifested both as a loss of bactericidal activity and the loss of ability to lyse antibody-sensitized erythrocytes. Their experiments allowed them to conclude that snake venom destroyed complement but had no effect on antibody. They also concluded that passive hemolysis by snake venom required complement. Work by Sachs and Omorokow (15) and Ritz (16) showed that cobra venom did not inactivate either of the two then identified components of complement and that therefore there must be a third component which was destroyed by cobra venom. There was yet another line of experimentation that led toward the conclusion that there must be a third component of complement. It began with the observation that bacteria and yeast destroyed mammalian complement activity (17). Just as with cobra venom treatment, serum incubated with yeast could be restored to full activity with either the first or second component of complement (18). Coca (19) drew these threads together and showed that cobra venom, yeast and certain bacteria all inactivated the same "third component." Browning and Mackie (20), in confirming these findings, also observed that serum depleted of complement by incubation with antibody-sensitized red cells still supported passive hemolysis induced by cobra venom. They prophetically concluded, "It is doubtful . . . if the assumption of an additional 'third component' can explain all the phenomena above described."

It later became apparent that there was a fourth component of complement (21) and that the "third" component was in fact six separate proteins (22-28). Prior to the delineation of these "late acting components," in the mid 1950's, Pillemer and his co-workers demonstrated the existence of a previously unrecognized serum protein, properdin (29), involved in the inactivation of complement by zymosan (a substance extracted from yeast cell wall). Two other proteins were identified in this system, factor A which was hydrazine sensitive (30) and factor B which was destroyed by heating to 50° (31). Magnesium ions (Mg^{++}) but not calcium were essential for activity of the system which was also activated by endotoxin, a wide variety of polysaccharides and perhaps other substances. The existence of this separate pathway was cast into doubt by the finding of natural antibody to zymosan and other polysaccharides in normal serum. It was, therefore, thought by many investigators that C3 consumption proceeded solely by the classical first three complement components (32). Several lines of investigation around 1970 led to a re-evaluation of the properdin pathway and its reacceptance by all in 1971: (1) On repeating the work of Pillemer and his group (29), it was found that with modern quantitative assays for individual complement components, C3 and later-acting components were consumed by endotoxin or zymosan without significant consumption of C1, C4 or C2 (33). (2) Studies of a patient with repeated bacterial infections and continuous consumption of C3 revealed normal levels of C1, C4, and C2 (34, 35), thereby suggesting "that there is an alternative physiological mechanism for the inactivation of C3 that bypasses the first three complement components" (34). (3) Antibodies of the IgG1 subclass in guinea pigs activated C3 with little consumption of C1, C4 or C2 (36). (4) Serum from guinea pigs with a hereditary deficiency of C4 supports C3 consumption by endotoxin (37) and, finally, (5) cobra venom-induced hemolysis and C3 consumption requires a protein which proved to be properdin factor B (38).

Our own work with the patient who appeared to have continuous activation of the alternative pathway led to the isolation and chemical characterization of factor B (39) and the first recognition of the enzyme which, in the presence of C3b, cleaves factor B (40). This enzyme is now known as factor D. When it became apparent that the patient had hereditary deficiency of the C3b inactivator (41, 42), it was possible to show that this protein served as an inhibitor of the properdin pathway.

The work of others defined the role of properdin in the alternative pathway as a stabilizer of its C3 convertase, $\overline{C3bBb}$ (43). Drs. Fearon and Austen give details of the modern view of the properdin pathway as well as observations on the initiating events of activation elsewhere in this book. Here it is enough to point out the continuity of science and our debt to our scientific forbears.

REFERENCES

1. W. Grohmann, Über die Einwirkung des zellenfreien Blutplasma auf einige pflanzliche Microorganismen (schimmel-, spross-, pathogene und nichtpathogene Spaltpilze), Dorpat. C. Mattiesen, 34 (1884).

2. G. Nuttal, Experimente über die bakterienfeindlichen Einflüsse des tierischen Körpers, Z. Hyg. 4, 353 (1888).

3. H. Buchner, Über die bakterientödtende Wirkung des zellenfreien Blutserums. Zbl. Bakt. 5, 817 (1889).

4. H. Buchner, Ueber die nähere Natur der bakterientödtenden Substanz im Blutserum, Zbl. Bakt. 6, 561 (1889).

5. R. Pfeiffer and R. Issaeff, Ueber die spezifische Bedeutung der Choleraimmunität, Z. Hyg. 17, 355 (1894).

6. E. Metchnikoff, Sur la destruction extracellulaire des bactéries dans l'organisme, Ann. Inst. Pasteur 9, 433 (1895).

7. J. Bordet, Sur l'agglutination et la dissolution des globules rouges par le sérum d'animaux injectés de sang défibriné, Ann. Inst. Pasteur 12, 688 (1898).

8. P. Ehrlich and J. Morgenroth, Zur Theorie der Lysin-wirkung, Berl. Klin. Wschr. 36, 6 (1899).

9. A. Ferrata, Die Unwirksamkeit der komplexen Hämolysine in salzfreien Lösungen und ihre Ursache, Berl. Klin. Wschr. 44, 366 (1907).

10. E. Brand, Über das Verhalten der Komplemente bei der Dialyse, Berl. Klin. Wschr. 44, 1075 (1907).

11. C. B. Ewing, The action of rattlesnake venom upon the bactericidal power of the blood serum, Lancet i, 1236 (1894).

12. J. W. W. Stephens and W. Myers, The action of cobra poison on the blood: a contribution to the study of passive immunity, J. Path. Bacteriol. 5, 279 (1898).

29. L. Pillemer, L. Blum, I. H. Lepow, O. A. Ross, E. W. Todd and A. C. Wardlaw, The properdin system and immunity. I. Demonstration and isolation of a new serum protein, properdin, and its role in immune phenomena, Science 120, 279 (1954).

30. J. Pensky, L. Wurz, L. Pillemer and I. H. Lepow, The properdin system and immunity. XII. Assay, properties and partial purification of a hydrazine-sensitive serum factor (Factor A) in the properdin system. Z. Immunitäetsforsch. Exp. Ther. 118, 329 (1959).

31. L. Blum, L. Pillemer and I. H. Lepow, The properdin system and immunity. XIII. Assay and properties of a heat-labile serum factor (Factor B) in the properdin system, Z. Immunitäetsforsch. Exp. Ther. 118, 349 (1959).

32. R. A. Nelson, Jr., An alternative mechanism for the properdin system. J. Exp. Med. 108, 515 (1958).

33. H. Gewurz, H. S. Shin and S. E. Mergenhagen, Interaction of the complement system with endotoxic lipopolysaccharide: consumption of each of the six terminal complement components, J. Exp. Med. 128, 1049 (1968).

34. C. A. Alper, N. Abramson, R. B. Johnston, Jr., J. H. Jandl and F. S. Rosen, Increased susceptibility to infection associated with abnormalities of complement-mediated functions and of the third component of complement (C3), N. Engl. J. Med. 282, 349 (1970).

35. C. A. Alper, N. Abramson, R. B. Johnston, Jr., J. H. Jandl and F. S. Rosen, Studies in vivo and in vitro on an abnormality in the metabolism of C3 in a patient with increased susceptibility to infection, J. Clin. Invest. 49, 1975 (1970).

36. A. L. Sandberg, A. G. Osler, H. S. Shin and B. Oliveira, The biological activities of guinea pig antibodies. II. Modes of complement interaction with γ_1 and γ_2 immunoglobulins, J. Immunol. 104, 329 (1970).

37. M. M. Frank, J. May, T. Gaither and L. Ellman, In vitro studies of complement function in sera of C4-deficient guinea pigs, J. Exp. Med. 134, 176 (1971).

38. O. Götze and H. J. Müller-Eberhard, The C3 activator system: an alternate pathway of complement activation, J. Exp. Med. 134, 90s (1971).

39. T. Boenisch and C. A. Alper, Isolation and properties of a glycine-rich β-glycoprotein of human serum, Biochim. Biophys. Acta 221, 529 (1970).

40. C. A. Alper and F. S. Rosen, Genetic aspects of the complement system, in Advances in Immunology, H. G. Kunkel and F. J. Dixon, eds., Academic Press, New York, p. 251 (1971).

41. N. Abramson, C. A. Alper, P. J. Lachmann, F. S. Rosen and J. H. Jandl, Deficiency of C3 inactivator in man, J. Immunol. 107, 19 (1971).

42. C. A. Alper, F. S. Rosen and P. J. Lachmann, Inactivator of the third component of complement as an inhibitor in the properdin pathway, Proc. Natl. Acad. Sci. (U.S.A.) 69, 2910 (1972).

43. D. T. Fearon and K. F. Austen, Properdin: binding to C3b-dependent C3 convertase, J. Exp. Med. 142, 856 (1975).

ALBUMIN: SEQUENCE, EVOLUTION AND STRUCTURAL MODELS

James R. Brown, Paula Shockley, and Patricia C. Behrens
Clayton Foundation Biochemical Institute, Department of Chemistry
University of Texas, Austin, Texas 78712

ABSTRACT

Human serum albumin is a single chain of 585 amino acids, crosslinded by 17 disulfide bridges. A single cysteine occurs at position 34. The spacing of cystine residues along the chain and pairing to form disulfide bridges occur in repeating patterns which, along with repeated sequence similarities have been explained as the result of gene duplication. It appears that the molecule evolved from a primordial protein of 77 residues containing a double loop formed by two adjacent disulfide bridges. Triplication and a major deletion of this gene gave a protein of about 195 residues. This gene further tripled to give a protein of about 585 residues, similar to human serum albumin. From the differences in sequence between the repeat units, it is estimated that this final stage of growth was reached about 700 million years ago. These repeated homology units revealed by the sequence further suggests that the protein is structurally orgainzed into three major independently folded units or domains and that each domain consists of a pair of similar subdomains. From the high helicity of albumin, restrictions imposed by disulfide bridges, and by the location of proline residues, a three dimensional model is proposed. The basic structural unit of the model is the subdomain which is a trough-like structure formed by three helical rods. A pair of subdomains face each other in a parallel or antiparallel fashion to form a domain which is like a cylinder formed by six parallel rods. A hole through the cylinder is lined with hydrophobic residues and is proposed as the binding site for fatty acids and other ligands containing hydrophobic groups. The outside surface of the cylinder is mainly polar. The model also revealed similarity in three dimensional structure and sequence between the subdomain and the G-H helix region of myoglobin. This led to the hypothesis that the primordial 77 residue protein arose from a gene fragment of a primitive globin.

INTRODUCTION

Albumin, the most abundant of the plasma proteins is a classic protein which has been the object of extensive research for many years, especially in the field of protein chemistry. Its versitility in binding a great variety of ligands such as fatty acids, bilirubin, drugs, dyes and many other organic anions is perhaps its most important property related to its physiological function and it is certainly its most unusual and intriguing property to be explained by its molecular structure. The amino acid sequence of albumin has provided several insites into the structural organization of this protein and has suggested three dimensional models that help explain its unusual binding properties (1-6). The sequence also reveals the evolutionary history of the molecule, indicating that it grew from a small protein of about 77 residues by successive gene duplication (1-7). This chapter will be focused on details of structure and evolution of serum albumin deduced mainly from amino acid sequence and disulfide bridges. Excellent reviews of albumin structure of broader scope than this paper by Joseph Foster (8) and by Theodore Peters and Roberta Reed (9, 10) are recommended. Other aspects of albumin can be found in recent books (11-13).

AMINO ACID SEQUENCE

The amino acid sequence of human serum albumin is given in Fig. 1. The single chain of 585 residues is crosslinked by 17 cystine bridges to form 8 double loops and one single loop. The single loop formed by residues 53-62 was probably part of a large double loop in the past until the bridge linking positions 8 and 54 was lost by mutations. The sequence is layed out so that the Cys-Cys sequences of the 5 large double loops are aligned vertically. The insides of the sequences closed by loops are filled in black to emphasize the similarity of the double loop folding that occurs along the sequence. The single cysteine residue occurs at position 34.

Evaluation of the Human Serum Albumin Sequence

The sequence results from various laboratories were previously summarized and evaluated (5). Subsequently, a large amount of sequence (292 residues, 50% of the molecule) was given by Meloun, Moravek, and Kostka in their summary report of the human albumin sequence (14). Although a number of differences exist between the sequences, they are in about 98% agreement. We are currently trying to resolve these differences and the sequence given in Fig. 1 is only partially updated. The main change from our previous sequence involves relocation of a Cys residue from position 282 to 279 to correspond with the sequence of Meloun and coworkers. Our evidence for the sequence 279-282 was weak and our recent investigation of this sequence has been inconclusive. The location of that Cys residue has important structural implications and the similarity with the other 7 double loops gives extr weight to the correctness of the Meloun sequence.

Proalbumin and Preproalbumin Sequences

When albumin is synthesized in liver it occurs as a precursor called proalbumin (15 It contains an N-terminal hexapeptide, namely Arg-Gly-Val-Phe-Arg-Arg (16, 17). These initial studies were done with rat proalbumin, but the same sequence was foun for the pro-piece of bovine proalbumin (18). Chicken proalbumin has also been studied, however, the sequence of the pro-piece, namely Arg-Asn-Leu-Gln-Arg-Met-Ala-Arg is somewhat different in containing two more residues, Met-Ala, before the C-terminal Arg, but it also contains three Arg residues with one at each end (19). The significance of this pro-piece as a signal peptide to direct albumin from ribosomes into the secretory pathway has been reviewed (20, 21). A further 18 residue N-terminal extension of sequence has been found when albumin is synthesized from messenger in a cell free system and the sequence has been determined as follow Met-Lys-Trp-Val-Thr-Phe-Leu-Leu-Leu-Leu-Phe-Ile-Ser-Gly-Ser-Ala-Phe-Ser-(pro-piece) (albumin) by Strauss and coworkers (22). This is referred to as preproalbumin and the 18 residue extension is called the pre-piece. Pre-pieces have been found similarly for several other secretory proteins such as insulin (23) and parathyroid hormone (24).

EVOLUTION

Albumin as a Molecular Clock for Studies of Evolution and Phylogenetics

The amino acid sequence of human serum albumin can be used in the study of evoluti and phylogenetics by comparing it with the sequence of serum albumin of other species. The amino acid sequences of homologous proteins from different animals serve as molecular clocks, the difference being related to the time of divergence since common ancestry (25). Albumin is well suited for such studies because of its

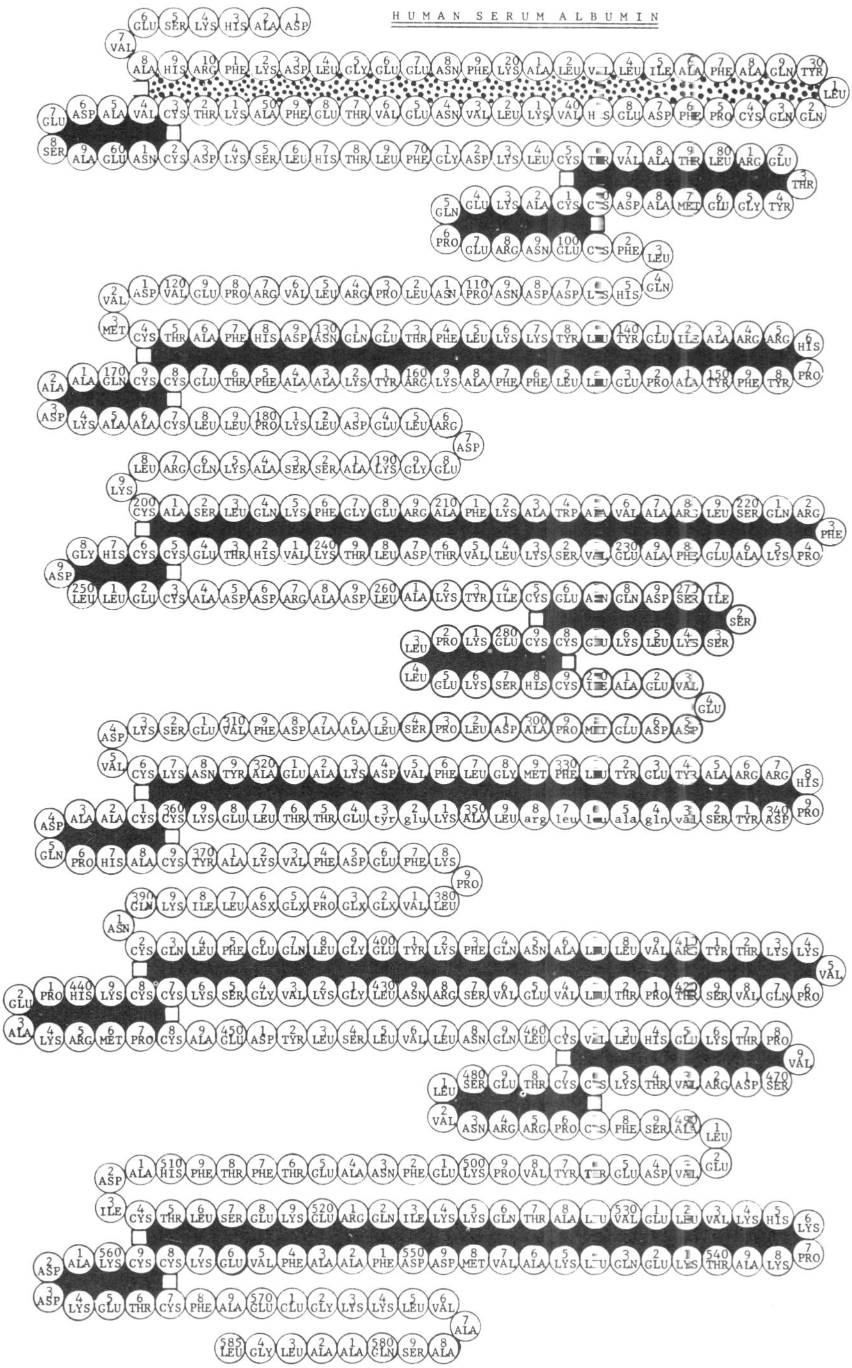

Fig. 1. Amino acid sequence of human serum albumin.

ease of preparation. Its relatively large size and moderately high rate of change make it particularly suited for studying closely related species. Its size is also a disadvantage because of the large amount of work required to complete a sequence At present only human and bovine serum albumins are effectively complete. Partial sequences have been determined for porcine (26, 27), ovine (28), chicken (29), equine (30), and rat serum albumins (31). The sequence of protein is of course much easier if the complete sequence of a closely related homologous protein is available for comparison, especially for overlapping, so that it should be possible to extend the sequence data in the future with less effort. However, albumin has been extensively used as a molecular clock in studies of evolution and phylogenetics based on immunological difference by Wilson and Sarich. This field has been reviewed recently by Sarich (30). From the difference between human serum albumin and bovine serum albumin, the rate of evolution has been calculated as 19 point acceptable mutations per 100 links per 100 million years (31).

Variant Albumins

Many variant forms of hemoglobin have been discovered and studied in detail. At least 25 electrophoretically distinguishable variants of human serum albumin have also been found, but no pathology has so far been related to these variants. The sites of variation have been determined for albumin Oliphant and albumin Ann Arbor by Winters and coworkers (32) as identical and involving the replacement of Glu which occurs at position 570 in normal albumin with a Lys residue. These variants are from unrelated families of German and Danish decent. These are the only variants analyzed so far, but with the complete sequence of human serum albumin available further studies of the site of variation should be encouraged. The field of albumin variants has been reviewed by Shell and Blumberg (33).

Molecular Evolution of Albumin

The most interesting evolutionary insite revealed by the sequence is the evolutionary history of the albumin molecule. The repeated pattern in the spacing of Cys residues along the sequence of bovine serum albumin was the key that lead to the hypothesis that this protein evolved from a small precursor by successive gene duplication that multiplied the structure 9 times (1). This was not apparent until the sequence was effectively complete because little repeated sequence was found except for several Cys-Cys sequences and a tetrapeptide sequence Arg-Arg-His-Pro which occurred twice. Little identical repeated sequence remains because the multiplication of the structure was complete about 700 million years and the repeated homology units have diverged 75 to 80%. The large and small double loops and connection segments in Fig. 1 form a pattern (large loop-small segment-small loop-long segment-large loop-long segment) which occurs three times. The three large homology units of about 195 residues correspond approximately to the three domains that will be described later. This unit was itself the result of triplication of a primordial protein of about 77 residues which corresponded to a single large double loop with some sequence on either side of the loop. A deletion of part of the middle loop and some of the connecting segment to the loop above produced the large-small-large loop pattern of the domain. Three-dimensional models of albumin, specifically the large loops which are proposed as consisting of two helical rods starting at the disulfide bridge and running antiparallel for 20-23 residues to the end of the loop where they are connected by the sequence which makes a hairpin turn, were discovered to be similar in three-dimensional structure to the G-H helix region of myoglobin (2, 3). Furthermore, the bend between the G and H helices has the sequence Arg-His-Pro, which is the same as the sequence at the tips of two of the loops of albumin (see positions 145-147 and 337-339 in Fig. in analogous structural positions. A comparison of the sequences of the albumin large loops with the G-H helix regions of sperm whale myoglobin and human alpha hemoglobin showed that the globin sequences were as close to albumin as they were to each other and this led to the hypothesis that albumin arose from a gene fragme of a primitive globin which was then multiplied by gene duplication (2, 4). The

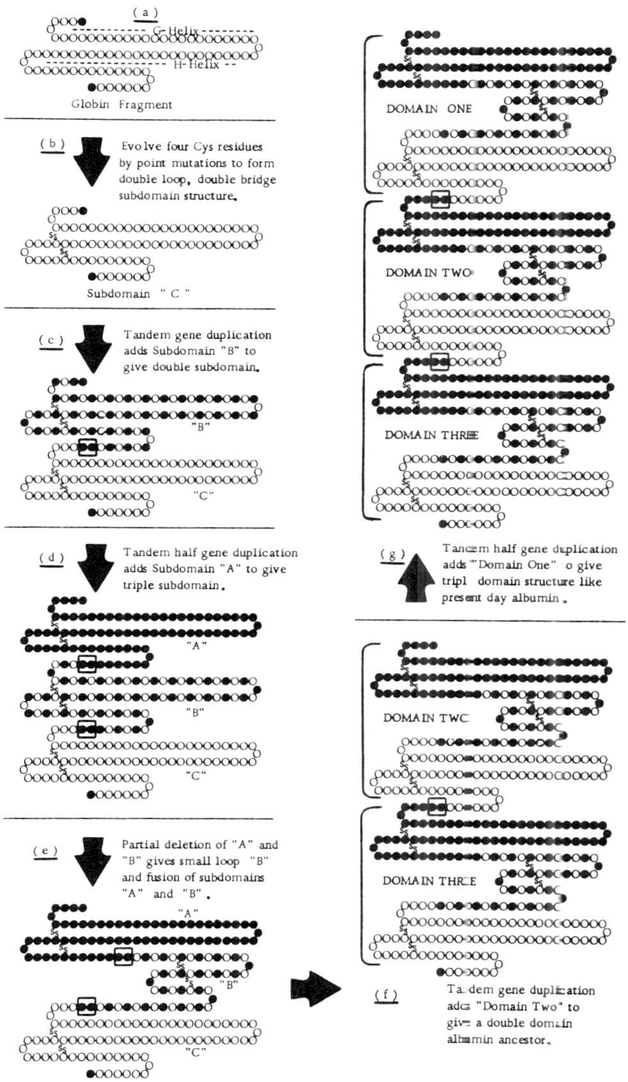

Fig. 2 Evolution of serum albumin

ı) I propose that albumin arose from the partial duplication of a primitive globin gene. This globin gene fragment orresponded to about 78 amino acid residues and included the G- and H-helix regions. (b) The original albumin recursor described above probably did not have the double Cys-bridge since this structure has not been found in present-ay globin molecules. Since many unrelated proteins contain the double Cys-bridge, it is reasonable to assume that ıis structure was introduced by convergent evolution after separation from the globin gene. (c) The basic subdomain ructure was doubled to give a two-subdomain structure shown here as subdomain "B" and "C". (d) A half gene duplication extended the structure to the triple subdomain. (e) The basic single domain structure consists of subdomain C ıd fused subdomains A and B. This resulted in a gene deletion corresponding to a small part of subdomain A and a ırge part of subdomain B. The deletion could have occured simultaneously with the previous duplication, so that the iple subdomain structure may never have existed. (f) Tandem duplication results in a double domain albumin ıcestor. (g) A tandem half gene duplication adds domain one, thus giving the triple domain structure of present-day lbumin. However, the great divergence of sequence between domains (about 80%) indicates that this final stage of ıplication was reached about 700 million years ago. (from Brown, Ref. 5) detailed scheme showing the steps in the evolution of albumin as proposed by Brown (5) is given in Fig. 2. McLachlan and Walker (7) have confirmed this scheme by computer comparison and statistical analysis, except for the common ancestry with myoglobin. They propose that the similarity between albumin and myoglobin is the result of structural convergence. We feel that insufficient similarity between the sequences to support a homologous relationship can in no way disprove that relationship. Many homologous sequences have diverged beyond the point of statistically significant similarity.

Common Ancestry of Albumin and α-Fetoprotein

Partial amino acid sequence of human alpha-fetoprotein has been determined and found homologous with human and bovine serum albumins by Ruoslahti and Terry (36). This is an abundant protein in fetal plasma, but drops to low levels after birth. The function of alpha-fetoprotein is not known, but it binds fatty acids (37) and bilirubin (38) and thus may in fact be a fetal albumin analogous to fetal hemoglobin. The sequences of human, bovine, chicken (29, 39), and alpha-fetoprotein are compared in Fig. 3. The number of differences for the 22 residues which inclu the chicken albumin sequence are as follows: HSA/BSA 4, HSA/CSA 10, BSA/CSA 9, AFP/HSA 12, AFP/BSA 11, AFP/CSA 14. The greater differences between AFP and the albumins than between chicken albumin and the mammalian albumins indicates that the gene duplication that separated albumin and alpha-fetoprotein occurred prior to the separation of birds and mammals. From the time of common ancestry of bovin

	204	5	6	7	8	9	210	1	2	3	4	5	6	7	8	9	220	1
HSA	Gln	Lys	Phe	Gly	Glu	Arg	Ala	Phe	Lys	Ala	Trp	(Ala)	Val	Ala	Arg	Leu	Ser	Gln
BSA	Gln	Lys	Phe	Gly	Glu	Arg	Ala	(Leu)	Lys	Ala	Trp	(Ser)	Val	Ala	Arg	Leu	Ser	Gln
AFP-I	(Lys)	(Asn)	Phe	Gly	(Thr)	Arg	(Thr)	Phe	(Gln)	Ala	(Ile)	(Thr)	Val	(Thr)	(Lys)	Leu	Ser	Gln

	222	3	4	5	6	7	8	9	230	1	2	3
HSA	(Arg)	Phe	Pro	Lys	Ala	Glu	Phe	(Ala)	Glu	Val	Ser	Lys
BSA	Lys	Phe	Pro	Lys	Ala	Glu	Phe	(Val)	Glu	Val	(Thr)	Lys
AFP-I	Lys	Phe	(Thr)	Lys	(Val)	(Leu)	Phe	(Thr)	Glx	(Ile)	(Gln)	
CSA	Lys	(Tyr)	Pro	Lys	Ala	(Pro)	Phe	(Ser)	Glu	Val	Ser	Lys

	262	3	4	5	6	7	8	9	270	1	2	3	4	5	6
HSA	Lys	Tyr	Ile	Cys	(Glu)	Asn	Gln	Asp	(Ser)	Ile	Ser	Ser	Lys	Leu	Lys
BSA	Lys	Tyr	Ile	Cys	(Asp)	Asn	Gln	Asp	Thr	Ile	Ser	Ser	Lys	Leu	Lys
AFP-II	(Ser)	Tyr	Ile	Cys	(Ser)	(Gln)	Gln	Asp	Thr	(Leu)	Ser	(Asn)	Lys	(Ile)	(Thr)

	277	8	9	280	1	2		3	4	5	6	7	8	9	290	1
HSA	Glu	Cys	Cys	(Glu)	Lys	Pro	Gap	Leu	Leu	Glu	Lys	Ser	His	Cys	Ile	Ala
BSA	Glu	Cys	Cys	Asp	Lys	Pro	Gap	Leu	Leu	Glu	Lys	Ser	His	Cys	Ile	Ala
AFP-II	Glu	Cys*	Cys*	(Lys)	(Leu)	(Thr)	Gap	(Thr)	Leu	Glu	(Arg)	(Gly)	(Gln)	Cys*	Ile	(Ile)
CSA	(Ile)	Cys	Cys	Asp	Lys	Pro	(Glx)	(Ile)	(Val)	Glu	(Arg)					

Fig. 3. Comparison of human, bovine, and chicken albumins and α-fetoprotein.

The numbering corresponds to the human serum albumin sequence. The ellipses point out the differences. AFP-I and AFP-II are fragments of alpha-fetoprotein isolated from the cyanogen bromide cleaved protein. *These residues were not well distinguished from Ser.

and human albumins of about 75 million years and of chicken and mammalian albumins of about 300 million years (25), we can make some estimates of the time since the gene duplication separated albumin and alpha-fetoprotein. If we convert the differences to PAMs (point acceptable mutations per 100 residues) according to Dayhoff (25) p. 95, the results are as follows: HSA/BSA 21, CSA/av. HSA and BSA 65, AFP/av. HSA, BSA, and CSA 98. If we take the difference of 65 PAMs between chicken and mammalian albumins as occuring in 300 million years, then the 98 PAMs for the alpha-fetoprotein/albumin difference corresponds to 450 million years. The 21 PAMs between HSA/BSA corresponds to 97 million years, which is a bit high. If we use the total 59 residues of AFP sequence, then the number of PAMs for HSA/BSA is 15 and for AFP/av. HSA and BSA is 93. Taking the 15 PAMs for HSA/BSA as the difference for 75 million years, the value of 93 PAMs for AFP/mammalian albumin corresponds to 465 million years. A more precise estimate of these times can be made when more data are available, but these results are fairly consistent.

STRUCTURAL MODELS

The repeated pattern of loops formed by the cystine bridges of serum albumin which was used to elucidate the evolutionary history of the molecule was also used to deduce details of structural organization (1-7). At the gross level it seems likely that the repeated homology units are similarly folded organized structures or domains. There is in fact much independent evidence that albumin contains domains. The most compelling is that limited proteolysis produces fragments (40-42) and these fragments retain secondary and tertiary structure as well as binding sites (43-47). Physical-chemical studies still earlier (1952-1956) led to the concept of albumin containing domains (48-50). This was perhaps the first protein to be proposed as having this type of structure. A prophetic model of albumin as consisting of two domains with each domain formed by two subdomains was proposed by Joe Foster in 1960 (51). This model is very similar to the model deduced from the sequence (2, 5).

Domains and Subdomains

If the sequence 8-62, which includes the one single loop, is considered structurally similar to a large double loop as it no doubt was in the past before the cystine bridge between positions 8 and 54 was lost, the albumin molecule consists of 9 double loops separated by connecting segments. The simplist hypothesis is that each double loop is organized independently, which leads to a model of albumin containing 9 domains (1). However, three of the double loops are small and the connecting segments are not all the same size. But these loops and connecting segments form a regular pattern that is repeated three times. This major repeat unit contains two large double loops with a small double loop between. It therefore seems likely that these three large units are independently but similarly organized and can be considered as domains. Each double loop within the domain may also be independently folded so that the domain may be formed by a specific association of three subdomains. However, three-dimensional models suggest that the small double loop became incorporated with the subdomain above it when it was formed by a deletion of its large loop precursor and part of the connecting segment above it. Therefore, the model proposed by Brown (5) considers the domain as containing two rather than three subdomains. While the domains and repeated homology units correspond to each other, they are conceptually different and may not have identical boundaries in the sequence. For example, the first homology unit should end at about residue 192, whereas, three-dimensional models suggest that the first domain may end at about 197 or right next to the start of the second domain at 199. The domain boundaries of course can only be certain when the three-dimensional structure is established.

Three-dimensional Models

From restrictions imposed by disulfide bridges, the locations of Pro residues, and the high helicity of albumin of as much as 68% (45), a three dimensional model has been proposed (2, 4-6). The basic structural unit of this model is the subdomain. It is a trough-like structure formed by three helices of about 20 residues each. The three helices are covalently linked at one end by the double Cys-bridge. The middle helix is antiparallel and making contacts along its length with the helices on either side. The Pro residues that occur at the tips of the five large loops (positions 147, 224, 339,416 and 537 in Fig. 1) form part of the bend that connects the two helices within the large loop. The trough-like geometry of the subdomain is based on the Cys-Cys sequence being helical so that there is 100° rotation between the linkages of the middle helix to the adjacent helices. A detailed description of the three-dimensional structures of the six subdomains of human serum albumin is given in Fig. 4. The geometry of the subdomain is illustrated as a view down the axes of the three helices which are depicted as wheels with lines joining adjacent residues in the sequence 100° apart. The heavy line through the three helices is a somewhat arbitrary division between the inside and outside of the subdomain. Examination of Fig. 4 reveals that the inside contains predominantly hydrophobic residues and the outside contains predominantly polar residues. It should be pointed out that the distribution of polar and nonpolar residues played no role in conceiving the model and the favorable distribution was discovered only after the models were built (5). Notable exceptions are in the "X" helices at positions 15 and 16, corresponding to 160° and 260° respectively, where hydrophobic residues are located on the outside. The structural location of any residue of interest in a helix can be found in Fig. 4, for example, the only Trp residue in human serum albumin is at position 214 and in Fig. 4 it occurs at position 15, at 60° in helix-"X"2A. The analogous sequences of the G and H helices of sperm whale myoglobin and human alpha hemoglobin are also included in Fig. 4 for comparison, G-helices with X-helices and H-helices with Y-helices. We believe that the similarities between the globin and albumin helices are striking. Photographic views of the inside and outside of a model of a subdomain of human serum albumin (residues 316-390 in Fig. 1) are given in Fig. 5.

The relationship of the sequence of human serum albumin to domains, subdomains, loops, helices, and connecting hinge segments is illustrated in Fig. 6. The secondary structure of bovine serum albumin has been calculated from the sequence by Reed and Peters (9) according to the method of Chou and Fasman (52). McLachlan and Walker (7) have made similar studies except that they have calculated the structure of the domain as averaged for all three domains of both human and bovine serum albumins. These results are fairly consistant with the model proposed by Brown (5).

Organization of Domains

It is coneivable that all six subdomains are fairly independent and perhaps they should be considered as domains. Fragments have been isolated which correspond to subdomains and some of these fragments retain binding properties (43-47) but it is possible that an isolated subdomain would dimerize to form a domain-like structure The three-dimensional models indicate that the subdomain has an exposed hydrophobic face and since this is thermodynamically unfavorable, a pairing of subdomains in a hydrophobic face to face arrangement seems likely. If a model of a domain is constructed in this way it has very interesting properties. It is a closed cylindrical structure formed by six helices and it has a channel running through it. The outside of the cylindrical surface is highly polar and the channel is lined with hydrophobic groups and appears to be the site for binding fatty acids.

There are however at least three plausible ways in which the subdomains can be paired. The first arrangement to be considered is parallel subdomains. In this structure the tips of the large loops are at one end and the double Cys-bridges are at the other end, similar to the way that the sequence is layed out in Fig. 1. A model of albumin with domains of this type is shown in Fig. 7. Since the first and third domains are connected to adjacent helices in the middle domain, the structure tends to be condenced, relatively spherical, and this does not agree

	HELIX "X"									HELIX "Y"									HELIX "Z"					
Degrees Rotation	1A 8	1C 124	2A 200	2C 316	3A 392	3C 514	HbG 91	MyG 97	Residue Number	1A 54	1C 167	2A 246	2C 361	3A 438	3C 559	HbH 136	MyH 142	Degrees Rotation	1AB 62	1C 177	2AB 253	2C 369	3AB 448	3C 567
100i	ALA	CYS	CYS	CYS	CYS	CYS	LEU	HIS	1	VAL	CYS	CYS	CYS	CYS	CYS	LEU	ILE	0i	CYS	CYS	CYS	CYS	CYS	CYS
200	HIS	THR	ALA	LYS	GLN	THR	ARG	LYS	2	CYS	CYS	CYS	CYS	CYS	CYS	VAL	ASP	100i	ASP	LEU	ALA	TYR	ALA	PHE
300	ARG	ALA	SER	ASN	LEU	LEU	VAL	ILE	3	THR	GLU	GLU	LYS	LYS	LYS	THR	LYS	200	LYS	LEU	ASP	ALA	GLU	ALA
40i	PHE	PHE	LEU	TYR	PHE	SER	ASP	PRO	4	LYS	THR	THR	GLU	SER	GLU	SER	ARG	300	SER	PRO	ASP	LYS	ASP	GLU
140	LYS	HIS	GLN	ALA	GLU	GLU	PRO	ILE	5	ALA	PHE	HIS	LEU	GLY	VAL	VAL	PHE	40i	LEU	LYS	ARG	VAL	TYR	GLU
240	ASP	ASP	LYS	GLU	GLN	LYS	VAL	LYS	6	PHE	ALA	VAL	THR	VAL	PHE	SER	LEU	140	HIS	LEU	ALA	PHE	LEU	GLY
-20i	LEU	ASN	PHE	ALA	LEU	GLU	ASN	TYR	7	GLU	ALA	LYS	THR	LYS	ALA	ALA	GLU	240	THR	ASP	ASP	ASP	SER	LYS
80i	GLY	GLN	GLY	LYS	GLY	ARG	PHE	LEU	8	THR	LYS	THR	GLU	GLY	ALA	LEU	LEU	-20i	LEU	GLU	LEU	GLU	LEU	LYS
180	GLU	GLU	GLU	ASP	GLU	GLN	LYS	GLU	9	VAL	TYR	LEU	TYR	LEU	PHE	PHE	ALA	80i	PHE	LEU	ALA	PHE	VAL	LEU
280	GLU	THR	ARG	VAL	TYR	ILE	LEU	PHE	10	GLU	ARG	ASP	GLU	ASN	ASP	LYS	LYS	180	GLY	ARG	LYS	LYS	LEU	VAL
20i	ASN	PHE	ALA	PHE	LYS	LYS	LEU	ILE	11	ASN	LYS	THR	LYS	ARG	ASP	ASP	ASN	280	ASP	ASP	TYR	PRO	ASN	ALA
120i	PHE	LEU	PHE	LEU	PHE	LYS	SER	SER	12	VAL	ALA	VAL	ALA	SER	MET	LEU	MET	20i	LYS	GLU	ILE	LEU	GLN	ALA
220	LYS	LYS	LYS	GLY	GLN	GLN	HIS	GLU	13	LEU	PHE	LEU	LEU	VAL	VAL	SER	ALA	120i	LEU	GLY	CYS	VAL	LEU	SER
320	ALA	LYS	ALA	MET	ASN	THR	CYS	ALA	14	LYS	PHE	LYS	ARG	GLU	ALA	ALA	GLY	220	CYS	LYS	GLU	GLX	CYS	GLN
60i	LEU	TYR	TRP	PHE	ALA	ALA	LEU	ILE	15	VAL	LEU	SER	LEU	VAL	LYS	HIS	GLN	320	THR	ALA	ASN	GLX	VAL	ALA
160	VAL	LEU	ALA	LEU	LEU	LEU	LEU	ILE	16	HIS	LEU	VAL	LEU	LEU	LEU	VAL	ALA	60i	VAL	SER	GLN	PRO	LEU	ALA
260	LEU	TYR	VAL	TYR	LEU	VAL	VAL	HIS	17	GLU	GLU	GLU	ALA	THR	GLN	ALA	ASP	160	ALA	SER	ASP	GLX	HIS	LEU
0i	ILE	GLU	ALA	GLU	VAL	GLU	THR	VAL	18	ASP	PRO	ALA	GLN	PRO	GLU	PRO	ALA	260	THR	ALA	SER	ASX	GLU	GLY
	ALA		ARG		ARG					PHE	ALA	PHE	VAL	THR	LYS	THR	GLY	0i	LEU	LYS	ILE	LEU	LYS	LEU
100i	PHE	ILE	LEU	TYR	TYR	LEU	LEU	LEU	19	PRO	TYR	GLU	SER	SER	THR	PHE	PHE	100i	ARG	GLN	SER	ILE	THR	
200	ALA	ALA	SER	ALA	THR	VAL	ALA	HIS	20	CYS	PHE	ALA	TYR	VAL	ALA	GLU	ASN	200	GLU	ARG	SER	LYS	PRO	
300	GLN	ARG	GLN	ARG	LYS	LYS	ALA	SER	21	GLN	TYR	LYS	ASP	GLN	LYS	ALA	GLY	300	THR	LEU	LYS	GLN	VAL	
40i	TYR	ARG	ARG	ARG	LYS	HIS	HIS	ARG	22	GLN	PRO	PRO	PRO	PRO	PRO	PRO	PRO	40i	TYR	LYS	LEU	ASN	SER	
140	LEU	HIS	PHE	HIS	VAL	LYS	LEU	HIS	23	32	157	224	339	416	537	114	120		84	199	275	391	470	585
240	GLN	PRO	PRO	PRO	PRO	PRO	PRO	PRO	24															
	32	147	224	339	416	537																		

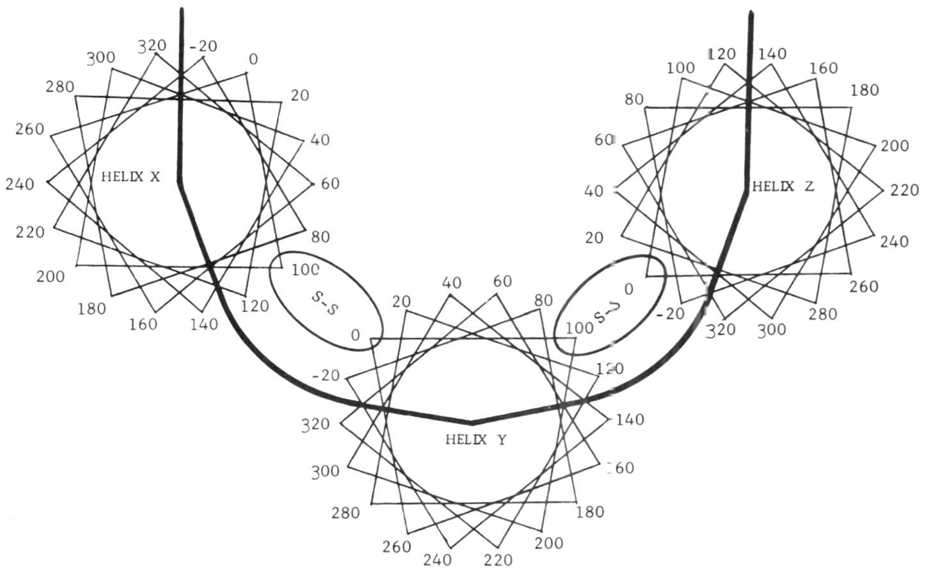

Fig. 4. Subdomain structure and helices of human serum albumin. The 18 helices of human serum albumin are aligned for comparison. The numbers at the top and bottom of the columns of sequence indicate the sequence locations of residues at the ends. The positions of amino acid residues indicated by the column "degrees rotation," correspond with the numbers in the helical wheel diagram of the subdomain, which is a view down the axes of the three helices starting from the Cys-bridges. Lines in the helical wheels connect adjacent residues 100° apart. The sequences of the G and H helices of human alpha hemoglobin (Hb) and sperm whale myoglobin (My) are aligned at their respective Pro residues 114 and 120.

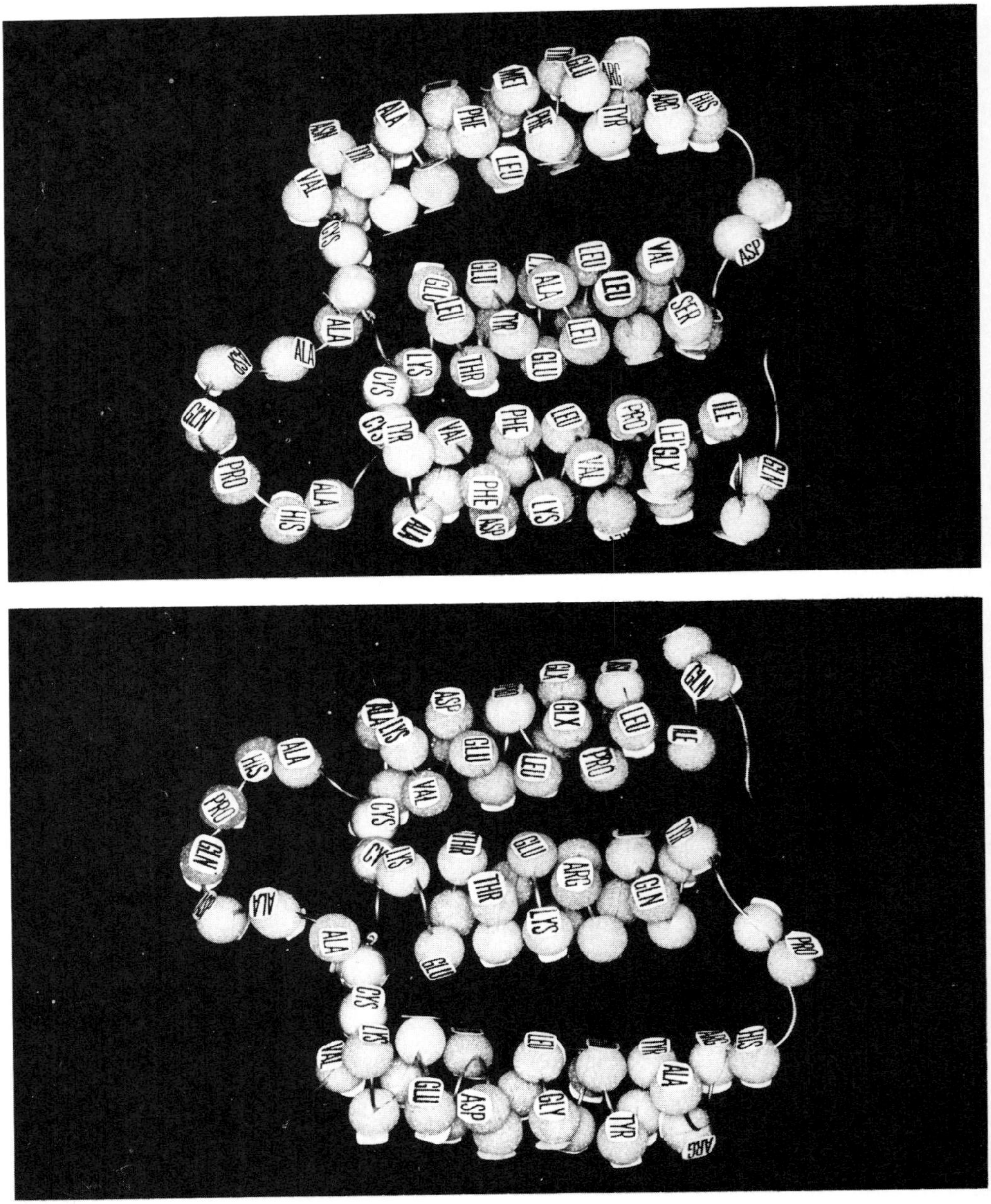

Fig. 5. Subdomain model

The subdomain model corresponds to residues 316-390 of human serum albumin. The upper view is facing the inside of the subdomain which is predominantly hydrophobic. The lower photograph is a view of the outside or backside of the subdomain and it is mainly polar.

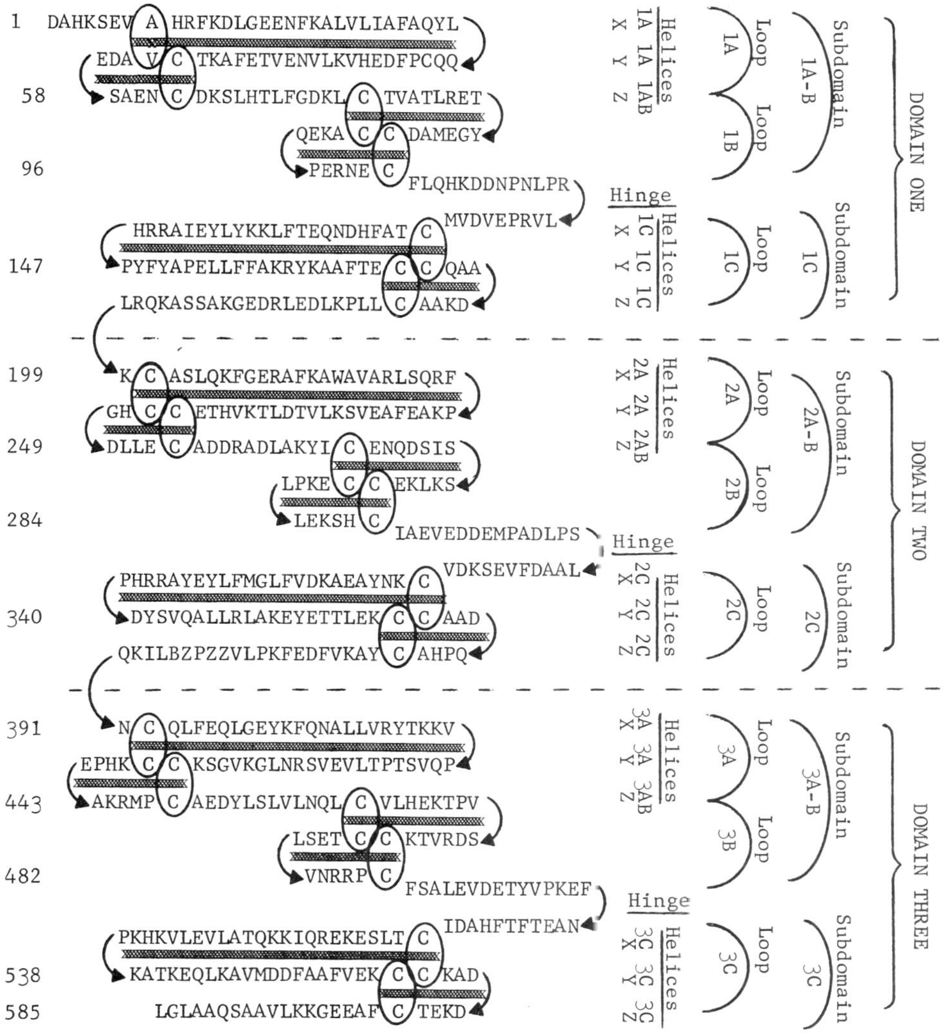

Fig. 6. Structural organization of human serum albumin.

The various structural units of human serum albumin are indicated relative to the complete sequence. The sequence layed out in this figure differs from Fig. 1 in that adjacent subdomains are antiparallel as depicted here.

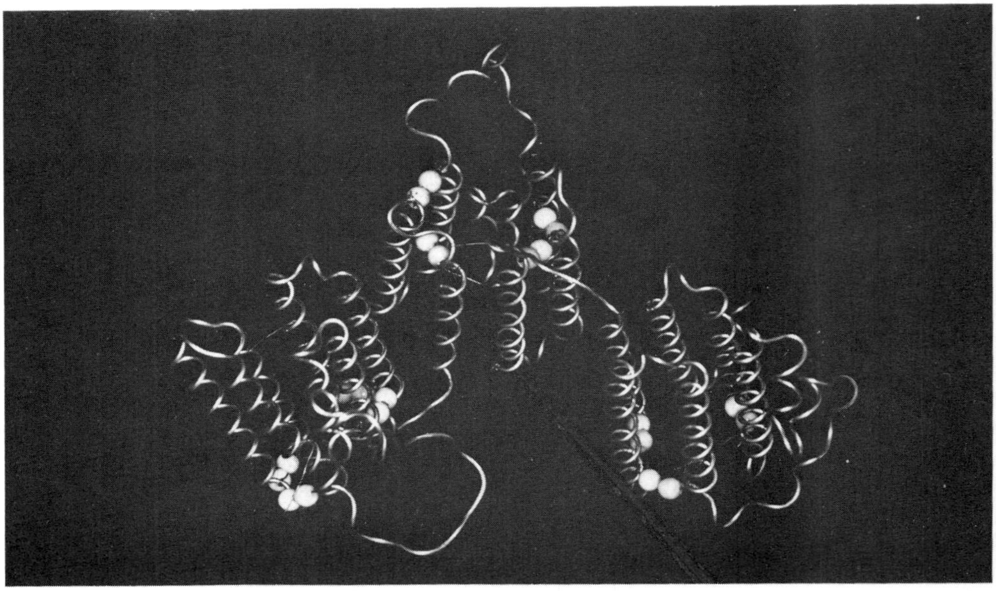

Figure 7. Parallel subdomain model of serum albumin.

with the dimensions of the molecule of about 140 x 40 A(9). A somewhat more extended structure can be formed by rotating the orientation of adjacent domains from parallel as shown to about 45°, but this seems to reduce the contact surface between domains.

Another arrangement is to pair subdomains in an antiparallel orientation, i.e. with the tips of the large loops of one subdomain facing the double Cys-bridge end of the other subdomain. Two views of a model of albumin with antiparallel subdomains are shown in Fig.8. In contrast to the parallel model, this structure nicely forms a linear orientation of the three domains which fits perfectly with the dimensions of the albumin molecule. The antiparallel domain has pseudosymmetry with a binding site at either end. We prefer this model but do not have any direct chemical evidence for it.

A third structural arrangement may also be considered. Since the molecule consists of six consecutive subdomains, it is possible that adjacent subdomains between the repeated homology units are paired. This would result in a two domain model with the first and sixth subdomains unpaired. Only the antiparallel orientation is possible. This would give four rather than 5 or 6 fatty acid binding sites as proposed by Spector and Fletcher (53) but it is possible that two fatty acids can occupy the same channel side by side. The first and sixth subdomains have not been shown to be in binding sites. If they are unpaired it would seem necessary to collapse the trough by rotating the Z-helix into the trough so that the hydrophobic surface would not be exposed.

Binding Sites

As mentioned above, the channels through the cylindrical domains appear to be tailor-made binding sites for fatty acids. The hydrocarbon chain of the fatty

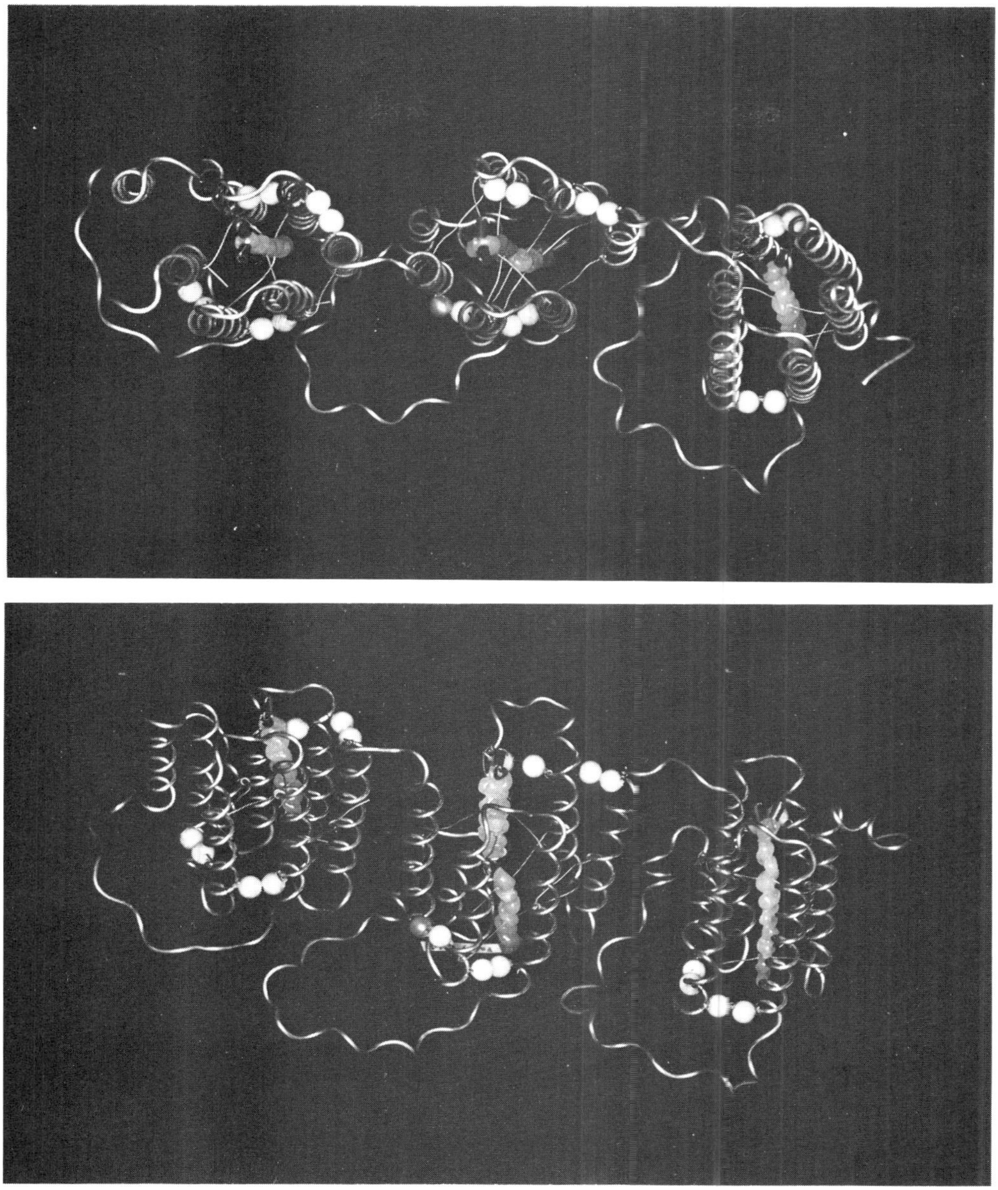

Fig. 8. Antiparallel subdomain model of human serum albumin.

This shows two views of a model of serum albumin with the subdomains facing each other within each domain in an antiparallel orientation. Several of the channels through the domains are occupied by fatty acids. Note that the middle domain contains two fatty acids, one at either end. The spheres represent the double Cys-bridges of the large double loops. For simplicity, the Cys-bridges of the small double loops are not shown.

acid should go into the nonpolar hole until its carboxylate group reaches the mouth where it forms electrostatic bonds with the positive charged groups at the tips of the long loops which are located at the mouth of the channel. Affinity labeling experiments support this model beautifully. McMenamy and coworkers (54, 55) have found that an affinity lable for the indol binding site, N-bromoacetyl tryptophan, reacts specifically with a His residue at position 146. This is at the tip of a large loop of the second subdomain of domain one at the mouth of a channel. These workers also found that dansyl chloride reacts with Lys-195 and blocks the indole binding site. This also fits beautifully with the model because Lys-195 is at or near the end of heliz-Z 1C and should be near His-146 at the mouth of the binding site. Andersson et al. (56) affinity labeled bovine serum albumin at Lys-220 (cf Arg-222 in HSA) with fluorescein isothiocyanate. Again, this supports model because that residue is also located at the tip of a large loop, at the mouth of a binding site in domain two. The analogous Lys-412 in bovine serum albumin (414 in HSA) in domain three was labeled specifically with trinitrobenzene sulfonic acid (5). Thus, affinity labels have gone to entrances of the channels in all three domains. Another related interesting study was done by Taylor (57) who identified Lys-220 of bovine serum albumin as a catalytic group in the degradation of a Meisenheimer complex. In human serum albumin the corresponding position 222 is replaced by Arg and is catalytically inactive. Taylor also studied this activity on fragments of albumin prepared as described by King (43). Using limited pepsin digestion in the presence of octanoate, King was able to cleave bovine albumin between residues 308-309 and isolate the two halves, the C-terminal half retained a binding site for octoanate. The two halves strongly associate to form a complex with molecular weight similar to bovine albumin. Taylor found that either fragment was catalytically inactive, but the complex of the two restored activity to 30% that of bovine albumin. This experiment strongly supports the three domain model. The cleavage by pepsin in the hinge peptide that joins the subdomains of domain two in effect cuts the middle domain in half. By allowing the two fragments to associate, the middle domain is reconstituted and catalytic activity is restored.

An interesting feature of the model of the domain is that the pair of subdomains are connected by a possibly flexible hinge segment. This could allow some movement of the subdomains in relationship to each other which could in effect allow some variability in the structure of the binding site and could explain how albumin is able to bind such a variety of ligands with high affinity. These hinge segments are quite different from other parts of the sequence by having a high concentration of Pro residues as illustrated in Fig. 9. These segments are about

Domain One (105–120)
HSA His-Lys-Asp-Asp-Asn-Pro-Asn-Leu-Pro-Arg-Leu-Val-Arg-Pro-Glu-Val
BSA His-Lys-Asp-Asp-Ser-Pro-Asp-Leu-Pro-Lys-Leu-Gap-Lys-Pro-Asp-Pro

Domain Two (295–310)
HSA Asp-Asp-Glu-Met-Pro-Ala-Asp-Leu-Pro-Ser-Leu-Ala-Ala-Asp-Phe-Val
BSA Lys-Asp-Ala-Ile-Pro-Glu-Asp-Leu-Pro-Pro-Leu-Thr-Ala-Asp-Phe-Ala

Domain Three (493–508)
HSA Val-Asp-Glu-Thr-Tyr-Val-Pro-Lys-Glu-Phe-Asn-Ala-Glu-Thr-Phe-Thr
BSA Pro-Asp-Glu-Thr-Tyr-Val-Pro-Lys-Ala-Phe-Asp-Glu-Lys-Leu-Phe-Thr
Chicken SA Tyr-Val-Pro-Pro-Pro-Phe-Asx-Pro-Asx-Met-Phe-Asx

Fig. 9. Hinge peptides of human, bovine, and chicken serum albumins.

the right length to correspond to Z-type helices of the middle double loop in each domain and the many Pro residues, not all of which are in homologous positions, may represent an adaptation to disrupt the tendency of these segments to be helical as they may have been in the past.

Fragments of Serum Albumin

Fragments of albumin prepared by limited proteolysis provide independent evidence for the domain-subdomain models of the albumin structure. The recent work by Peters and coworkers (44-46) is particularly notable as their fragments have been precisely located in the sequence and have been shown to retain secondary structure and binding sites. In this way they have been able to delineate some of the binding specificity. The cleavages by limited proteolysis generally have occurred in the connecting segments between domains, especially in the hinge segments. Many of the fragments thus correspond to subdomains or domains. A fragment corresponding to domain three was prepared by limited trypsin digestion and was found to contain a binding site for palmitate (44). Three fragments corresponding to subdomains also retain binding sites. All prepared from bovine serum albumin, fragment 115-184 corresponding to the second subdomain of domain one binds ANS; fragment 186-306 corresponding to the first subdomain of domain two binds bilirubin or bromcresol green; and fragment 307-385 corresponding to the second subdomain in domain two binds steroids (46,47). The presence of binding properties in subdomain fragments suggests that the subdomain may be an independent structure rather than associated in pairs as proposed for the domain structure. However, it seems plausible that the subdomain fragments dimerize to form a domain-like structure which has binding properties and enclosed hydrophobic faces. This remains to be tested experimentally. A novel and interesting use of fragments has been made by Teale and Benjamin (58) to analyze the mechanism of refolding of domains and subdomains.

Acknowledgment--Supported in part by NIH Grant No. HD02899.

References

(1) Brown, J. R. Structure of serum albumin: disulfide bridges, Fed. Proc. 33 1389 (1974).

(2) Brown, J. R. Structure of bovine serum albumin, Fed. Proc. 34, 591 (1975).

(3) Behrens, P. Q., A. M. Spiekerman, and J. R. Brown, Structure of human serum albumin, Fed. Proc. 34, 591 (1975).

(4) Brown, J. R., Structural origins of mammalian albumin, Fed. Proc. 35, 2141 (1976).

(5) Brown, J. R., Serum albumin: amino acid sequence, in Albumin Structure, Function and Uses, V. M. Rosenoer, M. Oratz, and A. Rothschild, Eds., Pergamon Press, Elmsford, N.Y., and Oxford, 27-51 (1977).

(6) Brown, J. R., Structure and evolution of serum albumin, in Albumin: Structure, Biosynthesis, Function, T. Peters, I. Sjoholm, Eds., Pergamon Press, Elmsford, N.Y., and Oxford, 1-10 (1978).

(7) McLachlan, A. D., and J. E. Walker, Evolution of serum albumin, J. Mol. Biol. 112, 543 (1977).

(8) Foster, J. F. Some aspects of the structure and conformational properties of serum albumin, in Albumin: Structure, Function and Uses, V. M. Rosenoer, M. Oratz, and M. A. Rothschild, Eds., Pergamon Press, Elmsford, N.Y., and Oxford, 53-84 (1977).

(9) Peters, T. and R. G. Reed, Serum Albumin: Conformation and active sites, in Albumin: Structure, Biosynthesis, Function, T. Peters, and I. Sjoholm, Eds., Pergamon Press, Elmsford, N.Y. and Oxford, 11-20 (1978).

(10) Peters, T., Jr., Serum albumin, in The Plasma Proteins, second edition, F. W. Putnam, Ed., Academic Press, N.Y. 1, 133-181 (1975).

(11) Rosenoer, V. M., M. Oratz, M. A. Rothschild, Albumin Structure, Function and Uses, V. M. Rosenoer, M. Oratz and M. A. Rothschild, Eds., Pergamon Press, Elmsford, N.Y., and Oxford, (1977).

(12) Peters, T., I. Sjoholm, Albumin: Structure, Biosynthesis, Function, T. Peters and I. Sjoholm, Eds., Pergamon Press, Elmsford, N.Y., and Oxford (1977).
(13) Sgouris, J. T., and A. Rene, Proceedings of the Workshop on Albumin, Bureau of Biologics, F.D.A. and National Heart and Lung Institute, Bethesda, Md. (1975).
(14) Meloun, B., L. Moravek and V. Kostka, Complete amino acid sequence of human serum albumin, FEBS Lett. 58, 134 (1975).
(15) Judah, J. D., M. Gamble and J. H. Steadman, Evidence for the existence of pro-albumin, Biol. Chem. J. 134, 1083 (1973).
(16) Urban, J., A. S. Inglis, K. Edwardes and G. Schreber, Chemical evidence for the difference between albumins from microsomes and serum and a possible precursor-product relationship, Biochem. Biophys. Res. Commun. 61, 444 (1974).
(17) Russell, J. H. and D. M. Geller, The structure of the rat proalbumin, J. Biol. Chem. 250, 3409 (1975).
(18) Patterson, J. E., and D. M. Geller, Bovine microsomal albumin: amino terminal sequence of bovine proalbumin, Biochem. Biophys. Res. Commun. 74, 1220 (1977).
(19) Rosen, A. M. and D. M. Geller, Chicken microsomal albumin: amino terminal sequence of chicken proalbumin, Biochem. Biophys. Res. Commun. 78, 1060 (1977).
(20) Peters, T., Intracellular Albumin Transport, in Albumin Structure, Function and Uses, V. M. Rosenoer, M. Oratz, and M. A. Rothschild, Eds., Pergamon Press, Elmsford, N.Y. and Oxford, 305-332 (1977).
(21) Judah, D. D., and P. S. Quinn, The biosynthesis of proalbumin and the mechanism of its conversion to albumin, in Albumin: Structure, Biosynthesis, Function, T. Peters and I. Sjoholm, Eds. Pergamon Press, Elmsford, N.Y., and Oxford, 21-30 (1977).
(22) Strauss, A. W., C. D. Bennett, A. M. Donohue, J. A., Rodkey and A. W. Alberts, Rat liver pre-proalbumin: complete amino acid sequence of the pre-piece. J. Biol. Chem. 252, 6846-6855 (1977).
(23) Chan, S. J., P. Keim, and D. F. Steiner, Cell free synthesis of rat preproinsulin, Proc. Natl. Acad. Sci. USA 73, 1964 (1976).
(24) Habener, J. F., J. T., Potts and A. Rich, Preproparathyroid hormone. Evidence for an early biosynthetic precursor of parathyroid hormone, J. Biol. Chem. 251, 3893 (1976).
(25) Dayhoff, M., Atlas of Protein Sequence and Structure, National Biomedical Research Foundation, Washington, D.C., (1972).
(26) Low, T., (Sup. J. R. Brown), Amino acid sequence of bovine serum albumin: cyanogen bromide fragments, Dissertation, Ph.D., University of Texas at Austin, (1970).
(27) Brown, J. R., T. Low, P. Behrens, P. Sepulveda, M. Parker and E. Blakeney, Amino acid sequence of bovine and porcine serum albumin, Fed. Proc. 30, 1241 (1971).
(28) Sepulveda, P. M., (Sup. J. R. Brown), Amino acid sequence of bovine serum albumin, Dissertation, Ph.D., University of Texas at Austin, (1972).
(29) Blakeney, E. W., (Sup. J. R. Brown), Amino acid sequence of chicken serum albumin: tryptic peptides, Dissertation Ph.D., University of Texas at Austin, (1972).
(30) Chincirini, C. and J. R. Brown, Amino acid enzyme of horse serum albumin: tryptic peptides, Fed. Proc. 35, 1621 (1976).
(31) Isemura, S., and T. Ikenaka, Fragmentation of rat serum albumin by cyanogen bromide cleavage and the amino acid sequences of four fragments, J. Biol. Chem., 79, 1183-1196 (1976).
(32) Sarich, V. M., Albumen phylogenetics, in Albumin Structure, Function, and Uses V. Rosenoer, M. Oratz, and M. A. Rothschild, Eds., Pergamon Press, Elmsford, N.Y., and Oxford, 85-112 (1977).
(33) Dayhoff, M., Atlas of Protein Sequence and Structure, Supplement 2, National Biomedical Research Foundation, Washington, D.C., (1976).
(34) Winter, W.P., L. R. Weitkamp, and D. L. Rucknagel, Amino acid substitution in two identical inherited human serum albumin variants: albumin Oliphant and albumin Ann Arbor, J. Biol. Chem. Vol. II, No. 5, 889-896 (1972).

(35) Schell, L. M., and B. Blumberg, The genetics of human serum albumin, in Albumin Structure, Function and Uses, V. M. Rosenoer, M. Oratz, and M. A. Rothschild, Eds., Pergamon Press, Elmsford, N.Y., and Oxford, 113-142 (1977).
(36) Ruoslahti, E. and W. D. Terry, α foetoprotein and serum albumin show sequence homology, Nature 260, 804 (1976).
(37) Parmelee, D. C., M. A. Evenson, and H. F. Deutsch, The presence of fatty acids in human α-fetoprotein, J. Biol. Chem. 253, 2114 (1978).
(38) Ruoslahti, E., T. Estes and M. Seppala, Binding of bilirubin by bovine and human alpha-fetoprotein, Biochem. Biophys., Acta, in press (1978).
(39) Brown, J. R., P. Shockley, R. Densen and E. W. Blakeney, Sequence of chicken serum albumin, unpublished.
(40) Weber, G. and L. B. Young, Fragmentation of bovine serum albumin by pepsin. II. Isolation, amino acid composition, and physical properties of the fragments, J. Biol. Chem. 239, 1424-1431 (1964).
(41) Peters, T. Jr. and C. Hawn, Isolation of two large peptide fragments from the amino- and carboxyl-terminal positions of bovine serum albumin, J. Biol. Chem. 242, 1566-1573 (1967).
(42) Pederson, D. N. and J. F. Foster, Subtilisin cleavage of bovine plasma albumin. Reversible association of the two primary fragments and their relation to the structure of the parent protein, Biochemistry 8, 2357-2365 (1969).
(43) King, T. P., Limited pepsin digestion of bovine plasma albumin, Arch. Biochem. Biophys. 156, 509-520 (1973).
(44) Peters, T. and R. C. Feldhoff, Fragments of bovine serum albumin produced by limited proteolysis. Isolation and characterization of tryptic fragments, Biochemistry 14, 3384-3391 (1975).
(45) Feldhoff, R. C. and T. Peters, Fragments of bovine serum albumin produced by limited proteolysis. Isolation and characterization of peptic fragments, Biochemistry 14, 4508-4514 (1975).
(46) Reed, R. G., R. C. Feldhoff, O. L. Clute and T. Peters, Fragments of bovine serum albumin produced by limited proteolysis. Conformation and ligand binding. Biochemistry 14, 4578-4583 (1975).
(47) Pearlman, W. H. and I. F. F. Fong, Steroid binding properties of some peptide fragments of bovine serum albumin obtained on peptic digestion. J. Biol. Chem. 247, 8078-8084 (1972).
(48) Weber, G., Polarization of the fluorescence of macromolecules. 2. Fluorescent conjugates of ovalbumin and bovine serum albumin, Biochem. J. 51, 155-167 (1952).
(49) Yang, J. T. and J. F. Foster, Changes in the intrinsic viscosity and optical rotation of bovine plasma albumin associated with acid binding, J. Am. Chem. Soc. 76, 1588-1595 (1954).
(50) Harrington, W. F., P. Johnson and R. H. Ottewill, Bovine serum albumin and its behavior in acid solution, Biochem. J. 62, 569-582 (1956).
(51) Foster, J. F., Plasma albumin, in The Plasma Proteins 1, F. W. Putnam, Ed., Academic Press, Inc., N.Y., 179-239 (1960).
(52) Chou, P. Y., and G. D. Fasman, Secondary structural prediction of proteins from their amino acid sequence, Trends Biochem. Sci 2, 128 (1977).
(53) Spector, A. A., and J. E. Fletcher, Fatty acid binding by serum albumin, in Albumin: Structure, Biosynthesis, Function, T. Peters and I. Sjoholm, Eds., Pergamon Press, Elmsford, N.Y. and Oxford, 51-60 (1977).
(54) Gambhir, K. K., R. H. McMenamy, and F. Watson, Positions in human serum albumin which involve the indole binding site, J. Biol Chem. 250, 6711 (1975).
(55) McMenamy, R. H., Albumin binding sites, in Albumin Structure, Function and Uses, V. Rosenoer, M. Oratz and M. A. Rothschild, Eds., Pergamon Press, Elmsford, N.Y. and Oxford, 143-158 (1977).
(56) Andersson, L. O., A. Rehnstrom and K. L. Eaker, Studies on non spacific binding. The nature of the binding of fluorescein to bovine serum albumin, Eur. J. Biochem. 20, 371-380 (1971).

(57) Taylor, R. P., Enzyme-like activities associated with albumin, in Albumin Structure, Function and Uses, V. Rosenoer, M. Oratz and M. A. Rothschild, Eds., Pergamon Press, Elmsford, N.Y. and Oxford, 183-201 (1977).

(58) Teale, J. M., and D. C. Benjamin, Antibody as immunological probe for studying refolding of bovine serum albumin, J. Biol. Chem. 252, 4521-4526 (1977).

THE MAPPING OF FUNCTIONAL SITES ON IMMUNOGLOBULIN G

R. H. Painter and K. J. Dorrington
Department of Biochemistry
University of Toronto
Toronto, Canada M5S 1A8

The primary activity of immunoglobulin G (IgG) is to combine specifically with its antigenic determinant, but the role of this protein in homeostasis depends on its ability to link antigen with the constitutive, non-specific elements of defence in the body to bring about the destruction and elimination of the antigenic material. The constitutive non-specific defence systems include the phagocytic cells, such as macrophages and granulocytes, and the classical complement components. Thus IgG is a protein capable of engaging in a remarkable number of varied interactions and is endowed with a multiplicity of functional sites which are believed to be discretely distributed to various parts of the molecule.

The immunoglobulin G molecule is formed from two identical light (L) and two identical heavy (H) polypeptide chains (1, 2). These chains are linked by interchain disulfide bridges from the carboxy-terminal ends of the light chain to the heavy chain and between the heavy chains in their mid-region. Repetitive homologous sequences can be recognized within each of these polypeptide chains, subdividing them into sections of about 110 residues, known as the homology regions (3). The amino-terminal homology region of each chain is distinct from the other regions of the chain and is known as the variable region (V_L and V_H) because the sequence differs between immunoglobulin molecules which are specific for different antigens. The sequence of the remaining, constant homology region of the light chain (C_L) and the regions of the heavy chain (Cγ1, Cγ2 and Cγ3) do not vary between molecules of different specificity except for differences associated with sub-class and allotype.

Amino acid sequence analyses of the L and H chains, together with high resolution X-ray diffraction studies (4), have provided a detailed picture of how a site is created having shape and features which permit the stereochemical recognition of antigen. It is wholly contained in the Fab fragment, a portion of the molecule consisting of a light chain and the N-terminal half of a heavy chain, and it is now clear that the site is further confined to that portion of the molecule which is made up from the variable regions of the polypeptide chains with the hypervariable regions creating the surfaces which are complementary to antigen. Recent studies suggest that there is some structural dependence on interactions between the C_L and Cγ1 regions of the light and heavy polypeptide chains respectively (5).

The constitutive, non-specific defence mechanisms of the body each possess recognition units for immunoglobulin which interact with specific sites on the H chains in the Fc region of the IgG molecule. Most of these interactions can be shown to occur with the isolated Fc fragment or can be inhibited by an excess of this protein fragment. Other properties of immunoglobulin, such as its transportation across the placenta and the regulation of its clearance from the circulation, are also dependent upon sites in the Fc fragment. The distribution of these different functions, adaptive and constitutive, onto separate parts of the molecule created problems in some therapeutic preparations of immunoglobulin (Immune Serum Globulin). Endogenous proteolysis caused cleavage of the Fab and Fc regions and the antibody activity contained in the Fab fragment was rapidly cleared from the circulation, thereby seriously reducing the effectiveness of the preparation (6).

The number and variety of specific sites identified on the Fc have stimulated a number of investigations to attempt a more precise mapping of the structural features involved in the individual interactions. Two major approaches have been used to date. In the first, a variety of subfragments of Fc, some corresponding to whole homology regions of the polypeptide chain, others representing smaller portions of the sequence, have been tested for their ability to interact with the particular constitutive element under test. In many cases the extent of interaction by the fragment has been measured by the inhibition of a standard reaction between the whole antibody and the constitutive element. This technique suffers from the difficulty that the loss of a particular property may be caused by the loss of conformational structure and not by the absence of the site in question. As a check on this possibility, various physical properties (such as circular dichroism) of the fragments have been observed and used to establish the integrity of the structure. In general, the fragments representing complete homology regions have been found to deviate only slightly from that which would be expected for the native structure.

Perhaps the most satisfactory application of this technique has been in relation to the location of the site which binds to Clq, particularly since this site appears to depend little upon conformation (7). Fragments corresponding to the Cγ3 domain have usually been found to be unable to react with Clq. However, a variety of fragments comprising the Cγ2 domain in one form or another have been shown to interact with Clq. Thus a CNBr fragment (8), a plasmin fragment corresponding to $F(ab')_2$ with Cγ2 attached (9) and trypsin fragments corresponding to the whole isolated Cγ2 domain (10,11) have all been shown to interact with Clq in a manner analogous to IgG. In the last mentioned study the molar binding activities of Cγ2 monomer, Cγ2 dimer, Fc and IgG were identical. Thus, although as a result of its symmetrical nature IgG possesses two potential Clq binding sites per mole, apparently only one can be occupied at a time.

The precise location of the site on the Cγ2 region for Clq binding is not known. Model compounds suggest that a hydrophobic centre with associated positive charges provides the essential elements of the site (11), and studies with synthetic peptides (12) have shown that sequences modelled on that around tryptophan 277 have significant activity. This is also consistent with chemical modification studies on tryptophan and lysine (13). Since tryptophan is normally a buried residue and not exposed to the solvent it has been suggested that the unusual structure of the Cγ2 domain, compared with the other domains, serves to keep a tryptophan exposed to the solvent (7). Thus the structures which interact with Clq may not be unique in themselves but only in that they are accessible. This is borne out by studies by Isenman et.al. (14). A dimer of Cγ3, pFc' shows no ability to bind Clq; however, a fragment, atCγ3, which is identical to pFc' except for the lack of seven residues at the carboxy-terminal end, binds Clq as effectively as the Cγ2 fragment. The development of the Clq binding property in Cγ3 seems to correlate with the exposure to the solvent of normally buried aromatic chromophores, especially tryptophan (detected by solvent perturbation difference spectroscopy).

Measurements of the ability of various fragments of IgG to mediate or inhibit reactions with the cellular elements with which IgG is known to interact have provided some information on the distribution of functional sites, although at the present time conflicting results have been reported by different groups of investigators. For example, data obtained in our laboratories indicate that the Cγ3 domain in a heterologous assay system can be as effective in inhibiting rosettes as whole Fc or IgG (11) and this is supported by reports from other laboratories using a fully homologous system (15, 16). Our experience with the homologous system shows the Cγ3 fragments to have 10% of the activity of the whole molecule, the fully active site presumably being dependent on structural support from the Cγ2 region. Others have failed to find any activity with the Cγ3 region and even report activity associated with the Cγ2 region in tests with macrophages (17, 18). At present the matter is unresolved. It is evident that these interactions are more complex than was at first thought, and this is illustrated by the recent paper in which Diamond et. al. (19) have reported finding two Fc receptors on mouse macrophage cells each having different specificities for Fc.

The other experimental approach for mapping functional sites is based on the change of structure brought about by reduction of the inter-heavy chain disulphide bonds. An examination of the associative properties of the subfragments has revealed that the Cγ3 homology region of the heavy chain shows a very strong tendency to form dimers through powerful non-covalent interactions. Thus all fragments representing the Cγ3 region of the molecule (pFc', Fc', atCγ3, etc.) occur as dimers. In contrast, peptide fragments derived from the Cγ2 region of the H chain exist in solution in monomeric form unless joined by the interheavy chain disulphide bonds (10). Recent X-ray crystallographic studies show that the Cγ2 regions of each heavy chain are separated by the carbohydrate chains and that there is no direct contact between the polypeptide chains in this region (20). Thus the close apposition of this part of the molecule is very dependent on the interheavy chain disulphide bonds. Reduction of these bonds should increase the segmental flexibility of the molecule, moving the fulcrum of this flexibility from the mid-point of the H chain, the "hinge region," to the beginning of the Cγ3 region. While the effects of this reduction are barely discernable by physical means (21,22), the effect on the biological properties of the molecule is profound. For example, mild reduction of antibody does not affect the ability of antibody to bind antigen but it completely destroys the ability to activate the complement cascade (23). Isenman et. al. (24) showed that mildly reduced antibody did not bind to Clq as measured in the Augener et. al. assay (25) and that the critical bonds were those between the heavy chains. This phenomenon was not evident with the reduced Fc fragment which interacted normally with Cl, suggesting that the Fab in some way interfered with the proper access of Cl in the more flexible reduced molecule.

Goers et. al. (26) have argued that Clq binding by IgG differs from binding by whole Cl and that in some way it is the interaction with Clr and Cls that is affected by reduction of the hinge disulphide. Certainly it would appear that complex formation between IgG and Clq as observed in the ultracentrifuge is not affected by reduction of the IgG. However, the concentration of IgG required to effect measurable change in the sedimentation rate of Clq is 10 to 40-fold greater than that at which changes in behaviour in the Augener et. al. Cl binding assay are observed, and it is likely that different aspects of the binding are being compared in these two techniques.

Isenman et. al. (24) observed that the Fc fragment from proteins belonging to the human IgG4 subclass (a subclass which normally does not interact with complement) behaved in the Cl binding assay in a manner identical to Fc from IgGl. These authors suggested that the fundamental difference in the IgGl and IgG4 subclasses lay not in the presence or absence of a Clq binding site in the Cγ2 region of these molecules but in the differing segmental flexibility of the molecules permitted by their individual hinge regions which regulated access by the Clq. Differences in the amino acid sequences of the proteins are only minor in the Cγ2 regions but extensive in the hinge region and therefore consistent with this hypothesis.

Further evidence for the increased flexibility produced by reduction of the hinge disulphides has been produced by Romans et. al. (27) who were able to convert so-called "incomplete" non-agglutinating IgG antibodies into complete hemagglutinins by reduction of the interchain disulphide bonds.

Striking changes occur also in the properties of IgG and Fc towards cell receptors following reduction of the hinge disulphide. Since in some cases these properties are lost also when the Fc fragment is reduced, other additional possibilities have to be considered. For example, there may be a need for the Cγ2 domains to be in close apposition for the Fc to be bound by the Fc receptor, there may be a need for structures in the interdomain region which are recognized by the cell receptor or, indeed, for conformation stability in the Cγ3 region to be maintained by the hinge disulphide through the Cγ2 region. At the present time, apart from the studies with isolated fragments, there is no information which allows one or the other of these considerations to be discarded.

The recent description by Huber et. al. (28) of the binding site of staphylococcal protein A in the junction region between Cγ2 and Cγ3, however, does provide an opportunity to examine the role of this region in the various Fc interactions. The ability of this protein and, in particular, its univalent tryptic peptide, Fragment B, to interfere with Fc function should be an indication of involvement of this interdomain region of Fc in the property under test. Such experiments are already in progress in our laboratories.

Recent observations on the effect of reduction on the ability of IgG or Fc to interact with the Fc receptors of different classes of cells have shown that not all Fc receptors are alike. For example, Figure 1 shows histograms representing the relative ability of the same preparations of IgG and Fc in either native form, or after reduction and alkylation, to inhibit rosette formation between anti D-coated D positive red cells and human peripheral blood granulocytes or monocytes. The concentrations of IgG and Fc were 10^{-5}M, a concentration at which inhibition by IgG is just maximal. Reduction and alkylation of the Fc has only slight effect as far as monocytes are concerned but granulocyte binding is severely impaired (29). Similar, though less striking, effects are observed with the whole protein. The Fab fragments serve as controls indicating the level of background inhibition produced by adding immunoglobulin protein, a phenomenon at present not understood.

These results, coupled with reports from a number of laboratories that many cells are believed to carry multiple Fc receptors, each having individual specificities, indicate that the situation is more complex than was at first thought.

Among the other properties of IgG, some are susceptible to reduction and alkylation, thus transplacental transport is prevented (30) while others, e.g., clearance from the circulation, appear not to be affected (11). Thus, the interheavy chain disulphides play an important role in maintaining the structure of Fc and the range of responses seen in the various systems with which Fc reacts indicates the variety of structures in Fc which are recognized by individual systems.

Summary

The modular structure of IgG, first predicted from the amino acid sequence, has been borne out in X-ray diffraction and electron micrographic studies. However, it does not appear that the functional sites on the molecule will be found to be as discretely differentiated as first thought.

While the concept that each domain fills an independent and separate function is attractive at first sight, it now seems evident that in many instances there is need for both domains, either because the site spans both regions of the protein or because of the structural support which one domain provides the other. It is intriguing that the complete separation of function found between Fab and Fc, and indeed within the domains of Fab, does not seem to occur in the Fc fragment.

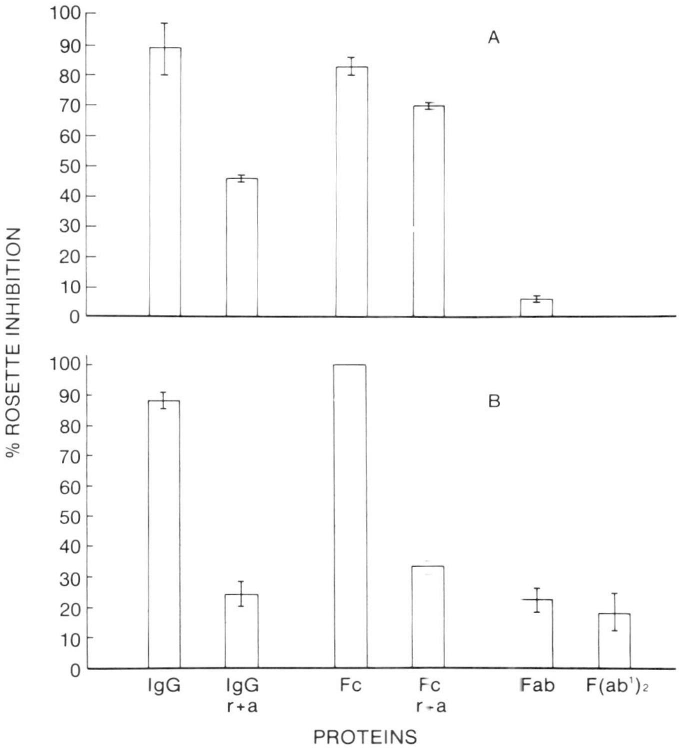

Fig. 1. Percentage inhibition of rosettes using IgG, Fc and their alkylated counterparts. All proteins are present at 10^{-5} molar concentration. The values represent the mean of duplicate determinations for one experiment. The bars show the range of values. These results are representative of a number of similar experiments.

A. Human peripheral blood granulocytes prepared by entrifugation through isopaque Ficol and purified by suspension in 4.5% dextran.

B. Human peripheral blood monocytes enriched by adherence on culture plates on which fibroplasts have previously been grown and detached. EA rosettes (human D positive cells coated with human anti-D immunoglobulin were stained before counting to ensure identity of rosetting cell.

REFERENCES

1. Edelman, G.M., Cunningham, B.A., Gall, W.E., Gottlieb, P.D., Rutishauser, U, and Waxdal, M.J., The Covalent Structure of an Entire γG Immunoglobulin Molecule, Proc. Nat'l Acad. Sci. U.S.A. 63, 78-85.

2. Fleischmann, N.B., Pain, R H., and Porter, R.R., Reduction of γ Globulins, Biochem. Biophys., Suppl. 1, 174 (1962).

3. Edelman, G.M., The Covalent Structure of Human γG Immunoglobulin XI Functional Implications, Biochemistry 9, 3197 (1970).

4. Davies, D.R., Padlan, E.A., and Segal, D.M., Three-Dimensional Structure of Immunoglobulin, A Rev. Biochem. 44, 639 (1975).

5. Klein, M., Kortan, C., Kells, D.I.C., and Dorrington, K.J., Equilibrium and Kinetic Aspects of the Interaction of Isolated Variable and Constant Domains of Light Chain with the Fd' Fragment of Immunoglobulin G, Biochemistry (in press), (1978).

6. Painter, R.H., Walcroft, M.J., and Weber, J.C.W., The Efficacy of Fragmented Immune Serum Globulin in Passive Immunization, Canad. J. Biochem. 44, 381 (1965).

7. Isenman, D.E., Painter, R.H., and Dorrington, K.J., The Structure and Function of Immunoglobulin Domains I. Studies with Beta 2-Microglobulin on the Role of the Intrachain Disulfide Bond, Proc. Nat'l. Acad. Sci. U.S.A. 72, 548 (1975).

8. Kehoe, J.M., Fougereau, M., Immunoglobulin Peptide with Complement Fixing Activity, Nature 224, 1212 (1969).

9. Connell, G.E. and Porter, R.R., A New Enzymic Fragment (Facb) of Rabbit Immunoglobulin G, J. Biochem. 123, 53P (1971).

10. Ellerson, J.R., Yasmeen, D., Painter, R.H., and Dorrington, K.J., Structure and Function of Immunoglobulin Domains III: Isolation and Characterization of a Fragment Corresponding to the Cγ2 Homology Region of Human Immunoglobulin G, J. Immunol. 116, 510 (1976).

11. Yasmeen, D., Ellerson, J.R., Dorrington, K.J., and Painter, R.H., The Structure and Function of Immunoglobulin Domains: IV. The Distribution of Some Effector Functions among the Cγ2 and Cγ3 Homology Regions of Human Immunoglobulin G, J. Immunol. 116, 518 (1976).

12. Johnson, B.J. and Thames, K.E., Investigations of the Complement-Fixing Sites of Immunoglobulins, J. Immunol. 117, 1491 (1976).

13. Cohen, S. and Becker, E.L., The Effect of Benzylation or Sequential Amidination and Benzylation on the Ability of Rabbit γG Antibody to Fix Complement, J. Immunol., 100, 403 (1968).

14. Isenman, D.E., Ellerson, J.R., Painter, R.H., and Dorrington, K.J., Correlation Between the Exposure of Aromatic Chromophores at the Surface of the Fc Domains of Immunoglobulin G and Their Ability to Bind Complement, Biochem. 16, 233 (1977).

15. Okafor, G., Hay, F.C., and Turner, M.W., Localisation of Monocyte Binding Site of Human Immunoglobulin G., Nature 248,228 (1974).

16. Ciccimara, F. Rosen, F.S., and Merler, E., Localisation of the IgG Effector Site for Monocyte Receptors, Proc. Nat'l Acad. Sci. U.S.A. 72, 2081 (1975).

17. Ovary, Z., Saluk, P.H., Quijada, L., and Lamm, M.E., Biologic Activities of Rabbit Immunoglobulin G in Relation to the Domains of the Fc Region, J. Immunol. 116, 1265 (1976).

18. Alexander, M.D., Andrews, J.A., Leslie, R.G.Q., and Wood, M.J., The Binding of Human and Guinea Pig IgG Subclasses to Homologous Macrophage and Monocyte Receptors, Immunol. 35, 115 (1978).

19. Diamond, B., Bloom, B.R., and Scharff, M.D., The Fc Receptors of Primary and Cultured Phagocytic Cells Studied with Homogeneous Antibodies, J. Immunol. 121, 1329 (1978).

20. Silverton, E.W., Navia, M.A., and Davies, D.R., Three-Dimensional Structure of an Intact Immunoglobulin, Proc. Nat'l Acad. Sci. U.S.A. 74, 5140 (1977).

21. Lapanje, S. and Dorrington, K.J., Influence of Subunit Interaction and Intersubunit Disulphide Bonds on the Unfolding of Immunoglobulin G by Guanidine Hydrochloride, Biochem. Biophys. Acta. 322, 45 (1973).

22. Venyaminov, S.Y., Rajnavolgyi E., Medgyesi, G.A., Gergely, G.A., and Zavodsky, P., The Role of Interchain Disulphide Bridges in the Conformational Stability of Human Immunoglobulin Gl Subclass. Hydrogen-Deuterium Exchange Studies. Eur. , J. Biochem. 67, 81 (1976).

23. Schur, P.H., and Christian, G.D., The Role of Disulphide Bonds in the Complement-Fixing and Precipitating Properties of 7S Rabbit and Sheep Antibodies, J. Exp. Med., 120, 531 (1964).

24. Isenman, D.E., Dorrington, K.J., and Painter, R.H., The Structure and Function of Immunoglobulin Domains. II. The Importance of Interchain Disulphide Bonds and the Possible Role of Molecular Flexibility in the Interaction Between Immunoglobulin G and Complement, J. Immunol. 114, 1726 (1975).

25. Augener, W., Grey, H.M., Cooper, N.R., Muller-Eberhard, H.J., The Reaction of Monomeric and Aggregated Immunoglobulins with Cl, Immunochemistry 8, 1011 (1971).

26. Goers, J.W., Ziccardi, R.J., Schumaker, V.N., and Glovsky, M.M., The Mechanism of Activation of the First Component of Complement by a Univalent Hapten-IgG Antibody Complex, J. Immunol. 118, 2182 (1977).

27. Romans, D.G., Tilley, C.A., Crookston, M.C., Falk, R.E., and Dorrington, K.J., Conversion of Incompatable Antibodies to Direct Agglutinins by Mild Reduction: Evidence for Segmental Flexibility within the Fc Fragment of Immunoglobulin G, Proc. Nat'l. Acad. Sci. U.S.A.74, 2531 (1977).

28. Deisenhofer, J., Jones, T.A., and Huber, R., Crystallization, Crystal Structure Analysis and Atomic Model of the Complex Formed by a Human Fc Fragment and B of Protein A from Staphylococcus Aureus, Hoppe-Seyler's Z. Physiol. Chem. 359, 975 (1978).

29. Foster, D.E.B., Dorrington, K.J., and Painter, R.H., The Structure and Function of Immunoglobulin Domains. VII. Studies on the Structural Requirements of Human Immunoglobulin G for Granulocyte Binding, J. Immunol. 120, 1952 (1978).

30. McNabb, T., Koh, T.Y., Dorrington, K.J., and Painter, R.H., Structure and Function of Immunoglobulin Domains. V. Binding of Immunoglobulin G and Fragments to Placental Membrane Preparations. J. Immunol., 117, 882 (1976).

ANTIBODIES: DIVERSITY AND GENES

Leroy E. Hood
Division of Biology, California Institute of Technology,
Pasadena, California 91125 U.S.A.

ABSTRACT

A variety of constraints imposed by structural, genetic and recombinant DNA studies of antibody genes and molecules are reviewed with regard to the question of antibody diversity. The general conclusion is that at least five different mechanisms may contribute to antibody diversity. The relative importance of the individual mechanisms for generating diversity is uncertain at this time.

INTRODUCTION

Speculations about the origin of antibody diversity and, accordingly, the organization of antibody genes have intrigued immunologists for the past 15 years. How can the vertebrate organism generate perhaps as many as 10^5 to 10^7 different antibody molecules? Two points of view have developed in response to this question. The _germ line theory_ postulates that most, if not all antibody genes are separately encoded in the zygote or germ line of the organism and that these genes arose by gene duplication and changed by mutation and selection during vertebrate evolution (1). This theory suggests that the diversity of antibody genes exists prior to the somatic differentiation of each individual; antibody synthesis therefore merely requires the activation of distinct antibody genes in each individual lymphocyte. In contrast, the _somatic mutation theory_ postulates a more limited number of germ line genes which diversify by some type of somatic mutational mechanism during the differentiation of each individual (2). Thus somatic mutation generates antibody diversity anew in each individual. A third model suggests that the rearrangement of antibody gene segments during differentiation also may generate antibody variability (3, 4, 5). As we shall see, perhaps each of these mechanisms contributes to antibody diversity.

GENERAL CONSTRAINTS ON THEORIES OF DIVERSITY

Cellular, genetic and molecular studies have placed important constraints on our understanding of the antibody problem.

Cellular Patterns

One antibody-producing cell is committed to the synthesis of a single antibody molecule. The clonal selection hypothesis suggests that at some time in ontogeny and independently of antigen, individual lymphocytes become committed to the expression of a single type of antigen-recognition domain (6). This commitment is expressed through antigen-specific receptors, presumably antibody, on the lymphocyte cell surface. Thus, when antigen is introduced into the vertebrate organism, it selects out those lymphocytes which already have receptors for the antigen on their surface. Presumably the interaction of surface-receptor molecules and antigen activates the specific lymphocytes and leads to clonal proliferation, differentiation and ultimately the secretion of antibody molecules with the same specificity as the original receptors. Thus antigen can select discrete units of information (clones of antibody-producing cells) for amplification and expression.

Homogeneous immunoglobulins are derived from single lymphocytes that have been clonally expanded. Single lymphocytes can be clonally expanded by neoplastic transformation (i.e., multiple myeloma) or by antigenic stimulation. The discovery that multiple myeloma can be induced in two laboratory strains of mice, BALB/c and NZB, by the injection of mineral oil into the peritoneal cavity is important because these strains are highly inbred and immunoglobulin genes of all individual mice from each strain should be very similar, if not identical (7). Most of the amino acid sequence analyses on the immunoglobulin molecules to be discussed subsequently have been carried out on myeloma proteins.

Genetic Patterns

Three genetically unlinked clusters or families of antibody genes are present in mammals (8). Two code for light chains, λ and κ, and a third codes for heavy chains. These gene families are comprised of two kinds of genes, variable (V) and constant (C). The gene families have been genetically mapped primarily by serological markers on their C regions.

Immunoglobulin Structure

The basic subunit of the immunoglobulin molecule is composed of two identical light (L) and two identical heavy (H) chains linked by disulfide bonds and non-covalent interactions. The existence of nonidentical subunits provides an important strategy, combinatorial association, for increasing antibody diversity as will be discussed subsequently.

All immunoglobulin polypeptide chains can be divided into an N-terminal portion, the variable (V) region, and C-terminal portion, the constant (C) region, which are defined by sequence variation or the lack thereof among chains of a similar class. These regions reflect a fundamental functional dichotomy of antibody molecules. Namely, the V regions comprise the antigen-binding site, whereas the C regions encode the effector functions such as complement fixation. This dichotomy also is reflected at the gene level in that V and C regions are encoded by separate genes. The constant regions of heavy chains (C_H) define the various classes and subclasses of immunoglobulins (C_μ-IgM; C_γ-IgG, etc.).

Immunoglobulin molecules can be divided into homology units which are approximately 110 amino acids in length. The V regions for both light and heavy chains are approximately one homology unit in length, whereas the C regions are one (C_L), three (C_γ), or four (C_μ) homology units in length (9). The V_L and V_H regions show amino acid sequence homologies to one another as do the C_L, C_H1, C_H2, and C_H3 homology units of an IgG molecule. Furthermore, X-ray analysis indicates that both the V and C regions fold into a very similar configuration designated the "immunoglobulin fold" (10). These homology units and similar three-dimension configurations suggest that all immunoglobulin genes probably evolved from the duplication of an ancestral gene coding for a primitive homology unit.

A comparative amino acid sequence analysis of many V_L and V_H regions reveal three and four segments, respectively, of extreme diversity. These are termed the hypervariable regions (3). X-ray analysis has shown that five or six of the seven hypervariable regions comprise the walls of the antigen-binding site of the antibody molecule. The nonhypervariable portions of the V region are remarkably constant in their three-dimensional structure and these have been termed the framework regions. Accordingly, the hypervariable regions are the antigen-binding site of the antibody molecule and should reflect selective pressures for binding-site diversity and any unusual genetic mechanisms for generating variability. For example, Kabat has postulated that the hypervariable and framework regions are encoded by separate minigenes that are joined at the nucleic acid level during the differentiation of antibody-producing cells (11).

A comparison of the V regions from a particular family of antibody polypeptide chains reveals related groups or subgroups of V regions that have similar amino acid sequences. The detailed amino acid sequence analysis of a set of 22 closely-related proteins has necessitated a new nomenclature (12). A group of V regions is defined as a set of proteins that share very similar amino acid sequences over their N-terminal 23 residues or so. A subgroup is denoted a set of immunoglobulins that share extensive amino acid sequence and homologous sequence gaps (insertions or deletions) throughout their entire V region. Every individual appears capable of producing the major subgroups (or groups). To generate two or more subgroups from a single germ line V gene would require multiple identical or parallel mutations. Since the hypothesis of identical mutations in separate lymphocyte lines is genetically unattractive, most immunologists agree that each subgroup is encoded by at least one germ line V gene. This reasoning is designated the argument of parallel mutation. Thus subgroups are convenient means of estimating the minimum number of germ line V genes.

Immunoglobulin Gene Organization

These observations have been made on mouse DNA using recombinant DNA techniques and DNA sequencing.

Lambda family. The organization of λ genes in embryonic (undifferentiated) mouse DNA appears different from that of myeloma (differentiated) DNA (Fig. 1) (13).

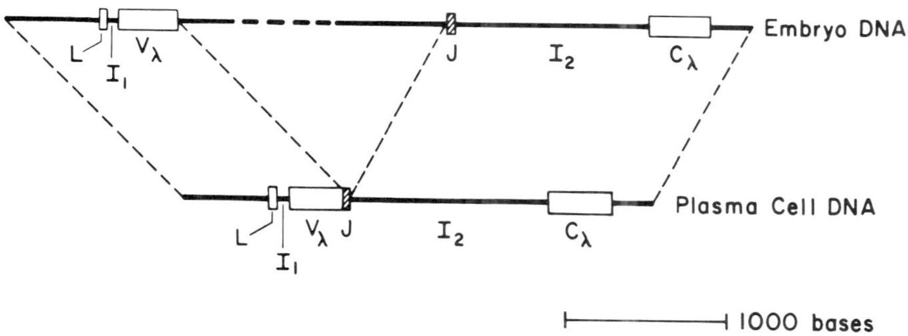

Fig. 1. The organization of mouse λ genes in undifferentiated (embryonic) and differentiated (myeloma) DNAs. Adapted from (13).

In the embryonic DNA, the lambda polypeptide is encoded by three distinct pieces of DNA, each separated by 1200 or more nucleotides: the V segment (approximately residues 1-98); the J segment (approximately residues 99-108); and the C segment (approximately residues 109-215). The V region of the polypeptide includes residues 1-108 and, accordingly, is encoded by the V and J segments. Thus the V segment differs from the V region by the length of the J segment. In myeloma DNA a rearrangement occurs which joins the V and J segments in contiguous alignment (Fig. 1). The 1200 nucleotides separating the J and C segments remain, presumably to later be removed by RNA processing of the nuclear transcript. Thus the differentiation of the antibody-producing cell appears to be accompanied by the rearrangement of antibody gene segments.

Kappa family. The mouse kappa genes also appear to be composed of three gene segments, V_κ, J_κ, and C_κ (12, 14). Attempts at counting V_κ genes have been carried out in the following manner. V_κ regions can be divided into groups based on the similarity of their N-terminal sequences. Depending on the criteria that are used, mouse myeloma κ chains currently can be divided into 25-40 groups (7), although the actual number may be considerably larger. DNA saturation hybridization and Southern blotting experiments suggest that each of three different groups of kappa chains are encoded by 6-8 germ line V genes (14, 15, 16). If this number is typical for most mouse κ groups, the mouse κ family will have somewhere between 175 to 280 germ line V genes. A possible mechanism for generating germ line or somatic V region diversity has been suggested by the electron microscopic analysis of multiple V gene clones isolated from a single group (17). The flanking DNA sequences for V genes within a group appear to be homologous whereas the flanking sequences for V segments of different groups appear distinct. This gene organization would promote crossing-over or gene conversion at meiosis or mitosis and, accordingly could account in part for the rapid expansion and contraction of gene families and/or somatic variation of antibody genes to be discussed subsequently.

SYSTEMS FOR THE ANALYSIS OF ANTIBODY DIVERSITY

Studies on groups of V regions from two antibody gene families of the mouse, λ and κ, have provided interesting insights into our understanding of mechanisms for antibody diversity.

The Mouse λ System

The sequences from mouse λ chains suggest that somatic mutation may play a role in generating antibody diversity. The V regions from 18 myeloma λ chains have been sequenced (18, 19). Twelve V regions are identical and the six variant sequences differ from the prototype sequence ($V_{\lambda I}$) by one to three amino acid substitutions, all of which are in the hypervariable regions. These data are compatible with the concept of somatic mutation; namely, there is a single germ line $V_{\lambda I}$ gene from which the variants arise by somatic mutation. Moreover, since all of the variation is observed in the antigen-binding site (i.e., the hypervariable regions), perhaps the variants are selected for improved fit to particular antigens (antigen-driven selection). This interpretation is supported by nucleic acid hybridization studies that suggest V_λ regions are encoded by one or a few germ line genes.

The Mouse V_κ21 System

This system suggests that the κ family is encoded by multiple germ line V genes and that the J segment may play a role in generating antibody diversity. In several screens of the N-terminal 23 residues of κ chains from BALB/c (20, 21) and NZB (22) mice, a particular sequence, later designated the V_κ21 group (20), was found repeatedly. We determined the complete V_κ21 sequences of four BALB proteins (23). Two V regions differed by only three residues and, accordingly, defined one subgroup whereas the other two V regions differed from each other and the subgroup prototype sequences more extensively. Recently McKean and his coworkers have analyzed four additional BALB/c $V_\kappa21$ sequences (24). Two of these are very similar to the two unpaired $V_\kappa21$ regions in the former analyses and thus permit us to define two additional subgroups. Once again two unpaired proteins were distinct from each other and those proteins in the three subgroups. Antisera were made that could specifically recognize the $V_\kappa21$ light chains (D. McKean, M. Potter, and M. Weigert, personal communication). The $V_\kappa21$ polypeptides constitute about 8% of both the myeloma and normal serum light chain populations (M. Weigert, personal communication). In collaboration with Dr. Weigert, our laboratory has determined the nearly complete V region sequences of 22 $V_\kappa21$ chains from the NZB mouse (Fig. 2) (12). Two important observations emerge from these data.

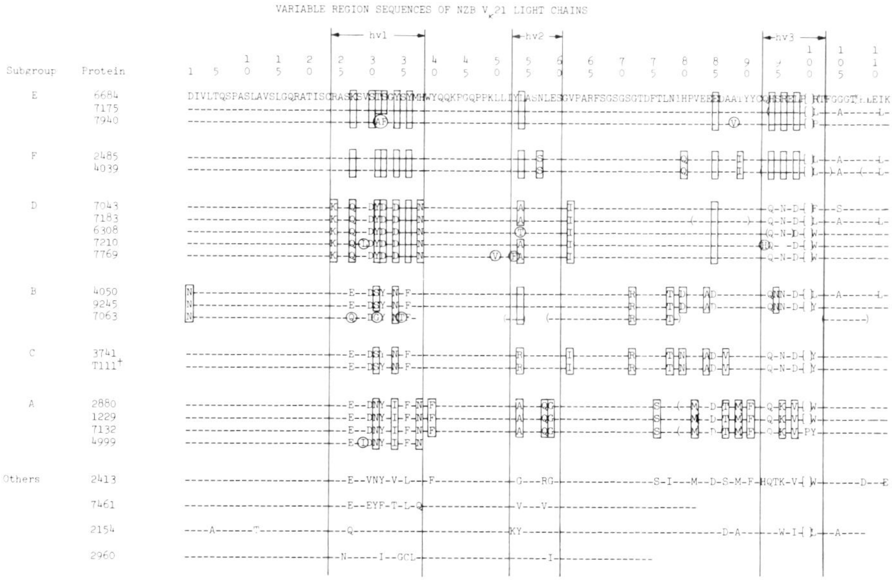

Fig. 2. The amino acid sequences of V regions from the mouse $V_\kappa21$ group. The sequences are divided into subgroups which are designated $V_\kappa21A$ through $V_\kappa21F$. Additional potential subgroups are indicated with question marks. The T111 sequence is a BALB/c protein (24), identical to PC3741, which permits the definition of subgroup $V_\kappa21C$. The subgroup-associated residues unique to to three or fewer subgroups are boxed. The intrasubset substitutions are circled. Amino acid compositional data are indicated by brackets. The three hypervariable regions are indicated as hv1, hv2, and hv3. The J segment extends from residue 100-112. From (12).

Eighteen of these $V_\kappa21$ regions may be divided into six subgroups. Subgroup-associated residues distinguish the members of a particular subgroup from members of most other subgroups (boxed residues in Fig. 2). The number of subgroups is, presumably, a minimal estimate of the number of germ line V genes in the κ21 group. DNA saturation hybridization experiments suggest that the number of germ line $V_\kappa 21$ genes is 5-6 (15). In spite of this striking agreement between these two approaches, one reservation must be emphasized. Four of the 22 $V_\kappa 21$ regions are unpaired and do not fall into any subgroup (Fig. 2). If additional $V_\kappa 21$ sequences are determined which pair with these unmatched proteins, additional $V_\kappa 21$ subgroups will be defined. If additional $V_\kappa 21$ subgroups are found, then two possibilities must be considered. First, the nucleic acid studies are underestimating the number of germ line $V_\kappa 21$ genes. Alternatively, a somatic mechanism may exist which permits a single germ line V gene to generate two or more subgroups of $V_\kappa 21$ regions.

A J segment is evident. The J segment appears to have started by position 101 because of the invariant association of a leucine at this position with an alanine and leucine at positions 105 and 111, respectively, in the J segment of six different $V_\kappa 21$ regions (Fig. 2). This repeated and invariant association of three residues suggests that positions 101 through 111 behave as a discrete genetic unit. The last subgroup-associated residue of the V segment is at position 98. Accordingly, the N-terminal boundary of the J segment may start somewhere between residues 99 and 101. Position 100 is an amino acid insertion in one κ chain (PC7132) and we have arbitrarily chosen the J segment to include this position, suggesting that the extra residue comes from a J segment one residue longer than the others. The C-terminal boundary of the J segment occurs at position 112, the C-terminal-most variable residue in κ chains (Fig. 2 - PC2413). Moreover, since the C region appears to be coded by one or a few C genes (25, 26), the variability in the J region is too great to be accounted for by multiple C_κ genes beginning at position 100.

The V and J segments associate independently with one another. In the 18 $V_\kappa 21$ regions with relatively complete sequence data between residues 100 and 112, there are 16 different V segments and 8 different J segments (Fig. 2). A particular J segment may be associated with V_κ segments from four different subgroups. Conversely, identical V segments may be associated with different J segments (e.g., PC6684 and PC7175, PC7043 and PC7183, and PC4050 and PC9245). The implication is that the V and J segments associate freely with one another and that particular V segments are not generally associated with certain J segments. Indeed, some of these same J segments are associated with non-$V_\kappa 21$ V segments of widely differing sequence. Thus, a particular J segment of the κ family may be capable of associating with any V segment of the κ family.

Nucleic acid studies on mouse λ and κ genes discussed earlier also suggest that there are V and J segments. Moreover, these nucleic acid studies suggest for the λ and κ families that the J segment extends into the third hypervariable region. Our $V_\kappa 21$ sequence data suggest the kappa gene family has two important organizational features: 1) The κ chain is encoded by three noncontinuous gene segments, V, J, and C. 2) Multiple V gene and J gene segments are present in the kappa gene family of each mouse.

The most attractive function for the J segment is that it may be involved in generating antibody diversity. Residues 100 and 101 constitute a portion of the third hypervariable region (24). Accordingly, if the J segment extends from positions 100-112, a single J segment may be joined in a combinatorial fashion to each V segment to provide another stage in the amplification of antibody diversity. We designate this process as combinatorial joining. Indeed, position 101 is among the most variable in the $V_\kappa 21$ regions examined (Fig. 2). This diversity might include sequence gaps (insertions or deletions) as well as nucleotide substitutions. The sequence gaps would result from J regions of different length (e.g., proline at position 100 in PC7132). If the mouse κ gene family has 200 V segments and 20 J segments, a combinatorial joining of V and J segments could generate 4000 different V regions.

FIVE MECHANISMS FOR STORING OR GENERATING DIVERSITY IN THE IMMUNE SYSTEM

The immune system of the vertebrate organism is capable of storing or generating a great deal of information--the information required to produce antibody molecules recognizing many different antigens. Five basic strategies for information storage and generation are given in Table 1.

TABLE 1 Strategies for Generating Antibody Diversity

Genetic	multiple germ line V genes somatic mutation combinatorial joining
Molecular	combinatorial association multispecificity

These basic strategies fall into two general categories. The genetic strategies amplify information by producing multiple antibody V genes, whereas the molecular strategies amplify information by employing certain fundamental characteristics of antibody molecules themselves. Unfortunately, molecular immunology has focused on the genetic mechanisms discussed above almost to the exclusion of the molecular mechanisms. Let us therefore discuss the molecular mechanisms.

Combinatorial association is possible because antibody molecules are made up of nonidentical subunits (light and heavy chains) (28). This mechanism suggests that a single light chain may associate with many different heavy chains to produce different antibody molecules. For example, if a thousand light and a thousand heavy chains can each associate freely with one another, 10^6 different antibody molecules would be produced. X-ray crystallographic studies suggest that appropriate residues are highly conserved at the sites of V_L and V_H interaction so that virtually any light chain might in theory associate with virtually any heavy chain (29). Furthermore, somatic cell hybrids formed between two different myeloma cells or a myeloma cell and an antibody-producing cell suggest that many different light-heavy chain combinations are permissible (30). For example, 9 out of a possible 11 light-heavy combinations were seen in various somatic cell hybrids created at Cambridge (C. Milstein, personal communication). Thus combinatorial association may be a powerful strategy for amplifying a given amount of germ line information.

Multispecificity indicates that a single antibody molecule may interact with a variety of different antigens, some presumably related in tertiary structure and others possibly unrelated (31, 32). The antigen-binding crevice is a shallow trough (33) and accordingly, there is room in the active site for many different molecular interactions. If individual antibody molecules may combine with 10 to 100 different antigenic determinants, a given number of antibody molecules may interact with a much larger number of different antigens.

Surprisingly few experiments have been directed towards assessing the relative contributions of combinatorial association and multispecificity to the antibody repertoire. These molecular strategies appear to offer extremely important mechanisms for information generation in multigene families. Clearly multispecificity and combinatorial association will have to be studied at the level of antibody molecules since their diversity arises as a result of the interaction of two nonidentical polypeptides, a relationship that does not exist at the nucleic acid level. It must be stressed that in a formal sense neither multispecificity nor combinatorial association have been established as fundamental mechanisms for generating information.

The goal with regard to theories of antibody diversity in the future will be to ascertain the relative contributions of 1) multiple germ line V genes, 2) somatic mutation, 3) combinatorial joining, 4) combinatorial association, and 5) multi-specificity to the functional repertoire of antibody molecules. It seems likely that all of these processes will occur in any multigenic family. The key question is "What is the relative contribution of each mechanism to the total functional diversity of vertebrate antibody molecules?"

ACKNOWLEDGEMENTS

This work was supported by NSF grant PCM-71-0070 and NIH grant AI-10781.

REFERENCES

(1) L. Hood, The genetics, evolution, and expression of antibody molecules, Stadler Genet. Symp. 5, 73-142 (1973).

(2) J. A. Gally and G. M. Edelman, The genetic control of immunoglobulin synthesis, Ann. Rev. Genet. 6, 1-46 (1972).

(3) T. T. Wu and E. A. Kabat, An analysis of the sequences of the variable regions of Bence Jones proteins and myeloma light chains and their implications for antibody complementarity, J. Exp. Med. 132, 211-250 (1970).

(4) J. D. Capra and T. J. Kindt, Antibody diversity: Can more than one gene encode each variable region?, Immunogenetics 1, 417-427 (1975).

(5) T. J. Kindt and J. D. Capra, Gene-insertion theories of antibody diversity: A re-evaluation, Immunogenetics 6, 309-321 (1978).

(6) M. Raff, T and B lymphocytes and immune responses, Nature (Lond.) 242, 19-23 (1973).

(7) M. Potter, Antigen-binding myeloma proteins of mice, Adv. in Immunol. 25, 141-211 (1977).

(8) R. Mage, R. Lieberman, M. Potter and W. D. Terry. (1973) In: The Antigens, I, (Ch. 4, pp. 300-376) Academic Press, New York.

(9) J. Gally. (1973) In: The Antigens, I, (pp. 161-298) Academic Press, New York.

(10) D. R. Davies, E. A. Padlan and D. M. Segal. (1975) In: Contemp. Topics Molec. Immunol., (Vol. 4, pp. 127-155) Plenum Press, New York and London.

(11) E. A. Kabat, T. T. Wu and H. Bilofsky, Variable region genes for the immunoglobulin framework are assembled from small segments of DNA - A hypothesis, Proc. Nat. Acad. Sci. USA 75, 2429-2433 (1978).

(12) M. Weigert, L. Gatmaitan, E. Loh, J. Schilling and L. Hood, Rearrangement of genetic information may produce immunoglobulin diversity, Nature in press, (1978).

(13) C. Brach, M. Hirama, R. Lenhard-Schuller and S. Tonegawa, A complete immunoglobulin gene is created by somatic recombination, Cell 15, 1-14 (1978).

(14) J. G. Seidman, A. Leder, M. H. Edgell, F. Polsky, S. M. Tilghman, D. C. Tiemeier and P. Leder, Multiple related immunoglobulin variable-region genes identified by cloning and sequence analysis, Proc. Nat. Acad. Sci. USA 75, 3881-3885 (1978).

(15) O. Valbuena, K. B. Marcu, M. Weigert and R. P. Perry, Nature, submitted.

(16) R. Perry, personal communication.

(17) J. G. Seidman, A. Leder, M. Nau, B. Norman and P. Leder, Antibody diversity. The structure of cloned immunoglobulin genes suggests a mechanism for gene-rating new sequences, Science 202, 11-17 (1978).

(18) I. M. Cesari and M. Weigert, Mouse lambda-chain sequences, Proc. Nat. Acad. Sci. USA 70, 2112-2116 (1973).

(19) M. Weigert and R. Riblet, Genetic control of antibody variable regions, Cold Spring Harbor Symp. Quant. Biol. 61, 837-846 (1977).

(20) L. E. Hood, M. Potter and D. J. McKean, Immunoglobulin structure. Comparison of amino terminal sequences of kappa chains derived from genetically similar mice (BALB/c), Science 170, 1207-1210 (1970).

(21) L. E. Hood, D. McKean, V. Farnsworth and M. Potter, Mouse immunoglobulin chains: A survey of the amino terminal sequence of kappa chains, Biochemistry 12, 741-749 (1973).

(22) E. Loh, B. Black, R. Riblet, M. Weigert, J. M. Hood and L. Hood, Comparisons of myeloma proteins from NZB and BALB/c mice: Structural and functional differences of light chains, Proc. Nat. Acad. Sci. USA, in press (1978).

(23) D. McKean, M. Potter and L. Hood, Mouse immunoglobulin chains: The pattern of sequence variation among kappa chains with limited sequence differences, Biochemistry 12, 760-771 (1973).

(24) D. J. McKean, M. Bell and M. Potter, Mechanisms of antibody diversity: Multiple genes encode structurally related mouse kappa variable regions, Proc. Nat. Acad. Sci. USA 75, 3913-3917 (1978).

(25) P. Leder, T. Honjo, D. Swan, S. Packman, M. Nau and B. Norman. (1975) In: Molecular Approaches to Immunology, Miami Winter Symposia, (Vol. 9, pp. 173-188) Academic Press, New York.

(26) T. H. Rabbitts and C. Milstein. (1977) In: Contemp. Topics Molec. Immunol., (Vol. 6, pp. 117-143) Plenum Press, New York and London.

(27) E. A. Kabat, T. T. Wu and H. Bilofsky. (1976) In: Tabulations and Analyses of Amino Acid Sequences, Beranek and Newman, Cambrige, Massachusetts.

(28) G. M. Edelman, Antibody structure and molecular immunology, Ann. N.Y. Acad. Sci. 190, 5-25 (1971).

(29) R. J. Poljak, L. M. Amzel, B. L. Chen, R. P. Phizackerley and F. Saul, Structural basis for the association of heavy and light chains and the relation of subgroups to the conformation of the active site of immunoglobulins, Immunogenetics 2, 393-394 (1975).

(30) J. Schwaber and E. P. Cohen, Pattern of immunoglobulin synthesis and assembly in a human-mouse somatic cell hybrid clone, Proc. Nat. Acad. Sci. USA 71, 2203-2207 (1974).

(31) J. Inman. (1974) In: The Immune System: Genes, Receptors, Signals, Academic Press, New York and London.

(32) F. Richard, W. Konigsberg, R. Rosenstein and J. Varga, On the specificity of antibodies, Science 187, 130-137 (1975).

(33) D. R. Davies, E. A. Padlan and D. M. Segal, Three-dimensional structure of immunoglobulins, Ann. Rev. Biochem. 44, 639-667 (1975).

VARIANTS OF MOUSE MYELOMA CELLS

W. Cook, B. Dharmgrongartama and M.D. Scharff
Albert Einstein College of Medicine, 1300 Morris Park Ave., Bronx, N.Y. 10461

INTRODUCTION

As has been described in the two preceding papers, much has been learned about the structure of the antibody molecule and the structure and organization of the immunoglobulin genes (1-5). These studies have led to important insights into the structural basis of antibody function and suggested very specific genetic mechanisms for the generation of antibody diversity. Furthermore studies with whole animals and with complex mixtures of cells in vitro have provided us with a great deal of information on the cellular interactions responsible for antibody production (6). In spite of all of this progress, it seems likely that additional approaches will be required if we are to discover the detailed molecular mechanisms involved in the rearrangement and expression of immunoglobulin genes and the generation of antibody diversity. At least at the outset, such studies will probably have to be carried out with homogeneous populations of cells producing specific antibodies. Mouse myeloma cells provide one such system. Cells from the many tumors available can be adapted to continuous culture, cloned to guarantee homogeneity, and manipulated biochemically and genetically (7). In addition, the myeloma cells have two unusual and useful characteristics: 1) they are very unstable in the expression of immunoglobulin genes and generate a wide variety of variants at a very high frequency (8,9); and 2) variant cells can be injected into the peritoneal cavity of BALB/c mice and the resultant ascites contains 1-10mgs/ml of the mutant immunoglobulin. This means that variants can be accumulated relatively easily and large amounts of the variant gene product can be collected and chemically characterized.

In fact, it has been possible to begin to analyze the somatic cell genetics of immunoglobulin production by mouse myeloma cells using approaches which are similar to those developed years ago by the microbial geneticists. Techniques were developed to clone the cultured myeloma cells at high efficiencies in soft agar (10). Fluctuation analyses were carried out and revealed that variants arose spontaneously at a frequency of 10^{-3}/cell/generation, or one in every 1000 cell divisions resulted in a variant (11). Some mutagenizing agents increased the frequency of variants 20 fold (11,12). When the same myeloma cells were examined for a variety of mutations in proteins other than immunoglobulin, the spontaneous and mutagen induced frequencies of such variants were orders of magnitude lower than the frequency of immunoglobulin variants (11). A number of variants with changes in their heavy or light chains have been characterized serologically and chemically. Milstein and his colleagues (9) and Francus and Birshtein (13) have examined the amino acid sequence of a number of variants.

Synthesis Variants

The general characteristics of most of the variants studied up to now are summarized in Table 1. For convenience, we have divided these into two groups based on

TABLE 1 Ig Mutants in Mouse Myeloma Cells

1. Synthesis variants
    - a. Loss variants
      H^-L^+, H^+L^-, H^-L^-
    - b. Quantitative variants
      $H^{\pm}L^-$, $H^+L^{\pm}$
2. Structural variants
    - a. Short heavy chains
      deletions, premature terminations
    - b. Recombinant (hybrid) molecules
      IgG_{2b}-IgG_{2a}, IgG_1-IgG_{2b}
    - c. Small changes in sequence
      point mutations, frameshifts

their phenotype. In the first group there is an obvious change in expression of the immunoglobulin heavy and/or light chains. In most cases this has resulted in the loss of expression of one or both chains. Many possible defects could result in this phenotype: chromosomes bearing structural or regulatory genes could have been lost; all or part of a structural or regulatory gene could have been deleted; the transcription or processing of messenger RNA might be defective; the translation of messenger in the cytoplasm may be blocked; or there might be rapid degradation of the newly synthesized polypeptide chain. Detailed studies on a few variants have revealed examples of some of these molecular defects (14,15,16). Studies from Pestka's (15), and our own laboratory (16) have shown that some loss variants do not contain detectable messenger RNA for the missing polypeptide chain. Cowan and Milstein have also described a variant which synthesizes light chain messenger RNA which associates with ribosomes but is apparently not translated (14). Other loss variants may have defects in initiation of the transcription or processing of messenger RNA. It is likely that continued studies on the many loss variants available will reveal defects in each of the other steps in immunoglobulin synthesis.

The identification of somatic cell variants which synthesize fewer heavy or light chains than their parental cell are of particular interest because they suggest the presence of regulatory mechanisms. We have studied two spontaneously arising variants which synthesized half as many light chains as the parent (17,18). In one case, revertants to wild type behavior arose at a high frequency (18). We have also identified variants which synthesize approximately 1/10 the amount of heavy chains as the parental cells (19). Similar sorts of variants have also been reported by Shubert and Cohn (20) and by Cowan et al. (14). In some cases there appear to be structural changes in the variant chain (14,17,20) while in others the chains are normal in size and do not differ in their peptide maps from the parental chain (19). It is not yet clear whether the decreases in synthesis observed are due to changes in gene dosage, rates of transcription of messenger RNA, messenger processing or due to changes in the rate of translation. Clearly, detailed molecular biological studies will be required before we know the significance of these "synthesis" variants.

Structural Variants

Variants which produce immunoglobulins that differ structurally from the parental protein also arise frequently. A number of approaches have been used to identify such variants. We have cloned the cells in soft agar, overlayed the clones with antibody against one or another part of the immunoglobulin molecule, and looked for clones which had lost the ability to secrete a serologically reactive molecule (10). Some of the variants identified in this way were loss variants while others continued to produce heavy chains but these heavy chains differed serologically and structurally from those of the parent (21,22,23). We have also cloned a mouse myeloma cell line whose immunoglobulin reacted with a known antigen, overlayed with antigen, and identified clones which produced immunoglobulin which had decreased antigen binding (24). Milstein and his colleagues have cloned a mouse myeloma cell line, and studied the products of 7000 clones by isoelectric focusing (25). Four variants with changes in the amino acid sequence of their heavy chains were identified and characterized (25,26,27).

A number of these structural variants have been characterized in some detail with the hope that they will provide information on the structure of the immunoglobulin genes. Since they arise so frequently, it is also possible that they could provide insights into the mechanisms responsible for antibody diversity. Those structural variants studied so far can be divided into three phenotypes (Table 1). There is a large number of spontaneous and mutagen induced variants whose heavy chains are smaller than the heavy chain of the parental clone. Adetugbo et al. have determined the amino acid sequence of three of these "short" chain mutants (9,26,27). Two have deletions at the C-terminal end of their heavy chain. Nucleic acid sequencing of the messenger RNA revealed that one of these was due to a frameshift and a premature termination while another was due to a point mutation to a terminating codon producing a premature termination (28). The third variant had an internal deletion similar to that seen in many human heavy chain disease proteins. Morrison has also identified a variant with an internal deletion (29). We have found that short chain mutants with C-terminal deletions come in a continuum of sizes (30,31).

We have described a second type of structural variant which has a normal sized heavy chain but contains the amino acid sequence and serology of a constant region which was not expressed in the parental cell (22,23). Since the variable region of the parental cell is still associated with this new constant region, we have for convenience call these "recombinant" variants (23). This sort of variant has also been identified by Liesegang et al (32). Similar variants have been reported in man by Kunkel and his colleagues (33). Francus and Birshtein (13) and Greenberg et al (34) have examined the amino acid sequence of a few of these recombinant variants. At the moment the simplest, though not necessarily correct, explanation of their origin is that crossing over has occurred between the IgG_{2b} and IgG_{2a} constant region genes in the mouse genome.

Finally, some of the structural variants are almost identical with the parental protein. For example, Adetugbo et al. have identified a variant which has a single amino acid substitution in its constant region (26). We have identified and studied a set of variants which have changes in antigen binding associated with small changes in the peptide maps of their heavy chains (24,30). These variants were generated from a cultured cell line of the S107 tumor. S107 cells produce an IgA kappa immunoglobulin which binds the hapten phsophocholine (PC) (35). The cells were cloned in soft agar and overlayed with PC attached to a protein (KLH). Most of the clones secreted the parental immunoglobulin into the surrounding agar where it reacted with PC-KLH to produce a precipitate that could be seen surrounding the clones using a low power inverted microscope (24). Clones that were not surrounded by precipitates were recovered from the agar and studied in detail.

Some of these had lost the ability to produce IgA heavy chains but most were secreting what appeared to be normal sized fully assembled immunoglobulin in the same amounts as the parent (24,30). However, when the immunoglobulin secreted by these 1st generation antigen binding variants was purified and reacted with antigen in agar diffusion, it did not react while equal amounts of the purified parental protein did (24,30) (Table 2). While the lack of reactivity in the original cloning

TABLE 2 Characterization of Antigen Binding Variants

Generation	Reactivity with PC-KLH (agar diffusion)	Hemagglutination Titer (PC-SRBC)[a]	Relative Binding[b] PC-KLH	Relative Binding[b] Site Specific Antibody	Difference in Peptide Analysis of Chains H	L
parent	+	8192	100%	100%		
1	-	128	9	8.7	yes	no
2	+	512	26	18	yes	no
3	-	-	<0.4	n.d.	yes	no

[a] 250 μg of purified antibody was used as starting material

[b] competition between purified parental or variant antibody and labelled parent was examined using a solid radioimmuno assay.

$$\frac{\text{(ng parent required for 50\% inhibition of binding of label)}}{\text{(ng parent required for 50\% inhibition of binding of label)}}$$

assay and in agar diffusion suggest a loss of antigen binding, the variant protein retained some affinity for the hapten (Table 2). This variant protein was 1/10th as effective as the parent in binding PC-KLH in a radioimmunoassay (24) (Table 2) and had a lower hemagglutinating titer than the parental protein (Table 2).

Second generation variants with binding that was intermediate between that of the parent and another 1st generation variant were isolated by recloning the 1st generation variant in agar, overlaying with antigen, and picking clones surrounded by a visible precipitate (24). Third generation variants with low antigen binding were obtained by looking amongst the 2nd generation subclones for unstained clones. The phenotype of each generation was confirmed by agar diffusion, hemagglutination, and radioimmunoassay of the purified immunoglobulin from each variant (Table 2). These variants also differed from the parent and from each other when they were examined serologically with antibody directed against the antigen binding site in the variable region (24) (Table 2).

An analysis of the tryptic peptides prepared from heavy (H) and light (L) chains showed that the light chains of 1st, 2nd, and 3rd generation variants were indistinguishable from the parental light chain (24,36). In contrast, each of the heavy chains differed from the parental heavy chains and from the variants by one or two tryptic peptides (24,36) (Table 2). While amino acid sequence analyses which are now in progress will be required to determine the exact nature of the differences, all of these findings suggest that the changes in antigen binding are due to small changes in the primary structure of the heavy chains.

Since each generation of variants arose spontaneously at a frequency of 0.1-2% from its immediate parent (24), we have concluded that primary sequence changes are occuring in the heavy chain variable region at a very high frequency. In fact, we appear to be generating antibody diversity in somatic cells. As already described above, constant region structural variants also arise at a very high frequency. Taken together, these results indicate that the expression and structure of the immunoglobulin genes are highly unstable in mouse myeloma cells. At the moment, it is not clear whether this instability is related to the normal mechanisms responsible for antibody diversity.

Finally, it is worth pointing out that these variant myeloma cells and the proteins produced by them are useful in studying the synthesis, assembly, glycosylation, and secretion of immunoglobulins and in examining structure-function relationships in the immunoglobulin molecule itself. For example, we have isolated and studied variants which produce non-glycosylated IgG immunoglobulins (37,38). Since these proteins are synthesized, assembled and secreted normally it was possible to conclude that the carbohydrate moiety on heavy chains was not required for the intracellular metabolism of mouse IgG.

CONCLUSION

In conclusion, cultured mouse myeloma cells have been shown to generate a wide variety of variants which differ from the parental cells in production and structure of the immunoglobulin molecules. Since these variants are stable and often produce mutant gene products with defects (deletions, frameshifts, amino acid substitutions) similar to those found in bacterial mutants, they would normally be assumed to have resulted from classical mutational processes. However, since the frequency of these variants is much higher than normally seen, the mechanism responsible for them will have to be determined and their relationship to normal events must be examined in detail.

ACKNOWLEDGMENT

This work was supported by grants from the NSF (PCM75-13609, NSF PCM77-25635) and the NIH (AI10702, AI5231-15). Wendy Cook is supported by a Fellowship from the Young Man's Philanthropic League.

REFERENCES

1. R. Painter, This Volume (1979).

2. L. Hood, This Volume (1979).

3. C. Brack, M. Hirama, R. Lenhard-Schuller, and S. Tonegawa, A complete immunoglobulin gene is created by somatic recombination, Cell 15, 1 (1978).

4. J.A. Seidman, A. Leder, M. Mace, B. Newman, and P. Leder, Antibody diversity: the structure of cloned immunoglobulin genes suggests a mechanism for generating new sequences, Science 202, 11 (1978).

5. E.A. Kabat, T.T. Wu, and H. Bilofsky (1976) Variable Regions of Immunoglobulin Chains, Bolb, Beranek, Newman, Cambridge, Ma.

6. Cold Spring Harbor Symposium on Quantitative Biology, 41 (1976).

7. M.D. Scharff, The synthesis, assembly, and secretion of immunoglobulin: a biochemical and genetic approach, Harvey Lectures 69, 125 (1975).

8. S.L. Morrison, R. Baumal, B.K. Birshtein, W.M. Kuehl, J.-L. Preud'homme, L. Frank, T. Jasek, and M.D. Scharff, The identification of mouse myeloma cells which have undergone mutations in Ig production. In Cellular Selection and Regulation in the Immune Response, ed. G.M. Edelman, p.233, Raven Press, New York.

9. K. Adetugbo, C. Milstein, and D.S. Secher, Nature 265, 299 (1977).

10. P. Coffino, R. Baumal, R. Laskov, M.D. Scharff, Cloning of mouse myeloma cells and detection of rare variants, J. Cell. Physiol. 79, 429 (1972).

11. R. Baumal, B.K. Birshtein, P. Coffino, and M.D. Scharff, Mutations in immunoglobulin-producing myeloma cells, Science 182, 164 (1973).

12. J.-L. Preud'homme, J. Buxbaum, and M.D. Scharff, Mutagenesis of mouse myeloma cells with "Melphalan", Nature 245, 320 (1973).

13. T. Francus and B.K. Birshtein, An IgG_{2a}-producing variant of an IgG_{2b}-producing mouse myeloma cell line. Structural studies on the Fc region of parent and variant heavy chains, Biochemistry 17, 4324 (1978).

14. N.J. Cowan, D.S. Secher, and C. Milstein, Intracellular immunoglobulin chain synthesis in non-secreting variants of a mouse myeloma: detection of inactive light-chain messenger RNA, J. Molecular Biol. 90, 691 (1974).

15. M. Green, P.N. Graves, T. Zehavi-Willner, J. McInnes and S. Pestka, Cell-free translation of Ig mRNA from MOPC 315 plasmacytoma and MOPC 315 NR, a variant synthesizing only light chain, PNAS 72, 224 (1975).

16. W.M. Kuehl, B.A. Kaplan, M.D. Scharff, M. Nau, T. Honjo, and P. Leder, Characterization of light chain and light chain constant region fragment mRNAs in MPC 11 mouse myeloma cells and variants, Cell 5, 139 (1975).

17. R. Baumal and M.D. Scharff, Immunoglobulin biosynthesis by the MOPC 173 mouse myeloma tumor and a variant clone, J. Immunol. 116, 65 (1976).

18. S.L. Morrison and M.D. Scharff, A mouse myeloma variant with a defect in light chain synthesis, European Journal of Immunology, In Press (1979).

19. S.L. Morrison, and M.D. Scharff, Heavy chain-producing variants of a mouse myeloma cell line, J. Immunol. 114, 655 (1975).

20. D. Shubert, and M. Cohn, Blocks in defective synthesis, J. Mol. Biol. 38, 273 (1968).

21. B.K. Birshtein, J.-L. Preud'homme, and M.D. Scharff, Variants of mouse myeloma cells that produce short immunoglobulin heavy chains, P.N.A.S. 71, 3478 (1974).

22. J.-L. Preud'homme, B.K. Birshtein, and M.D. Scharff, Variants of a mouse myeloma cell line that produce immunoglobulin having an altered serotype, P.N.A.S. 72, 1427 (1975).

23. T. Francus, B. Dharmgrongartama, R. Campbell, M.D. Scharff, and B.K. Birshtein, IgG_{2a}-producing variants of an IgG_{2b}-producing mouse myeloma cell line, J. Exp. Med. 147, 1535 (1978).

24. W.D. Cook, and M.D. Scharff, Antigen-binding mutants of mouse myeloma cells, P.N.A.S. 74, 5687 (1977).

25. R.G.H. Cotton, D.S. Secher, and C. Milstein, Somatic mutation and the origin of antibody diversity. Clonal variability of the immunoglobulin produced by MOPC21 cells in culture, Eur. J. Immunol. 3, 135 (1973).

26. K. Adetugbo and C. Milstein, Spontaneous missense mutation of an immunoglobulin in a mouse myeloma cell line, J. Mol. Biol. 115, 75 (1977).

27. K. Adetugbo and C. Milstein, Spontaneous somatic frameshift mutation in a mouse myeloma, J. Mol. Biol. 121, 239 (1978).

28. C. Milstein, K. Adetugbo, N.J. Cowan, G. Kohler, D.S. Secher and C.D. Wilde, Somatic cell genetics of antibody-secreting cells: studies of clonal diversification and analysis by cell fusion, CSHSQB 41, 793 (1976).

29. S.L. Morrison, Murine heavy chain disease, Eur. J. Immunol. 8, 194 (1978).

30. W.D. Cook, B. Dharmgrongartama, and M.D. Scharff, Variable and constant region variants of mouse myeloma cells, in Cells of Immunoglobulin Synthesis, ed. B. Pernis and H.J. Vogel, P & S Biomedical Sciences Symposia, Columbia Press, N.Y., In press (1979).

31. B. Dharmgrongartama and M.D. Scharff, In preparation.

32. B. Liesegang, A. Radbruch, and K. Rajewsky, Isolation of myeloma variants with predefined variant surface immunoglobulin by cell sorting, P.N.A.S. 75, 3901 (1978).

33. H.A. Kunkel, J.B. Natvig, and F.G. Joslin, A "Lepore" type of hybrid γ globin, P.N.A.S. 62, 144 (1969).

34. M.L. Greenberg, R. Campbell, and B.K. Birshtein, Fed. Proc. Fed. Am. Soc. Exp. Biol. 37, abstract no. 2704 (1978).

35. M.A. Leon, and N.M. Young, Six mouse IgA myeloma proteins with phosphoryl choline specificity, Fed. Proc. 29, 437 (1970).

36. W.D. Cook and M.D. Scharff, In preparation.

37. S. Weitzman, and M.D. Scharff, Mouse myeloma mutants blocked in the assembly, glycosylation and secretion of immunoglobulin, J. Mol. Biol. 102, 237 (1976).

38. S. Weitzman, S.G. Nathenson, and M.D. Scharff, Abnormalities in the glycosylation of immunoglobulin heavy chain and an H-2 transplantation antigen in a mouse myeloma mutant, Cell 10, 679 (1977).

MOUSE LAMBDA-2 LIGHT CHAINS: A MODEL SYSTEM FOR STUDYING IMMUNOGLOBULIN DIVERSITY*

Tom Cotner and Herman N. Eisen

Department of Biology and Center for Cancer Research
Massachusetts Institute of Technology, Cambridge, MA 02139

For over a decade the origin of diversity of the variable (V) regions of immunoglobulin (Ig) molecules has been a central question in immunology. Does the great number of these regions derive entirely from a large number of diverse genes in the germ line or from a much smaller number that become diversified during somatic development (1)? It has recently been found that there are probably 100 and perhaps as many as 1,000 genes for the V regions of κ chains in mouse embryo DNA and presumably, therefore, in germ cell DNA (2). However, for the V regions of λ1 chains, another type of mouse light (L) chain, there appears to be only a single embryonic or germ line gene (Vλ1) (3); hence the earlier finding that some mouse myeloma proteins have λ1 chains whose V regions differ in sequence from the putative germ line Vλ1 gene indicates that somatic variation of the deoxynucleotide sequence of the germ line gene can indeed occur (4,5).

With these recent findings, the central question is no longer whether V regions of Igs are encoded entirely by germ line V genes or entirely by somatic variants of these genes, but rather what proportion of V regions derived from one or the other source. As was noted above, mouse κ and λ1 L chains have already demonstrated their usefulness for approaching this question. We wish here to call attention to the advantages of another set of mouse L chains, called λ2. The λ2 set has until very recently been represented in a single Ig: the IgA protein, M315, made by the myeloma tumor MOPC-315 of BALB/c mice (5). Its L chain, L^{315}, has an amino acid sequence that establishes both its resemblance to the more common λ chains (λ1) and its uniqueness: the constant or C half of L^{315} differs from the corresponding half of λ1 chains at 29 of 110 positions. However their V regions differ at only 11-14 positions (7-10) (Fig. 1).

---

*Supported in part by a research grant (CA-15472) and by a Center grant to the M.I.T. Center for Cancer Research (CA-14051) from the National Cancer Institute, and by a training grant (GM 007 10) to the Department of Biology from the National Institute of General Medical Sciences, Department of Health, Education and Welfare.

ABBREVIATIONS: Abs, antibodies; BSA, bovine serum albumin; C, constant region of Ig chain; CM, carboxymethyl; CPA, carboxypeptidase A; Dnp, 2,4-dinitrophenyl; H, heavy Ig chain; Ig, immunoglobulin; KLH, keyhole limpet hemocyanin; L, light Ig chains; NP, 4-hydroxy-3-nitrophenylacetyl; Tnp, 2,4,6-trinitrophenyl; V, variable region of Ig chain or gene.

The L^{315} (λ2) chain offers several advantages for probing the origin of diversity. First, it can be split with pepsin to yield a fragment, called Fv, that consists of the complete V regions of L and H chains (V_L + V_H) (11). Linked noncovalently, these regions together contain all of the ligand-binding activity of the intact myeloma protein, and the fragment can be used to separate antibodies (Abs) to the C and V regions of L^{315}. These Abs, as noted below, permit the serological identification and analysis of other λ2 chains among normal and myeloma Igs (12). Second, with the mRNA for a mouse λ1 chain, Tonegawa et al. screened restriction endonuclease fragments from mouse DNA and identified a single gene for Vλ2 in the DNA of 12-day embryos (13). Hence there is probably a single Vλ2 gene in the mouse germ line. Its sequence differs from that of L^{315} at four positions in the V region: one in the "framework" at position 38 and three at contiguous positions -- 94, 95, 96 -- in the third hypervariable region (Fig. 1). Thus, comparison of amino acid or deoxynucleotide sequences for other λ2 chains or their genes (from Ig-producing cells) should reveal the frequency with which the V regions of λ2 chains are encoded by the germ line Vλ2 gene or by somatic cell variants of this gene.

How frequent are λ2 chains in normal mouse Igs? Chemical and serological approaches suggest that in the mouse about 1 in 100 Ig molecules have λ2 chains (12,14). As is shown in Fig. 2, the carboxy-terminal amino acids and the carboxy-terminal peptides expected in tryptic digests differ for κ, λ1, and λ2 (L^{315}) chains. Accordingly, L chains from normal mouse serum Igs (7S) were reduced and alkylated with iodoacetic acid and digested at pH 8 with carboxypeptidase A (CPA). As expected under these conditions the C-terminal carboxymethyl (CM)-cysteine of κ chains, which make up about 95% of L chains from mouse Igs (15), was not released; in addition, the C-terminal serine of λ1 chains was not found to a significant extent, probably because serine is released very slowly when next to a CM-cysteine (16). However, leucine, the C-terminal amino acid of λ2, was recovered at about 1 mmole per 100 mmoles of L chain, suggesting that about 1% of Igs have λ2 chains (12).

In another approach (14), the C-terminal peptides expected in a tryptic digest of the three types of L chains (Fig. 1) were synthesized by Dr. Kurt Blaser, who used them to develop a two-dimensional mapping procedure for separating the S-CM derivatives of these peptides (Fig. 3A). Tryptic digests of ^{14}C-CM-labeled κ (L^{460}) and λ2 (L^{315}) chains confirmed that the natural C-terminal peptides were indistinguishable from the synthesized ones (Fig. 3B). In tryptic digests of ^{14}C-iodoacetic acid-labeled L chains from normal serum Igs the predominant κ tripeptide and a much fainter λ1 tetrapeptide were evident; and the λ2 octopeptide was also distinctly recognizable (Fig. 3C). To confirm the identifications, each of these peptides was eluted from the peptide map and subjected to electrophoresis at two different pH values: in each case the S-^{14}C-CM-peptide from serum Igs co-migrated with the corresponding nonradioactive, synthesized S-CM peptide (Fig. 3D, E). On the assumption that all three ^{14}C-peptides were recovered to an approximately equal extent, it appeared from their ^{14}C content that λ2 chains account for about 1% of Ig L chains in BALB/c mice, λ1 accounts for about 5%, and κ chains for the rest (ca 95%) (14).

Serological analyses have been more useful than chemical ones for identifying λ2 chains. Besides being more rapid, sensitive, and quantitative, they permit independent measurements to be made of the concentration of L chains with the V and C regions of L^{315} (12). The strategy is outlined in Fig. 4. Goat antisera to protein M315 was adsorbed successively with the BALB/c myeloma proteins M460 (α,κ) to remove Abs to α chains and MOPC-104E (μ,λ1) to remove Abs that cross-react with λ1 chains. The remaining Abs, specific for L^{315} (and perhaps also for the idiotype of M315) were then adsorbed on an Fv-Sepharose column: the pass-through consisted of Abs to the C domain of L^{315} (anti-Cλ2) while the Abs that were adsorbed and then

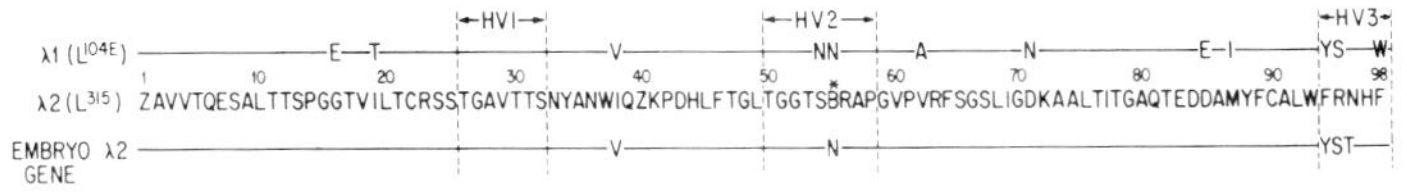

Fig. 1

Fig. 1 The amino acid sequences of V regions of λ L chains from mouse myeloma protein 104E (λ1, L^{104E}) and 315 (λ2, L^{315}) are compared with each other and with the deoxynucleotide sequence (expressed as amino acid sequence) of a λ gene from mouse embryo DNA. The sequences are shown from position 1 (the N-terminus) to 98 with the one-letter code for amino acids (see below). Horizontal lines show where the sequences for L^{104} and the λ gene are the same as L^{315}. HV1-HV3 are the three hypervariable regions. Asp at position 55 in the reported L^{315} sequence (8) is here given as Asx (B) to indicate some uncertainty. The one-letter amino acid code: A, ala; B, asx; C, cys; D, asp; E, glu; F, phe; G, gly; H, his; I, ile; K, lys; L, leu; M, met; N, asn; P, pro; Q, gln; R, arg; S, ser; T, thr; V, val; W, trp; Y, tyr; Z, glx.
Based on refs. 7-10 for the L chain sequences and 13 for the gene sequence.

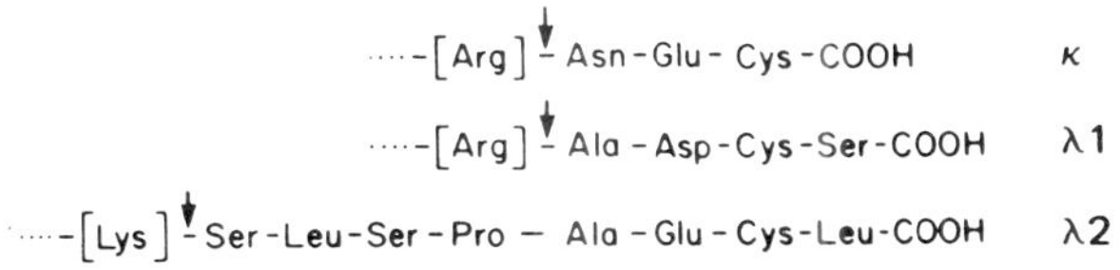

Fig. 2

Fig. 2 The carboxy-terminal peptides released by trypsin from κ, λ1, and λ2 chains. Arrows mark sites of proteolytic cleavage. These peptides were synthesized and their S-carboxymethyl (CM) derivatives were used as markers for peptide maps (see Fig. 3). Taken from ref. 14.

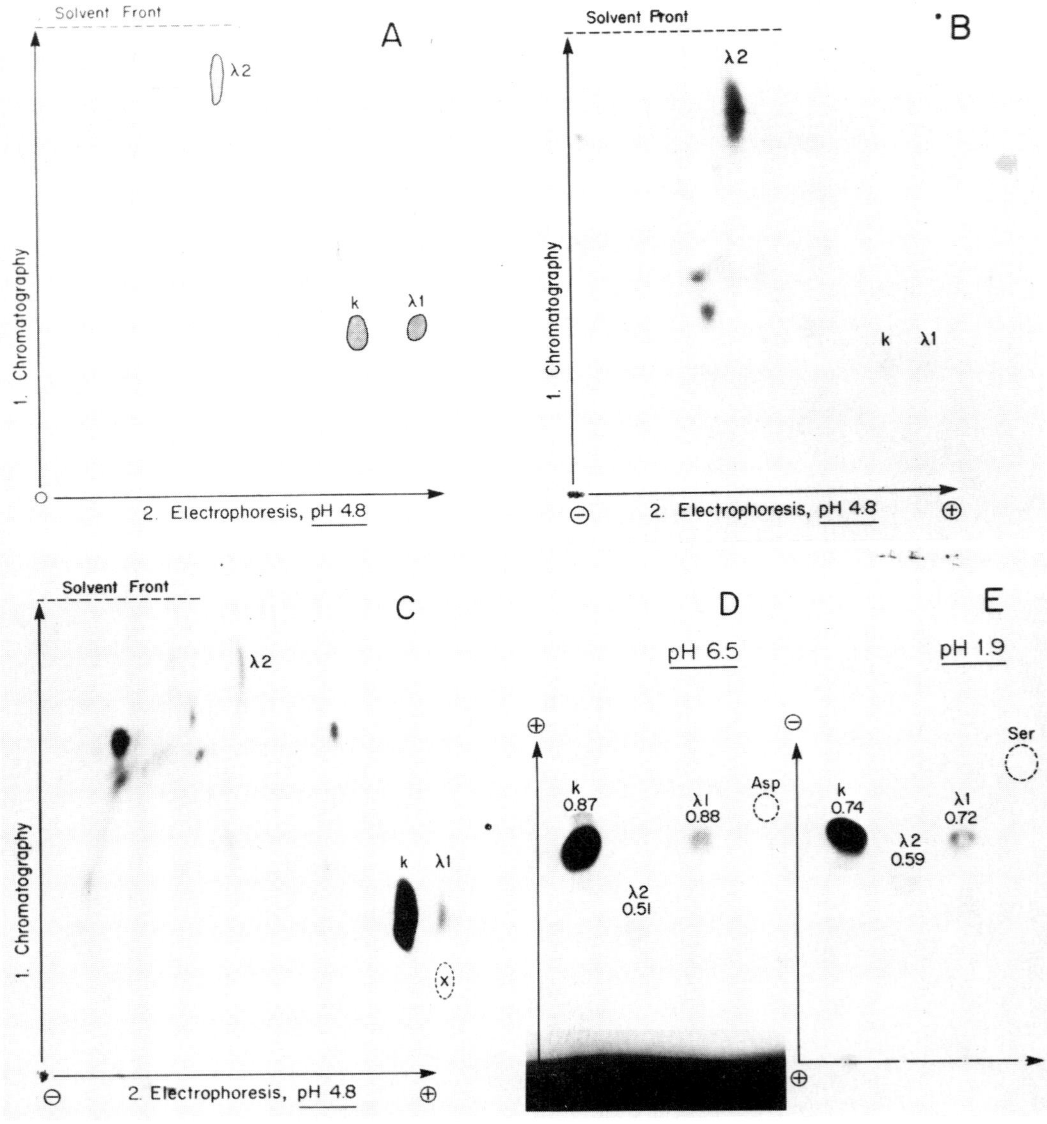

Fig. 3 Separation of synthetic C-terminal peptides (S-CM-derivatives) of κ, λ1, and λ2 chains in a peptide map (A). Radioautographs of peptide maps of tryptic digests of S-^{14}C-CM L chains reveal the λ2 peptide in L^{315} and in L chains of normal Igs (in B and C respectively). The three C-terminal peptides eluted from the map in panel C co-migrated with the corresponding synthetic peptides at pH 6.5 and 1.9 (D and E; numbers are R_F relative to marker amino acids). From ref. 14.

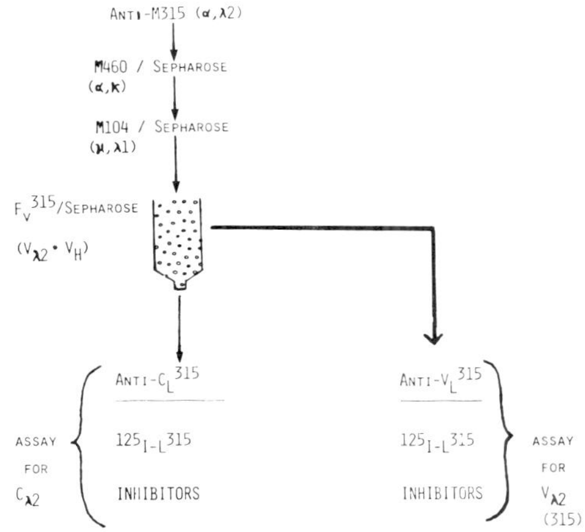

Fig. 4

Fig. 4 Preparation of Abs to C and V regions of L^{315} (anti-$C_L{}^{315}$ and anti-$V_L{}^{315}$, respectively). After adsorbing antisera to M315 to remove Abs that react with α chains and cross-react with λ1 chains, the remaining Abs were adsorbed on Fv (of M315): the pass-through is anti-$C_L{}^{315}$ and the acid-eluted Abs are anti-$V_L{}^{315}$. Based on ref. 12.

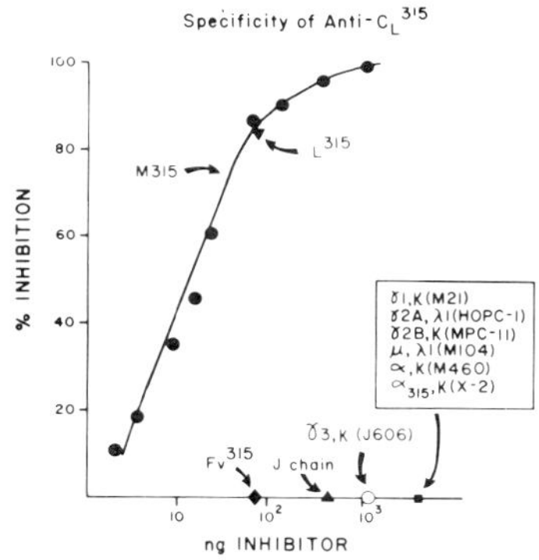

Fig. 5

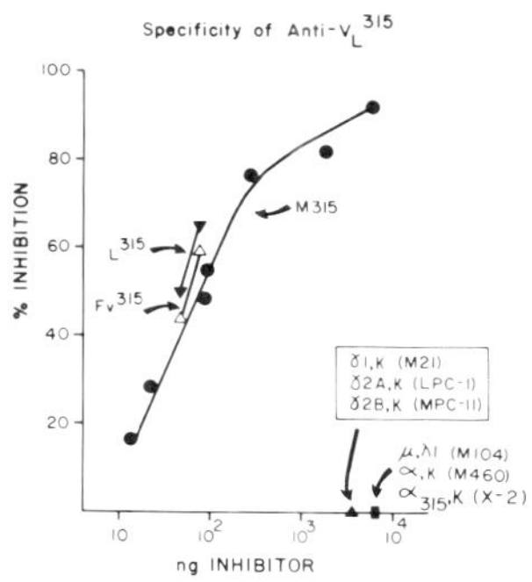

Fig. 6

Fig. 5 Specificity of the assay for Igs with the C domain of L^{315}. Note that 75 ng of L^{315} inhibited > 80% whereas an equivalent amount of Fv did not inhibit. Based on ref. 12.

Fig. 6 Specificity of the assay for Igs with the V domain of L^{315}. Note that equivalent amounts of Fv and L^{315} are equally effective. Based on ref. 12.

eluted (at low pH) were specific for the V domain of this chain (anti-V_L^{315}). Competition-radioimmunoassays were developed with each of these Ab preparations and with $^{125}I-L^{315}$ to measure respectively the concentration of λ2 chains (with anti-Cλ2) and chains with the V region of L^{315} (with anti-V_L^{315}). The specificity of each assay is illustrated in Figs. 5 and 6. Only L^{315} and approximately equivalent amounts of Fv fragments or M315 inhibited the assay for V_L^{315}; only intact M315 or isolated L^{315} (or other λ2-containing Igs or their isolated L chains, see below), but not Fv, inhibited the assay for Cλ2.

With the anti-Cλ2 assay, λ2 chains were found in sera from all of the over 35 inbred mouse strains tested (but not in serum from rabbit, horse, or human) (12). Because serum λ2-levels increase with age until a plateau is reached at 12-15 wks, the sera used to compare different strains were taken from old mice (over 15 weeks). The levels (expressed as μg Ig equivalents per ml) ranged from a low of 15-30 μg per ml in DBA/2, SJL, and BSVS mice to a high of 75-140 μg per ml in AL/N, NZB, BALB/c, and A/J mice (Table 1). No genetic linkage of λ2 levels to Ig heavy chain linkage group or to H-2 haplotype was evident. By testing isolated Igs (7S) it was evident that in the high-λ2 strains (e.g. BALB/c) λ2 chains are present in about 0.8% of all 7S Igs, while in low-λ2 strains (e.g. SJL) these chains are present in only about 0.3% of Igs. The latter value is clearly significant as it is still about 10-fold above the background found in control assays with myeloma proteins having λ1 or κ chains.

In serum Igs about 10% of all λ2 chains have V regions that are identical with or very similar to V_L^{315}. For instance, in BALB/c mice the average serum concentration of Igs with λ2 chains is about 85μg per ml and of Igs with V_L^{315} is about 5-20 μg per ml. The same ratio is evident in low-λ2 strains, such as SJL, where the level of serum Igs with λ2 is about 25-30 μg per ml and of Igs with V_L^{315} is about 1-3 μg per ml (Table 1). Stated otherwise, in high-λ2 strains about 1 in 100 Ig molecules have λ2 chains and about 1 in 1000 have the L^{315} type of V region. In low-λ2 strains the 10-fold difference is still present but the total λ2 level is reduced 3- or 4-fold. Thus in all strains there appear to be at least two subsets of λ2V regions: a minority where V is the same or very similar to that of L^{315} and a majority where V regions clearly differ. If there is indeed only a single germ line Vλ2 gene, as suggested by Tonegawa et al.(13), there must be somatic cell variants of this gene and λ2 chains would appear to be a promising set for analysis of V variants.

The analysis of variants requires information on the amino acid sequences of V regions of at least several λ2 chains or the deoxynucleotide sequences of the corresponding genes (from cells that produce the different λ2 chains). The obvious sources are hybridomas and myeloma tumors. To facilitate the production of hybridomas we have started to search for evidence that λ2-producing B lymphocytes might be preferentially stimulated by certain immunogens.

In the antisera elicited with conjugates of keyhole limpet hemocyanin (KLH) or chicken γ-globulin with Dnp (2,4-dinitrophenyl) or Tnp (2,4,6-trinitrophenyl) or NP (4-hydroxy-3-nitrophenylacetyl), marked increases in serum levels of λ2 were observed in some strains, e.g. (up to 400 μg per ml in C57Bl/6) (12). The elevated levels varied in different preparations of purified anti-hapten Abs: e.g., λ2 chains were present in 5-16% of purified anti-NP Abs and in an average of 5% of purified anti-Dnp molecules. Anti-Tnp Abs were roughly similar to anti-Dnp. High levels of λ1 chains in anti-NP Abs have been previously noted (18,19). Preliminary findings indicate that, overall, when a lot of Abs has an increased level of λ2, it also has an increased level of λ1 chains (measured by a λ1-specific radioimmunoassay). The only instance where λ1 is increased but not λ2 is in anti-dextran Abs of BALB/c mice (ref. 20; see also Table 2).

TABLE 1 Concentration of Serum Immunoglobulins with λ2 L Chains and with $V_L{}^{315}$, the V Region of L^{315}, in Mouse Strains with the Highest and Lowest Serum Levels of λ2.

Strain	Serum concentration of Igs (μg/ml) with*	
	λ2 Chains	V Region of L^{315}
AL/N	140	20
BALB/c	85	14
DBA/2J	28	3.3
SJL/5	25	1.2

*Values are averages for serum from mice that are 15 wks or older. From ref. 12.

TABLE 2 Some Immunogens that Elicit Antibodies Enriched for λ2 (or λ1) Chains*

Antisera or Purified Antibodies to:	Strain	Enriched for	
		λ1	λ2
Dnp†	BALB/c, AKR, B6	+	+
Tnp†	BALB/c, AKR	+	+
NP †	B6	+	+
Dextran (α1→3)	BALB/c	+	0
Phosphorylcholine	BALB/c	NT	0
KLH, bovine γ-globulin, chicken red blood cells, myoglobin, ribonuclease, streptococcal A vaccine	BALB/c	NT	0

+ = enriched, i.e., at least 3 times the average level in 7S Igs from normal serum from mice of the same strain and age as those that were immunized; zero means the same as, or less than, the level in normal 7S Igs; NT, not tested.

† Attached to KLH or chicken γ-globulin

* From refs. 12 and 17.

Enrichment for $V_L{}^{315}$ in some anti-hapten Abs was especially notable. On immunizing BALB/c mice with Dnp-KLH, Igs with $V_L{}^{315}$ increased 10-fold over the level in control mice immunized with KLH alone (12). Purified anti-Dnp and purified anti-NP Abs were, likewise enriched for $V_L{}^{315}$ (17). The extent of enrichment cannot be determined by radioimmunoassay, because in plots of the % inhibition vs. concentration of inhibitor Ig (see Figs. 5,6 as examples), the slopes obtained with purified Abs were not the same as the slope for the prototype protein M315. This could mean that anti-$V_L{}^{315}$ Abs recognize more than one $V_L{}^{315}$ determinant and only one (or a few) of these determinants are shared with λ2 chains from anti-NP and anti-Dnp Abs. (V regions of L^{315} and L^{104E}, a λ1 chain, have essentially the same first and second hypervariable regions but differ especially in the third hypervariable region and also at a few scattered framework positions (Fig. 1). Hence after Abs to $V_L{}^{315}$ are adsorbed with L^{104E} the remaining Abs, used in the assay for $V_L{}^{315}$, may well be specific primarily for the third hypervariable region. The radioimmunoassays suggest, therefore, that the V regions of L^{315} and the λ2 chains of anti-hapten Abs differ in their third hypervariable regions.)

Many hybridomas that produce λ2-containing Abs to Dnp or Tnp or NP will probably soon become available: currently we are growing two (anti-Tnp) that were isolated by Dr. M. Gefter and Dr. Ann Marshak-Rothstein. In the meantime, are there available any λ2-producing myelomas, besides MOPC-315? With the finding that about 1% of BALB/c Igs have λ2 chains we undertook to screen additional myeloma proteins for λ2. Because the frequencies of different classes of Ig chains are generally the same in normal and in myeloma Igs (21,22), the actual incidence of λ2-producing mouse myeloma tumors provides an opportunity to confirm the incidence of λ2 chains in normal mouse Igs. At the same time, the identification of new λ2 chains provides valuable material for comparison with L^{315} and the Vλ2 gene sequenced by Tonegawa et al. (13).

In collaboration with Dr. Michael Potter of the N.I.H. 260 myeloma sera were screened by radioimmunoassay for λ2 chains (23). Four new ones were identified. Two are IgA (ABPC-72, CBPC-49), one is IgG2A (SAPC-15), and the fourth is an H·L half-molecule (22) with one λ2 chain and an as yet unidentified H chain. SAPC-15 reacts with dextran sulfate and heparin (M. Potter, personal communication), and we found that it also binds Dnp_{29}-BSA and Tnp_{40}-BSA but not lightly substituted conjugates, such as Dnp_8-BSA or Tnp_{11}-BSA. Hence SAPC-15 appears to react with diverse high molecular weight polyanions and it is not specific for Dnp and Tnp. Neither are any of the other new λ2 myeloma proteins reactive with Dnp or Tnp or NP, and MOPC-315 remains the only one with high affinity and specificity for Dnp and Tnp ligands (24).

The purified λ2 myeloma proteins and their isolated L chains inhibit the anti-$C_L{}^{315}$ assay almost completely, with slopes and in amounts that are roughly comparable on a weight:weight basis with L^{315} (Fig. 7). None of these chains inhibits a sensitive λ1-specific competition-radioimmunoassay, and they inhibit a k-specific assay only to the extent that low levels of k-containing Igs are probable contaminants of the purified myeloma proteins (14% for SAPC-315 and 0-5% for the others). The carboxy-terminal amino acids were determined for three chains (ABPC-72, SAPC-15, and TEPC-952): the only amino acid released was leucine and it was obtained in yields of 0.28-0.64 moles per mole L chain (compared to 0.5 moles per mole L chain with L^{315}). In addition, all three chains have the carboxy-terminal tryptic peptide characteristic of L^{315} (Fig. 3) (23).

From the serological analysis of λ2 V regions it was concluded that there are at least two sets, with most of the chains having V regions that differ from L^{315} (12,25). Thus it might be anticipated that V regions of most of the other myeloma λ2 chains would also differ from L^{315}. That this is so is shown in Fig. 8. All

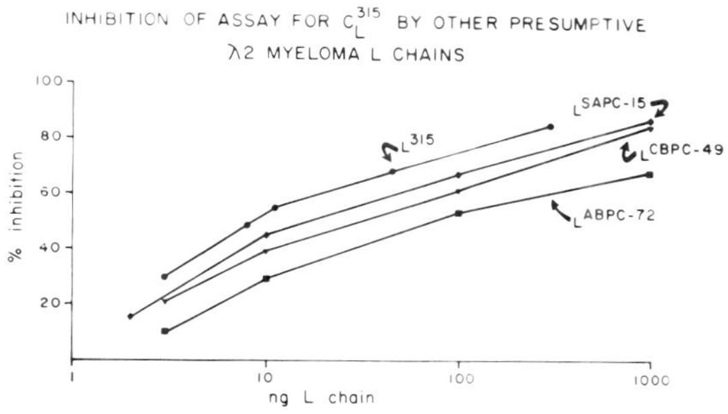

Fig. 7

Fig. 7 Evidence for λ2 light chains in several myeloma proteins from BALB/c mice. The differences between L^{315} and the other chains was essentially eliminated in a similar assay in which antiserum elicited with CBPC-49 was absorbed with the Fv of M315 and tested with $^{125}I-L^{315}$ as indicator. From ref. 23.

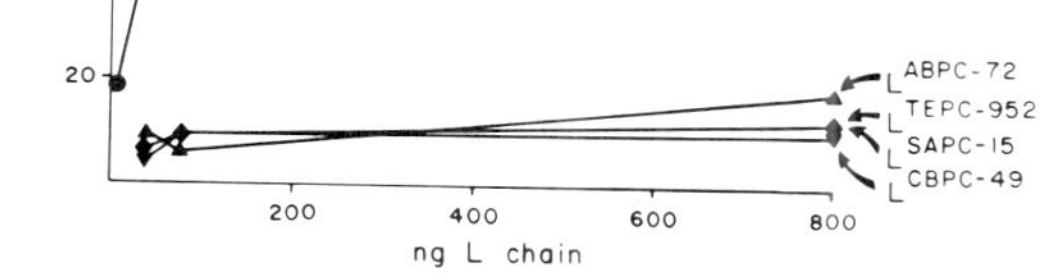

Fig. 8

Fig. 8 Evidence that the V regions of four new λ2-containing myeloma proteins differ from the V domain of L^{315}. From ref. 25.

four isolated chains (as well as the respective intact myeloma proteins) inhibited anti-V_L^{315} only weakly (about 10-14%). Evidentally only a small fraction of anti-V_L^{315} Abs recognize these new λ2 chains.

Amino acid composition data, obtained in collaboration with Dr. Lisa Steiner, also indicate that the new myeloma λ2 chains differ in their V regions from L315 (25). The L^{315} chain has two tyrosine residues, both in the V region (7). Each of the other λ2 chains has at least four tyrosines. If the C domain in these new proteins is exactly the same as that of L^{315} (as is suggested by peptide maps and CPA analysis, but not quite so clearly by the serological tests), they would also have all of their tyrosines in V regions, and each would have at least twice as many V-region tyrosines as V_L^{315} (25). Other amino acid compositional differences distinguish the other λ2 chains from each other as well as from L^{315}. Detailed comparison of amino acid sequences, particularly in the hypervariable regions, of the four new λ2 chains with L^{315} may suggest particular genetic mechanisms for the somatic diversification of the germ line λ2 V gene.

REFERENCES

1. Hood, L., E. Loh, J. Hubert, P. Barstad, B. Eaton, P. Early, J. Fuhrman, N. Johnson, M. Kronenberg, and J. Schilling (1977) Cold Spring Harbor Symp Biol 41 817
2. Seidman, J.G., A. Leder, M.H. Edgell, F.I. Polsky, S. Tilghman, D.C. Tiemeier and P. Leder (1978) Proc. Nat. Acad. Sci. USA 75 3881
3. Brack, C., M. Hirama, R. Lenhard-Schuller, and S. Tonegawa (1978) Cell 15 1
4. Weigert, M., I.M. Cesari, S.J. Yonkovich and M. Cohn (1970) Nature 228 1045
5. Weigert, M. and R. Riblet (1977) Cold Spring Harbor Symp. Quant. Biol. 41 837
6. Eisen, H.N., E.S. Simms and M. Potter (1968) Biochemistry 7 4126
7. Schulenberg, E.P., E.S. Simms, R. Lynch, R.A. Bradshaw, and H.N. Eisen (1971) Proc. Nat. Acad. Sci. USA 68 2623
8. Dugan, E.S., R.A. Bradshaw, E.S. Simms, and H.N. Eisen (1973) Biochemistry 12 5400
9. Appella, E. (1971) Proc. Nat. Acad. Sci. USA 68 590
10. Cesari, I.M. and M. Weigert (1973) Proc. Nat. Acad. Sci. USA 70 2112
11. Inbar, D., J. Hochman, and D. Givol (1972) Proc. Nat. Acad. Sci. USA 69 2659
12. Cotner, T. and H.N. Eisen (1978) J. Exp. Med. 148 1388
13. Tonegawa, S., A.M. Maxam, R. Tizard, O. Bernard, and M. Gilbert (1978) Proc. Nat. Acad. Sci. USA 75 1485
14. Blaser, K. and H.N. Eisen (1978) Proc. Nat. Acad. Sci. USA 75 1495
15. McIntire, K.R. and A.M. Rouse (1970) Fed. Proc. 29 704 (abstr.)
16. Ambler, R.P. (1967 Methods in Enzymology XI C.H.W. Hirs, ed. Academic Press, N.Y., 445
17. Cotner, T. and J. Kriedberg, unpublished observations
18. Jack, R.S., T. Imanishi-Kari, and K. Rajewsky (1977) Eur. J. Immunol. 7 559
19. Makela, O., and K. Karjalainen (1978) Eur. J. Immunol. 8 105
20. Blomberg, B., W.R. Geckeler, and M. Weigert (1972) Science 177 178
21. Natvig, J.B., and H.G. Kunkel (1973) Adv. Immunol. 16 1
22. Potter, M. (1972) Physiological Rev. 52 631
23. Cotner, T., K. Blaser, J. Kriedberg, M. Potter, and H.N. Eisen (manuscript in preparation)
24. Haimovich, J., H.N. Eisen, and D. Givol (1971) Ann. N.Y. Acad. Sci. 190 352
25. Cotner, T., L.A. Steiner, and H.N. Eisen (manuscript in preparation)

THE COVALENT STRUCTURE OF HUMAN FIBRINOGEN

R. F. Doolittle, H. Bouma, III, B. A. Cottrell, D. Strong, and K. W. K. Watt,
Department of Chemistry, Univ. Calif., San Diego, La Jolla, CA 92093 U.S.A.

Fibrinogen is a large molecular weight multi-subunit protein found in the blood plasma of all classes of vertebrates. Under certain conditions, thrombin is released into the plasma and proteolytically excises small portions of the fibrinogen molecule (the fibrinopeptides). As a result, the parent molecules spontaneously polymerize into a gel which is the fibrin clot. Under physiological circumstances, the clot is further stabilized by the factor XIII-catalyzed introduction of covalent crosslinks between neighboring units in the polymer. Factor XIII is a transglutaminase which is itself activated by thrombin. Fibrin clots are ultimately degraded by another protease, plasmin (fibrinolysin). Thus, the important phenomenologic features of the activated fibrinogen molecule are polymerization, stabilization and fibrinolysis. A general appreciation of these events has been at hand for the better part of a generation, but a genuine understanding has been thwarted by the fact that the structure of the starting molecule has resisted determination. Although the might of every conceivable physico-chemical technique and electron microscopy was long ago brought to bear on the problem, no general agreement could be reached on the overall structure (for a general review of these disagreements, see Ref. 1). Recently, however, the covalent structure of the molecule from human plasma has been determined. This accomplishment has--in our opinion--cleared up much of the previous controversy and confusion.

The covalent structure of a multi-subunit protein includes the amino acid sequences of its constituent polypeptide chains, the consequences of any post-translational modification such as glycosylation or phosphorylation, and the location of intra- and inter-subunit disulfide connections. In this regard, our knowledge of the covalent structure of human fibrinogen is virtually complete. The amino acid sequences of two of the three non-identical chains have been reported, and the sequence of the remaining chain (α-chain) is now at hand. The attachment points and compositions of the two different carbohydrate clusters are known, and one phosphorylation point has been identified and another possible phosphorylation target recognized. Finally, an arrangement for the 29 disulfide bonds has been proposed. In this article we will review some of the highlights revealed by these structural studies and then attempt to assess their significance with regard to the three-dimensional structure of the molecule, which is--after all--the key feature in appreciating how the molecule functions.

Overall Characteristics

Human fibrinogen is a typical vertebrate fibrinogen in that it is composed of three pairs of non-identical chains ($\alpha_2\beta_2\gamma_2$) interconnected by a complicated series of disulfide bonds. Its molecular weight as determined by traditional physico-chemical procedures is 340,000 ± 20,000, a value in good agreement with the molecular weight calculated from the observed amino acid sequences of the constituent chains and the composition of the covalently attached carbohydrate (Table 1). The molecule has a relatively high frictional ratio (f/f_0 = 2.34), suggesting an asymmetric structure and/or an excessive degree of hydration. Early electron micrographs made by shadow casting techniques gave rise to a depiction of the molecule composed of three globular regions connected by slender (unresolvable) strands (2). A number of subsequent physico-chemical and biochemical observations were reported which were entirely consistent with such a model (3,4,5). On the other hand, many other workers were unable to observe a three-globule structure in the electron microscope, and, combined with the equivocal nature of some other physico-chemical and biochemical observations, these results led to a contrary opinion which at the very least claimed the three-nodule structure was an artifact of the preparative procedure (6,7,8). As we shall see, however, the observed covalent structure strongly supports and extends the concept of a molecule composed of three interconnected domains. Moreover, a variety of considerations has led to the conclusion that the structure occupies some portion of a 90 x 450 A cylindrical volume.

Number and Sizes of Subunits

Quantitive amino-terminal analysis of fibrinogens from a variety of species revealed that there were characteristically three different endgroups, each occurring twice in every 340,000 molecule weight particle (9). The conclusion

TABLE 1. Some Key Features of the Human Fibrinogen Molecule[a]

Subunit	Number Residues	Molecular Weight[b]	Number Cysteines	Carbohydrate Attachments
α-Chain	600 ± 10	65,000 ± 1000	8	(none)
β-Chain	461	55,000	11	Asn-364
γ-Chain	410	47,000	10	Asn-52
αβγ	1470 ± 10	167,000 ± 1000	29	
$(\alpha\beta\gamma)_2$	2940 ± 20	334,000 ± 2000	58	

[a]Assembled from a variety of reports from three laboratories, including Blombäck's (16, 18), Henschen's (17, 19) and our own (20-22).

[b]Molecular weights calculated from the sum of amino acids based on amino acid sequence plus an estimated contribution determined from carbohydrate composition.

```
  1  Y V A T R D N C C I L D E R F G S Y C P T T C G I A D F L S
                                            *
 31  T Y Q T K V D K D L Q S L E D I L H Q V E N K T S E V K Q L
 61  I K A I Q L T Y N P D E S S K P N M I D A A T L K S R K M L
 91  E E I M K Y E A S I L T H D S S I R Y L Q E I Y N S N N Q K
121  I V N L K E K V A Q L E A Q C Q E P C K D T V Q I H D I T G
151  K D C Q D I A N K G A K Q S G L Y F I K P L K A N Q Q F L V
181  Y C E I D G S G N G W T V F Q K R L D G S V D F K K N W I Q
211  Y K E G F G H L S P T G T T E F W L G N E K I H L I S T Q S
241  A I P Y A L R V E L E D W N G R T S T A D Y A M F K V G P E
271  A D K Y R L T Y A Y F A G G D A G D A F D G F D F G D D P S
301  D K F F T S H N G M Q F S T W D N D N D K F E G N C A E Q D
331  G S G W W M N K C H A G H L N G V Y Y Q G G(T)Y S K A S T P
361  N G Y D N G I(I,W,A,T)K T R W Y S M K K T T M K I I P F N R
391  L T I G E G Q Q H H L G G A K Q A G D V
```

Fig. 1. Amino acid sequence of human fibrinogen γ-chain. A, Ala; B, Asx; C, Cys; D, Asp; E, Glu; F, Phe; G, Gly; H, His; I, Ile; K, Lys; L, Leu; M, Met; N, Asn; P, Pro; Q, Gln; R, Arg; S, Ser; T, Thr; V, Val; W, Trp; Y, Tyr. * = carbohydrate attachment site.

that there must be six chains per molecule was reinforced by the isolation of three different chains after disruption of disulfide bonds (10, 11). Molecular weight determination of the individual subunits in 6M guanidine gave rise to values of 47,000, 56,000 and 63,500, the sum of which was only half of the observed molecular weight of the native fibrinogen molecule (12). As it turns out, the agreement between these values and those calculated on the basis of amino acid sequences reported a decade later is remarkable (Table 1 and Figs. 1-3).

Determining the Covalent Structure

In general, three different strategies were employed in the determination of the covalent structure of human fibrinogen. First, conventional amino acid sequence studies were conducted on isolated α-, β- and γ-chains. Secondly, advantage was taken of the early observation that a set of core fragments results from the plasmin digestion of fibrinogen (13). These fragments, which were originally dubbed fragments A-E in correspondence with the order upon which they elute from a DEAE-cellulose column, have proved especially important for the determination of the disulfide bond arrangement of the molecule, as well as for general considerations about domainal structure. Finally, the third approach begins with the chemical fragmentation of the native fibrinogen by cyanogen bromide. This method was initially used by Blombäck's group, who were able to isolate a fragment after cyanogen bromide digestion which amounted to 15-20% of the mass of

```
  1 Q G V N D N E E G F F S A R G H R P L D K K R E E A P S L R
 31 P A P P P I S G G G Y R A R P A K A A A T Q K K V E R K A P
 61 D A G G C L H A D P D L G V L C P T G C Q L Q E A L L Q Q E
 91 R P I R N S V D E L N N N V E A V S Q T S S S S Q F Y M Y L
121 L K D L W Q K R Q K Q V K D N E N V V N E Y S S E L E K H Q
151 L Y I D E T V N S N I P T N L R V L R S I L E N L R S K I Q
181 K L E S D V S A Q M E Y C R T P C T V S C D I P V V S G K E
211 C E E I I R K G G E T S E M Y L I Q P D S S V K P Y R V Y C
241 D M N T E N G G W T V I Q N R Q D G S V D F G R K W D P Y K
271 Q G F G N V A T N T D G K B Y C G L P G E Y W L G B B K I S
301 E L T R M G P T E L L I E M E D W K G D K V K A H Y G G F T
331 V Q N E A N K Y Q I S V N K Y R G T A G N A L M D G A S Q L
             *
361 M G E N R T M T I H N G M F F S T Y D R D N D G W L T S D P
391 R K Q C S K E D G G G W W Y B R C H A A N P N G R Y Y W G G
421 Q Y T W D M A K H G T B D G V V W M N W K G S W Y S M R K M
451 S M K I R P F F P Q Q
```

Fig. 2. Amino acid sequence of β-chain from human fibrinogen. See legend to Fig. 1 for explanation of symbols.

the starting molecule, but contained almost 40% of its cystine (14). Eventually it was shown that this structure, which was called the "disulfide knot", also contained all six amino-terminals of the molecule. As such, the structure included the fibrinopeptides which are released by thrombin, it being previously known from endgroup studies that the fibrinopeptides A and B corresponded to the amino-terminal segments of the α- and β-chains respectively. It was demonstrated at about the same time that there was a large degree of immunologic cross-reaction between the "disulfide knot" and one of the core fragments generated by plasmin digestion (fragment E), and it was hypothesized that these coincidentally overlapping fragments (fragment E and DSK) corresponded roughly to the central ball in the three-nodule model of fibrinogen derived from the electron microscope studies (15, 16). This was an especially attractive hypothesis because the course of the plasmic digestion of fibrinogen indicated that the two principal core fragments, D and E, were present at a ratio of 2:1. Accordingly, it was supposed that the fragments D corresponded to the terminal nodules of the three-domained structure (3, 4). Everything we have learned since about the covalent structure of fibrinogen is consistent with such a scheme.

1 A D S G E G D F L A E G G G V R G P R V V E R H Q S A C K D

31 S D W P F C S D E D W N Y K C P S G C R M K G L I D E V N Q

61 D F T N R I N K L K N S L F E Y Q K N N K D S H S L T T N I

91 M E I L R G B F S S A B B R D N T Y N R V S E D L R S R I E

121 V L K R K V I Q K V Q H I Q L L E K N V R A Q L V D M K R L

151 E V D I D I K I R S C R G S C S R A L A R E V D L K N Y E B

181 Q Q K Q L E Q V I A K D L L P S R D R Q H L P L I K M K P V

211 P N L V P G N F K S Q L Q K V P P E W K A L T D M P Q M R M

241 E L E R P G G N E I T R G G S T S Y G T G S E T E S P R N P

271 G S A G S W N(P.G.S.T.G.G.A)R N P G S X G T G T(S.A)W K P G

301 S S G P G S T W N(P.G.S.T.Q*.N.P.G.S.T.S.G)R P G S T G T W N

331 P G S S E R G S A G H W T S E S S V S G S T G Q* W H S E S G

361 S F R P D S P(T.G.G)N A R P N N P D T G W G S F E E V S G N

391 V S P G T R R E Y H T E K L V T S K G D K E L R T G K E K V

421 T S G S T T T T R R(S)C S K T V T K T V I G P D G H K E V T

451 K E V V T S E D G S D C P E A Q M D L G T L S G I G T L D G

481 F R H R H P D E A A F F D T A S T G K T F P G F F S P M L G

511 E F V S E T E S R G S E S G I F T N T K E S S S H H P G I A

541 E F P S R G K Q F T S S Y N R G D S T F E S K S Y K M A D E

571 A G S E A D H E G T H S T K R G H A K S R P V

Fig. 3. Amino acid sequence of human fibrinogen α-chain. See legend to Fig. 1 for explanation of symbols; Z = Glx. * = cross-linking acceptor sites.

Sequence Studies on Individual Chains

During the past ten years or so, major sequencing efforts on all three chains have been conducted in laboratories in Stockholm, Munich and La Jolla, and numerous reports from all three laboratories have appeared dealing with the sequences of various portions of the molecule. A virtually complete sequence for the γ-chain was reported by the Munich workers (17) in 1977, and a combination of data from Stockholm (18) and Munich (19) provided a β-chain sequence not too long thereafter; the structure was independently determined by our group in La Jolla (20). We have previously published data covering much of the α-chain (21,22) and include an almost complete sequence in this article.

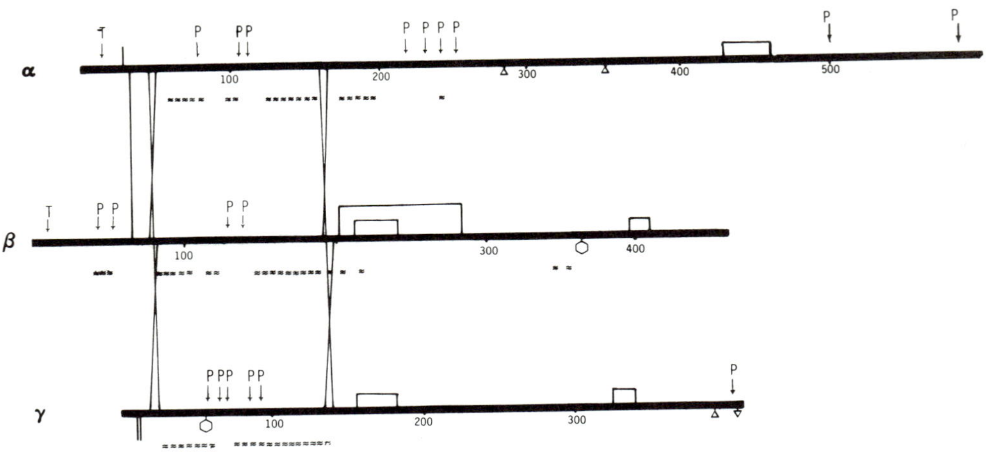

Fig. 4. Schematic alignment of α, β and γ-chains; thin solid lines indicate disulfide bonds. T, thrombin attack points; P, plasmin attack points; ▽ and Δ, crosslinking donor and acceptor sites; ⬡, carbohydrate; ≈, helix-permissive.

The most sigificant feature to emerge from the primary structure studies so far, we feel, is the extensive homology among the three non-identical chains. Clearly, all three chains have descended from a common ancestral polypeptide (23). Interestingly enough, the homology between pairs of the three chains in their amino-terminal "halves" is evident to about the same degree (average 15% identity), whereas in the carboxyl-terminal halves, the β-chain and γ-chains exhibit extensive homology, but the α-chain is different to an extreme (Table 2). With the exception of some faint homology near the very ends of the chains, the degree of resemblance of the α-chain with either the β- or γ-chain appears to be at a random level. It is as though some radical intrusion has taken place--a gene splice or a frame shift--and changed the entire character of the α-chain carboxyl-terminal half. There is also evidence of internal homology in this region of the α-chain, and the suggestion has been made that the chain has been elongated by a series of contiguous duplications 50-60 residues in length (22).

TABLE 2. Percent Identical Residues Observed in Best Alignments of the Three Non-Identical Chains from Human Fibrinogen

Carboxyl-Terminal "Half"	Amino-Terminal "Half"		
	α-Chain	β-Chain	γ-Chain
α-Chain	-	17	13
β-Chain	6	-	15
γ-Chain	5	35	-

egion of the α-chain seems to have been less restricted er portions of the molecule, and a good deal of species even in the size distribution as observed in SDS gels nt of the three non-identical chains is presented in

Bonds

molecule contains 58 cysteine residues, all of which bonds (24). They are distributed such that there are each β-chain and 10 in each γ-chain. As in the case owhere is the common evolutionary heritage of the non- evealed than with regard to the distribution of cys- ity of which occur in the same relative locations in the case of the β- and γ-chains, 9 of their 10 and 11 hed.

ds which exist in each fibrinogen molecule can be cate- First, there is general agreement that three of these f the molecule together (18); thirteen others occur once in each dimeric half). Assignments for all 29 ed (Fig. 5).

cyanogen bromide digestion of fibrinogen gave rise to a was very rich in disulfide bonds and which contained ns of all three pairs of chains (14). Interestingly non-identical chains contained braces of two cysteines cally according to the sequence Cys-Pro-X-X-Pro. logous nature of the sequences--registration of which ent of the chains--the particular constellation of amino cial structural significance. On intuitive grounds, ow all six cysteines in the three non-identical chains

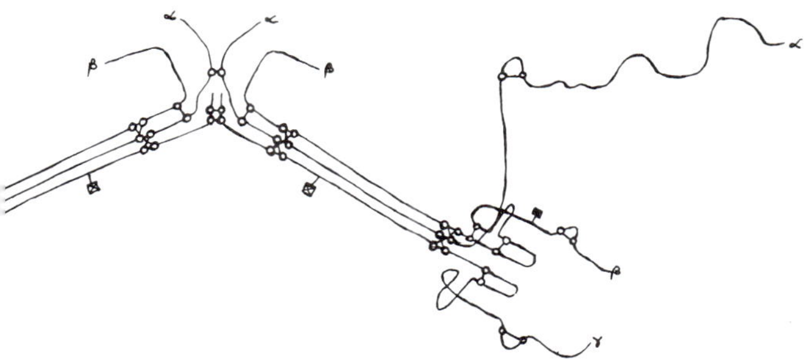

rangement of 29 disulfide bonds in human fibrinogen. resent cysteine residues; lines connecting circles de- ide bonds. Squares represent carbohydrate clusters 26).

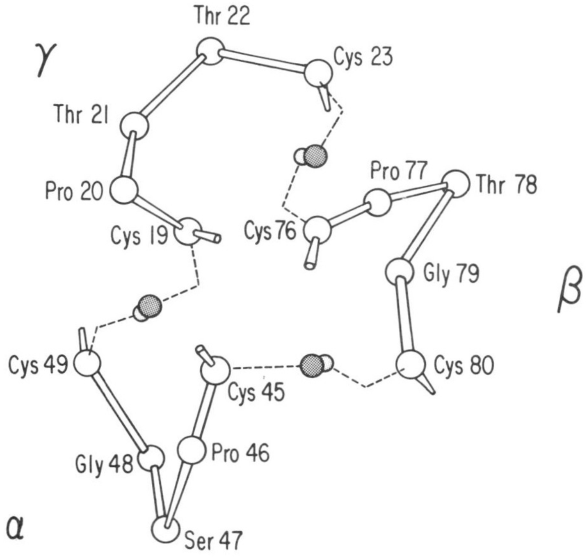

Fig. 6 (left) α-Carbon backbone diagram of one of the two disulfide rings found in each half of human fibrinogen molecule. The sidechains of the six cysteines are shown with broken lines and the six sulfur atoms are shaded. As seen from the amino-terminal end. (from Ref. 27).

could be interconnected to form a "disulfide swivel". Subsequently, we discovered that all three chains contain another brace of two cysteines, in all three cases the two cysteines again separated by exactly three residues. Moreover, the braces were the same distance away from the first set in all three chains, being separated by 111 residues in the case of the α- and γ-chains and (evidently) 112 residues in the case of the β-chain. What was more, the primary attack zone for the fragmentation by plasmin of fibrinogen into fragments D and E was situated almost exactly in the middle of the 111(112)-residue stretches between these cysteine braces (21, 25

The experimental delineation of the exact disulfide bridges linking these cysteines was a difficult and arduous task, primarily because of the nature of the particular amino acids occurring in the three-residue spaces (26). Being impatient by nature, we undertook an alternative approach while simultaneously proceeding with the systematic isolation of linked peptides. On theoretical grounds we reasoned that because of the high degree of homology among the three chains in these regions, the three pairs of cysteines ought to be structurally involved in equivalent modes, which is to say the system ought to have (pseudo) three-fold symmetry (27). In the primeval molecule, if all the chains were identical, there ought to have been only one possible arrangement. The first cysteine in a brace would have to be connected to the second of a neighbor, the first of that neighbor being connected to the second of the third chain, and the first of that last chain being attached to the second of the first-named, thereby closing the ring.

Accordingly, we constructed such a model, incorporating three-fold symmetry as much as possible, with the disulfides on the inside and inaccessible, and with parallel "inlets" and "outlets" for the three chains (27). The result was quite interesting in that all six cysteines fell roughly into the same plane, which itself was normal to the axis of the triad of (non-identical) chains emerging from either side (Fig. 6). It was our contention that all three chains are held together at these junctions by these "disulfide rings". Indeed, all our subsequent results on the actual disulfide attachments have been entirely consistent with the original proposal.

Nature of the Sequences Between the Disulfide Rings

Given the notion of two sets of disulfide rings holding all three chains together, what must be the nature of the three-chain involvement as the strands proceed from one ring to the next? In fact, the answer to this question may lie in some X-ray diffraction data collected more than 35 years ago. At that time, Astbury and his colleagues (29) showed that fibrinogen, even though it is a globular protein when classified by solubility properties, has a fiber diffraction pattern which is indistinguishable from keratin and myosin (k-m-e-f = keratin-myosin-epidermin-fibrinogen). The characteristic 5.1A spacing observed in those proteins was subsequently interpreted as being due to interwoven α-helices, or "coiled coils" (30,31). After the proposal was put forth that fibrinogen was a three-noduled structure, it was even suggested that the interglobular connectors would be logical places to expect the predicted "coiled coils" (32). Now, it is our contention that the 111-residue long stretches between the disulfide rings are in fact interdomainal connectors and do indeed have a nature consistent with sets of three coiled α-helices.

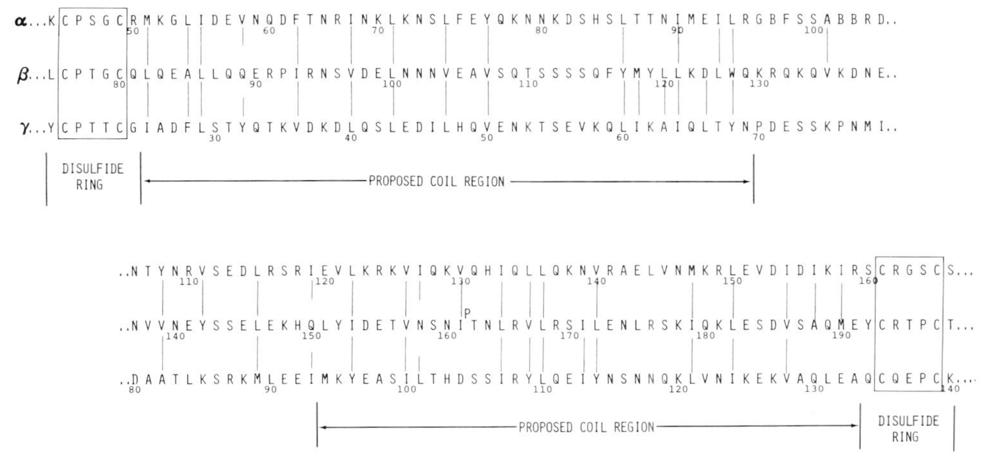

Fig. 7. Amino acid sequences of those portions of the α-, β- and γ-chains which exist between "disulfide rings." It is proposed that the three chains are supercoiled over two large segments. The middle region is thought to have a less defined structure; it is the primary interdomainal attack zone for plasmin. The vertical lines indicate nonpolar residues occurring in two or three chains in register. (adapted from Ref. 27).

In this regard, all three sequences have some unusual features. For example, there is a marked deficiency of the amino acids glycine and proline, there being only three and four of these residues respectively among the 334 residues situated between the rings, in contrast to the 32 and 17 which would be expected if this region were typical of the fibrinogen molecule as a whole. Glycine and proline residues are generally considered to be incompatible with α-helical conformations. Even more interesting, there is a definite rhythm to the occurrence of nonpolar amino acids in this region, their distribution being very much in synchrony in all three chains over large stretches (Fig. 7). Finally, a variety of computer programs designed to predict helicity indicated that these regions were highly helix-permissive. Moreover, no substantial regions of helix were located elsewhere in the molecule by this approach.

In order to test the proposition that the regions between the disulfide rings do indeed correspond to the coiled-coils which give rise to the keratin-like diffraction pattern, we constructed scale models of portions of each of the three chains. In each case we built α-helical backbones with suitable handedness and pitch, and then attached the sidechains corresponding to observed sequences. When the models of the three individual chains were fitted together to make a three-stranded rope, a not unexpected situation was observed; to wit, all the polar sidechains were directed outward and toward the solvent, and almost all the nonpolar sidechains were nestled in the interior (27).

It must be made clearthat we only constructed models of portions of each of the chains and not the entire 111-residue lengths. In fact, the helix-predictive schemes indicated that the very central region of these sequences was probably not helical. Coincidentally, this central region is also where the initial cleavages by plasmin occur during the inter-domainal attack by that enzyme. It seems reasonable that perfectly coiled helices might have an inherent stability which is relatively resistant to proteolytic attack, and the existence of a non-helical central portion may be an important feature for susceptibility and fibrinolysis.

A Model of Fibrinogen

Summing to this point, we feel there is a substantial body of evidence supporting a model of fibrinogen consisting of two terminal domains connected to a central domain by three-stranded interwoven helices. Moreover, this basic model can be refined in light of the amino acid sequence and disulfide attachment data now in hand. For example, the nature of the disulfides in the central domain suggestsa horsetail structure comprised of the amino-terminal segments of all six polypeptide chains (Fig. 8). Further, the boundaries of the inter-domainal connectors appear to be set by the disulfide rings. Knowing that there are 111-112 residues in each of the chains between these nodes, we can readily estimate the extended distance, assuming our designation of "coiled coils" for these regions is correct. Thus, the translational distance per residue in an α-helix is approximately 1.5A, and accordingly the interdomainal distance ought to be about 160A (Fig. 8). The terminal domains, as evidenced by the core fragments remaining after plasmic digestion and/or the specific disulfide connections, are primarily composed of the carboxy-terminal two-thirds of the β and γ-chains, with only a small section of the α-chain associated. The β and γ-chains are markedly homologous over these regions (about 35% identical), giving rise to the notion that a two-fold symmetry ought to exist throughout most of the terminal domain (Fig. 8). In contrast, the α-chain continues on an aberrational course, giving rise to an appendage which is readily excised by a variety of proteases (33,34). Preliminary physical studies (33), as well as computer predictions using the observed amino acid sequences, indicate that these polar,

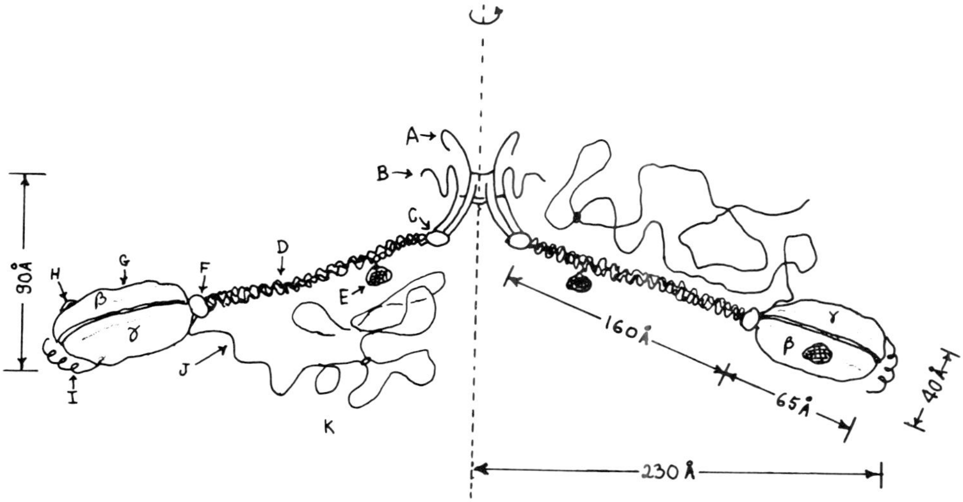

Fig. 8. Schematic model of fibrinogen indicating key features: A, Fibrinopeptide A; B, fibrinopeptide B; C, first disulfide ring; D, coiled-coil interdomainal connector; E, carbohydrate on γ-chain; F, second disulfide ring; G, terminal domain; H, carbohydrate on β-chain; I, γ-chain cross-linking site; J, protease-sensitive region; K, polar carboxy-terminal half of α-chain. Note proposed pseudosymmetry of the halves of the terminal domain contributed by β- and γ-chains respectively. (adapted from ref. 27).

exposed α-chain extensions have an undefined structure approximating a random coil.

Distribution of Amino Acids in Fibrinogen

Taken as a whole, the amino acid composition of the human fibrinogen molecule is unremarkable, all the usual amino acids being present in reasonable amounts (1). The individual chains are also rather ordinary in this regard, although they are recognizably different one from another. But when the three chains are examined segment by segment according to the domain in which they occur, a definite pattern becomes evident. Thus, the interdomainal connectors, as noted above, are markedly deficient in glycine and proline residues. Threonine and tryptophan residues are also significantly underrepresented. More than a third of the residues are nonpolar, however, consistent with the proposed packing arrangements whereby every third or fourth residue would be directed to the interior of the coiled-coil.

Tryptophan residues are definitely clustered in certain portions of the molecule. In the case of the β- and γ-chains, 21 of the 22 tryptophans occur in the carboxy- two-thirds of the chains which comprise the terminal domain. In the α-chain, 8 of 11 tryptophans are found within a 100 residue section near the middle of the chain. This same region is extraordinarily rich in glycine, serine, theonine and proline, and is virtually devoid of nonpolar amino acids

TABLE 3. Sidechain Charges on Human Fibrinogen

	Lysine Arginine	Histidine	Glutamate Aspartate	Sialic Acid	Phospho-Serine[a]	Approximate Net Charge[b]
α-Chain	78	15	78	0	1	+2
β-Chain	58	7	61	2	0	-5[c]
γ-Chain	44	10	54	2	0	-10
(αβγ)	180	32	193	4	1	-13
$(\alpha\beta\gamma)_2$	360	64	386	8	2	-26

[a]Phosphoserine occurs fractionally in at least two different places in α-chains.

[b]at pH 7.3. Histidine contribution based on an average pK of 6.7.

[c]The β-chain lacks a free α-amino group, giving the chain one additional unbalanced negative charge (α-carboxyl group).

other than tryptophan. The region is of considerable interest because it contains the primary α-chain cross-linking acceptor sites.

Charge Distribution on the Fibrinogen Molecule

Let us extend our discussion of amino acid fluctuations to include charge distribution, a property long thought to be involved in the conversion of fibrinogen to fibrin (35). The fibrinopeptides of most species bear a net negative charge, and it has been supposed from the outset that the spontaneous polymerization which ensues upon removal of the fibrinopeptides is at least partly due to the removal of mutually repulsive charge clusters.

If associated counter-ions are neglected for the moment, it can be estimated that the native fibrinogen molecule has approximately 26 extra negative charges at pH 7.3 (Table 3). This reckoning takes into account the contributions of α-amino and carboxyl groups, sidechain carboxyls, lysine amino and arginine guanidino groups, as well as contributions from phosphoserine and, finally, sialic acid associated with the four carbohydrate clusters.

The excess negative charge is not spread equally over the entire molecule, of course, and a careful consideration of where unbalanced charge clusters reside is quite revealing. In fact, a disproportionate amount of the excess negative charge is located on the central domain (Table 4). Removal of the two fibrinopeptides A, while reducing the overall negative charge on the molecule from -26 to -19, lowers the excess charge on the central domain from

-8 to -1. When the two fibrinopeptides B are cleaved away, the overall charge is lowered to about -13, whereas the central domain actually assumes a net positive charge (+5). Although these values must be regarded as approximations, it is interesting that the remainder of the molecule seems to maintain a local neutrality, compensatory positive and negative charges being present throughout. The coiled coil regions, for example, although quite polar, have approximately the same number of positively charged sidechains as negatively charged ones. In fact, their slight negative charge (Table 4) can be attributed to the sialic acids on the γ-chain carbohydrate cluster. This situation is all very much in keeping with the idea that the interdomainal connectors do not become involved in intermolecular interactions, but instead remain open and accessible for subsequent attack by plasmin even after the polymerization event.

The terminal domains do seem to have a net negative charge (-4 each), a feature which is compatible with a complementary interaction with a positively charged component during the polymerization process. It should be mentioned, however, that the terminal domains also contain tightly bound calcium ions which partly offset their net negativity (36-38). In the following section we would like to elaborate a scheme of events which seems altogether consistent with the notion of electrostatic facilitation leading to polymerization after the removal of negatively charged fibrinopeptides from the central domain. Although the scheme was originally suggested some time ago (1), a number of experiments has now been executed which seem to confirm its basic elements.

TABLE 4. ESTIMATED CHARGE DISTRIBUTION ON HUMAN FIBRINOGEN BY SECTOR[a]

	Native Fibrinogen	Fibrin: A Removed	Fibrin: B Removed
"Coiled Coils"	2 @ -3 = -6		
Terminal Domain	2 @ -4 = -8		
α-Chain 1st Ext.	2 @ -1 = -2		
α-Chain 2nd Ext.	2 @ -1 = -2		
Central Domain (dimer)	-8	-1	+5
Entire Molecule (dimer)	-26	-19	-13

[a]Includes contributions from amino acid sidechains and carbohydrate clusters. See Table 3 for additional details.

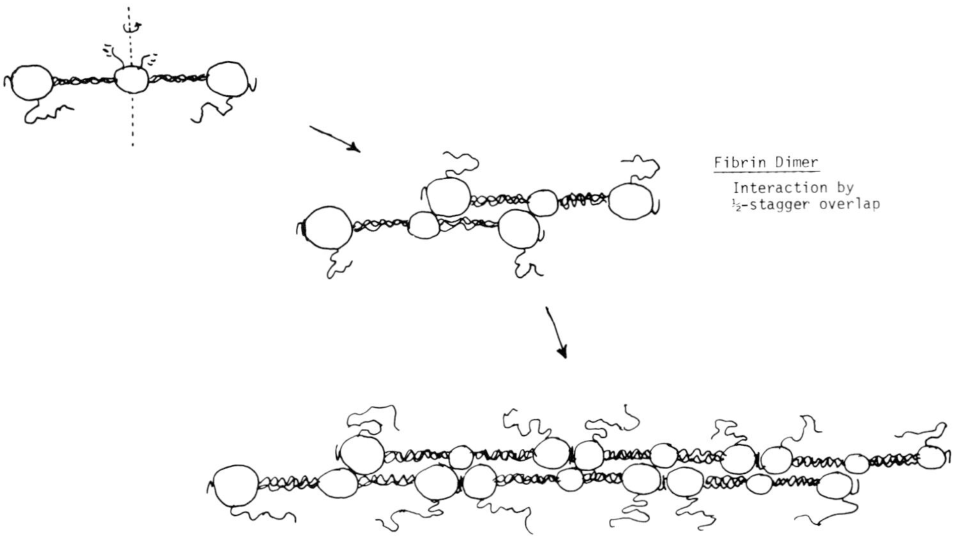

Fig. 9. Outline of initial events involved in polymerization of fibrin. Release of fibrinopeptide(s) from central domain allows complementary interaction with terminal domain of another fibrinogen molecule which has also lost fibrinopeptide(s). A second set of interactions comes into play when a third molecule is added, at which time γ-chains in neighboring molecules come into contact and can be covalently cross-linked by factor XIII (from Ref. 1).

The Conversion of Fibrinogen to Fibrin

Basically, the proposal (1) was that the thrombin-catalyzed release of fibrinopeptides from the central domain of a molecule like that posed in Fig. 8 allowed that region of the parent molecule to interact with the terminal domain of another fibrinogen molecule which had also been cleaved by thrombin (Fig. 9). The pairing of the two molecules was complementary, but--inasmuch as the molecules were dimeric to start with--the new dimer product was necessarily half-staggered. The contact sites involved in this polymerization were widely separated on a given molecule, one being at or near the amino-terminus of the α-chain and being unmasked by the removal of the fibrinopeptide A, and the other being always present (i.e., no need for unmasking) and on the terminal domain. It was also proposed that the next stage of the polymerization event, whereby the two molecule aggregate grew to three and more units, involved a different set of reciprocal contact sites, located exclusively on the terminal domains (Fig. 9). This interaction, which occurred whenever units were added to either end of the growing polymer, was consistent with a molecular orientation which could give rise to "γ-γ dimers" upon the incorporation of cross-links by factor XIII (39).

The oligomers which resulted from these two kinds of interaction were necessarily two molecules thick and had a periodicity consistent with a half-molecule overlap. In order for thick fibrin strands to develop, these intermediate polymers would themselves have to become involved laterally (Fig. 10). This stage of fibrin formation is well known to be influenced by the solution environment, including pH and ionic strength, suggesting that electrostatic factors are important. It has been suggested that this aspect of the process may be facilitated by the removal of the fibrinopeptide B, and also that cross-links involving α-chains can only be introduced subsequent to these lateral interactions (40). Finally, a necessary correlate of this mode of polymerizing a molecule of such a design is that the three-stranded interdomainal connectors remain exposed to solvent throughout, and the intermolecular space remaining after polymerization is sufficient to allow access for enzymes involved in subsequent fibrinolysis.

Experimental results which support such an interpretation of fibrin polymerization have been reported from several laboratories. For example, Kudryk et al. (41) found that fibrinogen could be adsorbed by fibrinogen bound to Sepharose, if the fibrinopeptides were first removed from the bound molecules by treatment with thrombin. They also found that fragment D could also be adsorbed by such columns, suggesting that polymerization sites were available on that plasmic fragment. At about the same time, Hudry-Clergeon et al. (42) reported the isolation of a D_2E complex from a plasmin digest of cross-linked fibrin. Implicit in their finding was the notion that the three components (two D and one E) were originally from three different fibrinogen molecules, a situation in exact conformity with the two stages of polymerization depicted in Fig. 9.

Finally, the proposal was tested by synthesizing small peptides corresponding to the amino-terminal segments exposed upon the release of the fibrinopeptides

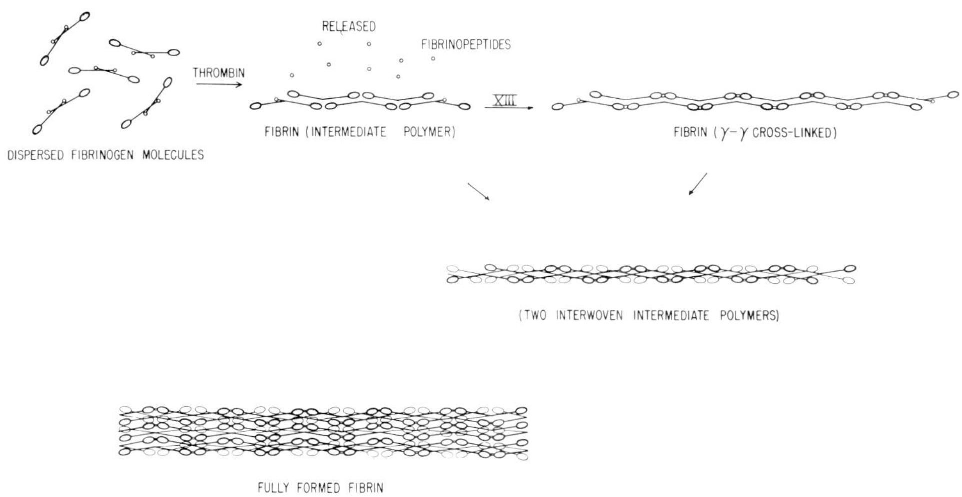

Fig. 10. Scheme of events in polymerization which leads to fully developed fibrin strands. The intermediate polymers are interwoven by a different set of molecular contacts than are involved in the initial interactions (from Ref. 28).

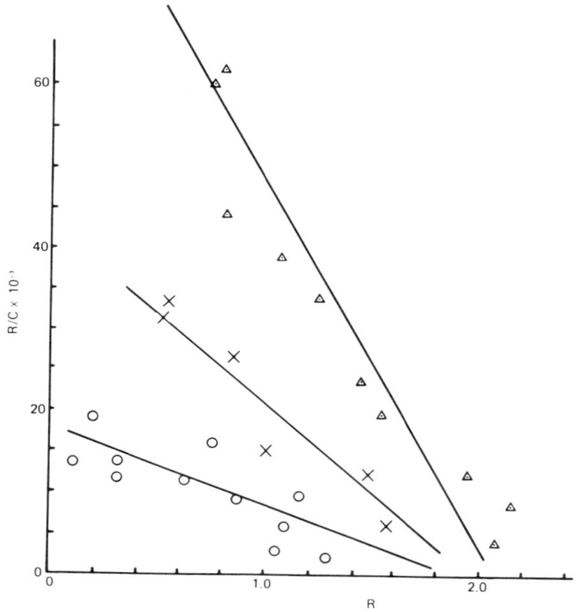

Fig. 11. Binding data (equilibrium dialysis) for radioactive peptides exposed to fibrinogen: △, Gly-Pro-Arg-Pro; ×, Gly-Pro-Arg; O, Gly-His-Arg-Pro. R = moles bound peptide/mole fibrinogen. (from Ref. 43).

(43). For example, peptides corresponding to the amino-terminus of the α-chain (Gly-Pro-Arg and Gly-Pro-Arg-Pro) were able to prevent fibrin polymerization by competing for the complementary contact sites on the terminal domains. A peptide corresponding to the β-chain amino-terminus, on the other hand, did not inhibit polymerization. These peptides were found to bind to native fibrinogen, consistent with the idea that the complementary sites are always exposed (Fig. 11). The number of such sites was found to be two for fibrinogen and, as expected, one for fragment D. The active peptides all have two essential positive charges, including the α-amino group on the terminal glycine residue and the guanidino group on the arginine at position 3. It is reasonable to expect that the complementary site on the terminal domain will involve negatively charged carboxyl-groups.

In summary, we have applied our knowledge of the covalent structure of fibrinogen not only to models dealing with the three-dimensional structure of that molecule, but also to the biochemical phenomena of polymerization, stabilization and fibrinolysis. In all these areas the picture seems entirely self-consistent and satisfying, although many details of the process remain to be explored. For example, do the calcium ions which are bound to the terminal domains facilitate the reciprocal interaction of those negatively charged domains? And how are the α-chain extensions oriented in space, and where do they end up in the polymerized system? These and other aspects remain mysterious and await further experimentation.

REFERENCES

(1) R. F. Doolittle, Structural aspects of the fibrinogen to fibrin conversion, Adv. Protein Chem. 27, 1 (1973).

(2) C. E. Hall and H. S. Slayter, The fibrinogen molecule: Its size, shape, and mode of polymerization, J. Biophys. Biochem. Cytol. 5, 11 (1959).

(3) E. Mihalyi, Review of the physicochemistry of bovine fibrinogen with special reference to its proteolytic fragmentation, Throm. Diath. Haem. Supp. 39, 43 (1970).

(4) V. J. Marder, Physicochemical studies of intermediate and final products of plasmin digestion of human fibrinogen, Thromb. Diath. Haem. Supp. 39, 187 (1970).

(5) J. W. Donavan and E. Mihalyi, Conformation of fibrinogen: calormetric evidence for a three-nodular structure, Proc. Natl. Acad. Sci., U.S.A. 71, 4125 (1974).

(6) G. Köppel, Electron microscopic investigation of the shape of fibrinogen nodules: a model for certain proteins, Nature (London) 212, 1608 (1966).

(7) G. Hudry-Clergeon, G. Marguerie, L. Pouit and M. Suscillon, Models proposed for the fibrinogen molecule and for the polymerization process, Thromb. Res. 6, 533 (1975).

(8) M. W. Mosesson, Fibrinogen structure after spraying on mica: assessing the electron microscopic basis for a trinodular model, Thromb. Res. 8, 737 (1976).

(9) B. Blombäck and I. Yamashima, On the N-terminal amino acids in fibrinogen and fibrin, Arkiv Kemi 12, 299 (1958).

(10) J. B. Clegg and K. Bailey , The separation and isolation of the peptide chains of fibrin, Biochem. Biophys. Acta 63, 525 (1962).

(11) A. Henschen, Peptide chains in S-sulfo-fibrinogen and S-sulfo-fibrin: isolation, methods, and general properties, Arkiv Kemi 22, 397 (1964).

(12) P. A. McKee, L. A. Rogers, E. Marler and R. L. Hill, The subunit polypeptides of human fibrinogen, Arch. Biochem. Biophys. 11, 271 (1966).

(13) V. Nussenzweig, M. Seligmann, J. Pelmont and P. Grabar, Les produits de dégradation du fibrinogène humain per la plasmine. I. Séparation et propriétès physico-chemiques, Ann. Inst. Pasteur 100, 377 (1961).

(14) B. Blombäck, M. Blombäck, A. Henschen, B. Hessel, S. Iwanaga and K. R. Woods, N-terminal disulphide knot of human fibrinogen, Nature (London) 218, 130 (1968).

(15) V. J. Marder, Identification and purification of fibrinogen degradation products produced by plasmin; considerations on the structure of fibrinogen, Scand. J. Haemat. Supp. 13, 21 (1971).

(16) B. Kowalska-Loth, B. Gårdlund, N. Egberg and B. Blombäck, Plasmic degradation products of human fibrinogen. II. Chemical and immunologic relation between fragment E and N-Dsk, Thromb. Res. 2, 423 (1973).

(17) A. Henschen and F. Lottspeich, Amino acid sequence of human fibrin. Preliminary note on the completion of the γ-chain sequence, Hoppe-Seyler's Z. Physiol. Chem. 358, 935 (1977).

(18) B. Blombäck, B. Hessel, and D. Hogg, Disulfide bridges in NH_2-terminal part of human fibrinogen, Thromb. Res. 8. 639 (1976).

(19) A. Henschen and F. Lottspeich, Amino acid sequence of human fibrin. Preliminary note on the completion of the β-chain sequence. Hoppe-Seyler's Z. Physiol. Chem. 358, 1643 (1977).

(20) K. W. K. Watt, T. Takagi and R. F. Doolittle, The amino acid sequence of the β-chain of human fibrinogen, Biochemistry, In Press.

(21) R. F. Doolittle, K. G. Cassman, B. A. Cottrell, S. J. Friezner and T. Takagi, Amino acid sequence studies on the α-chain of human fibrinogen. Covalent structure of the α-chain portion of fragment D, Biochemistry 16, 1710 (1977).

(22) B. A. Cottrell and R. F. Doolittle, The amino acid sequence of the carboxyl-terminal 142 amino acids of the α-chain of human fibrinogen, Thromb. Res. 12, 1135 (1978).

(23) R. F. Doolittle, The evolution of vertebrate fibrinogen, Federation Proceedings 35, 2145 (1976).

(24) A. Henschen, Number and reactivity of disulfide bonds in fibrinogen and fibrin, Arkiv Kemi 22, 355 (1964).

(25) T. Takagi and R. F. Doolittle, Amino acid sequence studies on plasmin-derived fragments of human fibrinogen: amino-terminal sequences of intermediate and terminal fragments, Biochemistry 14, 940 (1975).

(26) H. Bouma, III, T. Takagi and R. F. Doolittle, The arrangement of disulfide bonds in fragment D from human fibrinogen, Thromb. Res. 13, 557 (1978).

(27) R. F. Doolittle, D. M. Goldbaum and L. R. Doolittle, Designation of sequences involved in "coiled-coil" interdomainal connections in fibrinogen: construction of an atomic scale model. J. Mol. Biol. 120, 311 (1978).

(28) R. F. Doolittle, Structure and function of fibrinogen, Horizons Biochem. Biophys. 3, 164 (1977).

(29) K. Bailey, W. T. Astbury and K. M. Rudall, Fibrinogen and fibrin as members of the keratin-myosin group, Nature (London) 151, 716 (1943).

(30) L. Pauling and R. B. Corey, Compound helical configurations of polypeptide chains: Structure of proteins of the α-keratin type, Nature (London) 171, 59 (1953).

(31) F. H. C. Crick, The packing of α-helices: Simple coiled-coils, Acta Cryst. 6, 689 (1953).

(32) C. Cohen, An invited discussion at the 1960 Symposium on Protein Structure, J. Polymer Sci. 49, 144 (1961).

(33) T. Takagi and R. F. Doolittle, Amino acid sequence studies on the α-chain of human fibrinogen. Location of four plasmin attack points and a covalent cross-linking site, Biochemistry 14, 5149 (1975).

(34) E. J. Harfenist and R. E. Canfield, Degradation of fibrinogen by plasmin. Isolation of an early cleavage product, Biochemistry 14, 4110 (1975).

(35) J. D. Ferry, The mechanism of polymerization of fibrin, Proc. Natl. Acad. Sci., U.S.A. 38, 566 (1952).

(36) G. Marguerie, G. Chagniel and M. Suscillon, The binding of calcium to bovine fibrinogen, Biochim. Biophys. Acta 490, 94 (1977).

(37) F. Haverkate and G. Timan, Protective effect of calcium in the plasmin degradation of fibrinogen and fibrin products D. Thromb. Res. 10, 803 (1977).

(38) L. R. Purvis, G. G. Lindsey, G. Brown and J. Franks, Stabilization of the plasmin digestion products of fibrinogen and fibrin by calcium ions, Thromb. Res. 12, 473 (1978).

(39) R. Chen and R. F. Doolittle, γ-γ Cross-linking sites in human and bovine fibrin, Biochemistry 10, 4486 (1971).

(40) R. F. Doolittle, K. G. Cassman, R. Chen, J. J. Sharp and G. L. Wooding, Correlation of the mode of fibrin polymerization with the pattern of cross-linking, Ann. N. Y. Acad. Sci. 202, 114 (1972).

(41) B. J. Kudryk, D. Collen, K. R. Woods and B. Blombäck, Evidence for localization of polymerization sites in fibrinogen, J. Biol. Chem. 249, 3322 (1974).

(42) G. Hudry-Clergeon, L. Paturel and M. Suscillon, Identification d'un complexe (D-D)...E dans les produits de dégradation de la fibrine bovine stabilisée par le facteur XIII, Path. Biol. 22, suppl., 47 (1974).

(43) A. P. Laudano and R. F. Doolittle, Synthetic peptide derivatives that bind to fibrinogen and prevent the polymerization of fibrin monomers, Proc. Natl. Acad. Sci., U.S.A. 75, 3085 (1978).

SIMULTANEOUS MEASUREMENT OF THROMBIN AND PLASMIN PROTEOLYSIS OF FIBRINOGEN AND OF PLATELET RELEASE

Hymie L. Nossel and Karen L. Kaplan,
Department of Medicine, Columbia University College of Physicians and Surgeons, New York, New York 10032

ABSTRACT

Thrombin catalyzes the cleavage of fibrinogen in two steps. The products of the initial step are fibrinopeptide A (FPA) and fibrin I and those of the second step are fibrinopeptide B (FPB) and fibrin II. Plasmin proteolysis of fibrinogen or fibrin I proceeds in many steps. An early product of plasmin proteolysis is a peptide designated Bβ 1-42 which includes the FPB molecule. Radioimmunoassays have been used to measure FPA as an index of thrombin action on fibrinogen and Bβ 1-42 as an index of plasmin proteolysis of fibrinogen or fibrin I. In addition to its action on fibrinogen, thrombin induces energy-dependent secretion of platelet granular contents. Collagen, adenosine diphosphate and other agents can also induce this release reaction. Among the released materials are two platelet-specific proteins - platelet factor 4 (PF4) and β-thromboglobulin (βTG) and radioimmunoassays have been used to measure these proteins as an index of platelet secretion.

When thrombin is added to human blood without anticoagulant, cleavage of fibrinogen to yield FPA and platelet release both occur. Significant FPA is formed by 8×10^{-5} u/ml thrombin while detectable release of PF4 and βTG requires 2×10^{-2} u/ml. In contrast, during spontaneous coagulation of blood, formation of FPA and release of PF4 and βTG occur in parallel with a molar ratio of about 10:1:1. These data suggest that during spontaneous blood coagulation initial thrombin formation and action occur in proximity to the platelets, probably on the platelet membrane. FPB release by the second stage of thrombin action occurs during in vitro coagulation but plasmin proteolysis to yield Bβ 1-42 does not.

Sequential studies of in vivo coagulation in response to injury suggest the following sequence of reactions:

1. Thrombin proteolysis of fibrinogen as reflected by increasing FPA levels and thrombin-induced platelet release as reflected by increasing βTG and PF4 levels.

2. Plasmin proteolysis of fibrin I (or fibrinogen) as reflected by increasing Bβ 1-42 levels.

Bβ 1-42 was identified in plasma by its immunochemical behavior and its filtration pattern of Sephadex G-50. These studies suggest that plasmin cleavage of fibrin I to yield Bβ 1-42 and fragment X in preference to thrombin cleavage to yield FPB and fibrin II serves as a major mechanism controlling the type of fibrin formed in vivo.

INTRODUCTION

Understanding of the mechanism of blood coagulation at the molecular level is progressing rapidly. Significant advances have also been made in understanding the mechanism of platelet reactions important in hemostasis although these reactions cannot yet be described in molecular terms. This basic biochemical and physiological information comes at a time when the radioimmunoassay technique permits specific and quantitative measurement of very low concentrations of peptides in clinical blood samples. The application of the radioimmunoassay technique to the biochemical information permits analysis of the activation of the hemostatic system in vivo. The results of initial studies which provide information concerning molecular changes accompanying activation of hemostasis in vivo are reviewed in this manuscript. The information concerns the proteolysis of fibrinogen by thrombin and plasmin and the platelet release reaction.

FIBRINOGEN

1. Thrombin Action

Thrombin first cleaves the bond between arginine (Aα 16) and glycine (Aα 17) release fibrinopeptide A (FPA) - the remaining molecule being termed Fibrin I (1-5). Fibrin I polymerizes to form a visible clot composed of rather thin strands thought to represent end-to-end polymers resulting from the availability of a single polymerization site (6). Following the polymerization of Fibrin I, thrombin cleaves the bond between arginine (Bβ 14) and glycine (Bβ 15), to produce fibrinopeptide B and fibrin II (1, 4, 5). Fibrin II strands are considerably thicker than those of fibrin I. The thicker strands of fibrin II are thought to result from the uncovering of a second polymerization site and consequent lateral aggregation of fibrin molecules in addition to end-to-end aggregation (6, 7). Evidence for the two stage formation of fibrin is derived from measurements of the sequence of fibrinopeptide cleavage from fibrinogen by thrombin. The two stage cleavage of the fibrinopeptides was first described by Blomback and Vester-

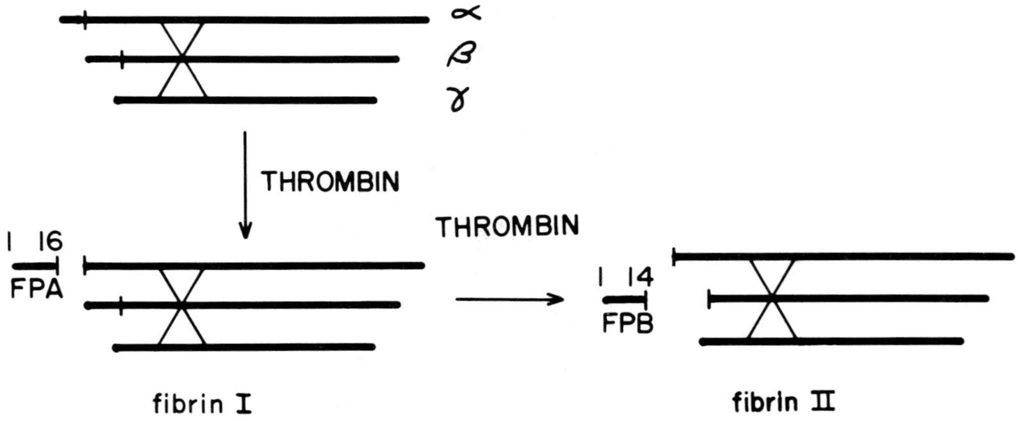

Fig. 1. Schematic representation of thrombin action on fibrinogen.

Half fibrinogen molecules are shown. Thrombin action on fibrinogen occurs in two stages. The products of stage 1 are fibrinopeptide A and fibrin I. The products of stage 2 are fibrinopeptide B and fibrin II.

mark (4) and confirmed by Bilezikian and colleagues (5) who used specific radioimmunoassays to measure the cleaved peptides. FPA cleavage is therefore a direct index of fibrin I formation and FPB cleavage of fibrin II formation (Fig. 1.).

2. Plasmin Action

Plasmin cleaves the fibrinogen molecule progressively to produce fragment X, then fragment Y and finally fragments D and E (8-10). The initial large molecular weight product, fragment X, is formed by removal of fragments from the carboxy-terminal end of the Aα chain and the amino- terminal portion of the Bβ chain (Fig. 2)(11, 12). Fragment X still polymerizes after addition of thrombin. Plasmin cleaves fragment X to remove a large molecular weight fragment termed D, the residual molecule being termed fragment Y. Fragment Y is further cleaved to form a second D fragment and a fragment termed E. Fragments D and E are the terminal large molecular weight derivatives of fibrinogen proteolysis by plasmin. Plasmin cleavage of the amino-terminal end of the Bβ chain occurs at multiple sites. Iwanaga and colleagues used Bβ chains derived from sulfitolyzed fibrinogen as substrate and found cleavages between amino acids 21 and 22, 22 and 23, 42 and 43, 47 and 48, 53 and 54, 54 and 55, 57 and 58, 58 and 59. The bond between amino

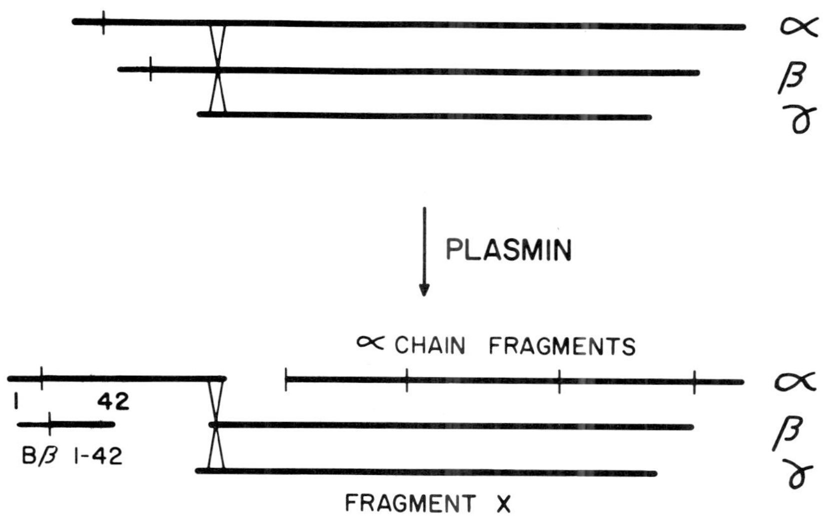

Fig. 2. Schematic representation of initial plasmin action on fibrinogen.

Half fibrinogen molecules are shown. A large fragment from the C-terminal and middle portions of the α chain is cleaved and a small fragment (including Bβ 1-42) from the N-terminal portion is cleaved. The remainder of the molecule is termed fragment X. A series of proteolytic cleavages occurs subsequently.

acids 14 and 15 - the thrombin sensitive site - was not cleaved (Fig. 3). Takagi and Doolittle studies the proteolysis of fibrinogen by plasmin. Based on the sequence of appearance of new amino-terminal amino acids (5 cycles were studied) the initial cleavage point on the Bβ chain was between arginine (42) and alanine (43) (11). Small molecular weight peptides corresponding to β chain residues,

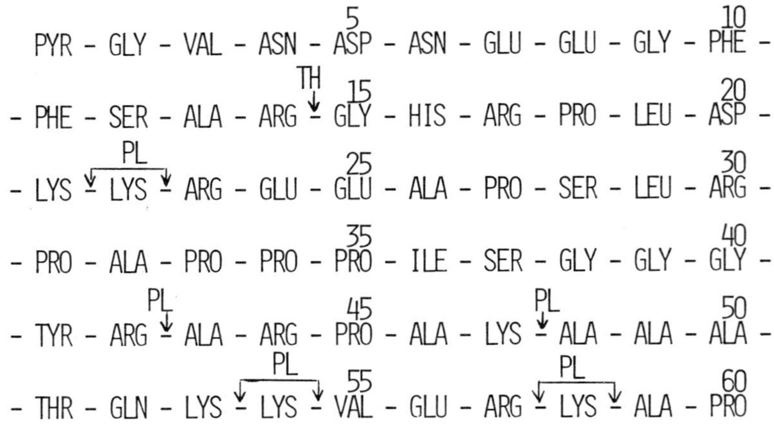

Fig. 3. Thrombin and plasmin cleavage sites on NH_2-terminal end of Bβ chain.

Amino acid sequence at the amino terminal end of the Bβ chain of fibrinogen. The thrombin (TH) and the plasmin (PL) cleavage sites are shown according to Iwanaga and colleagues (13).

22-42, 15-21 and fibrinopeptide B were identified implying cleavage of the 14-15 bond (14). The reason for the differences found by Iwanaga and colleagues and by Takagi and Doolittle is not clear.

ASSAYS OF FIBRINOPEPTIDE A (FPA), Bβ 1-42 AND FIBRINOPEPTIDE B (FPB)

1. Fibrinopeptide A

A radioimmunoassay for FPA has been developed in a number of laboratories (15-19). The assays are based on the use of two reagents, FPA with tyrosine coupled to the amino terminal alanine for use as a tracer and specific antibody generated by immunizing New Zealand white rabbits with FPA coupled to a protein carrier. Antibodies specific for the Aα chain sequence 10 through 16 discriminate very clearly between FPA and larger fibrinogen derived fragments which include the FPA sequence (20 , 64, 65). These larger fragments range in size between Aα 1-23 and fibrinogen. Although the antibodies can distinguish between FPA and fibrinogen the relative concentrations of these molecules are such that in order to measure FPA specifically in blood samples it is essential to completely remove fibrinogen from the plasma. This can be accomplished by ethanol precipitation or bentonite adsorption of the fibrinogen.

2. Fibrinopeptide B Assay

A specific radioimmunoassay for FPB was developed using the same principles as were used to develop the FPA assay. Since native FPB has a blocked N terminus an FPB analogue to which tyrosine could be coupled was used as a source for immunogen and tracer (5, 21). The analogue was prepared by solid-phase synthesis and glutamic acid was substituted for pyroglutamic acid. A number of major technical problems require solution before FPB can be measured in clinical blood samples. The first of these is that Bβ 1-42 is generated at a variable rate in plasma in vitro. Trasylol, heparin, EDTA, e-aminocaproic acid, soybean trypsin inhibitor, p-amino benzamidine, and a combination of heparin, trasylol, EACA, and benzamidine do not prevent such generation, nor does storage at various temperatures down to

-80°C as the cleavage appears to continue in the frozen state. It is possible that the cleavage is produced by plasmin adsorbed to fibrin I in the circulating plasma. Currently, in vitro cleavage is prevented by removing fibrinogen from the plasma within 1 hour of blood collection. A second problem in measuring FPB in plasma is cross-reactivity produced by Bβ 1-42. This problem can be solved by selectively adsorbing Bβ 1-42 from plasma with the appropriate concentration of bentonite without significantly removing fibrinopeptide B. A further problem concerns the degradation of FPB in blood. La Gamma and Nossel found that FPB added to blood lost 80-90% immunoreactivity very rapidly and at a variable rate in different blood samples (22). The loss of immunoreactivity was shown to result from cleavage of arginine (14) from fibrinopeptide B by carboxypeptidase B in plasma. In vitro loss of immunoreactivity is prevented by o-phenanthroline but there still remained the problem of in vivo degradation. This problem has been tackled by developing an assay for B 1-13, permitting plasma carboxypeptidase B to convert fibrinopeptide B in plasma to B 1-13 and measuring B 1-13. This procedure gives reasonably good recovery of fibrinopeptide B added to blood in vitro and it is hoped that it will permit measurement of fibinopeptide B in clinical blood samples.

3. Bβ 1-42 Assay

A specific assay for Bβ 1-42 is not available but the molecule cross-reacts in the FPB assay which can be used to identify Bβ 1-42 in plasma. Bβ 1-42 can be distinguished from fibrinopeptide B by three criteria.

1. Thrombin treatment of Bβ 1-42 results in a 10-fold increase in immunoreactivity in the fibrinopeptide B assay (using antiserum R22) whereas there is no increase in the immunoreactivity of fibrinopeptide B treated with thrombin (Table 1).

2. Bβ 1-42 is virtually completely adsorbed from a buffer solution by 3 mg/ml bentonite whereas 20 mg/ml bentonite adsorbs only 25% fibrinopeptide B.

3. The two molecular species are clearly separable by gel filtration on Sephadex G-50 with Bβ 1-42 eluting at 0.72 x the elution volume of fibrinopeptide B.

TABLE 1 Relative Molar Concentrations of Fibrinopeptide B (FPB) and Bβ 1-42 Required for 50% Inhibition of Binding of ^{125}I-FPB by Antiserum R22

FPB	FPB Treated With Thrombin	Bβ 1-42	Bβ 1-42 Treated With Thrombin
1 pmol.	1 pmol.	10 pmol.	1 pmol.

PLATELET RELEASE REACTION

There are no known defined cleavage products which reflect "platelet activation". The nearest approach to substances which reflect platelet activation are materials released from the platelet during its release reaction. The platelet release reaction is an energy dependent process during which the contents of certain granules inside the platelet are extruded to the exterior (23, 24, 25). At least two of the secreted materials appear to be specific for the platelet. These substances are a 31,000 M.W. polypeptide termed platelet factor 4 (26-28) and a 35,400 M.W. polypeptide termed beta thromboglobulin (29-35). Platelet factor 4 consists of 4 identical subunits composed of 70 amino acids the sequence of which has been determined (36-39). The carboxy-terminal portion of each subunit has 4 lysine residues in a 10 amino acid sequence which are probably responsible for the ability of platelet factor 4 to bind and neutralize heparin. The true physiological function is not known for either platelet factor 4 or beta thromboglobulin. Specific radioimmunoassays for platelet factor 4 and beta thromboglobulin have been developed in a number of laboratories(40-47). Uncoupled peptide has generally been used as the immunogen and since both polypeptides have tyrosine residues they may be directly radiolabelled.

STUDIES WITH ISOLATED FIBRINOGEN OR PLATELETS

Fibrinogen

Thrombin sequentially cleaves FPA and then FPB from fibrinogen. The Km for the FPA cleavage reaction was 2.99×10^{-6}M fibrinogen (48). This compares with Kms of 1.5×10^{-5} to 4.8×10^{-6}M for the thrombin-fibrinogen reaction reported by other workers (49-52). The Km for FPB cleavage has not been determined. The initial rate of the reaction at a substrate concentration of 7.35μM was 4.9×10^{-8} moles FPA cleaved per ml/min/unit of thrombin (48). Hogg and Blomback used a 20μM fibrinogen concentration and found an initial cleavage rate of 1.2×10^{-8} moles fibrinopeptide cleaved per ml/min/unit of thrombin (53).

Plasmin cleaves a peptide containing fibrinopeptide B from fibrinogen. The Km for this reaction has not been determined. At a substrate concentration of 1.32 μM the cleavage rate for the amino-terminal end of the Bβ chain was 188 pmol/ml/min/unit of plasmin (5). The exact cleavage point for this reaction is not known but based on Takagi and Doolittle's observations it presumably is the bond linking arginine (42) and alanine (43). In a purified system fibrinopeptide B containing peptide behaves immunochemically like FPB suggesting that plasmin cleaves Bβ 1-42 into FPB and Bβ 15-42. When streptokinase which converts plasminogen to plasmin is added to citrated or heparinized plasma, however, the peptide cleaved from the N-terminal end of the Bβ chain behaves like Bβ 1-42 immunochemically. Cleavage of FPA immunoreactivity is very much delayed but eventually occurs to a significant extent when isolated plasmin and fibrinogen are incubated together.

Crude extracts of leukocytes with proteolytic activity produce a quite distinct fibrinogen cleavage pattern. Neither fibrinopeptide A nor fibrinopeptide B is removed but instead larger peptides (<6,000 M.W.) which contain FPA or FPB are formed. The fibrinopeptide A containing peptide is removed more rapidly than the fibrinopeptide B containing peptide (54).

Platelets

Adenosine diphosphate (ADP) and collagen release platelet factor 4, beta thromboglobulin and C^{14}-labelled serotonin from platelets suspended in citrated plasma without cleaving fibrinopeptide A (45). Thrombin releases platelet factor 4, beta thromboglobulin and serotonin from gel-filtrated platelets and also cleaves fibrinopeptide A. The fibrinogen in this experiment is presumably derived from fibrinogen released from the platelets as well as residual plasma fibrinogen associated with the filtered platelets. Detectable release of platelet factor 4 and beta thromboglobulin in 3 minutes was observed with 2×10^{-2}u thrombin/ml(45)

EXPERIMENTS IN PLASMA AND WHOLE BLOOD IN VITRO

Thrombin cleaved detectable amounts of FPA at 5×10^{-4}u/ml during 3 minutes incubation with citrated platelet rich plasma but detectable release of platelet factor 4 and beta thromboglobulin occurred only at 1 x 10^{-1}u/ml. In whole blood without anticoagulant 8 x 10^{-5}u/ml thrombin cleaved 2.5 pmol FPA/ml in 3 minutes whereas platelet factor 4 and beta thromboglobulin release was only detected at 2 x 10^{-2}thrombin units per ml (Fig. 4). The greater sensitivity of platelet release in whole blood as compared with citrated plasma may be due to citrate inhibition of thrombin binding to platelets (45, 55). When blood was allowed to clot spontaneously (instead of adding thrombin) FPA cleavage and release of beta

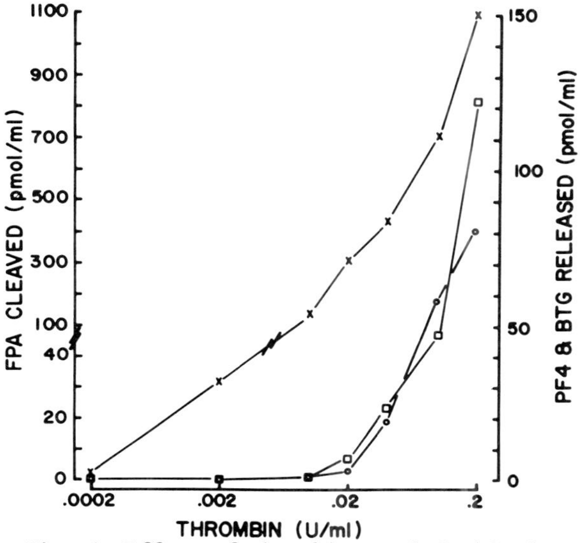

Fig. 4. Effect of thrombin on whole blood.

Effect of various concentrations of thrombin (units/ml plasma) on whole blood without anticoagulant. After 3 minutes incubation, heparin-trasylol or citrate, adenosine, and theophylline-hirudin was added and the plasma concentrations of fibrinopeptide A, platelet factor 4 and beta thromboglobulin were measured. (Reproduced from Kaplan, et al. (45))

thromboglobulin and platelet factor 4 occurred simultaneously with a molar ratio of 10 moles FPA cleaved per 1 mole platelet factor 4 and 1 mole beta thromboglobulin (Fig. 5) (46). Platelet release in spontaneously clotting whole blood is presumed to result from thrombin action (56). The difference between the relative sensitivities of platelets and fibrinogen to exogenous or spontaneously formed thrombin may be that in the latter instance thrombin first forms on the surface of the platelets and causes release at a lower concentration because of of its physical location. If so, the relative sensitivity of FPA cleavage and platelet release in vitro may be influenced by the method of activation of platelets and of blood coagulation. Simultaneous measurements of plasma FPA, beta thromboglobulin and platelet factor 4 levels in patients with disseminated intravascular coagulation, and venous and arterial thrombosis may then suggest the occurrence of specific activation mechanisms in these diseases.

In studies on the spontaneous clotting of blood very slow and episodic FPA generation occurs for 5-7 minutes and the rate then increases rapidly (57). Studies with a radioimmunoassay specific for thrombin showed a similar pattern of thrombin formation in spontaneously clotting whole blood (58). Thrombin formation and platelet factor 4 release occurred in parallel (59).

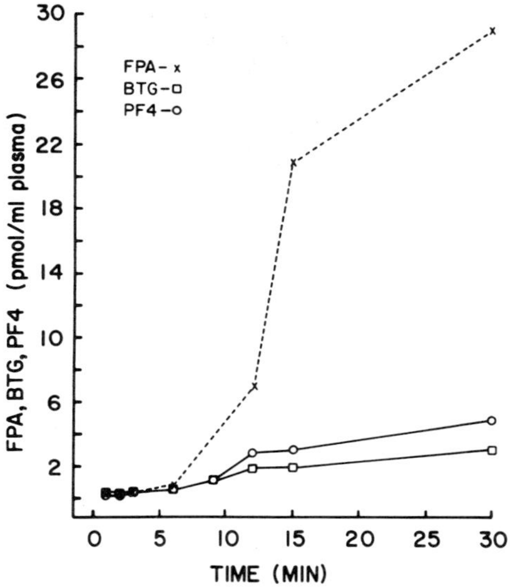

Fig. 5. PF4 and βTG release and FPA cleavage in whole blood.

Platelet factor 4 (PF4) and beta thromboglobulin (βTG) release and fibrinopeptide A (FPA) cleavage in whole blood allowed to clot spontaneously. Whole blood was incubated in plastic tubes at 37°. At 1, 2, 3, 6, 9, 12, 15, and 30 minutes following the beginning of blood flow into the syringe anticoagulant was added to the blood which after processing was assayed for PF4, βTG, and FPA. (Reproduced from Kaplan (46))

PLASMA LEVELS OF FIBRINOPEPTIDE A, Bβ 1-42, PLATELET FACTOR 4 AND BETA THROMBOGLOBULIN

Normal Ambulant Individuals

The mean normal plasma FPA level is 0.6 pmol/ml with an upper limit of about 1.3 pmol/ml. The results of different studies using different reagents and processing techniques have produced very similar results (16-19,48,57,60,62). In vivo infusion studies showed good recovery of FPA and a clearance rate equivalent to a $t_{1/2}$ of 3 minutes (57). Measurements of Bβ 1-42 immunoreactivity have not been reported but we have found a mean value of 1.8 pmol/ml in 10 normal individuals and estimate that the upper limit of normal may be about 3.5 to 4 pmol/ml. In vivo infusion and recovery studies have not yet been made. Fibrinopeptide B measurements in plasma have not been reported. Thus far we have not detected FPB in normal plasma with a detection limit of our assay of 1.5 pmol/ml. The normal plasma level of beta thromboglobulin is 18 ng/ml with an upper limit of 30 ng/ml. A mean normal level of 5 ng/ml has been reported for platelet factor 4 and an upper limit of 10 ng/ml. There is some variation between the results reported by different laboratories and these figures may well need revision in the future (61).

Studies in Venous Thromboembolism and Disseminated Intravascular Coagulation

The results of initial studies in venous thrombosis and in disseminated intravascular coagulation will be considered.

Venous Thromboembolism. FPA levels are elevated in patients with venous thromboembolism (16,57,62). In our own studies FPA levels >1.3 pmol/ml were found in 54 of 59 patients with documented venous thromboembolism, the mean level being 7.4 pmol/ml or 12 x the normal mean level. In patients with venographically proven venous thrombosis who had had symptoms for 6 days or less 29/30 had elevated FPA levels. Since FPA is cleared from the circulation with a t½ of 3 minutes, these data indicate that a sustained state of fibrin I formation often lasting 6 days is an almost invariable accompaniment of venous thromboembolism. Following intravenous infusion of heparin FPA levels began to drop immediately and in 25/26 patients were in the normal range within 15 minutes. FPA levels were normal in 42 of 48 patients with clinically suspect venous thromboembolism in whom the diagnosis was excluded by venography and lung scan. These data indicate that FPA levels have a very high negative predictive value. The positive predictive value is less since elevated FPA levels occur in many conditions not necessarily associated with deep venous thrombosis such as systemic lupus erythematosus, sepsis and neoplastic disease (17, 48). Hence fibrin I formation is not necessarily associated with thrombosis. In 10 patients so far studied Bβ 1-42 levels were normal or only slightly elevated in venous thrombosis without embolism but may be grossly elevated when pulmonary embolism is present. Limited studies reported elevated beta-thromboglobulin levels in about 50% of patients with post-surgical venous thrombosis diagnosed with the ^{125}I-fibrinogen uptake test (63). Simultaneous FPA and platelet protein measurements in the same patients with venous thromboembolism are too few for any conclusions.

Saline-Induced Abortion as a Model of In Vivo Coagulation. In studies on 10 patients before and at intervals following intrauterine infusion of hypertonic saline to terminate pregnancy we have observed a reproducible sequence of coagulation changes. A rapid linearly progressive increase in FPA concentration occurred reaching a peak at 1 hour with a mean level of 19 pmol/ml. The level remained steady till 2 hours after infusion, declined to a mean level of 12 pmol/ml at 4 hours and was within the normal range 24 and 48 hours later. Bβ 1-42 levels rose very slowly in the first hour but much more rapidly thereafter reaching a mean level of about 67 pmol/ml four hours after injection of saline. At 24 and 48 hours after injection of saline, the Bβ 1-42 level was in the normal range. Fibrinogen degradation product levels (FDP) showed no detectable change 1 hour after injection of saline but thereafter rose progressively to reach a mean of 40 μg/ml four hours after saline injection. The level was still markedly elevated at 24 hours - 20μg/ml and at 48 hours - 8μg/ml. The fibrinogen level decreased a mean of 0.4 mg/ml at 4 and 24 hours after saline injection but had returned to the pre-infusion level at 48 hours. In 4 patients studied during the first hour after injection of saline the FPA level began to rise significantly within 3 minutes of saline injection and in increased linearly at a rate of about 0.3pmol/ml plasma/minute to reach a mean of 17 pmol/ml at 1 hour after infusion of saline. Thrombin increasable FPB (Bβ1-42) increased from 0.7 to 2.3pmol/ml in the first hour, βTG levels rose from 27 to 58 ng/ml with the rate of increase paralleling the rate of FPA increase between 30 and 60 minutes. The βTG level fluctuated between 0 and 30 minutes showing no progressive change. The overall data suggest that thrombin is generated in vivo immediately after injection of hypertonic saline resulting in immediate formation of fibrin I. The finding that the βTG and FPA levels do not rise at exactly the same time could be due to slower diffusion into the blood of βTG released from platelets in an extravascular site or to an activation mechanism different from that which occurs when blood clots spontaneously in test tubes in vitro. The increase in Bβ 1-42 levels which follows the FPA increase implies formation of fragment X presumably by plasmin action on fibrin I. FPB levels are not known and the degree of fibrin II formation is therefore uncertain.

Based on these data and those of Blomback and colleagues (1), it is postulated that fragment X formation from fibrin I by plasmin is a major mechanism regulating the production of fibrin II. It is further postulated that the balance between fibrin I transformation into fibrin II or fragment X is of major pathophysiological significance in determining whether fibrin I formation is accompanied by thrombosis.

ACKNOWLEDGEMENTS

This work was supported by research grants HL15486, HL15596, and HL21006 from the National Institutes of Health. Dr. Kaplan is a senior investigator of the New York Heart Association.

REFERENCES

1. B. Blombäck, B. Hessel, D. Hogg, E. Therkildsen, A two-step fibrinogen-fibrin transition in blood coagulation, Nature 275, 501 (1978).

2. K. Bailey, F. R. Bettelheim, L. Lorand, W. R. Middlebrook, Action of thrombin in the clotting of fibrinogen, Nature 167, 233 (1951).

3. R. H. Herzig, O. D. Ratnoff, J. R. Shainoff, Studies on a procoagulant fraction of southern copperhead snake venom: the preferential release of fibrinopeptide B, J. Lab. Clin. Med. 76, 451 (1970).

4. B. Blomback, A. Vestermark, Isolation of fibrinopeptides by chromatography, Ark. Kemi. 12, 173 (1958).

5. S. B. Bilezikian, H. L. Nossel, V. P. Butler, Jr., R. E. Canfield, Radioimmunoassay of human fibrinopeptide B and kinetics of fibrinopeptide cleavage by different enzymes, J. Clin. Invest. 56, 438 (1975).

6. T. C. Laurent, B. Blombäck, On the significance of the release of two different peptides from fibrinogen during clotting, Acta Chem. Scand. 12, 137 (1958).

7. L. L. Shen, J. Hermans, J. McDonagh, R. P. McDonah, Role of fibrinopeptide B release: comparison of fibrins produced by thrombin and ancrod. Amer. J. Physiol. 232, H629 (1977).

8. V. J. Marder, N. R. Shulman, W. R. Carroll, High molecular weight derivatives of human fibrinogen produced by plasmin. I physico-chemical and immunological characterization, J. Biol. Chem. 244, 2111 (1969).

9. S. V. Pizzo, M. L. Schwartz, R. L. Hill, P. A. McKee, The effect of plasmin on the subunit structure of human fibrinogen, J. Biol. Chem. 247, 636 (1972).

10. M. W. Mosesson, J. S. Finlayson, D. K. Galanakis, The essential covalent structure of human fibrinogen evinced by analysis of derivatives formed during plasmic hydrolysis, J. Biol. Chem. 248, 7913 (1973).

11. T. Takagi, R. F. Doolittle, Amino acid sequence studies on plasmin-derived fragment of human fibrinogen: amino-terminal sequences for intermediate and terminal fragments, Biochemistry 14, 940 (1975).

12. B. Lahiri, J. R. Shainoff, Fate of fibrinopeptides in the reaction between human plasmin and fibrinogen, Biochim. et Biophys. Acta 303, 161 (1973).

13. S. Iwanaga, P. Wallen, N. J. Gröndahl, A. Henschen, B. Blombäck, On the primary structure of human fibrinogen. Isolation and characterization of N-terminal fragments from plasmic digests, European J. Biochem. 8, 189 (1969).

14. T. Takagi, R. F. Doolittle, Amino acid sequence studies on the α chain of human fibrinogen. Location of four plasmin attack points and a covalent cross-linking site, Biochemistry 14, 1549 (1975).

15. H. L. Nossel, L. R. Younger, G. D. Wilner, T. Procupez, R. E. Canfield, V. P. Butler, Jr., Radioimmunoassay of human fibrinopeptide A, Proc. Nat. Acad. Sci. USA 68, 2350 (1971).

16. C. Kockum, Radioimmunoassay of fibrinopeptide A: clinical applications, Thromb. Res. 8, 225 (1976).

17. M. Cronlund, J. Hardin, J. Burton, L. Lee, E. Haber, K. J. Bloch, Fibrinopeptide A in plasma of normal subjects and patients with disseminated intravascular coagulation and systemic lupus erythematosus, J. Clin. Invest. 58, 142 (1976).

18. W. B. J. Gerrits, O. T. N. Flier, J. van der Meer, Fibrinopeptide A immunoreactivity in human plasma, Thromb. Res. 5, 197 (1974).

19. A. Z. Budzynski, V. J. Marder, Determination of human fibrinopeptide A by radioimmunoassay in purified systems and in the blood, Thromb. Diath. Haemorrh. 34, 709 (1975).

20. H. L. Nossel, V. P. Butler, Jr., G. D. Wilner, R. E. Canfield, E. J. Harfenist, Specificity of antisera to human fibrinopeptide A used in clinical fibrinopeptide A assays. Thromb. Haemostas. 35, 101 (1976).

21. H. L. Nossel, R. Chatpar, V. P. Butler, Jr., R. E. Canfield, Radioimmunoassay of fibrinopeptide B, Blood 40, 955 (1972).

22. K. S. La Gamma, H. L. Nossel, The stability of fibrinopeptide B immunoreactivity in blood, Thromb. Res. 12, 447 (1978).

23. D. E. MacIntyre, The platelet release reaction: association with adhesion and aggregation, and comparison with secretory responses in other cells. In: Platelets in Biology and Pathology, edited by J. L. Gordon, North-Holland, Amsterdam, p. 61 (1976).

24. L. D. Witte, K. L. Kaplan, H. L. Nossel, B. A. Lages, H. J. Weiss, DeW. S. Goodman, Studies of the release from human platelets of the growth factor for cultured human arterial smooth muscle cells, Circ. Res. 42, 402, (1978).

25. S. Niewiarowski, D. P. Thomas, Platelet factor 4 and adenosine diphosphate release during human platelet aggregation, Nature 222, 1269 (1969).

26. S. VanCreveld, M. M. P. Paulssen, Isolation and properties of the third clotting factor in blood platelets, Lancet 1, 23 (1952).

27. R. Kaser-Glanzmann, M. Jakabova, E. F. Lüscher, Isolation and some properties of the heparin-neutralizing factor (PF4) released from human blood platelets, Experientia 28, 1221 (1972).

28. E. Deutsch, S. A. Johnson, W. H. Seegers, Differentiation of certain platelet factors related to blood coagulation, Circ. Res. 3, 110 (1955).

29. J. Salmon, Y. Bounameaux, Etude des antigenes plaquettaires et, en particulier, du fibrinogene, Thromb. Diath. Haemorrh. 2, 93 (1958).

30. G. Sokal, Etude methodologique des plaquettes snaguines et de la metamorphose visqueuse aux moyens d'antiserums fluorescents, antifibrinogenes et antiplaquettes. Acta Haematol. 28, 313 (1962).

31. R. L. Nachman, Immunologic studies of platelet protein, Blood 25, 703 (1965).

32. M. G. Davey, E. F. Luscher, Release reactions of human platelets induced by thrombin and other agents, Biochim. Biophys, Acta. 165, 490 (1968).

33. K. Dzoga, G. Stolotzner, R. W. Wissler, The production of a highly specific antiserum to human platelets, Lab. Invest. 27, 351 (1972).

34. S. Moore, D. S. Pepper, J. D. Cash, The isolation and characterization of a platelet-specific β-globulin (β-thromboglobulin)and the detection of anti-urokinase and anti-plasmin released from thrombin-aggregated washed human platelets, Biochim. Biophys, Acta. 379, 360 (1975).

35. S. Moore, D. S. Pepper, Identification and characterization of a platelet specific release product: β-thromboglobulin, In: Platetes in Biology and Pathology, edited by J. L. Gordon, North Holland, Amsterdam, p. 293 (1976).

36. T. F. Deuel, P. S. Keim, M. Farmer, R. L. Heinrikson, Amino acid sequence of human platelet factor 4, Proc. Natl. Acad. Sci. USA 74, 2256 (1977).

37. F. J. Morgan, C. N. Chesterman, J. R. McGready, G. S. Begg, Studies on the chemistry of human platelet factor 4, Haemostasis 6 53 (1977).

38. M. Hermodsen, G. Schmer, K. Kurachi, Isolation, crystallization and primary amino acid sequence of human platelet factor 4, J. Biol. Chem. 252, 6276 (1977).

39. D. A. Walz, V. Y. Wu, R. De Lamo, H. Dene, and L. E. McCoy, Primary structure of human platelet factor 4, Thromb. Res. 11, 898 (1977).

40. C. A. Ludlam, S. Moore, A. E. Bolton, D. S. Pepper, J. D. Cash, The release of a human platelet specific protein measured by a radioimmunoassay, Thromb. Res. 6, 543 (1975).

41. A. E. Bolton, C. A. Ludlam, D. S. Pepper, S. Moore, J. D. Cash, A radioimmunoassay for platelet factor 4, Thromb. Res. 8, 51 (1976).

42. A. E. Bolton, C. A. Ludlam, S. Moore, D. S. Pepper, J. D. Cash, Three approaches to the radioimmunoassay of human β-thromboglobulin, Br. J. Haematol. 33, 233 (1976).

43. S. Levine, L. Krentz, Development of a radioimmunoassay for human platelet factor 4, Thromb. Res. 11, 673 (1977).

44. C. N. Chesterman, J. R. McGready, F. J. Morgan, Radioimmunoassay of human platelet factor 4, Thromb. Haemostas. 38, 211 (1977).

45. K. L. Kaplan, H. L. Nossel, M. Drillings, G. Lesznik, Radioimmunoassay of platelet factor 4 and β-thromboglobulin: development and application to studies of platelet release in relation of fibrinopeptide A generation, Br. J. Haematol. 39, 129 (1978).

46. K. L. Kaplan, Proteins secreted by platelets: significance in detecting thrombosis. In: Thrombosis: Animal and Clinical Models, edited by H. J. Day, B. A. Molony, E. E. Nishizawa, R. H. Rynbrandt, Plenum, New York, p. 105 (1978).

47. R. I. Handin, M. McDonough, M. Lesch, Elevation of platelet factor 4 in acute myocardial infarction: measurement by radioimmunoassay, J. Lab. & Clin. Med. 91 ,340 (1978).

48. H. L. Nossel, M. Ti, K. L. Kaplan, K. Spanondis, T. Soland, V. P. Butler, Jr. The generation of fibrinopeptide A in clinical blood samples, J. Clin. Invest. 58, 1136 (1976).

49. W. J. Landis, D. F. Waugh, Interactions of bovine fibrinogen and thrombin, Arch. Biochem. & Biophys. 168, 498 (1975).

50. M. Bando, A. Matsushima, J. Hirano, Y. Inada, Thrombin-catalyzed conversion of fibrinogen to fibrin, J. Biochem. (Tokyo) 71, 897 (1972).

51. D. F. Waugh, B. J. Livingstone, Kinetics of the interaction of bovine fibrinogen and thrombin. J. Phys. Colloid Chem. 55, 1206 (1951).

52. B. Blomback, Fibrinogen to fibrin transformation. In: Blood Clotting Enzymology, edited by W. H. Seegers, Academic Press, New York, p. 143 (1967).

53. D. S. Hogg, B. Blomback, The specificity of the fibrinogen-thrombin reaction, Thromb. Res. 5, 685 (1974).

54. S. B. Bilezikian, H. L. Nossel, Unique pattern of fibrinogen cleavage by human leukocyte proteases, Blood 50, 21 (1977).

55. M. A. Shuman, P. W. Majerus, The perturbation of thrombin binding to human platelets by anions, J. Clin. Invest. 56, 945 (1975).

56. S. Jevons, P. G. Barton, Biochemistry of blood platelets. Interaction of activated factor X with platelets, Biochem. 10, 428 (1971).

57. H. L. Nossel, I. Yudelman, R. E. Canfield, V. P. Butler, Jr., K. Spanondis, G. D. Wilner, G. D. Qureshi, Measurement of fibrinopeptide A in human blood, J. Clin. Invest. 54, 43 (1974).

58. M. A. Shuman, P. W. Majerus, The measurement of thrombin in clotting blood by radioimmunoassay, J. Clin. Invest. 58, 1249 (1976).

59. M. A. Shuman, S. P. Levine, Thrombin generation and secretion of platelet factor 4 during blood clotting, J. Clin. Invest. 61, 1102 (1978).

60. V. Hofmann, P. W. Straub, A radioimmunoassay technique for the rapid measurement of human fibrinopeptide A, Thromb. Res. 11, 171 (1977).

61. H. L. Nossel, Secreted platelet proteins, Thromb. Haemostas. 40 (in press 1978).

62. I. Yudelman, H. L. Nossel, K. L. Kaplan, J. Hirsh, Plasma Fibrinopeptide A levels in symptomatic venous thromboembolism, Blood 51, 1189 (1978).

63. R. C. Smith, C. V. Ruckley, J. Duncanson, N. C. Allan, J. Dawes, D. S. Pepper, J. D. Cash, β-thromboglobulin and deep vein thrombosis in surgical patients. Thromb. Haemostas. 38, 166 (1977).

64. G. D. Wilner, H. L. Nossel, R. E. Canfield, V. P. Butler, Jr., Immunochemical studies of human fibrinopeptide A using synthetic peptide homologues, Biochem. 15, 1209 (1976).

65. R. E. Canfield, J. Dean, H. L. Nossel, V. P. Butler, Jr., G. D. Wilner, Reactivity of fibrinogen and fibrinopeptide A containing fibrinogen fragments with antisera to fibrinopeptide A, Biochem. 15, 1203 (1976).

STRUCTURE AND ASSEMBLY OF HUMAN SERUM LIPOPROTEINS

Charles Tanford and Jacqueline A. Reynolds
Whitehead Medical Research Institute and Department of Biochemistry,
Duke University Medical Center, Durham, N.C. 27710

ABSTRACT

Lipids by themselves do not form soluble particles and the formation of soluble lipoproteins must therefore be the result of structural features inherent to the polypeptide constituents of these proteins. The problem is complicated by the heterogeneity of the native proteins, and by the fact that some polypeptide constituents (the C-peptides) are transferred from one protein to another in the course of metabolic processes, but one can tentatively conclude that there are two fundamental core proteins: one consists of two A-I and two A-II polypeptides (total molecular weight 74,000) and is the nucleus for all proteins in the high density (HDL) class; the other consists of two B polypeptides (total molecular weight 510,000) and is the nucleus for all proteins in the low density (LDL) and very low density (VLDL) classes.

To find out how these core proteins organize themselves and how they combine with C-peptides and lipids into the ultimate lipoprotein molecules, one can use structural information derived from investigation of the intact native proteins (as initially done by J.L. Oncley in the laboratory of E.J. Cohn more than thirty years ago); or one can start with the purified polypeptide chains and determine by thermodynamic and structural methods the mode of their association with each other, with hydrophobic ligands in general, and with phospholipid and neutral lipids in particular. We have used the second approach and have fairly detailed data for the A-I polypeptide of HDL. The data show that A-I binds hydrophobic ligands in a manner unmistakably different from the binding of similar ligands to intrinsic membrane proteins and indicate that binding of various lipid constituents, formation of the HDL core protein, and subsequent assembly of complete HDL molecules probably have to occur in a unique sequence.

INTRODUCTION

The purpose of this paper is to discuss the molecular organization of the serum lipoproteins. What polypeptide chains combine to form the core protein structure of each molecule? How does the protein associate with lipid to create the assembled native molecules?

The problem is more complicated than for most other proteins because the lipoproteins are variable in composition. Variability with respect to the lipid component is an essential property because the physiological function of the lipoprotein is to transport lipids and to deposit them where they are needed, but there is also variability with respect to polypeptide chain composition, and some polypeptides are known to be transferred from one lipoprotein to another in the course of vascular circulation. At the same time there is an initially puzzling lack of variation where one would expect to find it; some of the grossly different native molecules obtained by fractionation on the basis of density or size turn out to have polypeptide chains in common, suggesting that they should perhaps be regarded as derivatives of the same core protein.

In discussing these problems we shall limit ourselves to the three major lipoprotein classes of normal human serum, the high density (HDL), low density (LDL) and very low density (VLDL) proteins. Minor lipoproteins and abnormal lipoproteins associated with certain clinical disorders will not be considered, nor will chylomicra which are usually classified as a fourth major lipoprotein component of normal human serum, but have proved difficult to study from a protein structural point of view because of their very low protein content (about 2% by weight). The discussion of the major lipoproteins will be organized into four sections:

(1) Roster of all known polypeptide chain constituents.

(2) Polypeptide chain and lipid compositions of the native proteins and definition of a small number of core proteins that may be considered to be structural nuclei for the generation of all major native molecules.

(3) Structural organization, as seen from experimental studies of intact native lipoproteins.

(4) Assembly of the native proteins, as seen from studies beginning with purified polypeptides. There are two aspects of this problem: association of polypeptides with each other and association between polypeptides and lipids.

Recent work from the laboratory of one of us (J.A.R.), relating to these problems, will be emphasized. There are many excellent reviews of earlier work, among which we have found the following especially useful: the review of Lewis (1977) on metabolic interrelationships, the review of Jackson et al. (1976) on structure, and the review of Osborne and Brewer (1977) on assembly.

POLYPEPTIDE CHAINS

The polypeptide chains that have been identified as lipoprotein constituents are listed in Table 1: one of them (D) is probably not a constituent of the major lipoproteins discussed in this paper. Amino acid sequences have been determined for five of the listed polypeptides, and accurate molecular weights have been measured for two others. An interesting feature of the sequences is that none of them contains long continuous segments of hydrophobic amino acids, such as have been found in the three intrinsic membrane proteins that have been sequenced so far (Nakashima and Konigsberg, 1974; Tomita and Marchesi, 1975; Fleming et al., 1978). What constitutes the fundamental difference between polypeptide chains that combine with lipid by entering into lipid bilayer membranes and those that combine with lipid to form soluble molecular complexes is one of the principal questions that characterization of the lipoproteins must answer, and it will be discussed further later in this paper.

It is difficult to understand why the molecular weight of the B polypeptide, measured several years ago by Smith et al. (1972) has not been accepted by some investigators (e.g. Scanu et al., 1975). The measurement was made on B chain that was purified to homogeneity in concentrated guanidinium chloride and reduced

TABLE 1 Major Polypeptide Chains of Human Lipoproteins

Polypeptide[a]	Amino acid sequence determined	Molecular weight from sequence	Molecular weight by ultracentrifuge[b]
A-I	Yes[c]	28,330[c]	28,300[d]
A-II	Yes[e]	8,710	9,100[d]
B	No	——	255,000[f]
C-I	Yes[g]	6,620	7,000[h]
C-II	Yes[i]	8,840	10,000[h]
C-III	Yes[j]	8,760	10,000[h]
D[k]	No	——	(18,000)[k]
E[l]	No		33,000[l]

(a) Nomenclature of Alaupovic et al. (1972).
(b) Theoretically rigorous measurements under conditions where dissociation to monomer state is virtually certain. All measurements except that for A-II were made before the amino acid sequence was known.
(c) There are some unresolved differences between sequences obtained by Baker et al. (1974) and Brewer et al. (1978). The molecular weight given in column 3 is based on the sequence of Baker et al.
(d) Makino et al. (1974). The molecular weight for A-II was determined for the disulfide-bonded dimer and divided in half.
(e) Brewer et al. (1972). In humans this polypeptide is always present as a disulfide-bonded dimer.
(f) Smith et al. (1972). The B peptide contains 7% carbohydrate which is included in the measured molecular weight.
(g) Shulman et al. (1972), Jackson et al. (1974).
(h) Brown et al. (1970). The measured molecular weight for C-III includes the contribution from carbohydrate.
(i) Jackson et al. (1977).
(j) Brewer et al. (1974). This polypeptide contains a carbohydrate side chain and exists in three forms containing respectively 0, 1 and 2 terminal sialic acid residues. The carbohydrate is not included in the molecular weight calculated from the sequence.
(k) There is no evidence to suggest that polypeptide D is incorporated into any of the principal native lipoproteins, as listed in Table 2 (McConathy and Alaupovic, 1976). The polypeptide contains 18% carbohydrate. The molecular weight is based on amino acid analysis and does not include the bound carbohydrate.
(l) Polypeptide E is a minor component of VLDL. The molecular weight was determined by Shelburne and Quarfordt (1974).

to break all disulfide bonds. Optical rotatory dispersion showed that the polypeptide was in the structureless random coil form that most proteins adopt in this solvent. A weak tendency for reversible self-association between randomly-coiled polypeptides may exist, but there are no known examples where the association is strong enough to prevent the major portion of the polypeptide from being in the monomeric state at the great dilutions used for molecular weight measurements. Indeed it is difficult to imagine how strong and essentially irreversible non-covalent association could occur without formation of structure detectable by optical methods. However, one does not actually have to rely on this argument to conclude that the B protein was unassociated under the conditions of the molecular weight measurement because Smith et al. measured the hydrodynamic radius independently of the molecular weight and found it to have the value expected for a linear continuous chain of molecular weight 255,000. An aggregate of smaller

TABLE 2 Analytical Data for Native Lipoproteins[a]

	Mol.wt.	Weight per cent protein	Weight per cent lipid	Constituent polypeptides[b]	Lipids (wt% of total lipid)[c] FL	FC	CE	TG
VLDL$_1$	32×10^6	6.4	93.6	B,C,E	11	6	8	75
VLDL$_4$	15×10^6	9.4	90.6	B,C,E	17	8	15	60
VLDL$_7$	8×10^6	13.2	86.8	B,C,E	23	10	26	41
LDL$_1$	4×10^6	18.0	82.0	B,C,E	29	7	28	36
LDL$_2$	2.7×10^6	21.0	79.0	B	29	10	53	8
HDL$_2$	360,000	40	60	A-I,A-II,C	53	10	29	8
HDL$_3$	175,000	55	45	A-I,A-II,C	54	8	28	10

(a) Data for VLDL are for representative subfractions from Patsch et al. (1978), for LDL they are from Lee (1976), and for HDL from Scanu (1971). Molecular weights are crude estimates from various sources.
(b) All three C-peptides are present when the presence of C is indicated.
(c) PL = phospholipid, FC = free cholesterol, CE = cholesteryl esters, TG = triglycerides.

polypeptides would have had considerably smaller dimensions, unless the aggregation occurred strictly end-to-end by means of a "bond" structurally indistinguishable from a peptide bond. While smaller molecular weight values for the B chain have sometimes been suggested (see Osborne and Brewer, 1977), the suggestion is in no case based on a valid measurement. On the other hand, there is support for a very high molecular weight from proteolysis experiments (Triplett et al., 1975; Triplett and Fisher, 1978; Ikai, 1976; Ikai and Yagisawa, 1977) which show that species of molecular weight above 100,000 are formed as initial proteolysis products.

NATIVE LIPOPROTEINS

The native lipoproteins are heterogeneous and each class of protein can be subfractionated by ultracentrifugation or gel exclusion chromatography into subfractions, which themselves are still heterogeneous but have a narrower distribution with respect to molecular size and composition. Analytical data for representative subfractions are shown in Table 2. It is seen from these data that C-peptides are present in all native proteins except LDL$_2$, but that A and B peptides never occur in the same molecule, the former being present only in HDL and the latter in LDL and VLDL. Recent data strongly suggest that the A and B peptides exist as two (and only two) core proteins, which are the nuclei for generation of all the major lipoprotein species other than chylomicra.

HDL core protein. Friedberg and Reynolds (1976) have made a careful study of the stoichiometry of association between A-I and A-II in native HDL, utilizing a method that avoids differential loss of the two peptides in fractionation procedures. Employing 10 different normal subjects, and examining both HDL$_2$ and HDL$_3$, they observed a constant 1:1 ratio between A-I and A-II polypeptides, suggesting the existence of a core protein as shown in Fig. 1. Molecular weights reported for native HDL$_3$ range from 148,000 to 186,000, about half of which is protein, indicating that each HDL$_3$ molecule contains one copy of the core protein. The molecular weight of HDL$_2$ is probably close to 360,000, with a protein content of 40%, indicating the presence of two copies of the core protein. Both forms contain C-peptides, but at a level of less than 10% by weight. The average content of C-peptides in HDL$_3$ corresponds to less than one polypeptide chain per

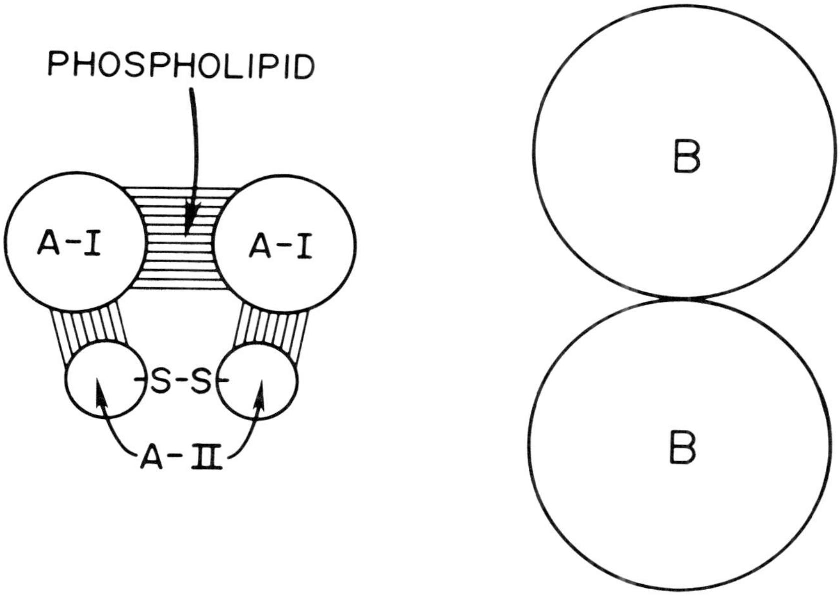

Fig. 1. Core proteins for HDL (left) and for LDL and VLDL (right). The A-II polypeptides in the HDL core protein are joined (in humans) by a disulfide bond. The shaded areas in the diagram for the HDL core protein are intended to symbolize an apparent requirement for the presence of diacyl phospholipids in the formation of this specific complex (see text).

molecule, so that some HDL_3 molecules undoubtedly contain only the core protein and lipid.

Support for the existence of a core protein of fixed composition comes from a recent study of Shepherd et al. (1977). By incubating whole HDL (mixture of HDL_2 and HDL_3) with radioactively labeled A-I polypeptide they were able to incorporate labeled A-I into the lipoprotein molecule. At low levels of incorporation, the labeled A-I displaced endogenous A-I on a mol per mol basis, i.e., the A-I: A-II stoichiometry remained fixed. When labeled A-I was added in large excess (10:1 molar ratio of A-I to HDL) release of endogenous A-I only partially compensated for incorporation of labeled A-I, i.e., there was a net increase in the A-I/A-II ratio in the lipoprotein. The product obtained was not fractionated to see whether the excess A-I was distributed uniformly among all molecules, and it is therefore possible that the product was a mixture of A-I-lipid complexes and of HDL molecules with unchanged A-I/A-II composition. Further studies are needed before it can be determined whether complete molecules containing a molar excess of A-I over A-II can be formed when A-I is present in large excess.

LDL and VLDL core protein. It has been shown by Schumaker (1973) and by Fisher et al. (1975) that variations in the molecular weight of LDL_2 between 2×10^6 and 4×10^6 probably arise from variations in the lipid content, the protein content remaining constant at 510,000 g/mol, i.e., two B polypeptides per molecule. The same is probably true for VLDL. For example, Kane et al. (1975) have used the insolubility of the B polypeptide in tetramethyl urea to determine the amount of B peptide in $VLDL_6$ samples from 43 normal human subjects, with a mean particle diameter of 364 Å, which corresponds to a mean molecular weight of 14.1×10^6. B peptide was found to represent 36.9% of the total protein. With a normal total protein content of 9% (Scanu et al., 1975), this corresponds to 470,000 g of B peptide per particle, not including the 7% carbohydrate normally part of the B peptide. If this is included, the total amount of B becomes 505,000. (The measured molecular weight of 255,000 for the B chain includes the carbohydrate moiety). In subfractions of VLDL (Kane et al., 1975; Patsch et al., 1978) the content of B peptide varies inversely with total molecular weight, such that the amount of B per particle remains constant to within the accuracy of analytical methods. The most compelling evidence for an invariant amount of B peptide in all VLDL and LDL molecules comes from studies of lipoprotein catabolism and lipid metabolism (Lewis, 1977), which show that there is a precursor-product relationship between VLDL and LDL_2, with a progressive decrease in C-peptides and lipids (primarily triglycerides). The smaller VLDL molecules have been called "remnant molecules" and LDL_2 is the ultimate remnant, containing no C-peptides and the least amount of lipid.

C-peptides. It is not yet known whether the C-peptides form core protein complexes of fixed stoichiometry. Since they are readily transferred between VLDL and HDL, they are certainly not tightly bound to the core protein formed by A or B polypeptides, but the stoichiometric ratio C-I: C-II: C-III is not the same in VLDL and in HDL (Osborne and Brewer, 1977), indicating that at least one of the chains must be transferred between VLDL and HDL as an independent entity. One of the peptides (C-II) is not simply a lipid transport protein, but has a separate physiological function in being a potent activator of the enzyme lipoprotein lipase.

The work of Kostner and Alaupovic (1972) and Alaupovic et al. (1972) purports to show that C-peptides form inherently independent lipoproteins, and that native VLDL and HDL molecules are created by weak complex formation between the C-containing lipoproteins and lipoproteins containing only A or B peptides. This is not an unreasonable possibility, but we do not find their experimental evidence compelling.

STRUCTURAL INFORMATION

It was shown by Oncley and coworkers more than thirty years ago that LDL, despite its high molecular weight and high lipid content, has a compact, nearly spherical shape, much like that of common compactly-folded globular proteins that do not contain lipid (Oncley et al., 1947). A similar result has since been obtained for VLDL and HDL as well, both by electron microscopy and by hydrodynamic studies (e.g., Nichols, 1969).

In another paper, Oncley et al. (1950) showed that the pH-dependence of the solubility of LDL resembles that of ordinary water-soluble proteins and could be ascribed to the titration of the acidic and basic groups of the protein moiety. Titration of most of these groups could be observed without indication of denaturation or other structural change, implying that most of the groups had to be at the surface of the native molecule, in contact with solvent. A similar inference can be made for HDL (at least for the amino groups) on the basis of their availability for succinylation (Scanu et al., 1968). Virtually all phosphate ester groups of phospholipid molecules in HDL and LDL are likewise accessible to solvent on the basis of shifts in the ^{31}P nmr spectrum induced by paramagnetic ions (Assmann et al., 1974; Yeagle et al., 1978), though an earlier report indicated that 50% of these groups are inaccessible in LDL (Henderson et al.,1975)

In HDL all phospholipid head groups have been shown to be available for cleavage by the enzyme phospholipase A_2 (Pattnaik et al., 1976). These results come as no surprise. The phospholipid head groups are ionic, and the titratable groups of proteins are ionic at neutral pH, and together they represent the most strongly hydrophilic parts of the molecular complex, which could be removed from contact with solvent only at great cost in terms of free energy (Tanford, 1962).

Dimensional considerations suggest that phospholipid head groups and protein polar groups completely fill the surface layer of a lipoprotein molecule, leaving no room for any part of the neutral lipid constituents (Shen et al., 1977). The neutral lipids thus occupy the internal space of the lipoprotein molecule, and this is not thermodynamically unreasonable. The ester groups of cholesteryl esters and triglycerides are only weakly hydrophilic in comparison with the charged groups present on ionic amino acid side chains of proteins and on phospholipid head groups. Moreover, the hydrophobic moieties on these molecules are extremely large; so that the free energy gained by their removal from contact with water far exceeds the free energy lost by removing the small hydrophilic groups along with them. A temperature-induced order-disorder transition has been observed in native LDL by several physical techniques (Deckelbaum et al., 1977a; Sears et al., 1976; Atkinson et al., 1977). It involves cholesteryl esters and has been interpreted as reflecting the presence of cholesteryl esters in LDL in a separate domain, with a molecular arrangement similar to that in pure cholesteryl esters. The presence of triglycerides lowers the temperature of the transition, indicating that triglycerides enter the same domain, being soluble only in the disordered phase. In VLDL, where the triglyceride content becomes very high, a transition can no longer be observed (Deckelbaum et al., 1977b).

The ^{31}P nmr studies of Yeagle et al. (1977,1978) also provide information about vicinal interactions of the phospholipid head groups. In LDL about 20% of the groups are immobilized by interaction with the protein, but the specific interaction with cholesterol, as normally seen in cholesterol-containing phospholipid bilayers, is absent, indicating that the OH group of unesterified cholesterol (like the ester groups of cholesteryl esters) may be located away from contact with solvent. In HDL there appear to be no immobilizing interactions between phospholipid head groups and protein.

It is sometimes claimed that x-ray and neutron scattering experiments (on lipoprotein <u>solutions</u>) can provide more detailed structural information, but this claim is not substantiated by the results and the elaborate model structures based on scattering data are perhaps best viewed as testimony to the power of human imagination. Two specific structures proposed for LDL (Mateu et al., 1972; Müller et al., 1978) require small symmetrically arranged protein "subunits", and contain no suggestions as to how these "subunits" might be derived from the two large B polypeptide chains known to be in the particle. One of the proposals (Mateu et al., 1972) confidently asserts that phospholipid is present as a spherical bilayer centered 75 Å from the center of the particle, a proposal that is not compatible with the accessibility of all phospholipid head groups to the solvent. A later paper by the same group (Tardieu et al., 1976) withdraws the claim for a phospholipid bilayer and is more modest in its conclusions than the earlier paper. However, even these more modest conclusions require unrealistic simplifying assumptions: for example, that the lipoprotein complex can be divided into two homogeneous and spherically symmetrical regions, one with low electron density ("hydrocarbon") and another with high electron density ("polar groups").

ASSEMBLY

The study of the assembly of the lipoproteins, starting with purified polypeptide chains, is easier for HDL than for LDL and VLDL because the A and C polypeptides are soluble in aqueous solutions in the absence of lipids. Furthermore, it has been shown that a lipoprotein particle closely resembling native HDL can be reconstituted by sonication of a mixture of HDL polypeptides and constituent lipids in appropriate relative amounts (Hirz and Scanu, 1970; Lux et al., 1972). The free B polypeptides, on the other hand, are not water-soluble and step-by-step reconstitution with thermodynamic analysis of each step becomes more difficult. For this reason analysi of the assembly process has progressed further with HDL than with LDL and VLDL, and the discussion in this section is thus confined to HDL.

One of the objectives of a study of assembly is to define the molecular basis for physiological function: in the case of HDL these include the ability to accept C-peptides from VLDL during conversion of the latter to LDL, the ability to take up cholesterol from the peripheral tissues (Glomset, 1968), and the ability to act as substrate for the enzyme lecithin-cholesterol acyltransferase in the interconversion of free cholesterol and cholesteryl esters. (These functions are reviewed succinctl by Lewis, 1977). From a purely chemical point of view, an added objective is to seek a molecular basis for the difference between lipoproteins and intrinsic membrane proteins, as was already noted in the Introduction.

Self-association of Apoproteins.

A-I and A-II polypeptides are independently soluble in aqueous solutions, as fairly compactly folded molecules called apoA-I and apoA-II. Circular dichroism studies indicate that the polypeptide chain conformation in both apoproteins is different from the conformations adopted by A-I and A-II when incorporated into native HDL (Lux et al., 1972): the most striking difference is in the near-ultraviolet part of the spectrum, probably ascribable to tryptophan residues in the A-I peptide (A-II has none). Both conformations have only marginal stability. The mid points for denaturation by guanidinium chloride are below 1 M, much lower than for typical water-soluble proteins (Reynolds, 1976). Thermal denaturation (studied for apoA-I only) sets in at 43°C (Gwynne et al., 1975; Tall et al., 1976); no transitio at such a low temperature is observed in native HDL or in most water-soluble protei

Both apoA-I and apoA-II self-associate in aqueous solution (Stone and Reynolds, 1975b; for comparison with other studies see Osborne and Brewer, 1977). In the case of apoA-I the equilibrium mixture contains monomers, dimers and higher aggregates, with no indication that the dimer, the state in which A-I occurs in the HDL core protein (Fig.1), has particular stability. Moreover, the association does not induce a change in conformation towards the state in which A-I exists in native HDL. In the case of apoA-II, the predominant form at equilibrium at moderate concentration is a tetramer (two disulfide-bonded dimers), whereas there is only a single disulfide-bonded dimer in the core protein. Preliminary experiments with mixtures of apoA-I and apoA-II do not indicate preference for formation of a comlex with the stoichiometry of the HDL core protein (Friedberg and Reynolds, unpublished results).

These results indicate that association products of the apoproteins in the absence of lipid are not related to the state of association observed in nature, but that they are instead ascribable to the existence of hydrophobic areas on the apoproteins, intended for binding of hydrophobic ligands, which, in the absence of hydrophobic ligands, can associate with each other. This supposition is supported by the observation that binding of simple hydrophobic ligands to apoA-I, which does drive the near-ultraviolet circular dichroism spectrum in the direction of the native state, results in dissociation of the associated forms of apoA-I. However, when diacyl phospholipids are bound to A-I, a homogeneous product with a molecular weight corresponding to an A-I dimer is formed, with an accompanying conformational state similar to that observed for simpler ligands (Reynolds et al., 1977). The formation of a native-like A-I dimer thus seems to be intimately linked to the presence of diacyl phospholipids. By inference, this suggests that the formation of the HDL core protein as a whole is dependent on the presence of diacyl phospholipids (as indicated in Fig.1), but appropriate experimental studies with mixtures of A-I and A-II have not yet been made.

The C-peptides also undergo self-association in the absence of bound hydrophobic ligands, but it is not known whether there is in this case a relation to possible associated forms existing in nature (Brown et al., 1970; Osborne and Brewer, 1977). ApoB cannot be studied in the absence of ligands because of its insolubility in aqueous solutions, but, in contrast to A-I and A-II, it has a strong tendency to exist as a dimer in detergents, even in a denaturing detergent such as Na dodecyl sulfate (Steele and Reynolds, 1979), indicating that formation of the B core protein (Fig. 1) is not dependent on the presence of diacyl phospholipids and may be an inherent property of the protein alone.

Binding of Simple Hydrophobic Ligands to A-I and A-II

It is generally assumed that the binding of lipids to lipoproteins involves sites or regions of the protein that are specifically designed to accommodate the hydrophobic moieties of the lipid. It then becomes useful to explore the nature of the binding sites by studying the association with simple hydrophobic ligands before an interpretation of binding data with the more complex endogenous lipids is attempted. A particularly important objective of such measurements is to define the difference between the hydrophobic binding sites of lipoproteins and of membrane proteins, the latter being designed for insertion into extended phospholipid bilayers without disruption of the bilayer organization, whereas lipoproteins are always found in nature as soluble particles. They come into frequent contact with cell membranes and transfer lipids to them, but the polypeptide chains always remain in solution.

Experimental binding data take the form of plots of the amount of bound ligand as a function of the free ligand concentration, and two types of binding are readily distinguishable in terms of the steepness of the binding isotherms (e.g. Tanford, 1973; Fig. 15-1). One is binding to discrete sites on the protein molecule, each site accommodating one ligand molecule more or less independently of other sites, which leads to a flat binding isotherm obeying the law of mass action for single site binding. The second mode of binding is <u>cooperative</u> binding in which many ligand molecules are bound simultaneously to binding sites or regions that are unable to form stable adducts with single or even a small number of bound ligands; this kind of binding is characterized by a very steep isotherm. A well-known example of discrete site binding is provided by serum albumin, which in its native state has about ten sites per molecule for individual hydrophobic ligands, most of the sites being specific for ligands with anionic head groups. Membrane proteins provide an example of cooperative binding: their tendency to insert into a phospholipid bilayer without disrupting the bilayer is reflected in their binding of micelle-forming amphiphiles, the amount bound often being close to the amount contained in a single micelle of the amphiphile (Tanford and Reynolds, 1976).

ApoA-I and apoA-II display <u>both</u> kinds of binding (Reynolds and Simon, 1974; Makino et al., 1974; Stone and Reynolds, 1975a; Haberland and Reynolds, 1975). Each protein has three or four discrete sites for binding single molecules of hydrophobic ligands. In contrast to serum albumin, there is no head group specificity. Cationic and anionic amphiphiles bind equally well, and even pure hydrocarbons can be accommodated, the free energy of binding being in each case consistent with what is expected on the basis that hydrophobic interactions alone are the determining

TABLE 3 Maximal Binding of Ligands to apoA-I[a]

Ligand	State of association	Maximal mols ligand per peptide chain	Molar volume of bound hydrophobic moiety per peptide chain (cm^3/mol)
$C_{12}H_{25}OSO_3Na$	monomer	138	24,900 ± 1000
$C_{14}H_{29}N(CH_3)_3Cl$	monomer	117	24,800 ± 1000
Lubrol WX[b]	monomer	80 ± 10	20,800 ± 2600
Palmitoyl lysoPC[c]	monomer	97	22,100 ± 2000
didecanoyl PC[c]	dimer	95 ± 10	25,000 ± 2600
Na deoxycholate[d]	monomer	27	9100

(a) Adapted from Reynolds et al. (1977).
(b) Lubrol WX is a mixture of hexadecyl and octadecyl ethers of polyoxyethylene glycol, with an average of 16 oxyethylene groups per molecule.
(c) PC = phosphatidylcholine.
(d) The "hydrophobic moiety" of deoxycholate is a steroid ring containing two OH groups, and thus differs from the pure hydrocarbon chains of the other ligands in the Table both in shape and in the possession of polar groups. The smaller volume bound indicates that the A-I binding area is specifically designed for hydrocarbon chains.

factor. Binding to the discrete sites induces a small conformational change in the protein, and cooperative binding of a large number of ligands occurs only after this change has occurred: synergistic effects have been noted, suggesting that occupancy of the discrete sites by any one ligand makes the cooperative sites available to all other ligands (Stone and Reynolds, 1975a). Cooperative binding, like binding to the discrete sites, does not seem to involve head group specificity. This indicates that polar interactions between the ligand head group and the protein play no part in the binding process, a result consistent with the nmr results for native HDL cited earlier, which show no immobilization of choline head groups of bound phospholipid.

Table 3 shows the maximal amount of ligand that can be bound to apoA-I in the cooperative mode. When the hydrophobic moiety of the ligand consists of pure hydrocarbon, fewer molecules of ligand can be bound as the size of the hydrophobic moiety increases, suggesting that the binding site is designed to accommodate a fixed volume of hydrocarbon, about 24,000 cm^3 per mol of polypeptide chain. This result is quite different from what has been observed with membrane proteins. While there are far too few studies of membrane proteins to permit a conclusive generalization, the few results obtained suggest that membrane proteins have a tendency to bind simple amphiphiles (without much specificity) as whole micelles. Since micelle size increases with increase in the size of the hydrophobic moiety, the maximal molar ratio would increase rather than decrease with increasing alkyl chain length. (Data for membrane proteins addressed directly to the effect of alkyl chain length are however not available).

A graphic visualization of the difference between binding to apoA-I and binding to membrane proteins is shown by the gel exclusion chromatography experiments in Fig. 2. The ligand for apoA-I is palmitoyl lysophosphatidylcholine, which, under the conditions of the experiment, forms large aggregated micelles emerging in the void volume of the column, whereas the apoprotein alone runs as a small particle with a Stokes radius (R_s) of 28 Å. When excess lysolipid is added to the protein, it is seen that a protein-lipid complex is formed which is larger than the lipid-

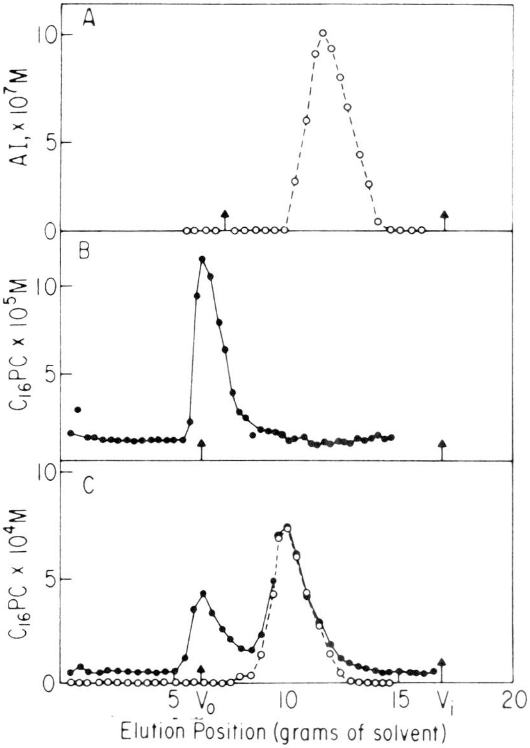

Fig. 2. Gel filtration chromatography on Sepharose 6B of apoA-I alone (A), palmitoyl lysophosphatidylcholine alone (B), and a mixture of the two (C). Open and filled circles represent analysis for protein and phospholipid, respectively, and arrows indicate void and total volume markers. From Haberland and Reynolds (1975).

free apoprotein (R_s = 35 Å), but much smaller than the pure micelle. Excess ligand appears in the void volume as before. Similar experiments done for at least one membrane protein (cytochrome b_5) show that the protein-ligand complex is always of the same size as or slightly larger than protein-free micelles (Robinson and Tanford, 1975).

Binding of Diacyl Phospholipids to ApoA-I

One quantitative binding study has been carried out using a diacyl phospholipid, di-decanoyl phosphatidylcholine (Reynolds et al., 1977). Apart from having shorter alkyl chains, this lipid is representative of the major class of endogeneous phospholipids in HDL. The maximal amount bound (Table 3) was found to be consistent with the fixed volume binding region found for simpler amphiphiles, and binding was accompanied by similar conformational changes. The actual binding isotherm (Fig. 3) was however found to be quite remarkable in that binding occurs at a free lipid concentration about 200-fold larger than the critical micelle concentration of the lipid (which in this case forms very large micellar aggregates), and is at the same time highly cooperative. This is a thermodynamically impossible result if the data represent what they are purported to represent. Binding of a micelle-forming ligand can be cooperative only below or near the critical micelle

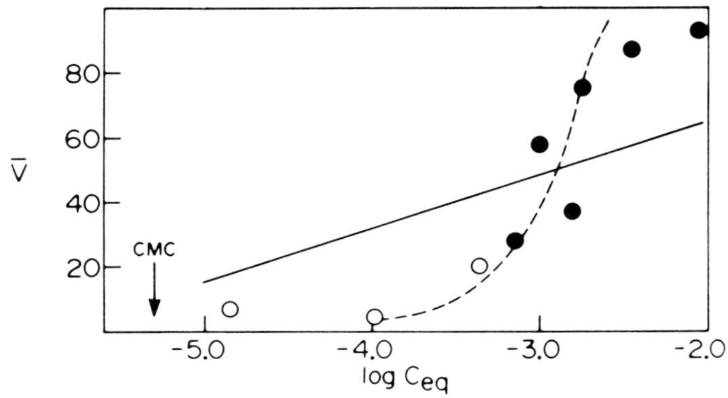

Fig.3. Binding isotherm for binding of di-decanoyl phosphatidylcholine to apoA-I, showing mols bound ($\bar{\nu}$) as a function of the unbound lipid concentration (C_{eq}). Open and filled circles indicate when the protein was found by parallel molecular weight measurements to be in the monomeric or dimeric state, respectively. The arrow indicates the critical micelle concentration of the lipid under the experimental conditions employed. The solid line is the theoretical binding isotherm for the reaction $2P + 190L \rightleftharpoons P_2L_{190}$, where P represents A-I and L represents the lipid. The dashed line is for the successive equilibria $P + 4Y \rightleftharpoons PY_4$, $2PY_4 + 190L \rightleftharpoons P_2Y_8L_{190}$, where Y represents either decanoate or decanoyl lysophosphatidylcholine, and 0.35% hydrolysis of the diacyl lipid to produce these molecules was assumed to have occurred. From Reynolds et al. (1977).

concentration of the ligand, when most of the added ligand is in monomeric form. If binding does not occur until the free ligand concentration is much above the critical micelle concentration, virtually all of the ligand being added is already in aggregated form (in this case at a higher state of aggregation than in the complex with protein),so that there cannot be an increase in the state of the aggregation of the ligand upon binding and the equilibrium isotherm cannot be cooperative, no matter what the mechanism by which the protein complex is formed.

The simplest explanation for this apparently impossible result is that there is a contaminant in the lipid being added, which enters into the reaction. The reason for the reaction requiring a concentration of diacyl lipid so much above the critical micelle concentration would then be that this is the concentration required to obtain a sufficiently high concentration of the contaminant. The most likely contaminants in aqueous solutions of diacyl phospholipids are low levels of lysolipid and fatty acid, arising from hydrolysis. There is moreover a plausible mechanism whereby a contaminant of this kind can enter into the reaction: we have seen that cooperative binding of simple single chain amphiphiles such as fatty acids or lysolipids is always triggered by noncooperative binding of 3 or 4 ligand molecules to sites designed to be occupied by single molecules. This binding process induces a conformational change, and cooperative binding occurs only after the conformational change has taken place. The data suggested also that binding of any one ligand with a single hydrocarbon chain to the discrete sites made it possible to bind any other ligand in the cooperative mode. If the discrete sites are in fact limited to single-chain ligands, so that diacyl phospholipids do not have sufficient affinity for binding (relative to the affinity for self-association in formation of pure micellar aggregates), then binding of simple single-chain amphiphiles would be an obligatory prerequisite for cooperative association with diacyl lipid. Assumption of a mechanism of this kind showed that as little as 0.35% hydrolysis of didecanoyl phosphatidylcholine in the experiments described by Fig. 3 would be enough to account quantitatively for the observed data. Actual addition of lysolecithin (10 mols palmitoyl lysophophatidylcholine per mol A-I) indicated that the binding isotherm of Fig. 3 was indeed moved to much lower concentrations of the diacyl lipid.

That apoA-I does not by itself bind significant amounts of diacyl phospholipids has been observed before (Assmann and Brewer, 1974), as has enhancement of the binding by lysolecithin (Verdery and Nichols, 1974; Nichols et al., 1974). In other previous investigations where direct association between apoA-I and diacyl phospholipids was observed, lysolipids or fatty acids must have been present in relatively large amounts; this is especially likely if the studies involved cosonication of the protein with the lipid.

Fig. 3 also shows the data for the spontaneous dimerization of A-I as the diacyl phospholipid is bound. Since both diacyl and monoacyl molecules appear to utilize the same binding region, and the volume of bound hydrocarbon is about the same for both (Table 3), the factor responsible for dimerization when diacyl phospholipids are bound may be the much greater separation between head groups for the same volume of hydrocarbon, i.e., the same factor that causes diacyl phospholipids alone to form extended bilayers instead of small soluble micelles (Tanford, 1973).

Other apoproteins. Many laboratories have shown that apoA-II and apoC proteins (singly and together) combine with phospholipid, sometimes specifically with phospholipid in bilayer form. The experiments usually involved cosonication of lipid and protein at high concentration, so that some lipid hydrolysis probably occurred. In no case was the binding studied as a function of progressively increasing lipid concentration (as in Fig. 3), so as to permit thermodynamic analysis. In one study, however, the combination of apoC-III with dimyristoyl phosphatidylcholine was shown to lead to disruption of the phospholipid bilayer and repackaging of the lipid to form particles smaller than vesicles (Novosad et al., 1976).

Amphipathic helics. A statistical survey of most known amino acid sequences has shown that lipoprotein polypeptides contain sequence segments that are capable of forming α-helical structures in which one face is hydrophobic while the opposite face is charged. Moreover, the charged faces so formed would contain positive and negative charges in about equal number in separate positive and negative strips (Segrest et al., 1974). Similar sequence segments occur in other proteins as well, but at a much lower frequency than in the lipoprotein polypeptide.

It has been pointed out that these hypothetical "amphipathic" helical regions would be ideally designed for interaction with zwitterionic phospholipids (90% of phospholipid head groups in plasma lipoproteins are in this category), and they would appear especially well adapted to associate with phospholipid in bilayer form. In fact, however, most of the phospholipid in plasma lipoproteins (at least in HDL and LDL) is not in bilayer form, and, as noted earlier, none of the polypeptides are ever found associated with bilayer membranes. Moreover, the hydrophobic binding area of the A-I polypeptide appears to bind simple amphiphiles with charged or uncharged head groups to the same extent as it binds phospholipids (Table 3) and nmr measurements show no perturbation of phospholipid head groups in native HDL. The functional significance of amphipathic helics (if, indeed, they are formed as postulated) is therefore at present obscure.

DISCUSSION

The binding studies and other data presented in this paper and elsewhere lead to the following suggested sequence of events in the assembly of the high density lipoproteins.

1. The nascent A-I polypeptide chain, synthesized in the liver, must combine with a small number of molecules of fatty acid or lysolipid before any further reaction can take place. In seeking a functional reason for this, it is tempting to speculate that location of fatty acid or lysolipid at unique positions in the protein is related to the fact that HDL uniquely serves as substrate for the enzyme lecithin-cholesterol acyltransferase, but there is no direct evidence to suggest this. Native HDL contains lysophosphatidylcholine, but so do the lipoproteins unable to serve as substrates for the enzyme (Skipski et al., 1967).

2. Combination with fatty acid or lysolipid induces a conformational change which permits the cooperative binding of larger amounts of hydrophobic ligand, and in particular the binding of diacyl phospholipids. The binding area of the protein is designed to accept a fixed volume of hydrocarbon. This gives an indication of what is likely to be the characteristic difference between proteins destined to be intrinsic membrane proteins and those destined to form soluble lipoprotein complexes. The former are designed to comicellize with micellar aggregates of any amphiphile in such a way as to cause minimal perturbation of the micellar aggregate. The lipoproteins on the other hand package lipids in an amount and manner of organization dictated by the protein.

3. Formation of the $(A\text{-}I)_2(A\text{-}II)_2$ core protein takes place only after cooperative binding of diacyl lipids has taken place. Experimental evidence for this so far exists only for the dimerization of A-I.

4. It is known that the neutral lipids (mostly cholesteryl esters in the case of HDL) do not combine with the protein until after diacyl phospholipids are bound (Sodhi and Gould, 1967; Scanu, 1972). The conformational adaptability of A-I and A-II is likely to be an important factor here, permitting association with variable amounts of neutral lipid, in contrast to the fixed amount of phospholipid that has to be associated with at least A-I.

5. Data on lipid binding of C-peptides is only qualitative at present, but they can certainly bind lipids independently. Whether C-peptides are transferred between VLDL and HDL with or without associated lipid cannot at present be decided.

There are no comparable data on the assembly of VLDL and LDL. It can however be stated with reasonable confidence that VLDL and LDL molecules each contain one copy of the same core protein, consisting of two non-covalently linked B-peptides, and the data suggest that the formation of this core protein is not dependent on the presence of lipid. It should be noted (Table 2) that the B_2 core protein has the remarkable property of being able to pull togther into a single lipoprotein particle as much as 50 times its own weight of lipid and small polypeptides. There are as yet no physical chemical data on which to base even a speculative model for how this is achieved.

Acknowledgment

The experimental work described in this paper has been supported in part by grant HL 14882, from the National Institutes of Health, U.S. Public Health Service.

REFERENCES

Alaupovic, P.D., D.M. Lee and W.J. McConathy (1972). Biochim. Biophys. Acta 260, 689.
Assmann, G., and H.B. Brewer (1974). Proc. Nat. Acad. Sci. U.S.A. 71, 989.
Assmann, G., E.A. Sokolski and H.B. Brewer, Jr.(1974). Proc. Nat. Acad. Sci. U.S.A. 71, 549.
Atkinson, D., R.J. Deckelbaum, D.M. Small and G.G. Shipley (1977). Proc. Nat. Acad. Sci. U.S.A. 74, 1042.
Baker, H.N., T. Delahunty, A.M. Gotto, Jr., and R.L. Jackson (1974). Proc. Nat. Acad. Sci. U.S.A. 71, 3631.
Brewer, H.B. Jr., S.E. Lux, R. Ronan and K.M. John (1972). Proc. Nat. Acad. Sci. U.S.A. 69, 1304.
Brewer, H.B. Jr., R. Shulman, P. Herbert, R. Ronan and K. Wehrly (1974). J. Biol. Chem. 249, 4975.
Brewer, H.B. Jr., T. Fairwell, A. LaRue, R. Ronan, A. Houser and T.J. Bronzert (1978). Biochem. Biophys. Res. Comm. 80, 623.
Brown, W.V., R.I. Levy and D.S. Fredrickson (1970). J. Biol. Chem. 245, 6588.
Deckelbaum, R.J., G.G. Shipley and D.M. Small (1977a). J. Biol. Chem. 252, 744.
Deckelbaum, R.J., A.R. Tall and D.M. Small (1977b). J. Lipid Res. 18, 164.
Fisher, W.R., M.G. Hammond, M.C. Mengel and G. Warmke (1975). Proc. Nat. Acad. Sci. U.S.A. 72, 2347.
Fleming, P.J., H.A. Dailey, D. Corcoran and P. Strittmatter (1978). J. Biol. Chem. 253, 5369.
Friedberg, S.J., and J.A. Reynolds (1976). J. Biol. Chem. 251, 4005.
Glomset, J.A. (1968). J. Lipid Res. 9, 155.
Gwynne, J., J.B. Brewer, Jr., and H. Edelhoch (1975). J. Biol. Chem. 250, 2269.
Haberland, M.E., and J.A. Reynolds (1975). J. Biol. Chem. 250, 6636.
Henderson, T.O., A.W. Kruski, L.G. Davis, T. Glonek and A.M. Scanu (1975). Biochemistry 14, 1915.
Hirz, R., and A.M. Scanu (1970). Biochim. Biophys. Acta 207, 364.
Ikai, A. (1976). J. Biochem. 79, 679.
Ikai, A., and H. Yagisawa (1977). J. Biochem. 81, 955.
Jackson, R.L., J.T. Sparrow, H.N. Baker, J.D. Morrisett, O.D. Taunton, and A.M. Gotto, Jr. (1974). J. Biol. Chem. 249, 5308.
Jackson, R.L., J.D. Morrisett, and A.M. Gotto, Jr. (1976). Physiol. Revs. 56, 259.
Jackson, R.L., H.N. Baker, E.B. Gilliam, and A.M. Gotto, Jr. (1977). Proc. Nat. Acad. Sci. U.S.A. 74, 1942.
Kane, J.P., T. Sata, R.L. Hamilton and R.J. Havel (1975). J. Clin. Invest. 56, 1622.
Kostner, G., and P. Alaupovic (1972). Biochemistry 11, 3419.
Lee, D., (1976). Low Density Lipoproteins (C.E. Day and R.S. Levy, eds.), Plenum Press, New York, p.3.
Lewis, B. (1977). Biochem. Soc. Trans. 5, 589.
Lux, S.E., R. Hirz, R.I. Shrager and A.M. Gotto (1972). J. Biol. Chem. 247, 2598.
Makino, S., C. Tanford and J.A. Reynolds (1974). J. Biol. Chem. 249, 7379.
Mateu, L., A. Tardieu, V. Luzzati, L. Aggerbeck and A.M. Scanu (1972). J. Mol. Biol. 70, 105.
McConathy, W.J., and P. Alaupovic (1976). Biochemistry 15, 515.
Müller, K., P. Laggner, O. Glatter and G. Kostner (1978). Eur. J. Biochem. 82, 73.
Nakashima, Y., and W. Konigsberg (1974). J. Mol. Biol. 88, 598.
Nichols, A.V. (1969). Proc. Nat. Acad. Sci. U.S.A. 64, 1128.
Nichols, A.V., T. Forte, E. Gong, P. Blanche and R.B. Verdery (1974). Scand. J. Clin. Lab. Invest. 33, 147.
Novosad, Z., R.D. Knapp, A.M. Gotto, H.J. Pownall and J.D. Morrisett (1976). Biochemistry 15, 3176.
Oncley, J.L., G. Scatchard and A. Brown (1947). J. Phys. and Colloid Chem.51,184.

Oncley, J.L., F.R.N. Gurd and M. Melin (1950). J. Am. Chem. Soc. 72, 458.
Osborne, J.C. Jr., and H.B. Brewer,Jr. (1977). Adv. Protein Chem. 31, 253.
Patsch, W., J.R. Patsch, G.M. Kostner, S. Sailer and H. Braunsteiner (1978). J. Biol. Chem. 253, 4911.
Pattnaik, N.M., F.J. Kezdy and A.M. Scanu (1976). J. Biol. Chem. 251, 1984.
Reynolds, J.A. (1976). J. Biol. Chem. 251, 6013.
Reynolds, J.A., and R.H. Simon (1974). J. Biol. Chem. 249, 3937.
Reynolds, J.A., C. Tanford and W.L. Stone (1977). Proc. Nat. Acad. Sci. U.S.A. 74, 3796.
Robinson, N.C., and C. Tanford (1975). Biochemistry 14, 369.
Scanu, A.M. (1971). Plasma Lipoproteins (R.M.C. Smellie, ed.), Biochem. Soc. Symp. No.33, Academic Press, New York, p. 29.
Scanu, A.M. (1972). Biochim. Biophys. Acta 265, 471.
Scanu, A.M., W. Reader and C. Edelstein (1968). Biochim. Biophys. Acta 160, 32.
Scanu, A.M., C. Edelstein and P. Klein (1975). The Plasma Proteins (F.W. Putnam, ed.), 2nd. ed., vol. 1, Academic Press, New York, ch. 7.
Schumaker, V.N. (1973). Acc. Chem. Res.6, 398.
Sears, B., R.J. Deckelbaum, M.J.Janiak, G.G. Shipley and D.M. Small (1976). Biochemistry 15, 4151.
Segrest, J.P., R.L. Jackson, J.D. Morrisett and A.M. Gotto, Jr. (1974). FEBS Lett. 38, 247.
Shelburne, F.A., and S.H. Quarfordt (1974). J. Biol. Chem. 249, 1428.
Shen, B.W., A.M. Scanu and F.J. Kezdy (1977). Proc. Nat. Acad. Sci. U.S.A. 74, 837.
Shepherd, J., A.M. Gotto, Jr., O.D. Taunton, M.J. Carslake and E. Farish (1977). Biochim. Biophys. Acta 489, 486.
Shulman, R., P. Herbert, K. Wehrly, B. Chesebro, R.I. Levy and D.S. Fredrickson (1972). Circulation 46, II-246.
Skipski, V.P., M. Barclay, R.K. Barclay, V.A. Fetzer, J.J. Good, and F.M. Archibald (1967). Biochem. J. 104, 340.
Smith, R., J.R. Dawson and C. Tanford (1972). J. Biol. Chem. 247, 3376.
Sodhi, H.S., and R.G. Gould (1967). J. Biol. Chem. 242, 1205.
Steele, J.C.H., Jr., and J.A. Reynolds (1979). J. Biol. Chem. in press.
Stone, W.L., and J.A. Reynolds (1975a). J. Biol. Chem. 250, 3584.
Stone, W.L., and J.A. Reynolds (1975b). J. Biol. Chem. 250, 8045.
Tall, A.R., G.G. Shipley and D.M. Small (1976). J. Biol. Chem. 251, 3749.
Tanford, C. (1962). J. Amer. Chem. Soc. 84, 4260.
Tanford, C. (1973). The Hydrophobic Effect, John Wiley, New York.
Tanford, C., and J.A. Reynolds (1976). Biochim. Biophys. Acta 457, 133.
Tardieu, A., L. Mateu, C. Sardet, B. Weiss, V. Luzzati, L. Aggerbeck and A.M. Scanu (1976). J. Mol. Biol. 101, 129.
Tomita, M., and V.T. Marchesi (1975). Proc. Nat. Acad. Sci. U.S.A. 72, 2964.
Triplett, R.B., and W.R. Fisher (1978). J. Lipid Res. 19, 478.
Triplett, R.B., G.L. Warmke and W.R. Fisher (1975). Fed. Proc. 34, 499.
Verdery, R.B., and A.V. Nichols (1974). Biochem. Biophys. Res. Commun. 57, 1271.
Yeagle, P.L., R.G. Langdon and R.B. Martin (1977). Biochemistry 16, 3487.
Yeagle, P.L., R.B. Martin, L. Pottenger and R.G. Langdon (1978). Biochemistry 17, 2707.

MECHANISMS OF LIPID TRANSPORT BY THE HUMAN PLASMA PROTEINS

Henry J. Pownall and Antonio M. Gotto, Jr.
Department of Medicine, Baylor College of Medicine
and The Methodist Hospital, 6516 Bertner Boulevard
Houston, Texas, U.S.A.

INTRODUCTION

In 1929 Macheboeuf reported that acidifying the supernatent from horse serum containing ammonium sulfate at 50% saturation gave a precipitate containing protein and cholesterol in the form of its fatty acid esters (1). He referred to this globulin fraction as C.A. (cenapses precipitated by acid) although we now know that he had isolated high density lipoproteins (HDL). With the development of electrophoretic techniques, Macheboeuf later showed that C.A. was an α-globulin (2). In 1947 Pedersen (3) showed that α- and β-globulin lipid-containing fractions could be separated on the basis of their different densities by high speed centrifugation. He found a floating fraction which he called X-protein and which is now known as the β-lipoproteins or low density lipoproteins (LDL). Shortly thereafter, Cohn and co-workers developed procedures for the large scale fractionation of human plasma using mixtures of ethanol and water (4). With these procedures serum lipids could be precipitated and separated into two fractions having α- and β-mobility. The fractions also differed in size, density and lipid composition.

Refinements in electrophoretic and ultracentrifugal techniques in the 1950's led to increased activity and discovery in lipoprotein research. Gofman and his associates at the Donner Laboratory of the University of California at Berkeley described a method using analytical ultracentrifugation which separated the plasma lipoproteins (5). These studies established the notion that serum lipoproteins appear in a specific density range and not at a single discrete density. They further proposed that an elevation of these substances in plasma predisposed the subject to coronary artery disease (6). In 1955, Havel et al. (7) developed preparative ultracentrifugal methods for the stepwise flotation of three different lipoprotein fractions through a buffer adjusted to increasing density with salt. At about the same time Dangerfield and Smith (8) showed that lipoproteins could be separated by paper electrophoresis. Following the discovery and partial characterization of the human plasma lipoproteins, workers attempted to identify specific metabolic roles for each lipoprotein class and searched for physiologic relationships between the different lipoprotein classes. Shore found similar but not identical protein constituents in LDL and HDL (9). Gitlin and Cornwall (10) demonstrated that LDL were derived from the very low density lipoproteins (VLDL) via the removal of triglycerides. It had been shown in the early 1940's that alimentary lipemia could be cleared by the intravenous administration of heparin (11). In 1955, Korn (12) isolated lipolytic activity from heart and adipose tissue; the activity was called lipoprotein lipase since its properties resembled those of the plasma clearing factor described by Hahn (11).

Subsequent clinical and epidemiological studies have supported the proposed connection between elevated lipid levels and coronary artery disease. With the accumulation of more information on lipoprotein structure and metabolism came the recognition of different forms of disorders of plasma lipid transport. Using the new electrophoretic methodology, Fredrickson and his colleagues (13) performed a comprehensive study which defined lipoprotein phenotypes. Initially five and later a sixth phenotype were defined. Phenotypes were found to be secondary to other diseases in some instances. Table 1 contains some clinical disorders associated with each of these phenotypes.

In addition to lipid transport disorders associated with hyperlipidemia several mutants have been described in which there may be a deficiency or absence of cer-

Table 1 Types of Hyperlipoproteinemias[1]

Phenotype		Plasma Lipids		Plasma Lipoprotein Fractions				Appearance of Plasma
Type	Definition	Ch[2]	Tg[2]	Chylomicrons	VLDL	LDL	HDL	
I	Hyperchylomicronemia, with absolute deficiency of LPL[2] or PHLA[2]	N[2] or ↑	↑↑	+	Mildly ↑, N, or ↓	N or ↓	0	"Cream" layer over a clear infranatant
IIa	Increased LDL	↑	N	0	N or ↓	↑	N	Clear
IIb	Increased LDL & increased VLDL	↑	↑	0	↑	↑	N	Clear or faintly turbid
III	Floating β-lipoproteins	↑	↑	+, may be ↑	↑	LDL_1, ↑; LDL_2, ↓	N or ↓	Usually turbid; may also be faint "cream" layer
IV	Increased VLDL	N or ↑	↑	0	↑	↓ or N	N or ↓	Usually turbid
V	Hyperchylomicronemia & increased VLDL, with LPL or PHLA present but reduced	N or ↑	↑↑	↑	↑	↓ or N	Usually ↓	"Cream layer"

[1]Adapted from Gotto (14).
[2]Abbreviations: Ch, cholesterol; Tg, triglyceride; N, normal; LPL, lipoprotein lipase; PHLA, post-heparin lipolytic activity

tain lipoproteins. These and some of their associated characteristics are given in Table 2.

Table 2 Types of Hypolipoproteinemias[1]

Disease	Major Clinical Findings	Laboratory Findings						
		Plasma Lipids mg/100 ml			Plasma Lipoprotein Fractions			
		Ch[2]	Tg[2]	Ph[2]	Chylomicrons	VLDL	LDL	HDL
Abetalipoproteinemia	Malabsorption of fat; acanthocytosis; retinitis pigmentosa; ataxic neuropathy	Low (35-54)	Low, <20	Low, <100	Absent	Absent	Absent	Present
Hypobetalipoproteinemia[3]	Generally asymptomatic	Low (55-164)	Low or N[2] (20-140)	Low or N (110-170)	N	Moderately reduced	Low: 1/8 - 1/10 of N	N
Tangier disease[4]	Cholesterol deposits in other tissues (reticular endothelial system); abnormal tonsils; splenomegaly; peripheral neuropathy	Low (30-125)	High (rarely N), (150-330)	Low (70-140)	N	Abnormal β-migrating VLDL	N or ↑	Very low & abnormal (HDL_T)

[1]Adapted from A.M. Gotto (15).
[2]Abbreviations: Ch, cholesterol; Tg, triglyceride; Ph, phospholipid; N, normal.
[3]Familial low density lipoprotein deficiency.
[4]Familial high density lipoprotein deficiency.

In abetalipoproteinemia (16), chylomicrons, VLDL and LDL are absent. The absence of these lipoproteins results in fat malabsorption, neuromuscular dysfunction and retinitis pigmentosa. In its less severe form, hypobetalipoproteinemia, clinical symptoms do not present and the levels of LDL are severely reduced (17). Tangier disease, discovered in a kindred of subjects by Fredrickson et al. (18), is characterized by the virtual absence of HDL. A characteristic of this disease is the localization of cholesteryl esters in other tissues (reticuloendothelial system) and peripheral neuropathy.

There are other disorders outside of the phenotypic descriptions in Tables 1 and 2.

In one of these, familial lecithin:cholesterol acyltransferase (LCAT) deficiency (19), plasma cholesteryl esters are virtually absent; anemia, renal insufficiency and ocular abnormalities present and plasma HDL levels are very low. A second disorder, obstructive liver disease (20), results in the formation of an abnormal lipoprotein called lipoprotein-X (LP-X). Patsch et al. (21) have identified three subfractions of LP-X and characterized their physical and chemical properties.

LIPOPROTEIN COMPOSITION, STRUCTURE AND METABOLISM

The individual protein components of lipoproteins were first referred to as apoproteins by Oncley (22). It is now known that HDL, LDL, and VLDL contain various amounts of several proteins; Table 3 lists the protein components of each density.

Table 3 Composition of Human Plasma Lipoproteins

Properties	Chylomicrons	VLDL	LDL	HDL
Density	< 0.95	0.95-1.006	1.006-1.063	1.063-1.210
Major apoproteins	ApoA-I ApoB[1] ApoC	ApoB ApoC-I ApoC-II ApoC-III ApoE	ApoB	ApoA-I ApoA-II
Minor apoproteins	ApoA-II ApoE[2] PRP[3]	ApoA-I ApoA-II ApoD[4]	ApoC	ApoC-I ApoC-II ApoC-III ApoD ApoE

[1]Also termed apoLDL.
[2]Also termed arginine-rich protein.
[3]Proline-rich protein.
[4]Also termed thin-line protein and apoA-III.

This table shows that there are some common apoproteins in each lipoprotein class. This fact originates from the metabolic relationships between different lipoproteins; lipoprotein composition and structure can be modified by plasma enzymes (23). As a consequence of the enzyme action the stability of the lipoprotein is altered to the point where some of its components may be transferred to another lipoprotein. Figure 1 contains a hypothetical scheme for some of these processes. Both HDL and VLDL derive, in part, from the liver, the former as a nascent disc-like structure and the latter as a triglyceride-rich particle. Nascent HDL contains apoE (24,25) which may be transferred to the VLDL as LCAT action converts the nascent particle to a spherical lipoprotein. Lipoprotein lipase (LPL) hydrolyzes VLDL-triglyceride, a process which is activated by a VLDL apoprotein, apolipoprotein C-II (apoC-II) (26). During lipolysis some of the surface components of VLDL, phospholipid and all of the apoC proteins, are transferred to the HDL (27). The remaining components, largely cholesteryl ester, apoB, phospholipids, and small amounts of triglyceride constitute LDL.

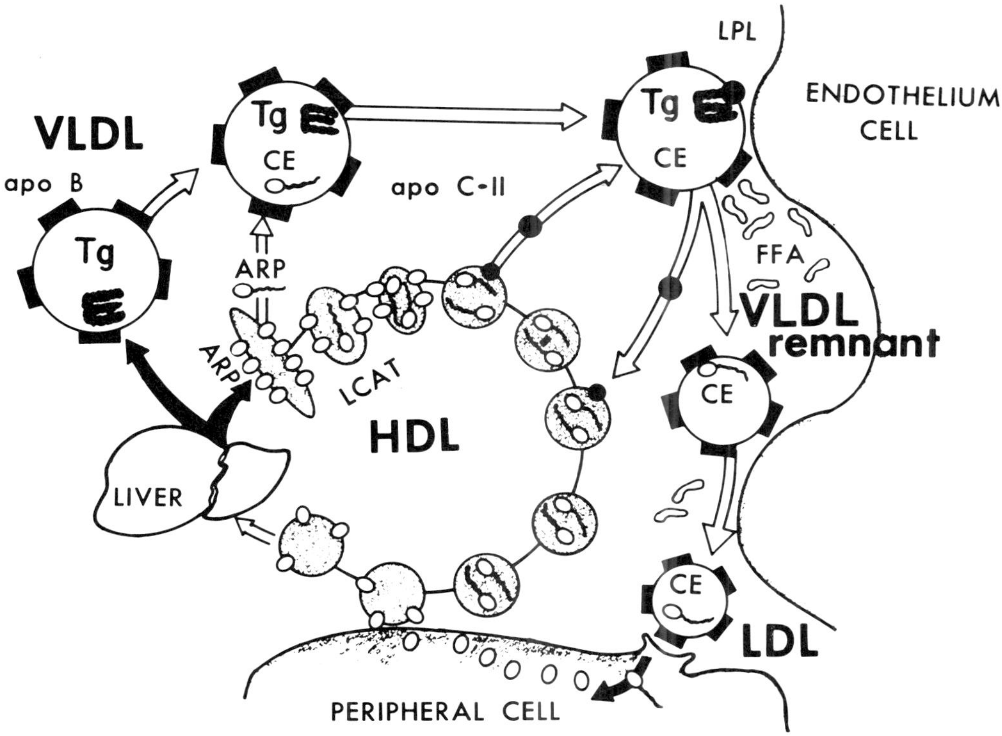

Fig. 1. Hypothetical scheme for the metabolic relationships among the human plasma lipoproteins.* (Permission granted by Baylor College of Medicine.)

Various models of lipoprotein structure have been proposed and sufficient evidence has accumulated suggesting that all lipoproteins may be viewed as a sphere having an apolar core and a surface containing the polar components (28). In the VLDL, the core is composed of about 70% triglyceride and 30% cholesteryl ester. The surface of VLDL contains apoB, the apoC proteins, cholesterol and phospholipids. Hydrolysis of VLDL-triglycerides and loss of apoC proteins by VLDL forms LDL. The core of LDL is largely cholesteryl esters and the surface contains phospholipid, cholesterol and apoB. Small and co-workers (29) found that the cholesteryl esters of LDL undergo a transition from an ordered smectic phase to an isotropic liquid at a temperature which is inversely related to the triglyceride content. This observation demonstrated that the cholesteryl esters exist in a separate phase which is believed to be in the core. HDL contains nearly equal amounts of lipid and protein and has been subfractionated into HDL_2 and HDL_3 which are distinguished on the basis of the higher molecular weight, lower density and lower protein content of the former. Figure 2 contains a schematic representation of the structure of HDL_2. The surface contains apoproteins, phospholipids, and cholesterol which surround a small apolar core of cholesteryl esters and triglycerides.

*Designed by J.R. Patsch, 1978.

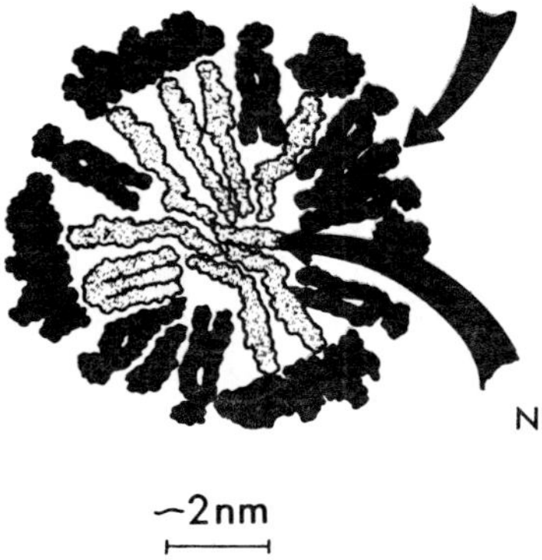

Fig. 2. The structure of HDL_2 obtained from space-filling models (adapted from Verdery and Nichols (30)). The surface contains the polar components, protein, phospholipid and cholesterol whereas the core contains the neutral lipids, mostly cholesteryl ester. (Permission granted by Baylor College of Medicine.)

CORRELATION OF THE STRUCTURE AND FUNCTION OF APOLIPOPROTEINS

The primary structures of apoA-I, apoA-II, apoC-I, apoC-II and apoC-III are known. This information, in conjunction with peptide synthesis and physical and chemical techniques, has been useful in identifying structure-function correlations in the plasma lipoproteins as well as in developing a model for a lipid-binding protein.

Sparrow and co-workers have synthesized a series of peptides which have been used to localize those respective regions of an apoprotein which are involved in lipid-binding and enzyme activation. This technique has been applied to several peptides but herein we shall focus on the studies of apoC-II and apoC-III since there is an abundance of physico-chemical information available concerning these two apoC proteins. The sequences of the apoC-II fragments synthesized by Sparrow and colleagues were based on the total sequence determination of Jackson et al. (31). The sequence and the synthetic fragments of apoC-II depicted in Fig. 3 were investigated as activators of LPL (32) and for their affinity for phosphatidylcholine (33). The results of these studies are summarized in Table 4. These data show little biological activity in fragments corresponding to residues 60-78. Fragment [55-78] activated LPL (32) as well as the whole peptide but does not associate with lecithin; thus, this sequence contains the minimum LPL-activating determinant, but a sufficient segment of the lipid-binding determinant is absent. Fragment 43-78 does bind to phospholipid (33) which indicates that at least a portion of the minimum lipid-binding determinant of the apoC-II resides in a part of the molecule that is not involved in LPL activation. This demonstrated, for the first time, that the lipid-binding and LPL activating regions of apoC-II could be assigned to different regions of the peptide.

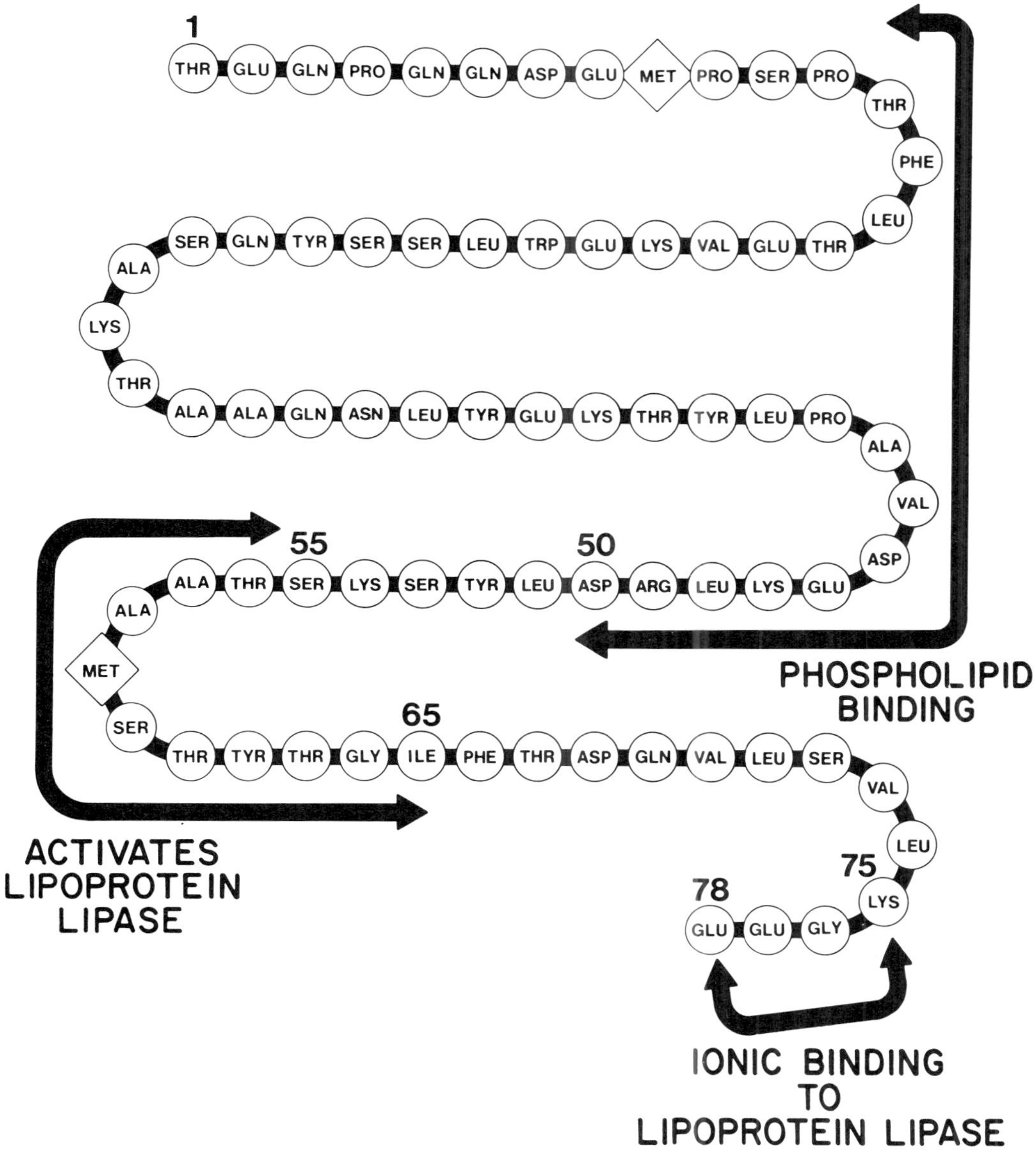

Fig. 3. Assignments of apoC-II functions to various regions of the peptide were based upon the activation of lipase and the lipid-binding studies conducted on synthetic and native fragments. (Permission granted by Baylor College of Medicine.)

Table 4 In Vitro Lipid-Binding and LDL Activation by Fragments of apoC-II

Fragment	LPL Activation	Lipophilicity[1]
1 - 78	++	++
43 - 78	++	++
50 - 78	++	-
55 - 78	+	-
60 - 78	-	-
60 - 78[2]	-	-

[1]Based upon isolation of a lipid-peptide complex by ultracentrifugation in a salt gradient.
[2]Cyanogen bromide fragment.

Studies on the structure and lipid-binding of apoC-III have contributed to our understanding of the physical chemistry of lipid-protein association (34). ApoC-III, the major C-apoprotein of VLDL and HDL, is composed of 79 amino acids whose sequence was determined by Shulman et al. (35). Thrombin cleavage of the protein gives two fragments composed of residues 1-40 ($C\text{-}III_A$) and 41-79 ($C\text{-}III_B$) which have been tested in various lipid-binding assays. The results demonstrated that $C\text{-}III_B$ spontaneously associates with lecithin to give a stable lipid-protein complex. This association occurs with a negative enthalpy and converts the peptide from a random to a helical conformation. A blue-shift in the intrinsic tryptophan fluorescence which accompanied binding suggested that the tryptophan was transferred from a polar to a nonpolar environment. Similar tests of $C\text{-}III_A$ revealed that no lipid-protein complex was formed nor were there any spectroscopic changes suggestive of a lipid-protein association. In Fig. 4 we have plotted some structural and thermodynamic parameters of apoC-III versus its sequence. In the upper portion of the figure we denote for each residue its probability of appearing in a β-pleated sheet or an α-helix (36). In the lower panel we have plotted the hydrophobicity (37) of each residue versus its sequence. Inspection of the structural and hydrophobicity correlations reveals that thrombin cleavage of apoC-III gives two peptides of similar size which are predicted to have very different properties. First, $C\text{-}III_A$ has a higher content of α-helix in solution than $C\text{-}III_B$. Secondly, when the respective hydrophobicity values of the amino acids composing $C\text{-}III_A$ and $C\text{-}III_B$ are summed and averaged, $C\text{-}III_B$ is found to be considerably more hydrophobic. Finally, a hydrophobic 20 residue segment corresponding to residues 41-60 binds to phospholipid while another hydrophobic fragment corresponding to residues 41-56 does not. These results permit us to formulate a number of rules identifying the properties of a good lipid-binding protein. These are:

1. The peptide need not have an α-helical structure in solution but must have the potential to form a helix; i.e., there should be no helix breakers.
2. The peptide must have a certain length which we refer to as the critical amphipathic length; this is approximately 20 residues.
3. Finally, as shown in Fig. 4, the peptide must have a high hydrophobicity and when arranged in a helical structure

(Fig. 5), the hydrophobic residues should appear on one face of the helix which, presumably, would penetrate the lipid matrix. In the 40-72 helical segment of apoC-III there is a distribution of the charged residues into one face of the helix with the hydrophobic residues appearing on the opposite face.

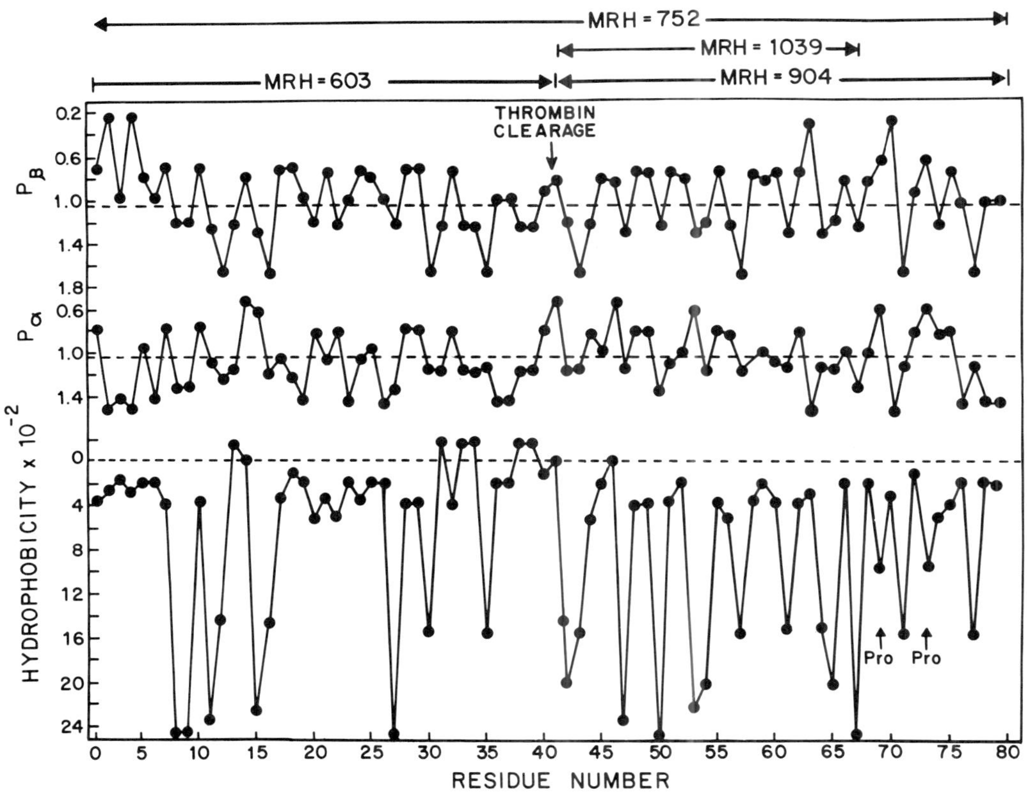

Fig. 4. Correlation of the hydrophobicity of each amino acid residue of apoC-III with its probability of appearing in a β-pleated sheet (P_β) or an α-helix (P_α). The probabilities and hydrophobicities are plotted as a function of the amino acid sequence. Values of P_α and P_β which are greater than those indicated by the dashed lines of the upper and middle panels, respectively, are predicted to exist in α-helical and β-pleated sheets. In the lower panel the hydrophobicity values appearing below the dashed line are predicted to partition into a hydrophobic environment. The lines at the top refer to the fragments discussed in the text and contain their respective hydrophobicities. (Permission granted by Baylor College of Medicine.)

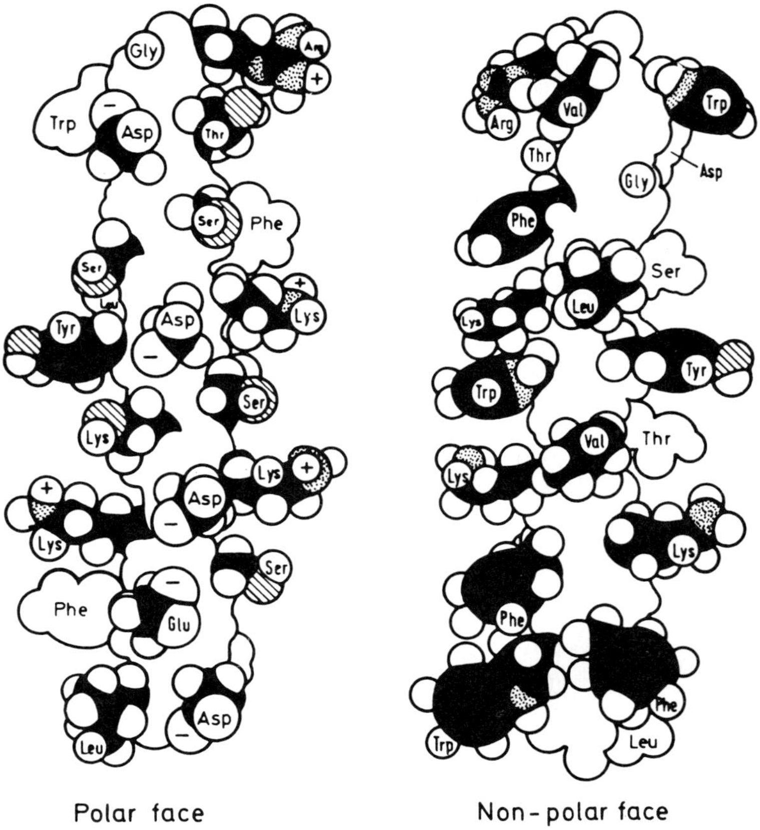

Fig. 5. Space-filling models of a fragment of apoC-III [40-72]. Note that polar and nonpolar amino acid side chains appear on the opposite sides of the helix. (Permission granted (38)).

MECHANISM OF LIPID-PROTEIN ASSOCIATION

The apoproteins of HDL spontaneously associate with phospholipids to give small lipid-protein complexes similar in size to HDL. The effects of temperature and cholesterol content on the rate of association of a model system composed of apoA-I and dimyristoylphosphatidylcholine (DMPC) has been studied in some detail (39). DMPC is a saturated phospholipid which undergoes a transition from an ordered quasi-crystalline phase to a disordered fluid phase at a transition temperature, T_c = 23.7° (40). The temperature dependence of the rate of binding to DMPC liposomes may be followed by measuring the rate of disappearance of liposomal turbidity. Figure 6 shows that the rate of association is very slow above and below T_c but at T_c the rate increases by about two orders of magnitude. The enhanced reactivity at T_c is assigned to the preferential insertion of apoA-I into matrix defects or "holes" at the borders of coexisting ordered and disordered phases. The addition of cholesterol to DMPC increases the number of defects and broadens the range of the order $\rightleftarrows$ disorder transition. Calorimetric studies have shown that cholesterol and DMPC form a separate phase composed of one sterol molecule for every three of DMPC. The maximum number of defects occurring between the 1:3 phase and a pure DMPC phase is predicted to be at that sterol:DMPC ratio where equal amounts of lipid appear in both phases. This corresponds to a sterol content of 12.5 mole %. The rate of association of apoA-I with DMPC is fastest at T_c, independent of sterol content and at 12.5 mole % cholesterol, independent of temperature. Figure 7 depicts a model of a DMPC:cholesterol matrix which would be consistent with the enhanced rate of binding at 12.5 mole % cholesterol. Therein we suggest that apoA-I penetrates a pre-existing hole between a 1:3 sterol:DMPC phase and a pure DMPC phase. It remains to be shown what molecular rearrangements occur after forming this initial lipid-protein complex. Similar though not identical behavior has been observed for apoA-II and the apoC proteins.

ALTERNATIVE MECHANISMS FOR LIPID TRANSPORT: DIFFUSION THROUGH THE AQUEOUS SPACE BETWEEN LIPOPROTEINS

Figure 8 shows the structure of a group of molecules that have been used to measure lipid transport in a number of real and artificial systems. A common feature of these molecules is that they contain pyrene, a fluorophore which is sensitive

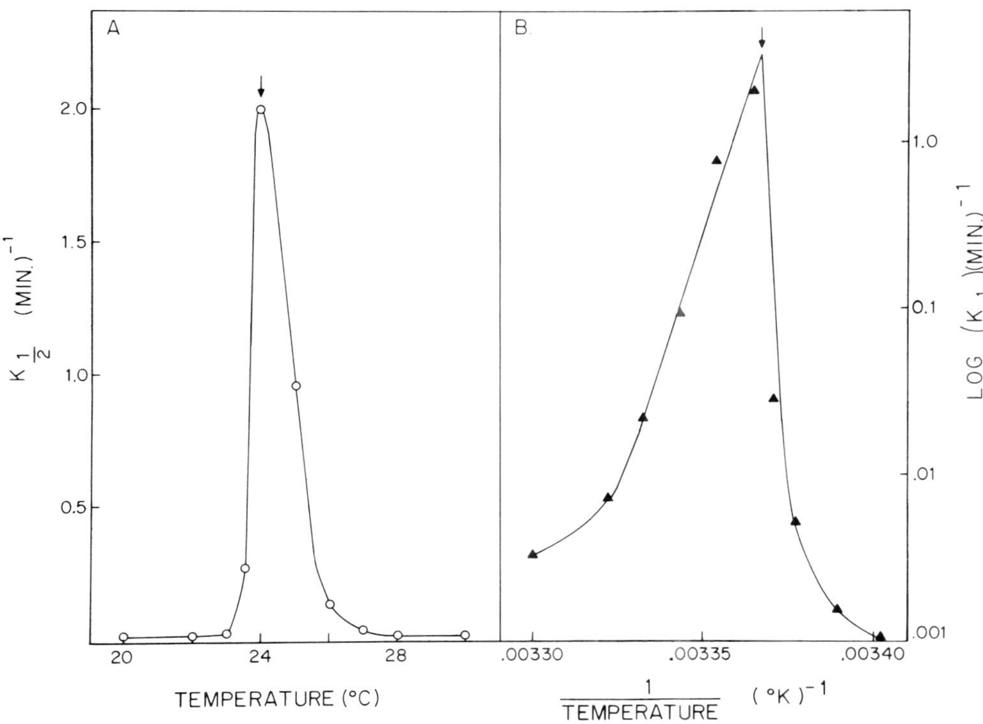

Fig. 6. Temperature dependence of the rate of association of apoA-I with DMPC. Panel A, linear plot; panel B, Arrhenius plot showing maximum at T_C. (Permission granted by Baylor College of Medicine.)

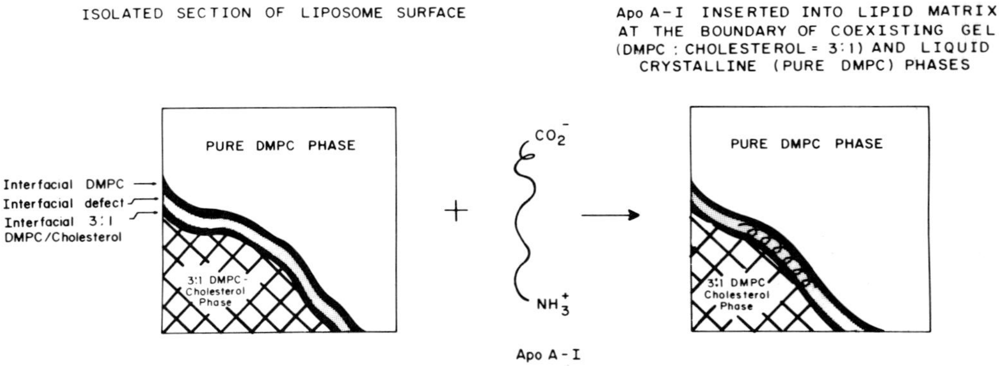

Fig. 7. A hypothetical model for the mechanism by which apoA-I associates with a lipid matrix. On the left is a section of the surface of a liposome in which a DMPC and a 1:3 cholesterol:DMPC phase coexist. Each phase is bounded by interfacial lipid and the interfacial lipid of each phase is separated from that of the other phase by a hole or channel defect. ApoA-I may insert into this defect to give the initial lipid-protein intermediate on the right. We have drawn the lipid matrix as a helical structure since it probably exists as such in HDL and in apoA-I:PC complexes. (Permission granted (50).)

to local order, viscosity and concentration (41,42). A useful property of this fluorophore is that it exhibits excimer fluorescence at ∿475 nm with an intensity that is proportional to its local concentration. Charlton et al. (43) first showed that the rapid (∿4 ms) rate of transfer of pyrene from one HDL to another must occur via the aqueous phase. This result obtained in spite of the relatively low solubility of pyrene in water (0.3 μM). Extension of this technique to lipid analogues covalently bound to pyrene has provided the rates of transfer of the cholesterol, phospholipid and fatty acid analogues of pyrene. These rates are summarized in Table 5. Also indicated in this Table are the critical micelle concentrations or solubilities of some representative lipids from which the pyrene analogues were derived. Although a quantitative relationship has not been derived it is clear that the rates of dissociation or transfer of these lipids decreases with the decrease in their critical micelle concentration. This correlation suggests that the free energy of transfer of lipids to the aqueous phase is an important determinant in the activation energy for this process. It is probable that some of these lipids, particularly the more soluble ones, are transferred between lipid domains via the aqueous phase.

HYDROPHOBICITY AND LIPOPROTEIN STABILITY

The hydrophobic effect has been suggested as an important determinant in the organization of biological membranes (45). Self-association of apolipoproteins and the organization of lipids into micelles, vesicles and liposomes are believed to be driven by the hydrophobic effect. Because many of the individual surface components of lipoproteins, primarily phospholipids, cholesterol and protein, self-associate, it is probable that their stability in the lipoprotein can be predicted from a modification of the theory of mixed micelles, i.e.,

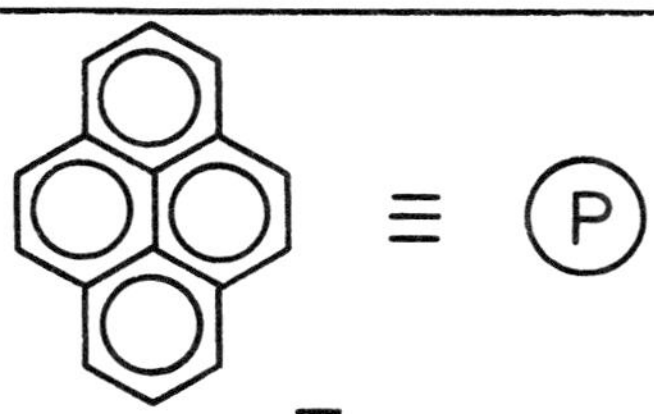

I

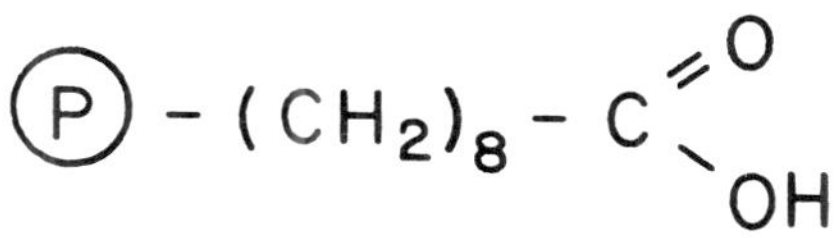

II

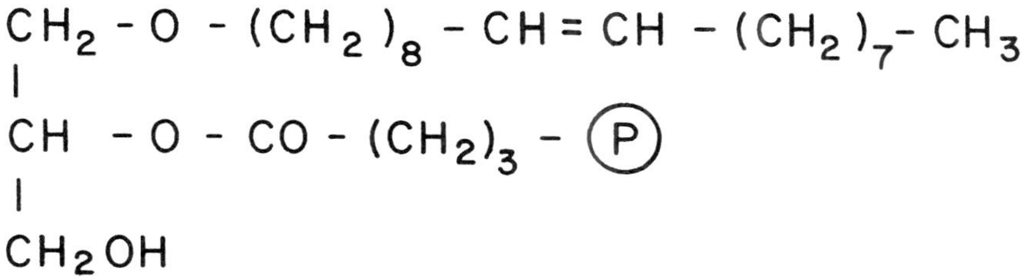

III

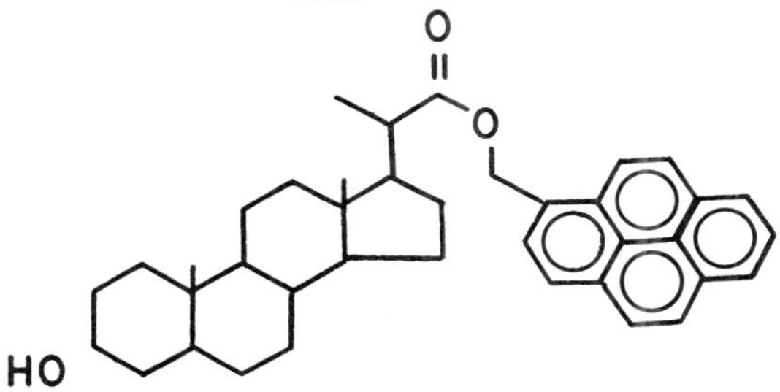

IV

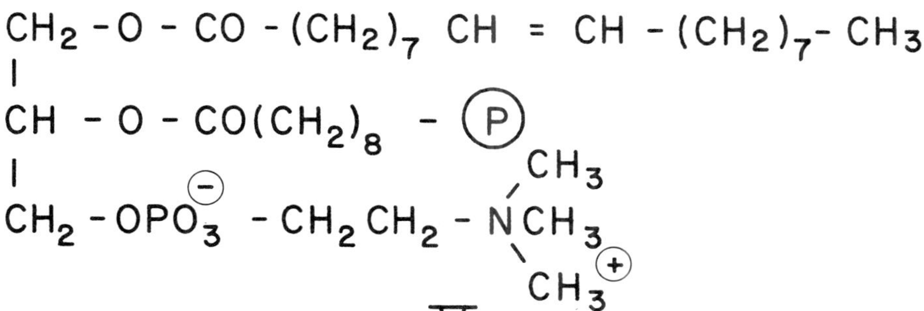

V

Fig. 8. Structure of pyrene and pyrene-containing molecules used to measure the rate of lipid transfer. I, pyrene; II, 9(3-pyrenyl)nonanoic acid; III, 1-oleyl-2-[4-(3-pyrenyl)butanoyl]glycerol (diglyceride analogue); IV, 3' pyrenemethyl-23,24-dinor-5-cholen-20-ate 3β-ol; V, 1-oleoyl-2[9-(3-pyrenyl)]nonanoyl lecithin. (Permission granted, Baylor College of Medicine.)

Table 5 Transfer Rates of Fluorescent Lipid Analogs Among the HDL

Compound[1]	Half-time for transfer between HDL	CMC (solubility)[3]	References
I	4 ms	3×10^{-7} M	42
II	40 ms	$\sim 1 \times 10^{-7}$ M	Unpublished[4]
III	140 ms	2.5×10^{-8} M	43
IV	75 s	3×10^{-9} M	Unpublished[4]
V	∿3 da[2]	5×10^{-10} M	Unpublished[4]

[1]See Fig. 8 for structure.
[2]Measured in DMPC instead of HDL.
[3]See Reference 44.
[4]Unpublished data from L.C. Smith and H.J. Pownall.

$$(1) \quad X_{i,w} = X_{i,LP}\ \mathrm{CMC}$$

where $X_{i,w}$ and $X_{i,LP}$ represent the mole fraction of the component i that is in the aqueous and lipoprotein phase respectively; CMC is the critical monomer or micelle concentration (CMC) of the ith component in the absence of other components. This equation suggests that the concentration of free amphiphile, lipid or protein, will always be less than its CMC. The studies of the transfer of pyrene-labeled lipids demonstrate that finite concentrations of a lipid in the aqueous phase co-exist in dynamic equilibrium with a certain concentration in the lipoprotein phase. The evidence to substantiate a similar equilibria for the distribution of apolipoproteins between the lipoprotein surface and the aqueous phase is less compelling but there is evidence which suggests a similar model. Long-term centrifugation of HDL and apoA-I:DMPC recombinants always results in the sedimentation of some free protein (46). This occurs in spite of the fact that under similar conditions, gel filtration of apoA-I:DMPC complexes reveals the loss of little or no protein (39, 47). These findings can be rationalized if one proposes that an apolipoprotein is in a state of dynamic equilibrium in which the apoA-I distributes between the lipoprotein and aqueous phase. During centrifugation, apoA-I in the aqueous phase will sediment thereby shifting the equilibrium causing more apoA-I to dissociate into the aqueous phase and to sediment to the bottom of the tube. Even more convincing evidence has been obtained from a recent study of HDL dynamics. Figure 9 shows some preliminary data (48) on the behavior of HDL labeled *in vitro* with [^{125}I]-apoA-I and total apoC proteins containing a [^{131}I]-label. Figure 9a shows the Sephacryl S-200 elution profile of HDL labeled with [^{125}I]-apoA-I. A large peak at tube #45 shows coelution of apoA-I and HDL-phosphorus. In addition a second small peak of free apoA-I elutes after HDL. This peak has an apoA-I concentration of ∿0.003 mg/ml, a value similar to that published by Scanu and co-workers (49) for the critical monomer concentration of apoA-I. Thus, it is possible that monomer apoA-I exists in plasma in equilibrium with apoA-I bound to HDL. This finding is not unexpected since apoA-I, unlike the HDL lipids, has a rather high aqueous solubility. In Fig. 9b we show that the addition of apoC proteins to HDL can displace apoA-I and form a new structure enriched in apoC and devoid of most

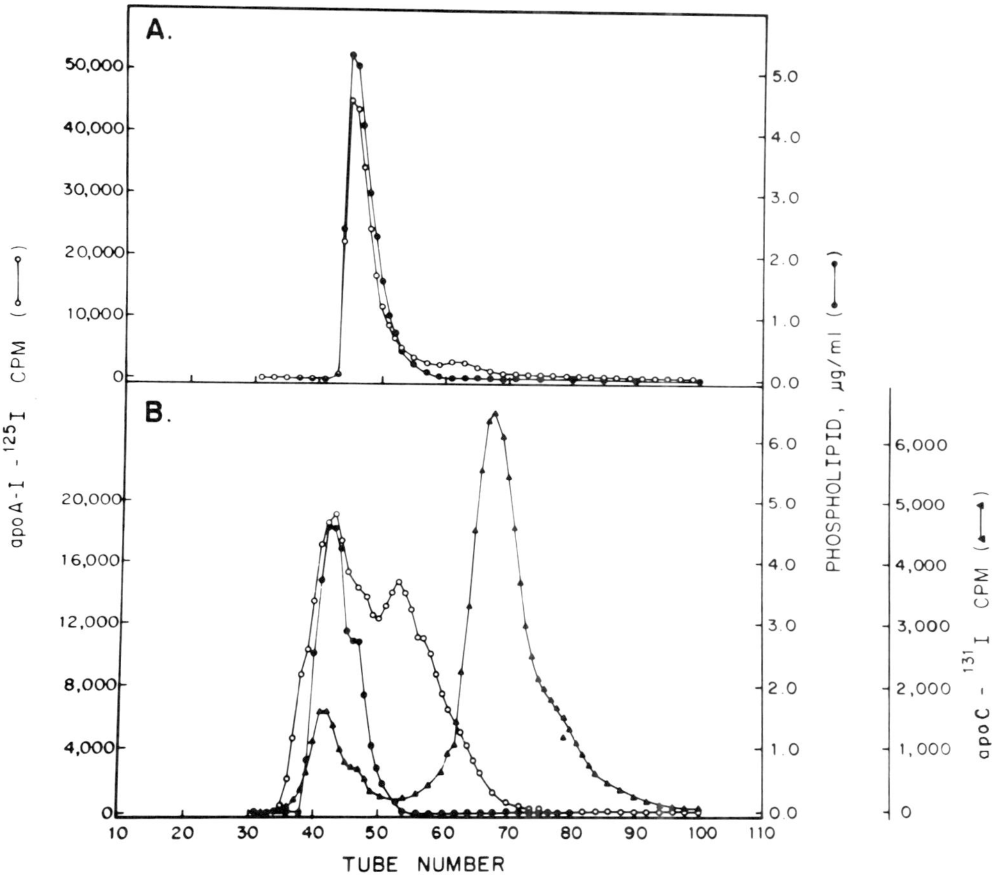

Fig. 9. A. Gel filtration profile of HDL (6.5 mg) phosphorus and [^{125}I]-apoA-I. B. Gel filtration profile of the products formed by the interaction of 6.5 mg HDL (containing [^{125}I]-apoA-I) and 5.5 mg total apoC proteins ([^{131}I]-labeled). The profile of the absorbance at 280 nm was approximately equal to the sum of the [^{125}I] and [^{131}I] profiles. (Permission granted (48).)

of its apoA-I. This new particle has a molecular weight of about 400,000. Since a C-protein displaces A-proteins, these results suggest that A and C proteins cannot be assigned to different families.

SUMMARY

Our understanding of the mechanism of lipid transport by the plasma lipoproteins has seen considerable refinement since the eras of Macheboeuf, Oncley, Cohn and Gofman. Much of the recent progress has been achieved through the orchestration of new technologies and well established *in vitro* and *in vivo* models. We anticipate that this approach will produce a better understanding of how changing life-styles and drug intervention can be used to alter lipoprotein structure and metabolism.

ACKNOWLEDGEMENTS

The authors gratefully acknowledge the work of their colleagues Joel D. Morrisett, Louis C. Smith, James T. Sparrow, William A. Bradley, Josef R. Patsch and Richard L. Jackson described in this manuscript and express their thanks to Ms. Kaye Shewmaker for preparation of the artwork and Ms. Barbara Allen for editorial assistance.

Work from the authors' laboratory described in this paper was supported in part by a grant from the National Institutes of Health for a National Heart and Blood Vessel Research and Demonstration Center (HL-17269).

H.J. Pownall is an Established Investigator of the American Heart Association.

REFERENCES

1. M.A. Macheboeuf, Recherches sur les phosphoaminolipides et les sterides du serum et du plasma sanguins; entrainement des phospholipides, des sterols et des sterides par les diverses fractions au cours du fractionnement des proteides du serum, Bull. Soc. Chim. Biol. 11, 268 (1929).
2. M.A. Macheboeuf, and P. Rebeyrotte, Studies of lipoprotein cenapses of horse serum, Discussions Faraday Soc. 6, 62 (1949).
3. K.O. Pedersen, Low density lipoproteins appearing in normal human plasma, J. Phys. Colloid. Chem. 51, 156 (1947).
4. E.J. Cohn, F.R.N. Gurd, D.M. Surgenor, B.A. Barnes, R.K. Brown, G. Derouaux, J.M. Gillespie, F.W. Kahnt, W.F. Lever, C.H. Liu, D. Mittleman, R.F. Mouton, K. Schmid, and E. Uroma, A system for the separation of the components of human blood. Quantitative procedures for the separation of the protein components of human plasma, J. Am. Chem. Soc. 72, 465 (1950).
5. J.W. Gofman, F.T. Lindgren, and H. Elliott, Ultracentrifugal studies of lipoproteins of human serum, J. Biol. Chem. 179, 973 (1949).
6. J.W. Gofman, F. Glazier, A. Tamplin, B. Strisower, and O. De Lalla, Lipoproteins, coronary heart disease and atherosclerosis, Physiol. Rev. 34, 589 (1954).
7. R.J. Havel, H.A. Eder, and J.H. Bragdon, The distribution and chemical composition of ultracentrifugally separated lipoproteins in human serum, J. Clin. Invest. 34, 1345 (1955).
8. W.G. Dangerfield, and E.B. Smith, An investigation of serum lipids and lipoproteins by paper electrophoresis, J. Clin. Pathol. 8, 132 (1955).
9. B. Shore, University of California Radiation Laboratory No. 3489 (1956).
10. D. Gitlin, and D.G. Cornwall, Plasma lipoprotein metabolism in normal individuals and in children with the Nephrotic Syndrome, J. Clin. Invest. 35, 706 (1956).
11. P.F. Hahn, Abolishment of alimentary lipemia following injection of heparin, Science 98, 19 (1943).
12. E.D. Korn, A heparin clearing factor: Activated lipoprotein lipase. I. Isolation and characterization of the enzyme from normal rat heart, J. Biol. Chem. 215, 1 (1955).
13. D.S. Fredrickson, R.I. Levy, and R.S. Lees, Fat transport in lipoproteins--an integrated approach to mechanisms and disorders, New Engl. J. Med. 276, 34, 94, 148, 215, 273 (1967).
14. A.M. Gotto, Part II, Hyperlipoproteinemias (Table), In Human Health and Disease (edited by P.L. Altman and D.D. Katz), p. 137, Federation of American Societies for Experimental Biology, Bethesda (1977).

15. A.M. Gotto, Part III. Hypolipoproteinemias (Table), In Human Health and Disease (edited by P.L. Altman and D.D. Katz), p. 139, Federation of American Societies for Experimental Biology, Bethesda (1977).
16. A.M. Gotto, R.I. Levy, K. John, and D.S. Fredrickson, On the protein defect in abetalipoproteinemia, New Engl. J. Med. 284 (1971).
17. D.S. Fredrickson, A.M. Gotto, and R.I. Levy, Familial lipoprotein deficiency, In The Metabolic Basis of Inherited Disease (edited by J.B. Stanbury, J.B. Wyngaarden, and D.S. Fredrickson), p. 493, McGraw-Hill, New York (1972).
18. D.S. Fredrickson, P.H. Altrocchi, and L.V. Avioli, Tangier disease, Ann. Int. Med. 55, 1016 (1961).
19. K.R. Norum, and E. Gjone, Familial plasma lecithin:cholesterol acyltransferase deficiency. Biochemical study of a new inborn error of metabolism, Scand. J. Clin. Lab. Invest. 20, 231 (1967).
20. S.-P. Noel and D. Rubinstein, Secretion of apolipoproteins in very low density and high density lipoproteins by perfused rat liver, J. Lipid Res. 15, 301 (1974).
21. J.R. Patsch, K.C. Aune, A.M. Gotto, and J.D. Morrisett, Isolation, chemical characterization, and biophysical properties of three different abnormal lipoproteins: $LP\text{-}X_1$, $LP\text{-}X_2$, and $LP\text{-}X_3$, J. Biol. Chem. 252, 2113 (1977).
22. J.L. Oncley, Lipid protein interactions, In Brain Lipids and Lipoproteins, and the Leukodystrophies (edited by J. Folch-Pi and H. Bauer), p. 1, Elsevier, Amsterdam (1963).
23. L.C. Smith, H.J. Pownall, and A.M. Gotto. The plasma lipoproteins: Structure and metabolism, Ann. Rev. Biochem. 47, 751 (1978).
24. R.L. Hamilton, M.C. Williams, C.J. Fielding, and R.J. Havel, Discoidal bilayer structure of nascent high density lipoprotein from perfused rat liver, J. Clin. Invest. 58, 667 (1976).
25. J.B. Marsch, Apoproteins of the lipoproteins in a nonrecirculating perfusate of rat liver, J. Lipid Res. 17, 85 (1976).
26. J.C. LaRosa, R.I. Levy, P. Herbert, S.E. Lux, and D.S. Fredrickson, A specific apoprotein activator for lipoprotein lipase, Biochem. Biophys. Res. Commun. 41, 57 (1970).
27. J.R. Patsch, A.M. Gotto, T. Olivecrona, and S. Eisenberg, Formation of high density lipoprotein_2-like particles during lipolysis of very low density lipoproteins in vitro, Proc. Natl. Acad. Sci. USA 75, 4519 (1978).
28. B.W. Shen, A.M. Scanu, F.J. Kezdy, Structure of human serum lipoprotein inferred from compositional analysis, Proc. Natl. Acad. Sci. USA 75, 837 (1977).
29. R.J. Deckelbaum, G.G. Shipley, D.M. Small, Structure and interactions of lipids in human plasma low density lipoproteins, J. Biol. Chem. 252, 744 (1977).
30. R.B. Verdery, and A.V. Nichols, Arrangement of lipid and proteins in human serum high density lipoproteins: A proposed model, Chem. Phys. Lipids 14, 123 (1975).
31. R.L. Jackson, H.N. Baker, E.B. Gilliam, and A.M. Gotto, Primary structure of very low density apolipoprotein C-II of human plasma, Proc. Natl. Acad. Sci. USA 74, 1942 (1977).
32. P. Kinnunen, R.L. Jackson, L.C. Smith, A.M. Gotto, and J.T. Sparrow, Activation of lipoprotein lipase by native and synthetic fragments of human plasma apolipoprotein C-II, Proc. Natl. Acad. Sci. USA 74, 4848 (1977).
33. J.T. Sparrow, and A.M. Gotto, Synthetic fragments of apolipoprotein C-II: Phospholipid binding studies, Circulation 58, II-77 (1978).
34. J.T. Sparrow, H.J. Pownall, F.-J. Hsu, L.D. Blumenthal, A.R. Culwell, and A.M. Gotto, Lipid-binding fragments of apolipoprotein C-III-1 obtained by thrombin cleavage, Biochemistry 16, 5427 (1977).
35. R.S. Shulman, P.N. Herbert, D.S. Fredrickson, K. Wehrly, and H.B. Brewer, Isolation and alignment of the tryptic peptides of alanine apolipoprotein, an apolipoprotein from human plasma very low density lipoproteins, J. Biol. Chem. 249, 4969 (1974).

36. P.Y. Chou, and G.C. Fasman, Conformation parameters for amino acids in helical, β-sheet, and random coil regions calculated from proteins, Biochemistry 13, 211 (1974).
37. H.B. Bull, and K. Breese, Surface tension of amino acid solutions; a hydrophobicity scale of the amino acid residues, Arch. Biochem. Biophys. 161, 665 (1975).
38. J.P. Segrest, J.D. Morrisett, R.L. Jackson, and A.M. Gotto, A molecular theory of lipid-protein interactions in the plasma lipoproteins, FEBS Lett. 38, 247 (1974).
39. H.J. Pownall, J.B. Massey, S.K. Kusserow, and A.M. Gotto, Kinetics of lipid-protein interactions: I. Interaction of apolipoprotein A-I from human plasma high density lipoproteins with phosphatidylcholine, Biochemistry 17, 1183 (1978).
40. S. Mabrey, and J. Sturtevant, Investigation of phase transitions of lipids and lipid mixtures by high sensitivity differential scanning calorimetry, Proc. Natl. Acad. Sci. USA 73, 3862 (1976).
41. H.J. Pownall, and L.C. Smith, Viscosity of the hydrocarbon region of micelles: Measurement by excimer fluorescence, J. Am. Chem. Soc. 95, 3136 (1973).
42. A.K. Soutar, H.J. Pownall, A. Hu, and L.C. Smith, Phase transitions in bilamellar vesicles. Measurement by pyrene excimer fluorescence and effect on transacylation by lecithin:cholesterol acyltransferase, Biochemistry 13, 2828 (1974).
43. S.C. Charlton, J.S. Olson, K.-Y. Hong, H.J. Pownall, D.D. Louie, and L.C. Smith, Stopped flow kinetics of pyrene transfer between human high density lipoproteins, J. Biol. Chem. 251, 7952 (1976).
44. S.C. Charlton, K.-Y. Hong, and L.C. Smith, Kinetics of rac-1-oleyl-2-[4-(3-pyrenyl)butanoyl]glycerol transfer between high density lipoproteins, Biochemistry 17, 3304 (1978).
45. Tanford, C., The Hydrophobic Effect, Wiley, New York (1973).
46. A. Kruski, and A.M. Scanu, Interaction of human serum high density lipoprotein apoprotein with phospholipids, Chem. Phys. Lipids 13, 27 (1974).
47. A. Jonas, D.J. Krajnovich, and B.W. Patterson, Interaction of human and bovine A-I apolipoprotein with 1-α-dimyristoylphosphatidylcholine and 1-α-myristoyl-lysophosphatidylcholine, J. Biol. Chem. 252, 2200 (1977).
48. H.J. Pownall, Q. Pao, M. Rohde, and A.M. Gotto, Lipoprotein-apoprotein exchange in aqueous systems: Relevance to the occurrence of apoA-I and apoC proteins in a common particle, Biochem. Biophys. Res. Commun. (in press).
49. L.B. Vitello, and A.M. Scanu, Studies on human serum high-density lipoproteins. Self-association of human serum apolipoprotein A-II in aqueous solutions, Biochemistry 15, 1161 (1976).
50. H.J. Pownall, J.B. Massey, S.K. Kusserow, and A.M. Gotto, Kinetics of lipid-protein interactions: II. Effect of cholesterol on the association of human plasma high density apolipoprotein A-I with α-dimyristoyl phosphatidylcholine, Biochemistry (in press).

THE INITIATION AND CONTROL OF BLOOD COAGULATION

Yale Nemerson and Margalit Zur
The Department of Medicine, Mount Sinai School of Medicine
New York, New York 10029

The commonly held view of blood coagulation is that it consists of two more-or-less independent proteolytic pathways which converge at the point at which factor X, a zymogen, is converted to activated factor X, an enzyme (Fig. 1). In recent years, this view has become somewhat less tenable owing to the fact that certain of the early reactions appear to depart from this formulation; for example, it has been shown that activated factor XII can activate factor VII, a component of the tissue factor pathway, and that factor VII can activate factor IX, a zymogen involved in the intrinsic pathway. Thus, the two pathways can no longer be viewed confidently as independent biochemical systems each resulting in the activation of factor X.

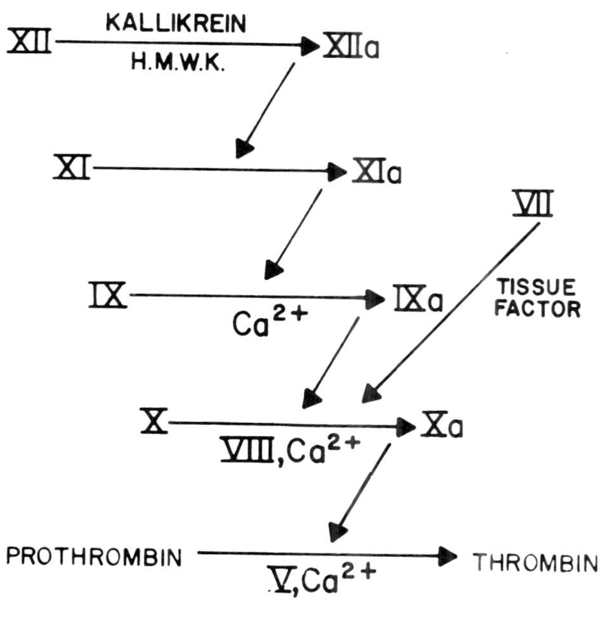

Fig. 1 The classical coagulation cascade

One of the major unsolved problems of coagulation is the mechanisms by which each of these pathways is initiated. Classically, it has been held that the coagulation proteins circulate as either zymogens of serine proteases or cofactors which accelerate the activation of zymogens. Yet when blood is shed from the body and collected into a tube, coagulation ensues. Under usual circumstances, a fibrin clot becomes visible in about 10 to 20 minutes. If small amounts of various tissues, particularly from lung, brain or placenta, are added to the blood, a remarkable acceleration of coagulation is observed: under appropriate circumstances a clot will form in about 12-15 seconds. While each of these sets of reactions involves proteins in common, there are also components which are unique to each. Each system may be described in part as a proteolytic cascade; in neither instance is the source of the initial proteolysis understood. The only reaction unique to the "tissue factor pathway" of coagulation is the activation of factor X catalyzed by factor VII. In this reaction, tissue factor acts as a cofactor, the effect of which is mainly on the k_{cat} which is enhanced some 3000-fold (1). Recently, another tissue factor dependent reaction has been described which will be discussed below.

Some years ago our laboratory was involved in a study which showed that various preparations of tissue factor, the lipoprotein in tissues responsible for the acceleration of the tissue factor or extrinsic pathway of coagulation, had demonstrable peptidase activity (2). However, further work by ourselves and others showed that as tissue factor was purified, the peptidase activity was diminished. Further, we showed the peptidase to be metal-dependent on a variety of synthetic substrates; its activity could be completely inhibited by the chelator orthophenanthrolene. Taking advantage of the low binding constant of this chelator for calcium ions, we were able to demonstrate that the coagulant activity of tissue factor was unaffected by concentrations of orthophenanthrolene which totally inhibited the associated peptidase. Thus, it became clear that the initiation of the tissue factor pathway of coagulation was independent of tissue factor-catalyzed proteolysis.

Some years ago, Williams demonstrated that partially purified factor VII was inhibited by the irreversible, active site-directed inhibitor diisopropylphosphoroflouridate (DFP) (3). At the time, it was uncertain whether the zymogen was being inhibited or whether factor VII was activated during purification thus leading to its reactivity with DFP. Subsequently, however, in collaboration with M.P. Esnouf, we showed that factor VII in fresh anticoagulated bovine plasma is rapidly inhibited by DFP, whereas several other coagulation factors are unaffected (4). This observation clearly indicates that either factor VII circulates in its activated, enzymic form, i.e., it is activated *in vivo* by an unknown mechanism, or that the zymogen form of factor VII is unusually reactive towards DFP. If the latter were the case, one could envision a possible mechanism for the initiation of coagulation that would not require proteolysis.

Subsequently, bovine factor VII was purified to homogeneity in our laboratory (5). It is a single chain glycoprotein with a molecular weight of 53,000 estimated from its mobility on SDS gels. Shortly thereafter, the protein was also purified by Kisiel and Davie (6); sedimentation equilibrium studies showed its molecular weight to be somewhat lower, 45,500; the difference is probably attributable to the inherent inaccuracies of gel electrophoresis plus the well known effect of carbohydrate on proteins which leads to erroneously high molecular weights when estimated by electrophoretic techniques. Both laboratories, however, agreed on the amino-terminal sequence of factor VII which showed a high degree of homology with that of prothrombin and the other vitamin K-dependent zymogens of blood coagulation (6,7). Unlike the other zymogens, however, factor VII incorporated DFP and was rendered inert by this reagent.

Dr. Robert Radcliffe made detailed studies of this protein in our laboratory:

when judged by its coagulant activity, approximately a 50-fold enhancement of activity was noted when the protein was cleaved at a specific Arg-Ile bond (5). Two enzymes were identified which rapidly catalyze this cleavage: activated factor X (the enzyme generated by the attack of factor VII on factor X) and activated Hageman factor (factor XII) the first enzyme generated by the intrinsic system. The latter studies were performed in collaboration with Drs. A. Bagdasarian and R.W. Colman of the University of Pennsylvania (8); independently E.W. Davie and his collaborators also demonstrated the activation of factor VII by factor XIIa (9). The finding that factor VII has a more active form, factor VIIa, leads to an interesting question: is the activity associated with the single chain zymogen form of factor VII endogenous to the zymogen or is it due to contamination with a small amount of the more active enzyme? This question appears to us to be critically important to the theory of coagulation because if the zymogen has significant coagulant activity, then coagulation can be initiated simply by exposing the blood to tissue factor. If, on the other hand, proteolysis of factor VII is an absolute requirement for the initiation of coagulation, then an unidentified enzyme present in tissues must be invoked as an absolute requirement for the initiation of coagulation.

We therefore addressed ourselves to the issue of the endogenous activity of the zymogen form of factor VII. Several approaches have been used, the first of which involves the kinetics of inhibition by DFP. We first showed that the single-chain form of factor VII and the more active two-chain, "enzymic" form of the molecule each incorporated the same amount of DFP: approximately 0.9 moles of inhibitor per mole of protein (based on a molecular weight of 53,000) (7). Second, we demonstrated that the same peptide in each species was labelled when ^{32}P-DFP was utilized. Third, using tritiated DFP we showed that the pseudo-first order rate constant for incorporation into the enzyme exceeded that of the zymogen only by a factor of four; this is in marked contrast to the rate constants for the incorporation of DFP into other enzyme-zymogen pairs in which the constants differ by several orders of magnitude (10). It should be noted that in these experiments trace contamination of factor VII by activated factor VII is irrevelant; the sensitivity of the experiment is such that only incorporation into the bulk species would be observed. On the basis of these data alone, it is obvious that factor VII is uniquely reactive in its zymogen form.

Knowing the rate constants for the incorporation of DFP into the zymogen and enzyme forms of factor VII, it was possible to use the kinetics of inhibition of factor VII to approach the question of the endogenous coagulant activity of the zymogen. DFP was added to an apparently homogeneous form of activated factor VII and the rate of inhibition exactly paralleled the rate of incorporation of the assay. The rate of inhibition exactly paralleled the rate of incorporation of the inhibitor into the enzyme. Next, we determined the rate of inhibition of the zymogen using the same techniques. Here, instead of observing an apparent first-order decay of activity, a curvilinear decay was observed when the log of activity was plotted vs. time, the expected result if two first-order processes were summed. The results were analyzed based on this assumption according to the following expression:

$$Y = C1 \times e^{-k_1 t} + C2 \times e^{-k_2 t}$$

where Y is the observed activity at time, t, and k_1 and k_2 are the first order rate constants describing the incorporation of labelled DFP into the enzyme and zymogen, respectively. By an iterative curve fitting technique, we solved for C1 and C2 which are coefficients describing the fractional contribution of the two species to the observed activity. Based on this analysis, we concluded that about one-third of the observed activity of the zymogen is a function of the zymogen itself and the remainder of the activity is a function of contamination of the zymogen with a small amount of the enzyme.

Owing to the nature of coagulation assays, however, we are uncertain as to the precise interpretation of these results. To assay for factor VII, the protein is added to factor VII-deficient plasma and clotting times are determined in the presence of saturating amounts of tissue factor. During the course of the assay, activated factor X is formed, which at least in principle, could convert factor VII into its two-chain form during the course of the measurement. The conversion of factor VII to activated factor VII would have to be at a rate which would yield the results alluded to above; this seems unlikely and highly coincidental, but nonetheless introduces a disquieting uncertainty to the results.

To deal with these uncertainties, we have pursued the activity of the zymogen utilizing different techniques. First, an ester was used to assay for factor VII. Owing to the minimal esterase activity of both forms of this protein, it was necessary to synthesize an extremely sensitive substrate, N^{α}-benzyloxycarbonyl-L-arginine p-nitrobenzyl ester (11). Utilizing this approach we found the zymogen indeed exhibited esterase activity with a Km about one order of magnitude higher than that determined for activated factor VII and a k_{cat} almost exactly 50% of that of the enzyme. We feel that these data, while not proving the proteolytic activity of the zymogen, again emphasize the unusual activity of this protein.

Finally, we have turned to an assay for factor VII developed in our laboratory to address the issue of the endogenous activity of the zymogen. The assay is based on determining the rate of activation of factor X in a pure system. We have taken advantage of the fact that the activation peptide of this zymogen contains most of the carbohydrate on the molecule. Thus, following established techniques we have tritiated the sialic acid residues on the molecule by mild periodate oxidation followed by reduction with tritiated $NaBH_4$ (12). The release of the peptide, which occurs *pari passu* with the appearance of enzymic activity, is conveniently measured by estimating TCA-soluble radioactivity as a function of time. Owing to the fact that activated factor X catalyzes the activation of factor VII, we have chemically modified the tritiated factor X by limited succinylation thereby generating a product which is readily cleaved as a substrate but which yields only about 1/2000 of the proteolytic activity of native factor X_a. Combining this assay with the kinetics of inhibition of DFP, we have again concluded that the zymogen is contaminated with a small amount of enzyme but that a considerable portion of the observed activity is attributable to endogenous activity of the zymogen form of factor VII. Inasmuch as we have not shown in an altogether convincing manner that factor VII is not activated during the course of this assay, these results must be viewed as provisional. These data taken together, however, have led us to conclude that in all likelyhood the zymogen form of factor VII has sufficient proteolytic activity to account for the initiation of coagulation in the presence of tissue factor.

A significant problem with respect to the theory of coagulation is the existence of two pathways involving considerable redundancy (see Fig. 1). Clearly, each leads to the formation of activated factor X and thus indirectly to thrombin formation. Based on this formulation, it is difficult to understand why patients lacking factors XI, IX or VIII, proteins unique to the intrinsic system, have hemorrhagic symptoms. Likewise, in the presence of an intact intrinsic system, hemorrhagic symptoms associated with factor VII deficiency are equally difficult to explain. An even greater peculiarity is the lack of symptoms accompanying a deficiency of factor XII, prekallikrein or high molecular weight kininogen, all required for the normal *in vitro* coagulation of blood.

Quite recently, Østerud and Rapaport (13) demonstrated that human factor VII activates factor IX in a tissue factor-dependent reaction. We have confirmed their conclusions with respect to the bovine system. Further, a kinetic analysis of this reaction showed it to proceed at favorable rates (14). However, under all conditions we have tested, the rate of activation of factor X exceeds the rate of activation of factor IX. Thus, this finding alone does not ameliorate the problems associated with the redundant pathways. However, the description of this new tissue factor-dependent reaction does allow a hypothetical model of coagulation quite different from the classical cascade (Fig. 2).

If one assumes that the activation of Hageman factor is an in vitro artifact, a possibility supported by the symptomless patients, then one could postulate two sites of initiation of coagulation, each catalyzed by tissue factor and factor VII. This formulation obviates the difficulties engendered by a model in which the initiation of the intrinsic system is catalyzed by Hageman factor, but for it to make physiological sense, the following requirements must be met: 1) a biological "switch" modulating the action of tissue factor-factor VII between the activation of factor X and the activation of factor IX; and 2) a mechanism for the activation of factor XI independent of Hageman factor. The latter is required because patients lacking factor XI may bleed abnormally. A platelet-dependent mechanism for the activation of factor XI has been proposed by Walsh (15).

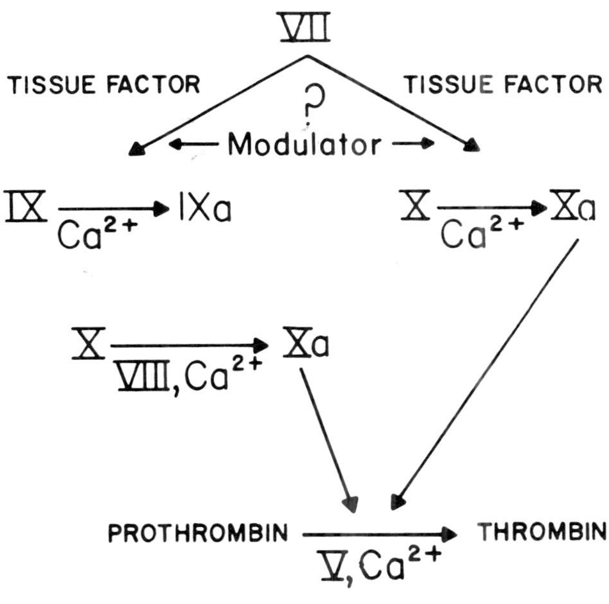

Fig. 2 A proposed reinterpretation of the coagulation cascade

No mechanism for modulating the activity of tissue factor-factor VII has been described. Owing to the fact that there are evidently no plasma inhibitors of factor VII or factor VIIa, it seems unlikely that such modulation would be a function of a plasma protein. Further, unpublished observations from our laboratory indicate that in a whole plasma system, factor IX is activated at almost the same rate as is factor X. Alternatively, one could postulate the existence of two different tissue factors, each specifically accelerating one reaction. However, we have found that the most purified preparations of tissue factor available seem to be equally active in these two reactions. Another possibility to be considered is that inhibitors of tissue factor exist which exhibit specificity towards the activation of either factor IX or factor X. Finally, modulation might be explicable on kinetic grounds. If such modulation exists, a model such as the one proposed in Fig. 2 would be physiologically tenable.

References

1. S.A. Silverberg, Y. Nemerson, and M. Zur, Kinetics of the activation of bovine coagulation factor X by components of the extrinsic pathway, J. Biol. Chem. 252, 8481 (1977).
2. F.A. Pitlick, Y. Nemerson, A.J. Gottlieb, R.G. Gordon, and W.J. Williams, Peptidase activity associated with the tissue factor of blood coagulation, Biochemistry 10, 2650 (1971).
3. W.J. Williams (1965). In Biophysical Mechanisms in Vascular Homeostasis and Intravascular Coagulation (Ed. P.N. Sawyer) p. 192. Appleton-Century-Crofts, New York.
4. Y. Nemerson and M.P. Esnouf, Activation of a proteolytic system by a membrane lipoprotein: mechanism of action of tissue factor, Proc. Natl. Acad. Sci. USA 70, 310 (1973).
5. R. Radcliffe and Y. Nemerson, Activation and control of factor VII by activated factor X and thrombin, J. Biol. Chem. 250, 388 (1975).
6. W. Kisiel and E.W. Davie, Isolation and characterization of bovine factor VII, Biochemistry 14, 4928 (1975).
7. R. Radcliffe and Y. Nemerson, Mechanism of activation of bovine factor VII, J. Biol. Chem. 251, 4797 (1976).
8. R. Radcliffe, A. Bagdasarian, R. Colman, and Y. Nemerson, Activation of bovine vactor VII by Hageman factor fragments, Blood 50, 611 (1977).
9. W. Kisiel, K. Fujikawa, and E.W. Davie, Activation of bovine factor VII (proconvertin) by factor XIIa (activated Hageman factor), Biochemistry 16, 4189 (1977).
10. P.H. Morgan, N.C. Robinson, K.A. Walsh, and H. Neurath, Inactivation of bovine trypsinogen and chymotrypsinogen by diisopropylphosphorofluoridate, Proc. Natl. Acad. Sci. USA 69, 3312 (1972).
11. M.Zur and Y. Nemerson, The esterase activity of coagulation factor VII, J. Biol. Chem. 253, 2203 (1978).
12. L. VanLenten and G. Ashwell, Studies on the chemical and enzymatic modification of glycoproteins, J. Biol. Chem. 246, 1889 (1971).
13. B. Østerud and S.I. Rapaport, Activation of factor IX by the reaction product of tissue factor and factor VII: additional pathway for initiating blood coagulation, Proc. Natl.Acad. Sci. USA 74,5260 (1977)
14. M. Zur, K. Shastri, and Y. Nemerson, Kinetics of the tissue factor pathway of coagulation: activation of factor IX, Blood 52 (Suppl. 1), 198 (1978)
15. P.N. Walsh, The effects of collagen and kaolin on the intrinsic coagulant activity of platelets, Br. J. Haematol. 22, 393 (1972).

HUMAN THROMBIN: PREPARATIVE EVALUATION, STRUCTURAL PROPERTIES, AND ENZYMIC SPECIFICITY

J. W. Fenton, II[1], B. H. Landis[1], D. A. Walz[2], D. H. Bing[3], R. D. Feinman[4], M. P. Zabinski[1], S. A. Sonder[1], L. J. Berliner[5], and J. S. Finlayson[6]
[1]Division of Laboratories and Research, New York State Department of Health, Albany, NY 12201; [2]Department of Physiology, Wayne State University School of Medicine, Detroit, MI 48201; [3]Center for Blood Research, Boston, MA 02115; [4]Department of Biochemistry, State University of New York Downstate Medical Center, Brooklyn, NY 11203; [5]Department of Chemistry, Ohio State University, Columbus, OH 43210; and [6]Bureau of Biologics, Food and Drug Administration, Bethesda, MD 20014

SUMMARY

Human α-thrombin (M_r =36,600) with high coagulant activity (~3 U/μg) can be produced in gram quantities, approaching enzymic homogeneity, from Fraction III paste obtained from large-scale plasma fractionation by the Cohn procedures. This form is the prothrombin activation product which possesses all known thrombin associated activities. It consists of a 36-residue A chain (M_r=4,600 activation peptide) and a 259-residue B chain (M_r=32,000 serine-protease moiety) joined by a disulfide bridge between the midportions of the two chains. Amino acid substitutions among human and bovine thrombins, as well as their prothrombin fragments, are compatible with structural predictions. The human enzyme is sparingly soluble in water (≤0.3 mg/ml), has limiting pH (~5-10.3) and thermal ($T_{½}$ = 51°C, 9 salts extrapolate to I = 0) boundaries, exhibits solute-solvent stability dependencies, and autolytically degrades.

Essentially noncoagulant (~1 U/mg), enzymically active forms arise from α-thrombin by proteolysis (autolytic or tryptic digestion) or may be made by selective chemical modification. Those produced by proteolysis include three-chain β- and subsequently four-chain γ-thrombin forms. The proximity of the A chain to the benzamidine binding site has been shown for both α- and γ-thrombins by exosite affinity labeling and is not related to clotting activity. Both thrombins react similarly with antithrombin III (± heparin), displacing proflavine to form covalent complexes, and fibrinogen does not interfere with γ-thrombin reactions. In contrast, α- and γ-thrombins form noncovalent complexes with hirudin, causing immobilization of active-site spin labels; binding affinities (K_i=0.063 vs. 13 nM for α- and γ-thrombins, respectively) correlate with clotting activity. These data, unlike contiguous sequences of thrombin susceptible bonds in proteins, provide evidence for specific protein binding/recognition sites, such sites are implicated in receptor interactions of α-thrombin with platelets and mitogenically responsive cells. In contrast to the related pancreatic enzymes with digestive functions, α-thrombin, with central functions in various events of hemostasis, is a bioregulatory protease.

INTRODUCTION

Thrombin (EC 3.4.21.5) is the serine protease which is generated by proteolytic activation of its circulating zymogen (prothrombin, coagulation Factor II) in the final preclotting event of the blood coagulation cascades. Like related serine proteases, human thrombin has more than one known enzymically active form (1, 2). These are the parent two-chain α-thrombin, the derivative three-chain β-thrombin, and the subsequent derivative, four-chain γ-thrombin (Fig. 1). The derivative forms arise by autolytic degradation or limited proteolysis with trypsin-like enzymes, where cleavages occur within the thrombin B chain to give rise to noncovalently associated fragments.

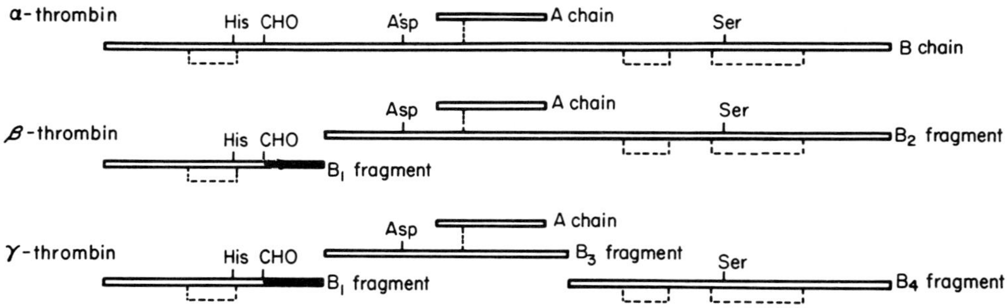

Fig. 1. Polypeptide structures of human α-, β-, and γ-thrombins. Structures are based on amino acid sequence data for human thrombin (6, 7), where the disulfide bridges (----), active-site residues of the charge relay system (His, Asp, and Ser), and the carbohydrate attachment (CHO) are assigned by homologies with bovine thrombin (3). Cleavage sites in the formation of human β- and γ-thrombin are based on the NH_2-terminal sequences of the B-chain fragments (2), where the CO_2H-terminal portion of the B_1 fragment is blackened to indicate the segment where additional cleavages occur (see text).

The thrombin B chain furthermore exhibits a high degree of amino acid sequence homology with other serine proteases and contains residues essential for catalysis (3-7). The derivative forms, in particular γ-thrombin, are of interest since the residues comprising the charge relay system (His_{43}, Asp_{99}, and Ser_{205}), as well as the activation salt bridge (Ile_1 and Asp_{204}), are separated in noncovalently associated B-chain fragments (Fig. 2). Human α- and β-thrombins are homologues of the corresponding bovine forms (8), whereas human γ-thrombin has no bovine counterpart (2).

Although β- and γ-thrombin retain estero/amidolytic and certain other activities, α-thrombin is the only human form with high clotting activity (1, 2). It not only hydrolyzes fibrinopeptides from fibrinogen to form clottable fibrin monomers but also activates the fibrin stabilizing factor (Factor XIII), interacts with preceding coagulation factors (e.g., activates Factors V and VIII; possibly inactivates others), stimulates platelets (e.g., secretion and aggregation reactions), reacts with protease inhibitors in plasma (e.g., antithrombin-III, α_2-macroglobulin), and may participate in other physiologic processes (e.g., actions on complement C3 and C5; binding to cell receptors; mitogenic stimulation). Thus, α-thrombin may be regarded as a bioregulatory protease, in contrast to serine proteases which have primarily digestive functions (9). Whether β- and γ-thrombins are formed *in vivo* and whether they have physiologic functions are unknown. These nonclotting derivative thrombins have nevertheless been exceedingly useful in assessing requirements for enzymic activity. The proteolytic specificity of α-thrombin and other biological properties have suggested that its

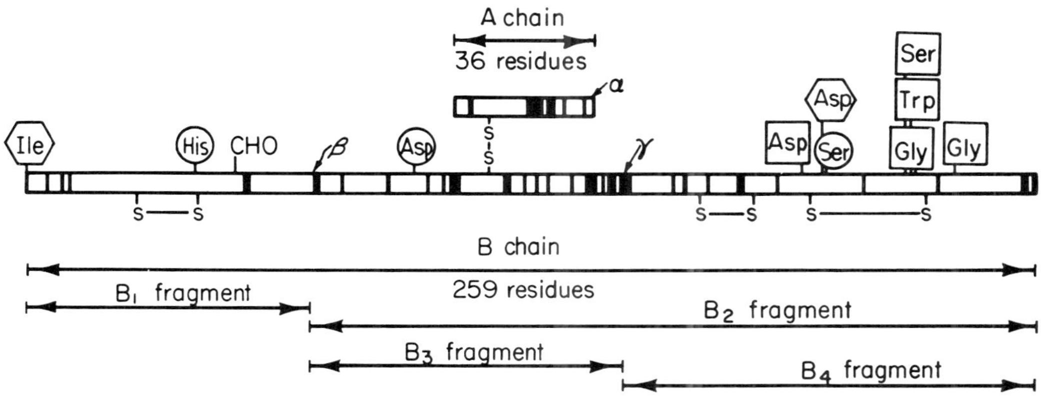

Fig. 2. Overall structure of human thrombin. Polypeptide chains are drawn to scale based on amino acids sequence (see Fig. 1), where the charge relay residues (O), activation salt-bridge residues (⬡), primary binding site residues (□), disulfide bridges (-S-S-), carbohydrate attachment (CHO), cleavage sites of the thrombin forms (α, β, and γ), and amino acid substitutions between human and bovine thrombins (■) are shown.

active site contains unique structural features not found in other serine proteases.

The complete amino acid sequences of bovine (3, 4) and human (5-7, 10) prothrombins have been reported. Notably, the NH_2-terminal third of prothrombin, which corresponds to Fragment F_1, contains the majority of carbohydrate in prothrombins; it also contains the ten vitamin K-dependent γ-carboxyglutamate residues, which are believed to participate in the binding of divalent cations in prothrombin activation (3, 4, 10, 11).

Under physiologic conditions, prothrombin concentrations greatly exceed those of preceding coagulation zymogens, and prothrombin is believed to form complexes with Ca^{2+}, phospholipids, activated Factor V (Factor V', believed to be a non-enzymic associating protein), and the protease Factor Xa. The latter cleaves prothrombin between the NH_2-terminal Fragment $F_{1.2}$ half (pro-piece) and the CO_2H-terminal thrombin half (prethrombin-2) and between the thrombin portions forming its A and B chains (cf. 3, 12). During the coagulation of whole human blood, $F_{1.2}$ is essentially the only NH_2-terminal fragment detected; it is therefore the prothrombin activation polypeptide (12). However, $F_{1.2}$ is degraded to Fragments F_1, F_2, and F_1-derivatives when prothrombin is activated at high concentrations, as in preparing thrombin (9, 10, 11, 13, 14). Under preparative activation conditions, human thrombin also loses a 13-residue peptide (Fragment F_3) from its A-chain NH_2-terminus (6, 7, 15, 16) to form α-thrombin which has been isolated (1, 2). Whether F_3 is lost during physiologic activation is not known. Bovine α-thrombin, which has a lysine at its A-chain position 13 instead of an arginine (7, 16) retains the corresponding peptide, but loses the peptide in converting to its derivative forms (8). The slight difference in size of human ($\underline{M}_r$ 36,600) vs. bovine ($\underline{M}_r$ 38,000) thrombin is in agreement with the size of missing human peptide, which is clearly not required for high coagulant activity (1).

The zymogens involved in the final events of coagulation and fibrinolysis (prothrombin and plasminogen) are relatively abundant, and both are present in human plasma at concentrations of approximately 100 mg/liter (17). Unlike prothrombin, plasminogen can be efficiently isolated from plasma by lysine-affinity chromatography techniques (18). A liter of human plasma should yield 40-50 mg of thrombin, assuming no procedural losses, but in practice about 8-10 times the volume of plasma is needed to produce this amount of thrombin (1, 2). Although human thrombin has been prepared from plasma (19) or clinical concentrates (15), this does not constitute efficient utilization of blood resources.

In the large-scale fractionation of human plasma by the Cohn procedure (20, 21), kilogram quantities of Fraction III paste are produced as a by-product of immunoglobulins (Fraction II). This paste is a rich source of the prothrombin-associated (vitamin K-dependent) coagulation factors (Factors II, VII, IX, and X), plasminogen, certain complement components, and other plasma proteins (22). Historically, in the mid-1940s, crude thrombin preparations were made by activating the prothrombin subfraction III-2, and such preparations are still used for clotting assay reference purposes (23, 24). However, not until the late 1950s and early 1960s, was Fraction III *per se* used as a prothrombin source in preparing thrombin. Procedures pioneered by Miller and associates (25-27) led to our current methods (1, 2), which have produced more than 40 g of human α-thrombin. These thrombin preparations and by-product fractions have been used for a variety of purposes (1, 2, 6, 10, 13, 14, 17, 29-107, *inter alia*). That these thrombin preparations have approached criteria for enzymic homogeneity has demonstrated the value of by-product fractions from the Cohn procedures.

PREPARATION AND EVALUATION

1. *Fraction III as a prothrombin source*. One of the major problems in utilizing Fraction III is that of solubilizing the desired proteins without forming emulsions, which cannot be clarified by conventional centrifugation or filtration. In the method of Miller and Copeland (26), Fraction III pastes were lyophilized and extracted with chloroform and methanol to remove lipids as well as to denature plasminogen. The extracted and dried Fraction III was then suspended in 0.15 M NaCl containing sodium citrate to extract prothrombin and enable recovery of prothrombin as its barium citrate complex in the subsequent step. In order to use the pastes as obtained from fractionators, we incorporated PEG 6,000 (see *Abbreviations*) into prothrombin extraction mixtures to prevent emulsions (27). This usage of PEG 6,000 led to the findings that low concentrations of the polymer greatly enhanced immunoprecipitin (108) and clotting (109) reactions. This use of PEG 6,000 in clotting assays contributed substantially to the development of our preparative procedure (1). At 40 g/liter, the polymer was also found to minimize extraction of plasminogen from Fraction III pastes (1), although it is now known that trace amounts of plasmin(ogen) may be carried through the procedure (see below). Plasmin, which can arise in pastes, will degrade prothrombin and thus prevent its activation to thrombin (110). However, most lots of freshly prepared Fraction III or those stored at $\leq$-50°C contain very little plasmin. Furthermore, high-purity thrombin preparations can be made from pastes containing considerable amounts of plasmin if the pastes are stored at low temperatures. Thrombin-like materials, which presumably arise from prothrombin degradation and adsorb to Amberlite CG-50 resin, are removed by CG-50 resin prior to activation (28). Nevertheless, Fraction III pastes which have deteriorated to the point where they give poor prothrombin recovery should be discarded.

Although the extraction of Fraction III paste is probably the least efficient step (~15-30%, Ref. 1), losses may be compensated for by increasing the preparation size. Furthermore, the extracted pastes are a rich starting material for preparing plasminogen (cf. 18), enabling the utilization of Fraction III for more than one product (1).

In the subsequent step, we have found barium citrate adsorption (26) to be preferable to DEAE-cellulose adsorption (27) for recovering the extracted prothrombin. The latter method is more cumbersome and spontaneous activation of prothrombin may occur in the presence of poly cations (e.g., polylysine). In the former method, Miller and Copeland (26) dissociated barium citrate complexes with CG-50 resin; we found dissociating the complexes with $(NH_4)_2SO_4$ to be simpler. However, the resulting solution includes thrombin-like materials, which are not obtained when large excesses of the resin are used. Therefore, we have dialyzed the prothrombin solution against 0.15 M NaCl and passed it through a column of CG-50 resin to remove such materials (28). As a consequence, only thrombin derived from the activation of prothrombin in the subsequent step is adsorbed to CG-50 resin. Prothrombin concentrates produced by our procedure are not only rich in prothrombin but also contain several times the normal plasma concentrations of Factors VII, IX, and X (Ref. 1). We have purposely not purified prothrombin to homogeneity, as in other procedures (19), because the Factors VII and X are required for activation with thromboplastin.

2. Prothrombin activation and thrombin isolation. Control of prothrombin activation is essential for preparing high purity α-thrombin; it must be both rapid and quantitative to prevent formation of extraneous products. We have used "bioactivation" employing human brain thromboplastin (26) adsorbed with bovine serum as a Factor V source, and routinely obtain complete activation within 30-60 min (1). Alternatively, Taipan snake venom activation (19, 48, 49) can be used to produce the same thrombin product (1). Activation in 25% sodium citrate is not recommended because prolonged times are needed and autolytic degradation of thrombin is promoted by high Na^+ concentrations (see below).

Amberlite CG-50 resin (polymethyl acrylic acid) has a high capacity for thrombin and quantitatively adsorbs it from 0.15 M NaCl. The nonadsorbed fraction from activation mixtures is a rich source of the prothrombin Fragments F_1 and F_2 (10, 11, 13, 14, 69). Although Miller and Copeland (26) eluted thrombin from CG-50 resin with a $CaCl_2$ salt gradient, we elute it with 0.75 M NaCl in order to obtain high protein concentrations (1, 27, 28). More recently, we have found that β- and γ-thrombins are eluted from the resin before α-thrombin (Fig. 3) and have modified our procedure to include stepwise washes of increasing salt concentration. We have also found it desirable to separate the initial from latter thrombin fractions.

Our preparations normally contain 2-8 mg of thrombin per ml (>100 preparations). As eluted with 0.75 M NaCl, thrombin preparations have a pH of ~6. At this pH, α-thrombin does not autolyze to any significant extent, and the preparations may be stored directly by freezing at $\leq$-50°C for periods well in excess of a year (1). Freeze-thawing of the enzyme will cause denaturation. Salt-free α-thrombin can be prepared by diluting to protein concentrations of about 0.3 mg/ml with water, dialyzing against water, centrifuging, and lyophilizing. Such thrombin stored at -20°C can be reconstituted to approximately 0.3 mg/ml in water or 2 mg/ml in 0.15 M NaCl (111). Highly concentrated thrombin solutions (10-12 mg/ml) can be made by precipitating with two volumes of saturated $(NH_4)_2SO_4$, centrifuging, and redissolving the pellet in 0.75 M NaCl. Such thrombin solutions, however, are very prone to autolytic degradation ($t_{1/2}$ = 50 min, 23°C; Ref. 111).

3. Derivative and modified thrombins. By employing conditions (e.g., ~2 mg/ml of thrombin in 3 M NaCl, pH 8, 23°C for ~2 days), which promote autolytic degradation of α-thrombin (1, 2, 111) and monitoring loss of clotting activity (109), large amounts of autolyzed thrombin can be made. The resulting mixtures are rich in β-thrombin form (e.g., 23% α-, 48% β-, and 29% γ-thrombin; ~20% the original clotting activity). The α-thrombin can be separated from these mixtures by its chromatography on CG-50 resin with a linear salt gradient (Fig. 3a), but we have

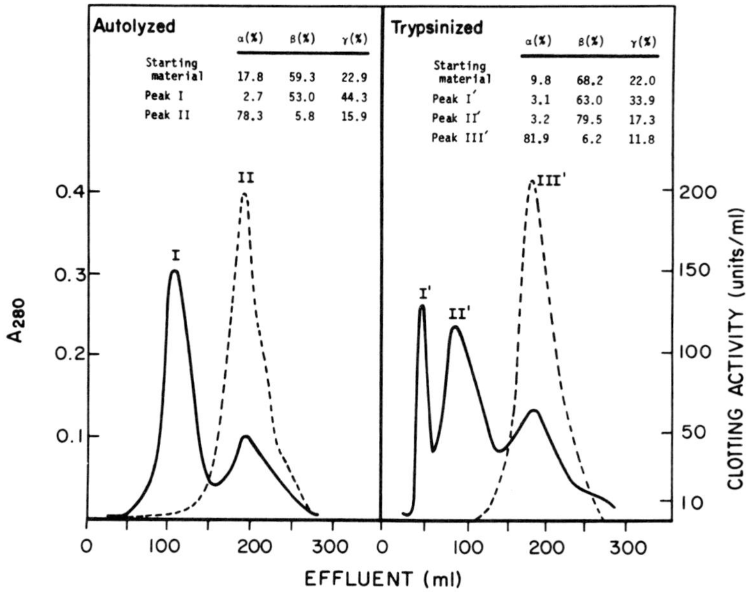

Fig. 3. Salt-gradient elution from Amberlite CG-50 resin of autolyzed and tryptic digests of human thrombin. Approximately 12 mg of thrombin digests were applied to 0.8 x 28 cm columns of CG-50 resin equilibrated in 0.2 M NaCl and were eluted with a linear gradient from 0.2 to 0.6 M NaCl at a flow rate of ~1 ml/min. The autolytic digest was prepared by incubating α-thrombin in 3.0 M NaCl at pH 8 and 23°C for 24 hours, whereas the tryptic digest was made by passing α-thrombin in 0.68 M NaCl, buffered with 10 mM Mes at pH 6.1, through a 1.3 x 3.0 cm column of trypsin-Sepharose 4B at ~1.25 ml/min. The A_{280} (——) and clotting activity (----) of eluates are drawn; the determined compositions of α-, β- and γ-thrombins are presented for the peak fractions in the respective inserts.

so far been unable to resolve β- from γ-thrombin under nondenaturing conditions (112). Attempts to subfractionate human thrombin by chromatography on SP-Sephadex (113) have been unsatisfactory (114). Nevertheless, autolytic mixtures of known compositions have been useful in assessing the enzymic properties of β-thrombin (e.g., reactions with antithrombin-III; Ref. 115).

Essentially complete conversion of α- to γ-thrombin can be achieved by controlled digestion with trypsin-Sepharose (pH 6, 23°C) under conditions in which thrombin does not autolyze (2, 29, 58). Such preparations contain 85-95% γ-thrombin and have 75-95% of the estero/amidolytic activities but only 0.2-0.05% of the specific clotting activities (>30 preparations). Because of their low α-thrombin contents (0-5%), these preparations have been valuable for studying noncoagulant thrombins (2, 29, 40, 54-59, 62, 73, 77, 91, 94, 101, 115). Recently, we have subfractionated the tryptic β- and γ-thrombins into two classes of β/γ-thrombins by their elution from CG-50 resin (Fig. 3b). The [^{14}C]DFP-labeled fragments of the β-thrombins from either class, as well as the γ-thrombins, coelectrophorese in SDS polyacrylamide gels with the corresponding autolytic forms (112), implying that their respective B_2 and B_4 fragments are the same (Fig. 1). This finding suggests more than one cleavage site on the CO_2H-terminus of the B_1 fragment as occurs in bovine thrombin (8, 116). Moreover, two B_1 fragment fractions with identical NH_2-termini (>3 cycles) but differing compositions have been isolated from the tryptic digests of human thrombin (117).

Essentially noncoagulant thrombin forms can also be made by selective chemical modification (113, 118-120). For example, human α-thrombin nitrated with tetranitromethane (121, 122) retains <2% clotting activity and 60-80% esterase activity (10 preparations). Such preparations have about 4 nitrotyrosines/thrombin by amino acid analysis (117), similar to nitrated bovine thrombin (119). Human γ-thrombin can also be nitrated to similar extent (122). Various noncatalytic forms of thrombin have been made by conjugation at the active-site serine (Ser_{205}) with a variety of reagents (e.g., DFP, MSF, PMSF, spin-labeling and fluorescent probe reagents; cf. Refs. 55, 56, 78, 91, 111). Thrombin can be affinity labeled at the active-site histidine (His_{43}) with TLCK (116) or at residues outside the classical active site with exosite reagents (57-59). Furthermore, fluorescein-labeled and photoaffinity-labeled α-thrombin can be made with retention of biological activities (123).

4. Thrombin purity and use. Although we have strived for producing preparations with the highest achievable enzymic activities without significantly sacrificing protein homogeneity or concentration, absolute homogeneity has not been obtained (1, 2). No single criterion is satisfactory for describing purity of thrombin preparation, and the criteria used should depend on the intended usage (Table 1).

TABLE 1 Considerations for Using Thrombin Preparations

Preparative Purity

Specific clotting activity -- U.S. "NIH" Units/mg protein
Active site titration -- % esterase sites/total enzyme
SDS electrophoresis -- protein homogeneity
Thrombin forms -- % α-thrombin by [^{14}C]DFP labeling
Contaminants -- plasmin(ogen), clotting factors, etc.

Storage Methods

Low-temperature freezing -- experimental uses
Freeze-drying -- reference purposes

Experimental Conditions

Storage Additives -- assay effects, toxicity, etc.
Enzymic stability -- pH, temperature, salts, etc.
Other proteins -- proteases, inhibitors, etc.
Significance -- physiologic counterpart of recovered enzyme

Since α-thrombin is the only human form with any significant coagulant activity (1, 2), specific clotting activities should ideally describe the purity of α-thrombin preparations. However, even with PEG-enhanced clotting assay, which minimizes most technical errors (1, 51, 109), specific activities of preparations are not completely reliable. Active-site titration with NPGB (28, 124) measures not only α-, but also β- and γ-thrombin, as well as possible contaminant plasmin or Factor X_a (cf. 1). It is particularly useful for estimating the total active enzyme content (e.g., relative to denatured thrombin). Staining with Coomassie blue after electrophoresis of [^{14}C]DFP-labeled preparations in SDS-10% polyacrylamide gels affords a qualitative assessment of protein homogeneity, whereas the radioactivity distribution of sectioned gels gives a quantitative ratio of the labeled forms (e.g., α-, β-, and γ-thrombins; serine proteases; Ref. 1). We have not routinely assessed preparations for trace contaminants. Some preparations may contain plasmin (ogen) which is detectable at high concentrations (125, 126). Certain preparations, when examined at about 10 units/ml, exhibited streptokinase-activatable fibrinolytic activity after 24 hours incubation at 37°C (127). In approximately two-thirds of the examined preparations streptokinase caused 0.05-0.5% incorporation of [^{14}C]DFP into plasmin relative to that incorporated into thrombin (111). Human thrombin will not activate plasminogen (111, 128). On the other hand, high concentrations of human thrombin are both caseinolytic and fibrinolytic (1).

In using a thrombin preparation (Table 1), it is important to know how the material has been stored and subsequently handled since the initial characterization data may no longer pertain. High purity preparations are prone to decomposition and care must be exercised in their handling and storage. Knowledge of thrombin stability under the conditions studied is also of paramount importance. Proteases and inhibitors in the biological system under study may inactivate the enzyme or alter its behavior. In general, experiments performed with greater than ten U.S. "NIH" clotting units/ml are of questionable physiologic significance (cf. 12), even though normal human plasma contains 130-160 units/ml of prothrombin (1,2).

STRUCTURES AND PROPERTIES

1. Prothrombin relationships. The covalent two-chain product of prothrombin activation, α-thrombin, is the enzyme form with high clotting and most other biologic activities (1, 2). The isolated human enzyme (M_r 36,600) consists of its 36-residue A chain (M_r 4,600) and 259 residue B chain (M_r 32,000). Now that the completed amino acid sequences have been reported for bovine and human prothrombins, it is apparent that the NH_2-terminal nonenzymic half (Fragment F1.2 moiety) and the CO_2H-terminal enzymic half (thrombin moiety) of this proenzyme are structurally unrelated (Fig. 4). The nonenzymic half contains the two so-called "kringle structures," which are each formed by three sets of disulfide bridges (Fig. 4a) and are homologous to the five "kringle structures" comprising the NH_2-terminal nonenzymic heavy-chain portion of plasminogen (3, 4). Unlike the NH_2-terminus of plasminogen, that of prothrombin begins with a peptide segment which precedes the first "kringle structure" and contains the ten vitamin K-dependent γ-carboxyglutamate residues. These residues explain the vitamin K biosynthetic dependence of prothrombin (c.f. coagulation Factors VII, IX, and X and other proteins) and account for its unique divalent metal binding properties, as well as the requirement for Ca^{2+} in its biologic activation. The divalent metal binding properties of prothrombin enable its isolation by adsorption with barium salts (see above). In contrast to the NH_2-terminal half, the prothrombin CO_2H-terminal half, corresponding to the thrombin B chain, is homologous with other serine proteases, notably the pancreatic digestive enzymes (3-5). The contrasting biologic functions of the prothrombin halves are reflected not only in their amino acid sequences but also in their distinctly different properties (Table 2).

2. Thrombin A chain. Since the thrombin A chain corresponds to the position peptides released from activation of the pancreatic serine proteases, it may be considered to be an activation peptide. However, its amino acid sequence is not homologous with those of the pancreatic enzymes, and it is covalently attached to the homologous enzyme moiety (thrombin B chain) by a disulfide bridge, so that the A chain must be considered a part of the functional enzyme (Figs. 1, 2, 4). Compared with that of bovine α-thrombin the A chain of the isolated human enzyme is missing a 13-residue NH_2-terminal peptide (see above). Its removal occurs autocatalytically by cleavage of the human enzyme at the arginine which replaces Lys_{13} of the bovine A chain (15, 16). In the formation of bovine β- and γ-thrombins, the 13-residue NH_2-terminal peptide is lost, in addition to a 9-residue CO_2H-terminal peptide (8). In contrast, no evidence has been obtained for the latter cleavage in human thrombins (2, 58), and all forms appear to share the same A chain (Fig. 1).

Comparison of the amino acid sequences of bovine and human thrombins indicates that the residues adjacent to the A/B-chain disulfide bridge are conserved. On the other hand, substitutions occur to either side of these conserved segments in

TABLE 2 Human Prothrombin Fragment $F_{1.2}$ and α-Thrombin Properties

Property	Fragment $F_{1.2}$ (Refs. 10, 12)	α-Thrombin (Refs. 1, 2, 6, 7, 111)
Polypeptides	One	Two (A + B)
Amino acid residues	273	295 (36 + 259)
Molecular weight	~35,000	36,600 (4,600 + 32,000)
Absorption coefficient at 280 nm, pH ~7 ($ml\ mg^{-1}\ cm^{-1}$)	1.29	1.73
Water solubility (mg/ml)	>1	<0.3 Increases with salt concentration
pH stability	Broad range	~5-10.3 Precipitates at pH 5 Catalytic optimum pH ~8.3
Thermal stability	100 (15 min)	~51 ($T_{½}$ 5 min, pH 8.3, IO) Precipitates with denaturation; salt-dependent
Autolytic stability	Stable	Autolysis depends on concentration, pH, temperature, and solute/solvent effects
Adsorption properties	Group IIa salts (γ-carboxyglutamic acids)	Negatively charged and hydrophobic surfaces/resins
Immunochemical properties	Predominant immunogenic determinants	Unrelated
Biologic properties	Activation peptide cleaved to F_1 and F_2	Bioregulatory protease

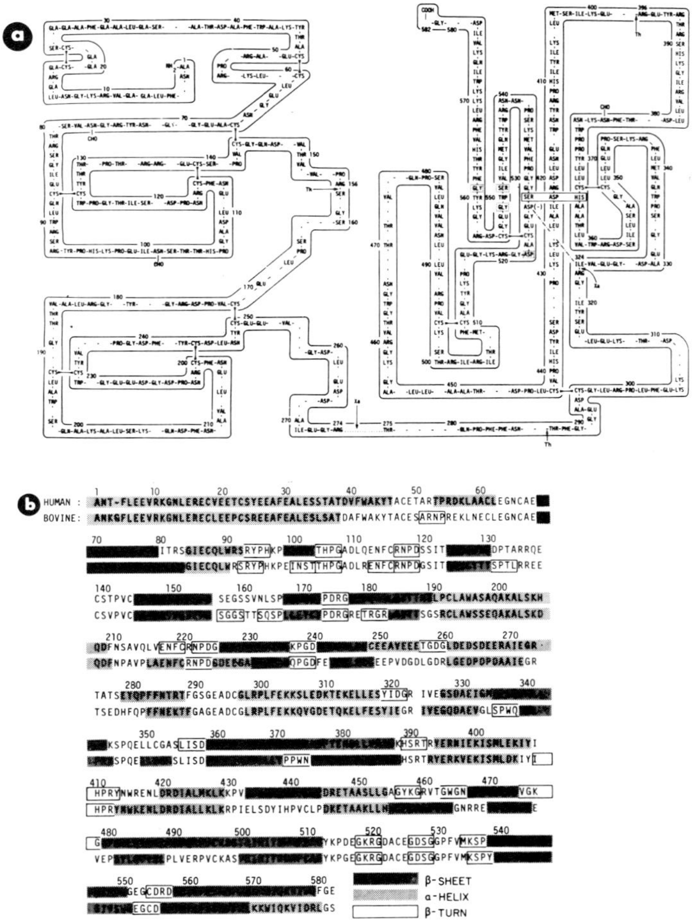

Fig. 4. Structural comparisons of human and bovine prothrombins. Data are based on the reported sequences for the human (6, 7, 10) and bovine (3, 4) zymogens and are selected for greatest homologies, where uncertain residues occur (117). a) The two halves of prothrombin are drawn with connecting disulfide bridges and carbohydrate attachments (CHO) established for the bovine zymogen (3, 4). Only the conserved residues are shown where spacings indicate substituted residues. Cleavage sites in the generation of human α-thrombin are shown by arrows for the Factor Xa cleavages (Xa) and the thrombin cleavages (Th). Residues comprising the charge relay system in thrombin are boxed; those of the activation salt bridge are joined by a line-dot line; and those forming the primary binding site are dotted rectangles. The overall prothrombin structure is drawn to illustrate the proximity of these active-site residues. b) Linear amino acid sequences and predicted peptide structures are compared for the two prothrombins. Predicted peptide structures are based on the Chou and Fasman method (148). Residues 1-156 correspond to Fragment F_1, 157-273 to Fragment F_2, 274-323 to the thrombin A chain, and 324-582 to the B chain.

both the A and B chains. These substitutions occur in clusters (Fig. 2), suggesting that the peptide segments are of lesser structural importance. One of the major clusters occurs between the disulfide bridge and CO_2H-terminus of the A chain and extends through the NH_2-terminus of the B chain. Since this portion derives from the zymogen, which contains one of the two Factor X_a cleavage sites, it undoubtedly represents an accessible or surface region in prothrombin (Fig. 4). Similarly, the substitution clusters surrounding the other Factor X_a cleavage site at the CO_2H-terminus of Fragment $F_{1.2}$ and the NH_2-terminus of the A chain (including the missing 13-residue F_3 peptide) must also occur in surface regions (Fig. 3). This further suggests that both the NH_2- and CO_2H-termini of the A chain have little structural importance to thrombin, whereas the central disulfide bridge segment may be of considerable importance.

The A/B-chain disulfide bridge in thrombin replaces the "serine loops" disulfide bridge found in the pancreatic serine proteases (2-7). The conserved peptide segments in this region may thus contribute to the conformational stability of the thrombin B chain (Fig. 2). However, the thrombin active-site serine (Ser_{205}) is not stabilized by the disulfide bridge of the pancreatic enzymes. This may be related to certain differences between thrombin and homologous proteases, such as the instability of thrombin at low pH (Ref. 2). On the other hand, the proximity of the A chain to the thrombin active site is predicted by homologies with the pancreatic enzymes, and this proximity has been shown by the labeling of the thrombin A chain with 1.7-nm exosite affinity-labeling reagent. Since the A chain labels to the same extent in both α- and γ-thrombins, its relative location does not change with B-chain fragmentation and loss of accompanying clotting activity (57-59).

3. <u>Thrombin B chain</u>. Unlike the thrombin A chain, the larger B chain is homologous with the pancreatic serine proteases (2-7). Residues comprising the charge relay system (His_{43}, Asp_{99}, and Ser_{205}) and the activation salt bridge (Ile_1 and Asp_{204}) are located in widely separated portions of the B chain, whereas residues homologous to those involved in substrate binding for the pancreatic enzymes are clustered within the CO_2H-terminal segment (Fig. 2). Residues contiguous with these active-site residues, like those surrounding disulfide bridges, are the same in both bovine and human thrombins.

A short conservative peptide contains the salt bridge Ile_1 and is followed by a variable peptide segment. The latter appears to represent a continuation of the replacement cluster of the A chain CO_2H-terminus (see above). This variable segment is then followed by a long conservative segment containing the "histidine loops." This segment is of major importance because it contributes the charge relay His_{43} (Ref. 116), and, by homologies with the pancreatic enzymes, constitutes a "hair-pin peptide" which forms the central core of the enzyme (129, 130). As such, it should contribute substantially to noncovalent structural stability, and may explain why the B_1 fragments of β- and γ-thrombins are retained by noncovalent association (Figs. 1 and 2) unless subjected to dissociating conditions (e.g., SDS, urea, etc.).

Beyond this disulfide bridge, but still within the conserved histidine segment, is the carbohydrate attachment site. No counterpart is found in the related pancreatic enzymes. The thrombin carbohydrate side chain has no known biologic function, and large portions of it can be removed without destroying clotting activity (131). Nevertheless, it contains labile sialic acid residues (6), which may account for the isoionic heterogeneity of otherwise homogeneous human α-thrombin (1, 2). The carbohydrate side chain is of further interest, since it must be attached to a surface residue in prothrombin to permit its biosynthetic elaboration, and must also be exposed in thrombin to enable enzymic removal (cf. 131). In pancreatic enzymes, a surface peptide extends from the "histidine loop" core and wraps around the back of the enzyme turning inward to contribute the aspartic acid of the charge relay system (129, 130). In the corresponding thrombin segment, a few substitutions occur between the carbohydrate attachment site and Asp_{99} but this entire peptide is notably conservative (Fig. 2). This thrombin segment

TABLE 3 Molecular Weights of [^{14}C]DFP-Labeled Chains of Human Thrombins[a]

Thrombin	Nonreduced				Reduced			
form	M_r	Chains	ΔM_r	Chains	M_r	Chains	ΔM_r	Chains
α	(38,500 ± 700)[b] 36,600 ± 1,000[c]	A + B	--	--	32,000 ± 2,000	B	--	--
β	~28,000	A + B_2	~8,600	B_1	23,000 ± 2,000	B_2	9,000 ± 2,800	B_1
γ	~12,000	B_4	~16,000 ~11,400[d]	A + B_3 B_3	12,500 ± 2,000	B_4	10,500 ± 2,800	B_3

[a]Molecular weights determined from isotope distribution following electrophoresis in SDS polyacrylamide gels (1, 58).

[b]Nonreduced α-thrombin migrate abnormally.

[c]Sum of reduced A (M_r 4,600 ± 200) and B (M_r 32,000 ± 1,000) chains.

[d]The A + B_3 difference (ΔM_r ~16,000) less the A chain (M_r 4,600).

contains an unusually high content of arginines and lysines, the spacing of which suggests that it might form a positively charged surface region. Thrombin notably binds to negatively charged surfaces (e.g., glass), and cationic exchange resins (e.g., CG-50 resin) are used in its purification (see above). That this arginine/-lysine-rich segment is highly conserved might suggest that it has an underlying significance, such as forming salt bridges within the zymogen.

The arginine/lysine-rich segment moreover contains sites which are cleaved to form β-thrombins (2, 8). In the human system, formation of β-thrombin is prerequisite for forming γ-thrombin (1, 2, 29), implying that conformational shifts occur upon cleavage within the arginine/lysine-rich segment. It is now known that cleavage occurs at more than one site for β-thrombin, giving rise to more than one subform of β-thrombin (Fig. 3; see above). However, the [^{14}C]DFP-labeled Ser_{205} fragments of the respective forms coelectrophorese in SDS polyacrylamide gels (Table 3). Thus, the B_1 fragments containing His_{43} may vary in size as the consequence of additional cleavages (117), similar to those cleavages originally described for bovine thrombin (116). Whether the initial cleavage produced by trypsin is the same one that occurs during autolysis is not known, but is is apparent that trypsin can generate at least two forms of β-thrombin (Fig. 3). It is of interest that hirudin complexing with α-thrombin not only prevents autolytic degradation according to substrate depletion but also prevents tryptic conversion to β- and γ-thrombins (hirudin does not inhibit trypsin, Ref. 111). This implies that hirudin binding masks the prerequisite cleavage site or causes a conformational shift to render it inaccessibile (111).

Following the charge relay Asp_{99} is a variable cluster which precedes the conserved A/B-chain disulfide bridge segment at the center of the B chain (Fig. 2). This conservative segment is of structural importance not only because of the disulfide bridge, but also because the attached A chain is located in proximity to the active site (see above). Exosite affinity labeling experiments have shown that B_1 fragments, as well as the A chain, of β- and γ-thrombins are labeled (58), suggesting that extended active-site regions of this fragment may also be in proximity to the A chain. Since the A chain is joined to the B_3 fragment in γ-thrombin (B_2 in β-thrombin, Figs. 1 and 2), the B chain segment surrounding the disulfide bridge is either inaccessible to the reagent or does not contain reactive residues for the labeling reagent.

The conserved A/B-chain attachment segment is followed by a long segment which contains the majority of the residues which differ between bovine and human B chains. This segment notably includes the cleavage site for human γ-thrombin, which has been tentatively located at positions 154-155 (Ref. 2), in agreement with [^{14}C]DFP-labeling patterns (Table 3). Since Lys_{154} in the human chain (7) is replaced by Glu_{154} in the bovine B chain (3), human γ-thrombin does not have a bovine counterpart. The unique feature of human γ-thrombin is that its B-chain fragmentation separates not only the residues comprising the charge relay system but also the activation salt bridge (Figs. 1 and 2). This form, like β-thrombin, must be held together by noncovalent associations in order to retain enzymic activity. The relatively large amounts of γ-thrombin made by carrying tryptic conversion essentially to completion (see above) has enabled the study of this form (2, 29, 40, 54-59, 62, 73, 77, 91, 94, 101, 115).

The CO_2H-terminal third of the B chain has relatively few substitutions (Fig. 2). This portion contains the two remaining disulfide bridges and the remaining active site residues. The latter includes the active site Ser_{205}, the activation salt bridge Asp_{204}, and the residues believed to participate in substrate binding. The presence of these residues in the portion of the B chain corresponding to the B_4 fragment of γ-thrombin may explain why α-, β-, and γ-thrombin behave similarly with small molecule substrates and inhibitors, despite their gross differences in clotting activities (2). In order to retain similar catalytic efficiencies with simple substrates, the functional residues of β- and γ-thrombins must remain in their proper orientations. It is apparent that the noncovalent core structure of thrombin is of major importance for the functional enzyme.

4. Thrombin structural stability. Loss of clotting activity of α-thrombin can result from adsorption, denaturation, and/or proteolytic degradation. Of these, adsorption, such as to negatively charged or hydrophobic surfaces, is primarily a technical problem in handling thrombin preparations (1, 51). However, it also has practical implications for "biocompatible materials" used in medical devices (e.g., dialysis machines) and may have biological counterparts (e.g., thrombin adsorption by fibrin clots and cellular surfaces). If adsorbed thrombin is inactive, whereas the desorbed enzyme is reactivated, then perturbation of equilibria becomes important. Such enzyme inactivation is perhaps analogous to processes governing solubility and those involved in denaturation.

Denaturation is characterized by loss of enzymic activities without change in the enzyme covalent structure. As such, denaturation may be reversible, partially reversibile, irreversible, or even differential (e.g., nonparallel changes in activities). Freeze-thaw denaturation of human α-thrombin may be an example of partial differential denaturation (cf. 1, 2). Low ionic-strength and low pH denaturation occurs with precipitation of the enzyme and is essentially irreversible. Thrombin is, however, very soluble in 1 M acetic acid but is completely inactive and precipitates upon removal or titration of the acid (1, 6, 50). Contrastingly, human α-thrombin does not precipitate above pH 9, where there is a sharp loss of clotting and esterase activities (half loss at pH 10.3), accompanied by a marked increase in tyrosine exposure (1). Below this pH boundary condition, however, the enzyme undergoes increasing autolytic degradation with increased pH (see below).

Thermal denaturation occurs rapidly above 40°C with associated precipitation and complete loss of enzymic activities without changes in the electrophoretic behavior in SDS polyacrylamide gels. Such denaturation depends upon solute-solvent conditions, such as individual salts and their concentrations (2). In increasing concentrations of Group Ia chlorides (except for >1.5 M LiCl), human α-thrombin becomes more stable, correlating with the cation lyotropic numbers for increasing water structure (111). Since NMR spectra for $^{23}Na^+$ and $^{85}Rb^+$ have indicated that they have low binding affinities for α-thrombin (K_d = 0.28 and 0.39 M, respectively), it is doubtful that their binding contributes directly to enzyme stability (132). In contrast, increasing concentrations of Group IIa chlorides decrease thermal stability, suggesting that these divalent cations may interact with thrombin to reduce its structural stability (also Li^+ at high concentrations, 111, 132). Regardless of the salt, the half extrapolated inactivation temperatures have a common intercept at zero ionic strength ($T_{1/2}$ = 51 ± 0.7°C for 5 min heating in 10 salts, Refs. 2, 111).

Whereas NaCl increases thermal stability, $NaNO_3$ decreases it, demonstrating that anions as well as cations alter denaturation processes (Fig. 5). The half inactivation temperatures of α- and γ-thrombins in the various salts essentially parallel one another, suggesting that similar salt effects are exerted on the two thrombin forms. That γ-thrombin is less stable (5 min $T_{1/2}$ = 41°C at zero ionic strength) is consistent with its noncovalent structure (Fig. 1). Estimates of thermal stabilities indicate that the noncovalent form is about 12.5 kJM^{-1} less stable than the covalent form (494 kJM^{-1} for 0.36 M NaCl). This is presumably an estimate of the energy necessary to hold the catalytic apparatus of γ-thrombin intact.

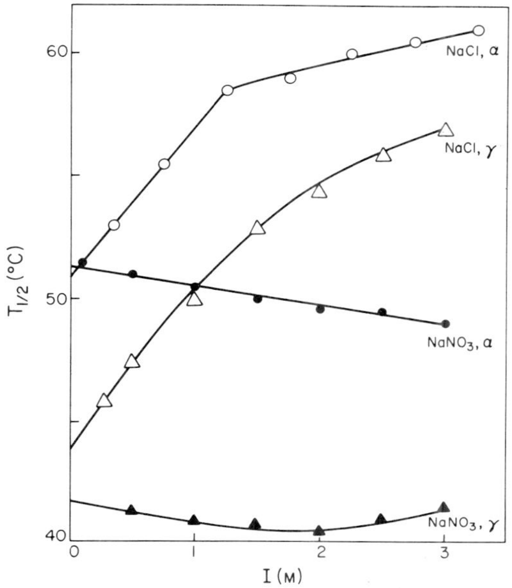

Fig. 5. Thermal denaturation of human α- and γ-thrombins in a stabilizing (NaCl) and denaturing ($NaNO_3$) salt. Samples of 20 μM enzyme were incubated at various temperatures for 5 min in varying salt concentrations buffered with 10 mM Tris at pH 8.3 and containing 5 mg/ml of PEG 6,000 to prevent thrombin surface adsorptions. The samples were subsequently quenched in an ice bath, and their relative activities with 1 mM TAME were measured by pH-stat in 0.15 M NaCl, pH 8.3. Temperatures ($T_{\frac{1}{2}}$ °C) for half initial activity are plotted with respect to salt concentrations.

The reduced structural stability of γ-thrombin can also be demonstrated with protein dissociating agents. With Ser_{205} conjugated spin labels (cf. 55, 56), the mobility of the labels increases; the half maximal changes occur in approximately 1 and 3 M urea or 0.4 and 1 M guanidine HCl for γ- and α-thrombins, respectively (133). When TAME hydrolysis activity is measured in urea, much higher transition concentrations are observed (~2 and ~4 M for γ- and α-thrombin, resp.). Renaturation of thrombin from high urea concentrations (e.g., 3.5 or 6.0 M) can be shown by dilution and measuring regained activity. The α-thrombin regains its initial TAME activity within 2-5 min, whereas γ-thrombin requires 6 to 24 hours. On the other hand, α-thrombin does not regain its full clotting activity (e.g., <50% from 6 M urea), suggesting differential renaturation (133).

Degradation of α-thrombin (i.e., proteolytic fragmentation of the B chain; see above), can occur autocatalytically or by limited proteolysis with trypsin (and to much lesser extents with plasmin or Factor Xa, Ref. 2). It is characterized by the loss of clotting activity, but retention of most activities with small-molecule substrates and inhibitors (Table 4). The loss of clotting activity parallels the conversion of α- to β- and subsequently to γ-thrombins. This can be quantitated by the ratios of [^{14}C]DFP-labeled chains upon electrophoresis in SDS polyacrylamide gels (cf. Table 3). Within the boundary conditions for denaturation, thrombin autolysis increases with the square of the active enzyme concentration, as well as pH, temperature, and certain solute concentrations (2, 111). The square relationship for the enzyme concentration results from the fact that thrombin is both the catalyst and the substrate. Although autolysis is relatively

TABLE 4 Human α- and γ-Thrombin Interactions with Synthetic Substances

Compound	Parameter	α-Thrombin	γ-Thrombin	Ref.
TAME	K_m (μM)	10.4 ± 1.1	10.0 ± 0.2	111
Tos-Arg-OMe	k_{cat} (sec^{-1})	3.52 ± 0.35	2.41 ± 0.05	
BAEE	K_m (μM)	41	40	94
Bz-Arg-OEt	k_{cat} (sec^{-1})	30	30	
S-2160	K_m (μM)	77	148	94
Bz-Phe-Val-Arg-pNA	k_{cat} (sec^{-1})	49	24	
Proflavine	K_m (μM) λ 466 nm	7.0 ± 0.6	8.5 ± 1.1	111

insignificant at pH 6, which is used to stabilize thrombin preparations (see above), it becomes significant as the pH approaches that for optimal catalytic efficiency (pH 8.0-8.5). Because thermal denaturation becomes important at 37°C in the presence of certain salts, autolysis at pH 8.3 has been studied at room temperature (23°C). In direct contrast to their effects on thermal stability, increasing concentrations of Group Ia chlorides (except for LiCl) enhance autolytic degradation, whereas Group IIa chlorides (and LiCl) have inhibitory effects (2, 111). For the Group Ia cations (other than Li^+), the autolytic rate correlates with lyotropic number, indicating that their effects are due to ordering of water structure (see above). On the other hand, the K_ms and k_{cat}s for α-thrombin hydrolysis of TAME correlate inversely with the cation lyotropic numbers, whereas the k_{cat}/K_m ratios are unaffected (decreased deacylation rate, k_3; Refs. 111, 132). These effects suggest that salts may alter thrombin catalysis by decreasing the accessibility of water. This could promote protein-protein interactions, as required for the autolytic process, and/or could cause protein conformational changes which render the cleavage sites more susceptible to autolytic degradation (132).

Knowledge of the conditions which affect thrombin stability is important for understanding its enzymic integrity and for carrying out meaningful experiments (cf. Table 1). One of the hazards of highly active α-thrombin preparations at high protein concentrations is their inherent instability. The effects of concentration are perhaps best illustrated by α-thrombin half lives (pH 8.3, 23°C): 2-3 days for approximately 1 mg/ml concentrations in 0.75 M NaCl vs. approximately 50 min for 10-12 mg/ml solutions reconstituted from $(NH_4)_2SO_4$ precipitates (111).

5. Thrombin active-site regions. In the absence of a three-dimensional crystallographic structure for α-thrombin, active-site structural features must be inferred from the pancreatic serine proteases and from the geometries of substrates and inhibitors. Like other proteases with arginine and/or lysine specificities, thrombin must have a primary cationic binding site. By homology with trypsin, this site is in proximity to the functional residues of the charge relay system (His , Asp_{99}, and Ser_{205}) and has an aspartic acid counterion (Asp204 in Figs. 2 and 4). This site not only binds and/or accommodates the arginine and lysine side chains of susceptible peptide bonds but also binds benzamidine and related compounds. Simple cations are not effective competitive inhibitors of thrombin (e.g., butylamine, K_i = 155 mM; 2-aminoethylbenzene, K_i = 82 mM); benzylamine (K_i = 55 mM) and phenylguanidine (K_i = 12.4 mM) are relatively poor inhibitors, unlike benzamidine (K_i = 0.75 mM) and p-chlorobenzylamine (K_i = 0.93 mM) (Fig. 6). Benzamidine is a planar compound; its amidine cation and benzene moieties are in resonance

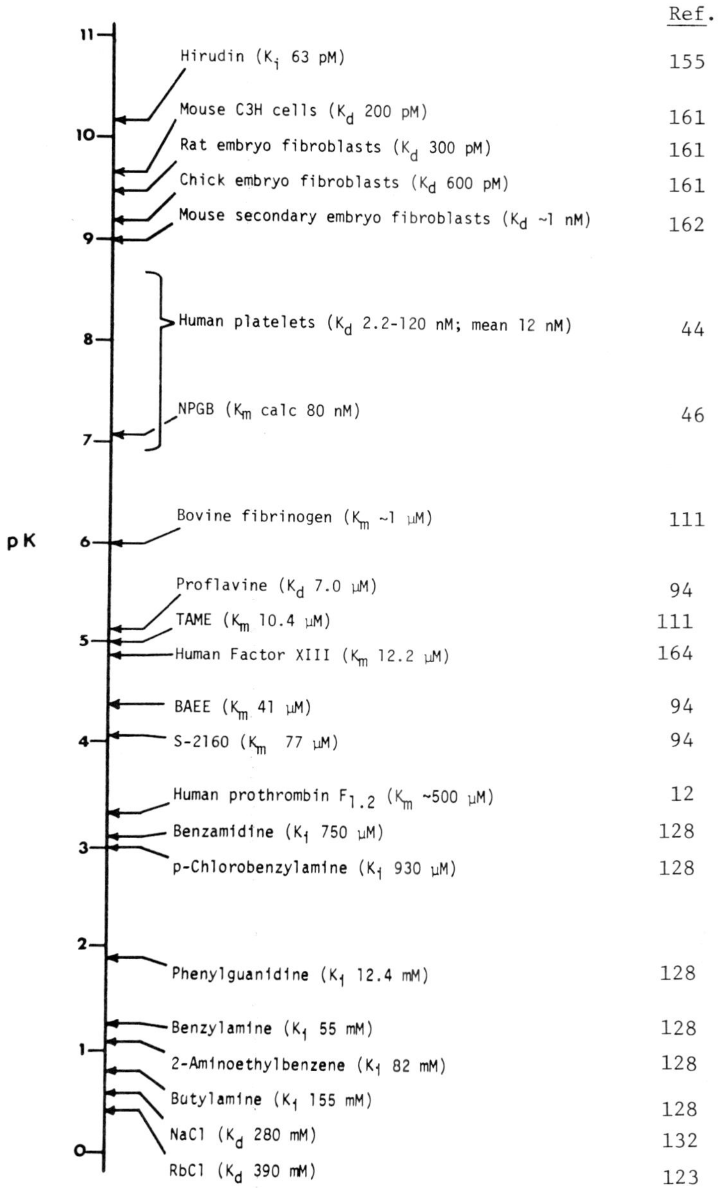

Fig. 6. Relative binding affinities of human α-thrombin. Binding affinities are expressed as pKs, the negative log of K_i, K_d, or K_m values.

conjugation with one another, and both are believed to contribute to binding. Both *meta* and *para* substituted side chains on benzamidine greatly enhance binding properties through additivity of secondary binding interactions, and these are among the more potent competitive synthetic inhibitors known (e.g., micromolar K_is, Refs. 58, 134, 135). The high potency of dansylarginine-4-ethylpiperidine amide and related compounds (136, 137) is also attributable to secondary binding interactions outside the classical active-site region (see below).

The potency of certain inhibitors, such as p-amidinophenylpyruvic acid (138), is accounted for by interactions with the catalytic apparatus (e.g., "transition state analogous"). Active-site titrants, such as NPGB (124), form semi-stable acyl-enzyme intermediates (e.g., slow deacylation rates, k_3) and are thus very effective inhibitors (Fig. 6). Inhibitors such as DFP, PMS, Ser_{205} spin labels and fluorescent probes (55, 56, 91) take advantage of the chemical reactivity of the active-site serine. Classical affinity-labeling reagents, such as TLCK (116), as well as exosite affinity-labeling reagents (57-59), are analogous to competitive inhibitors in that they initially form reversible active-site complexes, but subsequently react to form a covalent bond with the enzyme. These reagents react selectively because of their localization within the enzmye and their reactive substituents. The titrant NPGB may thus be considered an affinity-labeling reagent, as well as a "deacylation rate-limiting substrate."

From comparing ligand properties, it has become apparent that good inhibitor ligands are by and large poor substrate ligands, and vice versa. For example, benzamidine is a much better thrombin inhibitor than phenylguanidine (see above); p-amidinobenzoate ethyl ester behaves as an inhibitor (K_i = 2.3 mM), whereas p-guanidinobenzoate ethyl ester is a substrate (128). In contrast to NPGB, p-nitrophenyl-p'-amidinobenzoate is not a titrant substrate for thrombin (K_m 102 μM, k_{cat} = 0.0024 sec^{-1}), although it is a titrant for trypsin (K_m 0.1 μM, k_{cat} = 0.007 sec^{-1}; Ref. 128). Bulky substituents on the guanidino group of NPGB greatly decrease the reactivity with thrombin much more than with trypsin or chymotrypsin (28). This has suggested that the cationic binding site region of thrombin has a more limited bulk tolerance or cannot readily adapt to ligand substitutions (2).

Whereas NPGB can be considered an arginine ester analogue, the corresponding lysine ester analogue NPMT is an "acylation (k_2)-rate-limiting substrate" with thrombin in contrast to with trypsin or plasmin (32, 46). That is, NPMT binds thrombin with approximately the same affinity as NPGB but it is acylated only 1/60 as fast (46). Such differences in reactivity further emphasize the importance of geometric considerations between the ligand cation and the susceptible carbonyl bond for active site binding and catalytic cleavage, respectively. Decreasing structural rigidity and hydrophobicity of ligands lessens the affinity of thrombin for substrates and inhibitors (128).

The lack of an absolute requirement for cationic ligand is illustrated by the fact that N_α-benzyloxycarbonyl-L-tyrosine p-nitrophenyl ester is a good substrate for thrombin, as well as for chymotrypsin, trypsin, plasmin, Factor Xa, and complement Cls (57, 139). This ester is more readily hydrolyzed by thrombin than the corresponding phenylalanine ester (140), suggesting contributions from the phenolic hydroxyl group. In contrast to these aromatic amino acid esters, which are moderately stable at pH 8, the corresponding arginine ester cyclizes to form the lactam, and the lysine ester must be used at pH <6 to avoid spontaneous hydrolysis (139). The L-lysine ester is furthermore a better thrombin substrate than the p-nitrophenyl ester of ε-aminocaproic acid (128). This suggests that thrombin, like with other serine proteases (141), has a requisite for hydrogen binding through an α-amino group in an L configuration. However, the possible binding contributions of large α-amino blocking groups cannot be ignored (cf. 136, 137). In these regards, simple arginine substrates for thrombin (e.g., TAME and BAEE in Table 4), as well as tripeptide chromogenic substrates (e.g., S-2160 in Table 4), have relatively large α-amino blocking groups.

Like trypsin and chymotrypsin, but unlike plasmin (46), thrombin binds the acridine dye proflavine at or near its classical active site (30, 56, 142). Since human γ- compared with α-thrombin has only a very slightly lower affinity for the dye (Table 4), it is apparent that the proflavine binding site region is not significantly modified during B chain fragmentation nor is this region responsible for the loss of clotting activity (see above). Because active site-directed compounds, as well as protein inhibitors of thrombin (antithrombin-III and hirudin, see below) displace proflavine, its displacement can be used for monitoring active site reactions and measuring dissociation constants (30, 56, 67). Proflavine also causes immobilization of Ser_{205} conjugated spin labels, further localizing its binding within the vicinity of the classical active site. However, proflavine is displaced by indole and other apolar compounds (e.g., dioxane, tryptamine), which, unlike benzamidine, do not inhibit TAME hydrolysis but rather enhance hydrolysis in the absence of salt (56, 143). This has suggested that proflavine binding overlaps the benzamidine site as well as an apolar indole binding site (56). Such an apolar binding site beyond the catalytic active site may account for the tight binding of thrombin to p-chlorobenzylamido-ε-aminocaproyl agarose (6, 50). Moreover, secondary apolar sites are involved in the biologic specificity of thrombin (see below).

With Ser_{205}-conjugating spin-labeling reagents, six reagents have shown no detectable differences between α- and γ-thrombins, whereas five reagents display greater immobilization for γ-thrombin, and an ortho-substituted reagent does not label either thrombin (144). Failure of the ortho reagent to conjugate with Ser_{205} is consistent with the limited bulk tolerance exhibited by thrombin (see above). The differences found for the five reagents which distinguish between the two thrombins suggest that the portions of the active site of γ-thrombin are more constrained than these of α-thrombin (144). Such constraints in γ-thrombin might be the consequence of conformational changes from B chain fragmentation and must be at some distance from the active site region involved in TAME hydrolysis (Table 4) but must be sufficiently close to this region to immobilize certain Ser_{205} conjugated spin labels.

Differences between the two thrombins have also been detected in the rates of hydrolysis of certain tripeptide chromogenic substrates; γ-thrombin is a poorer enzyme (54, 77; S-2160 in Table 4). Although small, these differences may reflect differences between the thrombin forms in their interactions on the NH_2-terminal side of the susceptible arginine-anilide bond. On the other hand, the better thrombin substrates (S-2238 and Tos-Chromozym TH, Ref. 54) do not show significant differences, a finding which is of practical importance in the choice of chromogenic substrates for antithrombin-III measurements, because α-, β-, and γ-thrombins react similarly with antithrombin-III (115).

In contrast to their very similar reactivity with antithrombin-III (Table 5), γ-thrombin binds hirudin with a two to three orders of magnitude lower affinity than α-thrombin (101), consistent with the low specific clotting activity of γ-thrombin (e.g., <0.1-0.5% that of α-thrombin). The exceptionally high binding affinities of α-thrombin with hirudin and cellular receptors further implies that thrombin has unique protein binding/recognition sites which cannot be accounted for by its classical active site (see below).

BIOLOGIC SPECIFICITES AND FUNCTIONS

1. Susceptible bonds in proteins. As discussed in the preceding section, thrombin cleaves a variety of synthetic arginine and lysine ester or amide analogues in a manner similar to trypsin and related serine proteases. In general, thrombin is a less catalytically efficient enzyme than trypsin (2, 145). Evidence that the active site of thrombin has a more limited bulk tolerance than that of trypsin and is less able to adapt to substrate ligands has also been presented (see above). These active-site limitations may thus be related to the preferential specificity

TABLE 5 Human α- and γ-Thrombin Reactions with Proteins

Protein	Behavior	Parameter	α-Thrombin	γ-Thrombin	Ref.
Fibrinogen $\underline{M}_r$ ~330,000	Substrate	K_m (M) k_{cat} (sec^{-1})	~1 x 10^{-6} ~3	- -	111
Antithrombin-III $\underline{M}_r$ ~65,000	Covalent inhibitor	k_{2nd} (M^{-1} sec^{-1})	1.9 x 10^{-3}	2.0 x 10^{-3}	94
Antithrombin-III + heparin $\underline{M}_r$ ~65,000 + ~11,000		k_{2nd} (M^{-1} sec^{-1})	5.1 x 10^{-5}	4.9 x 10^{-5}	
Hirudin $\underline{M}_r$ ~7,400	Noncovalent inhibitor	K_i (M)	6.3 x 10^{-11}	1.2 x 10^{-8}	155

of thrombin for arginine vs. lysine bonds in protein substrates. Thrombin can hydrolyze 2-aminoethyl-S-cysteine-bonds in modified proteins but does so less efficiently than it cleaves lysine bonds (145).

More than 20 thrombin-susceptible bonds have been identified in proteins or peptides of known amino acid sequences. Tabulations of these sequences (113, 146, 147) have revealed no unique sequences or unique spacing patterns of individual amino acid residues. This absence of residue correlations led to the hypothesis (2, 58) that thrombin was a catalytically inefficient, trypsin-like enzyme, those apparent specificity resulted from the accessibility of certain bonds (e.g., the Aα-cleavage site in fibrinogen). It further led to the examination of the predicted secondary peptide structures (e.g., α-helix, β-sheet, β-turn, and random coil; Ref. 148) to determine if secondary rather than primary structures could explain thrombin specificity (149). Such structural analyses (up to 20 residues on either side of susceptible residues) predicted an incidence of 30-40% α-helix, on the NH_2-terminal side of susceptible arginines or lysines, correlating with the presence of hydrophobic residues. On the CO_2H-terminal side, up to 70% β-sheet was predicted immediately adjacent to the susceptible residues (149). Nevertheless, inspection of individual structures revealed no apparent restrictions for thrombin cleavage (see below).

Thrombin specificity traditionally has been thought of in terms of fibrinogen. The K_m for human α-thrombin with fibrinogen is in the micromolar range (Table 5), and fibrinogen ranks in the middle of the relative binding scale for the enzyme (Fig. 6). It is now established that α-thrombin hydrolyzes the Aα-chain of fibrinogen prior to the Bβ-chain and that the initial phase of clotting is attributable to the removal of fibrinopeptide A (Ref. 150). The predicted secondary structures of the Aα- and Bβ-chains are distinctly different. The former cleavage is adjacent to a random coil segment, and the latter, within an extended α-helix (149). The predicted Aα-chain structure begins with a random coil (Residues 1-4); this is followed by an α-helix (Residues 5-12) and then a short random coil (Residues 13-16) preceding the cleavage site. On the other side is a short β-turn segment (Residues 1-4 in the α-chain of fibrin), which is followed by a long random coil (Residues 5-16) and a subsequent β-turn segment (Residues 17-20...). The random coil segments neighboring are perhaps important since they should be flexible segments, which allow access to the cleavage site. The α-helix and β-turn segments might on the other hand contribute to substrate binding properties. The preference of thrombin for readily accessible bonds is further suggested by the high incidence of proline immediately preceding a susceptible residue (cf. Table 1 in Ref. 147). These prolines are primarily preceded by random coil segments or disrupt preceding α-helix segments in their predicted secondary peptide structures (149). Proline is furthermore a cyclic, apolar amino acid residue, which may thus participate in binding (see above), and such adjacent prolines (or proline analogues) have been incorporated into the design of certain chromogenic substrates (cf. 54, 147). In these regards, the Bβ-cleavage site of fibrinogen has neither a preceding random coil segment nor an adjacent proline, which may be why fibrinopeptide B is less readily cleaved by thrombin than is fibrinopeptide A.

The overall importance of the secondary and tertiary structure of proteins for thrombin susceptibility is indicated by the finding that some bonds which are not hydrolyzed in the intact protein are cleaved after disruption of disulfide bridges (146). Widely separated, noncontiguous residues are most likely involved in thrombin interaction with proteins. Although it might be concluded from the foregoing that thrombin is not an uniquely specific enzyme, the very high binding affinities of α-thrombin with hirudin and cellular receptors (Fig. 6; see below) suggest that this enzyme indeed has unique protein binding or recogntion sites, which are presumably involved in its biological proteolytic functions.

2. Protein inhibitors. Unlike trypsin, plasmin, Factor Xa, and other proteases, thrombin is not inhibited by protease inhibitors of plant origin or by certain pancreatic inhibitors. For example, the pancreatic inhibitor, aprotinin, which inhibits trypsin and plasmin, does not inhibit the clotting or TAME hydrolytic activity of human α-thrombin or the TAME activity of γ-thrombin, nor does it prevent the autolytic decomposition of α-thrombin (111). In contrast, hirudin, the anticoagulant from leeches (151), does not inhibit trypsin or plasmin and is the most potent thrombin inhibitor known (Fig. 6). However, crude hirudin preparations may contain an inhibitor of trypsin or plasmin (152), and caution therefore should be exercised in assessing thrombin functions with impure hirudin preparations.

Of the protease inhibitors in plasma, antithrombin-III (heparin cofactor) is correlated with thrombotic tendencies (153). This inhibitor is a plasma protein (M_r ~65,000) which reacts with a variety of proteases (e.g., activated coagulation factors, plasmin, etc.) to form complexes stable in SDS. It is unique among protein inhibitors in that its reactions are accelerated by heparin. Human α- and γ-thrombins react in an identical manner with antithrombin-III (94), in the presence or absence of heparin (Table 5). The γ-thrombin complex, moreover, electrophoreses in SDS polyacrylamide gels at the rate predicted for the size of an acyl complex with the Ser_{205} Fragment B (Figs. 1 and 2); this complex is dissociated in SDS by hydroxylamine (94). Human β-thrombin, which is essentially devoid of clotting activity like γ-thrombin, reacts with antithrombin-III in the fashion as α- and γ-thrombins, hence antithrombin-III measurements obtained from thrombin inhibition assays with synthetic chromogenic substrates are not affected by the relative concentration of the noncoagulant forms in the thrombin preparation used. By contrast, clotting inhibition assays give antithrombin-III values that are decreased in proportion to the content of β- and γ-thrombins relative to that of coagulant α-thrombin (115). The portion of the thrombin active site required for the reaction with antithrombin-III, therefore, is less extensive than that involved in fibrinogen recognition and/or hirudin binding (Table 5). Since antithrombin-III forms a covalent, presumably an acyl, complex with thrombin (94), this inhibitor might be thought of as the protein equivalent of an affinity-labeling reagent or active-site titrant (see above). Furthermore, since its reaction with thrombin is irreversible, it can inactivate the affinity enzyme even though it may initially combine with less affinity than do high-affinity noncovalent inhibitors (e.g., hirudin).

Heparin nonstoichiometrically enhances the reaction of antithrombin-III with thrombin, suggesting that heparin has a catalytic function (41, 42). Heparin may thus accelerate the formation of an initial, dissociable complex, or alternatively, of the nondissociable complex. Regardless of the kinetic mechanism, the finding that heparin increases the second order reaction rates with both α- and γ-thrombins to essentially the same extents (Table 5) supports other evidence that heparin interacts with antithrombin-III (41). Antithrombin-III can therefore be considered a general protease inhibitor whose bioregulation of thrombin and other plasma protease is enhanced by heparin (153).

In contrast to antithrombin-III, which is about twice the size of thrombin and is a general protease inhibitor that forms covalent complexes, hirudin is approximately one-fifth the size of thrombin and is an exceptionally specific inhibitor of thrombin, forming noncovalent complexes (151, 154, 155). Hirudin inhibits TAME hydrolysis by human α-thrombin stoichiometrically (1:1, although stoichiometry may be slightly nonlinear at high inhibitor to enzyme ratios); it has a functional M_r of 7,400 (M_r 7,100 calc. from amino acid sequence in Ref. 154; Ref. 155). Hirudin furthermore displaces proflavine from α-thrombin, demonstrating its involvement with the active site (155). Because of the exceedingly high binding affinity (Table 5), hirudin reactions with α-thrombin are essentially irreversible, although the complex is disrupted by SDS or heating. Since hirudin is very resistant to denaturation (151), it can be recovered with high specific activity from its complex by denaturing the thrombin moiety (155).

In contrast, hirudin was observed to be a less effective inhibitor of γ- than α-thrombin in assessing biologic functions (156, 157). Subsequent studies showed that hirudin inhibition of TAME hydrolysis by α-thrombin displays significant substrate concentration dependence, indicative of the dissociability of the complex (101). The K_i obtained for competitive inhibition of α-thrombin, moreover, is about 200-times that for γ-thrombin (Table 5). Hirudin was also found to complex with both α- and γ-thrombins which were conjugated with spin labels at Ser_{205}, where it caused very pronounced immobilization of the spin labels with α-thrombin and almost as much with γ-thrombin (111, 133). These experiments thus demonstrate that hirudin binding does not require the intact catalytic apparatus, yet it binds in proximity to the active site. The reduced binding affinity of γ-thrombin for hirudin (compared with α-thrombin), which correlates with loss of clotting activity, indicates that the hirudin binding site corresponds to a major portion of the fibrinogen recognition site. In this regard, nitrated human α-thrombin, which retains esterase activity but not clotting activity, also has a reduced hirudin binding affinity similar to that of γ-thrombin (158).

3. Cellular receptors. High purity α-thrombin is one of the most potent platelet stimuli known (65). Although its stimulatory activity is difficult to compare with that of collagen, it is qualitatively more potent on a weight basis. However, it is unquestionably more potent than trypsin or other proteases and several times more potent than ADP or epinephrine on a molar basis (34, 36). The binding of ^{125}I-labeled human α-thrombin to platelets is characterized by rapid equilibrium processes, a continuum of high to low affinity binding sites exist (44, 49, 65), and interaction with platelet membrane components (80, 97). The active enzyme is required for stimulation, indicating that thrombin has a catalytic function (cf. 34, 65). It not only causes the more generally studied aggregation and release reactions but also induces protein phosphorylation (35), endoperoxide production (70, 75), and arachidonic acid metabolism (82). These three metabolic events may represent a sequence of events, but the thrombin initiated step most likely preceding them is unknown.

Human γ-thrombin also stimulates platelets but has less stimulatory activity than α-thrombin (62, 159). This has enabled studies on platelet reactions in whole blood without the interference from the clotting of fibrinogen (62). Furthermore, γ-thrombin has been used to provide evidence for a specific step in the secretory pathway between thrombin binding and adenyl cyclase regulation (159).

Although active-site derivatized α-thrombin (e.g., with DFP, PMSF, MSF, TLCK) does not stimulate platelets, such thrombin derivatives bind platelets similarly to the active enzyme (114, 159, 160), and PMS-thrombin is similarly displaced from the high affinity sites with hirudin (160). In this regard, the binding affinity of α-thrombin for hirudin is about two orders of magnitude greater than for high-affinity platelet receptors (Fig. 6), and it follows that hirudin should displace the enzyme if a common portion of its protein binding site is involved. Preliminary attempts to identify receptors by photoaffinity labeling of [^{125}I] α-thrombin have indicated that a protein component ($\underline{M}_r$ ~35,000, reduced) from platelet associates with thrombin (123, 159).

In parallel with its action on platelets, α-thrombin is the most potent of the proteases known to stimulate cellular proliferation of mitogenically responsive chick embryo fibroblasts in tissue culture (38, 56, 93). Although α-thrombin is now established to be mitogenic with several cell lines (38, 76, 84, 86, 88, 92, 93, 102, 123, 161), some types of cell are not stimulated (e.g., bovine vascular endothelial cells), whereas others (e.g., human vascular endothelial cells), are synergistically stimulated in the presence of specific growth factors (85, 99). The resistance of vascular endothelial cells to the thrombin-induced mitogenic responses (85, 99) may be an important evolutionary adaptation since these cells are likely to be exposed to thrombin generated during hemostatic events. On the other hand, endothelial cell prostacyclin production is stimulated by thrombin (107), and such thrombin initiated processes, like those in platelets, may be important in hemostasis.

In serum-free media, addition of α-thrombin at very low concentrations is sufficient to intiate embryonic fibroblast proliferation (88, 93). Although the enzyme is internalized by cultured fibroblasts (76, 84, 102), α-thrombin covalently conjugated to inert beads (in the absence of detectable leakage from such beads) will induce the mitogenic response, suggesting that a catalytic process at the cellular surface is sufficient (92, 162). Inactivation of α-thrombin (e.g., with DFP, PMSF, etc.) destroys mitogenic activity, and high-affinity receptors for thrombin have been demonstrated on chick fibroblasts and other cells (123, 161). These receptors, in contrast to those of platelets, behave as a single class for individual cell lines and have higher binding affinities, approaching that of α-thrombin for hirudin (Fig. 6). Photoaffinity labeling experiments have further shown that human α-thrombin associates with protein component ($\underline{M}_r$ ~43,000; reduced) from mouse secondary embryonic cells (123). This receptor component is presumably analogous to that of platelets. Since hirudin displaces [^{125}I]α-thrombin from mitogenically responsive cells (123, 161), as well as from platelet high-affinity sites (160), it appears that a common region of thrombin is involved in specific protein binding and cellular recognition.

4. Biologic mechanisms. How thrombin, an enzyme with restricted proteolytic specificity, initiates cellular responses can only be hypothesized. It might, upon contact with cellular surfaces (e.g., receptors), generate protein fragments (e.g., low $\underline{M}_r$ growth factors, hormones), which stimulate cellular activities. Alternatively, it might activate a proenzyme (e.g., possibly the receptor itself), whose enzyme might in turn activate another proenzyme to effect an amplification cascade. If such cellular enzyme cascades exist, they are probably more primitive than those of the fluid phase of blood coagulation. The coagulation cascades may have reached maximum evolutionary complexity, so that compensating addition and subtraction of components occur. Nevertheless, the coagulation cascades seem to represent a redundancy of membrane-associated events with more primitive cellular origins. The ability to isolate individual components of the coagulation system has enabled the unraveling of various pathways which have become models for understanding protease bioregulation (cf. 9).

As the final protease in preclotting events, α-thrombin is generated in higher concentrations than preceding coagulation enzymes. This is the consequence of the higher concentration of its circulating zymogen (prothrombin) and the amplification by preceding events in its activation cascade. In further contrast with other coagulation enzymes, thrombin seemingly has a broad spectrum of biological activities which are not restricted to blood clotting. Whether the derivative β- and γ-thrombins are formed in vivo is not known; however, it is apparent that only α-thrombin has high activity in clotting and most other biologic systems.

The diverse biologic activities of thrombin, the spectrum of proteins known to be hydrolyzed by this enzyme, and the lack of definitive residue requirement surrounding susceptible bonds in such proteins have suggested that thrombin is not an absolutely specific protease but rather is one with reduced enzymic capability. The fact that trypsin is, in general, a more effficient enzyme than thrombin further suggests that thrombin is a bioregulatory enzyme which as such does not require the catalytic diversity of a digestive enzyme. Bond accessibility in proteins may therefore be of major importance in governing thrombin specificity. On the other hand, the high-affinity binding of α-thrombin with hirudin and cellular receptors strongly suggest that the enzyme has a unique protein binding or recognition site which is distinct from its classical active site. The combination of such a binding/recognition site and the apparently limited catalytic efficiency of the enzyme may create the highly effective biologic specificity of α-thrombin.

ADDENDUM

Since this manuscript has been in preparation, additional studies are known to have been published. These should be included among those utilizing preparations and cited for contributions in understanding thrombin functions (164-168).

ACKNOWLEDGEMENTS

We are indebted to numerous persons who, over the past ten years, have conveyed information regarding the use, performance, and problems encountered with thrombin preparations. This information has been invaluable (see communications cited and those in Refs. 1, 2). We are also indebted to various fractionators (see Ref. 1) for the Fraction III pastes used in producing human thrombin. In particular, we would like to acknowledge the large amounts of materials obtained during the past five years from Armour Pharmaceutical Company, Kankakee, Illinois, through Drs. Robert. M. Silverstein and Fred Feldman.

The present studies were supported in part by National Institutes of Health Research Grants AM 17351 (D. H. Bing), HL 13160 (J. W. Fenton II) and HL 14992 (R. D. Feinman); National Science Foundation Grant PCM 76-18640 (L. J. Berliner); American Heart Association National Grant 76-981 (L. J. Berliner); and American Heart Association chapter grants from the Northeastern New York Chapter (J. W. Fenton II) and the Michigan Chapter (D. A. Walz). Both D. H. Bing and L. J. Berliner are recipients of Established Investigatorship Awards from the American Heart Association; R. D. Feinman is recipient of the Career Development Award HL 00406 from the National Institutes of Health.

ABBREVIATIONS

Those used are: ADP, adenosine diphosphate; TAME, N_α-tosyl-L-arginine methyl ester; BAEE, N_α-benzoyl-L-arginine ethyl ester; DEAE, diethylaminoethyl; DFP, diisopropylfluorophosphate; MSF, methylsulfonyl fluoride; NPGB, p-nitrophenyl-p'-guanidinobenzoate; NPMT, p-nitrophenyl-α-amino-p-toluate; PEG, polyethylene glycol; PMSF, phenylmethylsulfonyl fluoride; SP, sulfopropyl; SDS, sodium dodecyl sulfate; and TLCK, N_α-tosyl-L-lysine chloromethyl ketone. Abbreviations used for equilibrium and kinetic constants are: K_d, dissociation constant; K_i, inhibition constant; K_m, apparent Michaelis-Menten constant; k_{cat}, catalytic rate constant; and k_{2nd}, second order rate constant.

REFERENCES

1. J. W. Fenton, II, M. J. Fasco, A. B. Stackrow, D. L. Aronson, A. M. Young, and J. S. Finlayson, Human thrombins. Production, evaluation, and properties of α-thrombin, J. Biol. Chem. 252, 3587-3598 (1977).
2. J. W. Fenton, II, B. H. Landis, D. A. Walz, and J. S. Finlayson, Human thrombins, Chemistry and Biology of Thrombin (R. L. Lundblad, J. W. Fenton, II, and K. G. Mann, eds.) Ann Arbor Science Publishers, Michigan, pp. 43-70 (1977).
3. S. Magnusson, T. E. Petersen, L. Sottrup-Jensen, and H. Claeys, Complete primary structure of prothrombin: isolation, structure, and reactivity of ten carboxylated glutamic acid residues and regulation of prothrombin activation by thrombin, Proteases and Biological Control (E. Reich, D. B. Rifkin, and E. Shaw, eds.) Cold Spring Harbor Laboratory, New York, pp. 123-149 (1975).
4. S. Magnusson, L. Sottrup-Jensen, T. E. Petersen, G. Dudek-Wojciechowska, and H. Claeys, Homologous "kringle" structures common to plasminogen and prothrombin. Substrate specificity of enzymes activating prothrombin and plasminogen. Proteolysis and Physiological Regulation (D. W. Ribbons and K. Brew, eds.)

Miami Winter Symposia, Vol. 11, Academic Press, New York, pp. 203-238 (1976).

5. J. Elion, M. R. Downing, R. J. Butkowski, and K. G. Mann, Structure of human thrombins: comparison with other serine proteases, Chemistry and Biology of Thrombin (R. L. Lundblad, J. W. Fenton, II, and K. G. Mann, eds.) Ann Arbor Science Publishers, Michigan, pp. 97-111 (1977).
6. A. R. Thompson, D. L. Enfield, L. H. Ericsson, M. E. Legaz, and J. W. Fenton, II, Human thrombin partial primary structure, Arch. Biochem. Biophys. 178, 356-367 (1977).
7. R. J. Butkowski, J. Elion, M. R. Downing, and K. G. Mann, The primary structure of human prothrombin 2 and α-thrombin, J. Biol. Chem. 252, 4942-4957 (1977).
8. H. S. Kingdon, C. M. Noyes, and R. L. Lundblad, Some aspects of the primary structure of alpha, beta, and gamma thrombins, Chemistry and Biology of Thrombin, R. L. Lundblad, J. W. Fenton, II, and K. G. Mann, eds.) Ann Arbor Science Publishers, Michigan, pp. 91-96 (1977).
9. H. Neurath and K. A. Walsh, Role of proteolytic enzymes in biological regulation (a review), Proc. Natl. Acad. Sci. USA 73, 3825-3832 (1976).
10. D. A. Walz, D. Hewett-Emmett, and W. H. Seegers, Amino acid sequence of human prothrombin fragments 1 and 2, Proc. Natl. Acad. Sci. USA 74, 1969-1972 (1977).
11. D. L. Aronson, A. P. Ball, B. R. Franza, Jr., T. E. Hugli, and J. W. Fenton, II, unpublished data.
12. D. L. Aronson, L. Stevan, A. P. Ball, B. R. Franza, Jr., and J. S. Finlayson, Generation of the combined prothrombin activation peptide (F 1.2) during the clotting of blood and plasma, J. Clin. Invest. 60, 1410-1418 (1977).
13. A. P. Ball, J. Fenton, D. L. Aronson, B. R. Franza, and A. M. Young, Purification and characterization of activation fragments F_1 and F_2 from human prothrombin. Thromb. Diath. Haemorrh. (Stuttgart) 34, 591 (1975).
14. D. A. Walz, D. Hewett-Emmett, and W. H. Seegers, Primary structure of the amino terminal (vitamin K-dependent) region of human prothrombin, Life Sci. 20, 79-84 (1977).
15. M. R. Downing, R. J. Butkowski, M. M. Clark, and K. G. Mann, Human prothrombin activation, J. Biol. Chem. 250, 8897-8906 (1975).
16. D. A. Walz, D. Hewett-Ennett, J. Reuterby, and W. H. Seegers, Human thrombins amino acid sequence of the autocatalytically removed 13 reside A peptide, Thromb. Res. 9, 289-292 (1976).
17. S. Chandra, N. U. Bang, and C. Marks, Radiolabeled ATIII as a probe for the detection of activation of blood coagulation in vivo, Thromb. Res. 9, 9-23 (1976).
18. D. G. Deutsch and E. T. Mertz, Plasminogen, purification from human plasma by affinity chromatography, Science 170, 1095-1096 (1970).
19. G. F. Lanchantin, J. A. Friedmann, and D. W. Hart, Two forms of human thrombin: isolation and characterization, J. Biol. Chem. 248, 5956-5966 (1973).
20. E. J. Cohn, L. E. Strong, W. L. Hughes, Jr., D. J. Mulford, J. M. Ashworth, M. Melin, and H. L. Taylor, Preparation and properties of serum plasmin proteins. IV. A system for the separation into fractions of the protein and lipoprotein components of biological tissues and fluids, J. Am. Chem. Soc. 68, 459-475 (1946).
21. J. L. Oncley, M. Melin, D. A. Richert, J. W. Cameron, and P. M. Gross, Jr., The separation of the antibodies, isoagglutinins, prothrombin, plasminogen, and β -lipoprotein into subfractions of human plasma, J. Am. Chem. Soc. 71, 541-550 (1949).
22. R. B. Pennell, Fractionation and isolation of purified components by precipitation methods, The Plasma Proteins (F. W. Putnam, ed.) Academic Press, New York, Vol. 1, pp. 9-50 (1960).
23. Minimum Requirement; Dried Thrombin, Division of Biological Standards, National Institutes of Health, Bethesda, Maryland, 2nd Revision (September 4, 1946).
24. D. L. Aronson, personal communication (1976).

25. K. D. Miller and W. H. Copeland, Isolation of human thrombin, Proc. Soc. Exp. Biol. Med. 111, 512-514 (1962).
26. K. D. Miller and W. H. Copeland, Human thrombin: isolation and stability, Exp. Mol. Pathol. 4, 431-437 (1965).
27. J. W. Fenton, II, W. P. Campbell, J. C. Harrington, and K. D. Miller, Large-scale preparation and preliminary characterization of human thrombin, Biochim. Biophys. Acta 229, 26-32 (1971).
28. M. J. Fasco and J. W. Fenton, II, Specificity of thrombin. I. Esterolytic properties of thrombin, plasmin, trypsin, and chymotrypsin with N -substituted guanidino derivatives of p-nitrophenyl-p'-guanidinobenzoate, Arch. Biochem. Biophys. 152, 802-812 (1973).
29. M. J. Fasco and J. W. Fenton, II, Human α-, $\beta_{(T)}$-, $\gamma_{(T)}$-thrombins. Fed. Proc. 34, 355 (1975).
30. E. H. H. Li, C. Orton, and R. D. Feinman, The interaction of thrombin and heparin. Proflavin dye binding studies, Biochemistry 13, 5012-5017 (1974).
31. D. A. Mills and S. Karpatkin, The molecular components and fibrinolytic activity of human thrombin, Haemostasis 2, 181-188 (1974).
32. T. J. Ryan and J. W. Fenton, II, Thrombin, plasmin, and trypsin specificities for arginyl and lysyl p-nitrophenyl ester analogs, Fed. Proc. 34, 681 (1975).
33. A. R. Thompson, L. H. Ericsson, and D. L. Enfield, Partial primary structure of human thrombin, Circulation 49, Suppl. III, 292 (1974).
34. T. C. Detwiler, B. M. Martin, and R. D. Feinman, Stimulus-response coupling in the thrombin-platelet reaction, Ciba Foundation Symp. 35, 77-100 (1975).
35. R. M. Lyons, N. Stanford, and P. W. Majerus, Thrombin-indueced protein phosphorylation in human platelets, J. Clin. Invest. 56, 924-936 (1975).
36. B. M. Martin, R. D. Feinman, and T. C. Detwiler, Platelet stimulation by thrombin and other proteases, Biochemistry 14, 1308-1314 (1975).
37. S. A. Silverberg and Y. Nemerson, The control of prothrombin conversion. Kinetic control by mechanism inherent in two activation pathways. Biochemistry 14, 2636-2644 (1975).
38. J. M. Buchanan, L. B. Chen, and B. R. Zetter, Protease-related effects in normal and transformed cells, Cancer Enzymology (J. Schultz and F. Ahmad, eds.) Miami Winter Symp., Academic Press, New York, Vol. 12, pp. 1-24 (1976).
39. B. A. Cottrell and R. F. Doolittle, Amino acid sequences of lamphrey fibrinopeptides A and B and characterization of the junctions split by lamphrey and mammalian thrombins, Biochim. Biophys. Acta 453, 426-438 (1976).
40. R. B. Credo, M. J. Fasco, and J. W. Fenton, II, Activation of fibrin-stabilizingfactor (factor XIII) by human α- and γ-thrombins, Fed. Proc. 35, 648 (1976).
41. E. H. H. Li, J. W. Fenton, II, and R. D. Feinman, The role of heparin in the thrombin-antithrombin III reaction, Arch. Biochem. Biophys. 175, 153-159 (1976).
42. E. H. H. Li, J. W. Fenton, II, and R. D. Feinman, Kinetics of the antithrombin-thrombin reaction and the role of heparin, Circulation 54, Suppl. II, 121 (1976).
43. A. P. Lobo, J. D. Wos, S. M. Yu, and W. B. Lawson, Active site studies of human thrombin and bovine trypsin: peptide substrates, Arch. Biochem. Biophys. 177, 235-244 (1976).
44. B. M. Martin, W. Wasiewski, J. W. Fenton, II, and T. C. Detwiler, Equilibrium binding of thrombin to platelets, Biochemistry 15, 4886-4893 (1976).
45. E. B. Ong and A. J. Johnson, Protamine, a substrate, for thrombolytic agents and enzymes of similar specificity, Analyt. Biochem. 75, 568-582 (1976).
46. T. J. Ryan, J. W. Fenton, II, T-L Chang, and R. D. Feinman, Specificity of thrombin: evidence for selectivity in acylation rather than binding for p-nitrophenyl-α-amino-p'-toluate, Biochemistry 15, 1337-1341 (1976).
47. F. Sachs and R. D. Feinman, Spin-labeled human platelets, Thromb. Res. 8, 43-50 (1976).
48. M. C. Shuman and P. W. Majerus, The measurement of thrombin in clotting blood by radioimmunoassay, J. Clin. Invest. 58, 1249-1258 (1976).
49. M. C. Shuman, D. M. Tollesen, and P. W. Majerus, The binding of human and bovine thrombin to human platelets, Blood 47, 43-51 (1976).

50. A. R. Thompson, High affinity binding of human and bovine thrombins to p-chlorobenzylamido-ε-aminocaproyl agarose, Biochim. Biophys. Acta 422, 200-209 (1976).
51. W. Wasiewski, M. J. Fasco, B. M. Martin, T. C. Detwiler, and J. W. Fenton, II, Thrombin adsorption to surfaces and prevention with polyethylene glycol 6,000, Thromb. Res. 8, 881-886 (1976).
52. G. Albrecht-Buehler and L. B. Chen, Local inhibition of centripetal particles transport where LETS protein patterns appear on 3T3 cells, Nature 266, 454-456 (1977).
53. T. Aogaichi and G. W. E. Plaut, Assay of the esterase activity of thrombin, plasmin and trypsin with a chromogenic substrate p-nitro-benzyl-p-toluene-sulfonyl-L-arginine, Thrombo. Haemostas. (Stuttgart) 37, 253-261 (1977).
54. N. U. Bang and L. E. Mattler, Thrombin sensitivity and specificity of three chromogenic peptide substrates, Chemistry and Biology of Thrombin (R. L. Lundblad, J. W. Fenton, II, and K. G. Mann, eds.) Ann Arbor Science Publishers, Michigan, pp. 305-310 (1977).
55. L. J. Berliner and Y. Y. Shen, Probing active site structure by spin-label (ESR) and fluorescence methods, Chemistry and Biology of Thrombin (R. L. Lundblad, J. W. Fenton, II, and K. G. Mann, eds.) Ann Arbor Science Publishers, Michigan, pp. 197-216 (1977).
56. L. J. Berliner and Y. Y. L. Shen, Physical evidence for an apolar binding site near the catalytic center of human α-thrombin, Biochemistry 16, 4622-4626 (1977).
57. D. H. Bing, J. M. Andrews, and M. Cory, Affinity labeling of thrombin and other serine proteases with an extended reagent, Chemistry and Biology of Thrombin (R. L. Lundblad, J. W. Fenton, II, and K. G. Mann, eds.) Ann Arbor Science Publishers, Michigan, pp. 159-177 (1977).
58. D. H. Bing, M. Cory, and J. W. Fenton, II, Exo-site affinity labeling of human thrombins. Similar labeling of the A chain and B chain/fragments of clotting α- and nonclotting γ/β-thrombins, J. Biol. Chem. 252, 8027-8034 (1977).
59. D. H. Bing, J. W. Fenton, II, and M. Cory, Exo-site affinity labeling of human α-(clotting) and γ/β-(nonclotting) thrombin with m-[o-(2-chloro-5-sulfonyl-fluorophenylureido)phenoxybutoxy]benzamidine (m CP(PBA)-F), Thrombo. Haemostas. (Stuttgart) 38, 148 (1977).
60. J. M. Buchanan, L. B. Chen, T. Hamazaki, E. Lenk, and D. F. Waugh, The early development of fibrin clot structure, Chemistry and Biology of Thrombin (R. L. Lundblad, J. W. Fenton, II, and K. G. Mann, eds.) Ann Arbor Science Publishers, Michigan, pp. 263-273 (1977).
61. S. Chandra and N. U. Bang, Analysis of primary and secondary complexes between antithrombin III, thrombin and factor Xa, Chemistry and Biology of Thrombin (R. L. Lundblad, J. W. Fenton, II, and K. G. Mann, eds.) Ann Arbor Science Publishers, Michigan, pp. 421-429 (1977).
62. I. F. Charo, R. D. Feinman, and T. C. Detwiler, Interrelations of platelet aggregation and secretion, J. Clin. Invest. 60, 866-873 (1977).
63. L. B. Chen, R. C. Gudor, T-T. Sun, A. R. Chen, and M. W. Mosesson, Control of a cell surface major glycoprotein by epidermal growth factor, Science 197, 776-778 (1977).
64. R. W. Colman, J. Kuchibhotla, and A. D. Schreiber, Effects of heterologous antiplatelet antibody on human platelets: a new pathway to platelet alteration, Blood 50, 575-585 (1977).
65. T. C. Detwiler and W. W. Wasiewski, The equilibrium reaction of thrombin with platelets, Chemistry and Biology of Thrombin (R. L. Lundblad, J. W. Fenton, II, and K. G. Mann, eds.) Ann Arbor Science Publishers, Michigan, pp. 465-478 (1977).
66. V. H. Donaldson and J. Kleniewski, Kinin release from high molecular weight kinonogen, Fed. Proc. 36, 329 (1977).
67. R. D. Feinman, T-L. Chang, S. M. Wilson, and E. H. H. Li, Application of rapid kinetic methods to thrombin reactions with substrates and antithrombin III, Chemistry and Biology of Thrombin (R. L. Lundblad, J. W. Fenton, II, and

K. G. Mann, eds.) Ann Arbor Science Publishers, Michigan, pp. 217-232 (1977).
68. J. W. Fenton, II, J. S. Finlayson, M. J. Fasco, B. H. Landis, M. P. Zabinski, and D. L. Aronson, Human α-thrombin preparations, Thromb. Haemostas. (Stuttgart) 38, 147 (1977).
69. M-C. Guillin, D. L. Aronson, A. Bezeaud, D. Menache, N. Schiegel, and M. Amar, The purification of human carboxy prothrombin. Characterization of its derivatives after thrombin cleavage, Thromb. Res. 10, 223-233 (1977).
70. R. I. Handin and P. Bockenstadt, Modulation of platelet endoperoxide synthesis by thrombin, Chemistry and Biology of Thrombin (R. L. Lundblad, J. W. Fenton, II, and K. G. Mann, eds.) Ann Arbor Science Publishers, Michigan, pp. 507-518 (1977).
71. T. E. Hugli, Complement factors and inflammation: effects of α-thrombin on components C3 and C5, Chemistry and Biology of Thrombin (R. L. Lundblad, J. W. Fenton, II, and K. G. Mann, eds.) Ann Arbor Science Publishers, Michigan, pp. 345-360 (1977).
72. M. B. Hultin, F. S. London, S. S. Shapiro, and W. J. Yount, Heterogeneity of Factor VIII antibodies further immunochemical and biologic studies, Blood 49, 807-817 (1977).
73. L. Lorand and R. B. Credo, Thrombin and fibrin stabilization, Chemistry and Biology of Thrombin (R. L. Lundblad, J. W. Fenton, II, and K. G. Mann, eds.) Ann Arbor Science Publishers, Michigan, pp. 311-323 (1977).
74. A. B. Malik and H. Van der Zee, Thrombin induced pulmonary insufficiency, Thromb. Res. 11, 497-506 (1977).
75. A. J. Marcus, S. T. Silk, L. B. Safier, and H. L. Ullman, Superoxide production and reducing activity in human platelets, J. Clin. Invest. 59, 149-158 (1977).
76. B. M. Martin and J. P. Quigley, Binding and uptake of thrombin: possible role in the thrombin-induced mitogenesis of chick embryo fibroblasts, Chemistry and Biology of Thrombin (R. L. Lundblad, J. W. Fenton, II, and K. G. Mann, eds.) Ann Arbor Science Publishers, Michigan, pp. 531-550 (1977).
77. L. E. Mattler and N. U. Bang, Serine protease specificity for peptide chromogenic substrates, Thromb. Haemostas. (Stuttgart) 38, 776-792 (1977).
78. D. B. McKay, L. M. Kay, and R. M. Stroud, Preliminary crystallization and x-ray diffraction studies on human thrombin, Chemistry and Biology of Thrombin (R. L. Lundblad, J. W. Fenton, II, and K. G. Mann, eds.) Ann Arbor Science Publishers, Michigan, pp. 113-121 (1977).
79. S. Niewiarowski, E. P. Kirby, and K. Stacher, Thrombocytin - a novel platelet activating enzyme from Bothrops atrox venom, Thromb. Res. 10, 863-869 (1977).
80. D. R. Phillips and P. T. Azin, Platelet plasma membrane glycoproteins. Identification of a proteolytic substrate for thrombin, Biochem. Biophys. Res. Commun. 75, 940-947 (1977).
81. M. E. Rick and L. W. Hoyer, Thrombin activation of Factor VIII. The effect of inhibitors, Brit. J. Haematol. 36, 585-597.
82. S. Rittenhouse-Simmons and D. Deykin, The mobilization of arachidonic acid in platelets exposed to thrombin or Ionophore A23187, J. Clin. Invest. 60, 495-498 (1977).
83. S. S. Shapiro and D. B. Anderson, Thrombin inhibition of normal plasma. Chemistry and Biology of Thrombin (R. L. Lundblad, J. W. Fenton, II, and K. G. Mann, eds.) Ann Arbor Science Publishers, Michigan, pp. 361-374 (1977).
84. B. R. Zetter, L. B. Chen, and J. M. Buchanan, Binding and internalization of thrombin by normal and transformed chick cells, Proc. Natl. Acad. Sci. USA 74, 596-600 (1977).
85. B. R. Zetter and D. Gospodarowicz, The effect of thrombin on endothelial cell proliferation, Chemistry and Biology of Thrombin (R. L. Lundblad, J. W. Fenton, II, and K. G. Mann, eds.) Ann Arbor Science Publishers, Michigan, pp. 551-560 (1977).
86. B. R. Zetter, T-T. Sun, L. B. Chen, and J. M. Buchanan, Thrombin potentiates the mitogenic response of cultured fibroblasts to serum and other growth promoting agents, J. Cell. Physiol. 92, 233-240 (1977).

87. A. Bagdasarian and R. W. Colman, Subcellular localization and purification of platelet α-antitrypsin, Blood 51, 139-156 (1978).

88. J. B. Baker, J. B. Barsh, D. H. Carney, and D. D. Cunningham, Dexamethasone modulates binding and action of epidermal growth factor in serum-free cell culture, Proc. Natl. Acad. Sci. USA 75, 1882-1886 (1978).

89. P. G. Barton, Effects of a polyoxyethylene detergent (BRIJ 58) on platelet aggregation, release and clottivity, Biochim. Biophys. Acta 539, 98-113 (1978)

90. J. S. Bennett, R. F. Colman, and R. W. Colman, Identification of adenine nucleotide binding proteins in human platelet membranes by affinity labeling with 5'-p-fluorosulfonylbenzoyladenosine, J. Biol. Chem. 253, 7346-7354 (1978).

91. L. J. Berliner and Y. Y. L. Shen, Active site fluorescent labeled dansyl and anthraniloyl human thrombin, Thromb. Res. 12, 15-25 (1978).

92. D. H. Carney and D. D. Cunningham, Cell surface action of thrombin is sufficie to initiate division of chick cells, Cell 14, 811-823 (1978).

93. D. H. Carney, K. C. Glenn, and D. D. Cunningham, Conditions which affect initiation of animal cell division by trypsin and thrombin, J. Cell. Physiol. 95, 13-22 (1978).

94. T-L. Chang, R. D. Feinman, B. H. Landis, and J. W. Fenton, II, Antithrombin reactions with α- and γ-thrombins, Circulation 58, Suppl. II, 137 (1978).

95. L. B. Chen, A. Murray, R. A. Segal, A. Bushnell, and M. L. Walsh, Studies on intercellular LETS glycoprotein matrices, Cell 14, 377-391 (1978).

96. R. B. Credo, C. G. Curtis, and L. Lorand, Ca^{2+}-related regulatory function of fibrinogen, Proc. Natl. Acad. Sci. USA 75, 4234-4237 (1978).

97. H. Y. Chuang, S. F. Mohammad, and R. G. Mason, Affinity chromatographic demonstration of a thrombin binding protein from the platelet plasma membrane, Res. Commun. Pathol. Pharmacol. 21, 379-382 (1978).

98. A. E. Davis, III, R. D. Rosenberg, J. W. Fenton, II, D. H. Bing, F. S. Rosen, and C. A. Alper, Is Factor D of tha alternative pathway a fragment of thrombi J. Immunol. 120, 1771 (1978).

99. D. Gospodarowicz, K. D. Brown, C. R. Birdwell, and B. R. Zetter, Control of proliferation of human vascular endothelial cells. Characterization of the response of human umbilical vein endothelial cell to fibroblast. Growth fact epidermal growth factor, and thrombin, J. Cell. Biol. 77, 774-788 (1978).

100. C. Kettner and E. Shaw, Synthesis of peptides of arginine chloromethyl ketone Selective inactivation of human plasma kallikrein, Biochemistry 17, 4778-4784 (1978).

101. B. H. Landis, M. P. Zabinski, G. J. M. Lafleur, D. H. Bing, and J. W. Fenton, II, Human α- and γ-thrombin differential inhibition with hirudin, Fed. Proc. 37, 1445 (1978).

102. B. M. Martin and J. P. Quigley, Binding and internalization of I thrombin in chick embryo fibroblasts: possible role in mitogenesis, J. Cell. Physiol. 96, 155-164 (1978).

103. E. Mihalyi and J. W. Donovan, Role of calcium in a slow conformational change in fibrin, Fed. Proc. 37, 1443 (1978).

104. R. Nachman, R. Levine, and E. Jaffe, Synthesis of actin by cultured guinea pi mecakaryocytes. Complex formation with fibrin, Biochim. Biophys. Acta 543, 91-105 (1978).

105. M. J. Polley and R. Nachman, The human complement system in thrombin-mediated platelet function, J. Exp. Med. 147, 1713-1726 (1978).

106. M. E. Rick and L. W. Hoyer, Thrombin activation of factor VIII. II. A comparison of purified factor VIII and the low molecular weight factor VIII procoagulant, Brit. J. Haematol. 38, 107-119 (1978).

107. B. B. Weksler, C. W. Ley, and E. A. Jaffe, Stimulation of endothelial cell prostacyclin production by thrombin, trypsin, and the ionophore A23187, J. Clin. Invest. 62, 923-930 (1978).

108. J. C. Harrington, J. W. Fenton, II, and J. H. Pert, Precipitation of antigen-antibody complexes with water-soluble polymers: the "precipiplex" reaction, Immunochemistry 8, 413-421 (1971).

109. J. W. Fenton, II and M. J. Fasco, Polyethylene glycol 6,000 enhancement of the clotting of fibrinogen solutions in visual and mechanical assays, Thromb. Res. 4, 809-817 (1974).
110. A. P. Ball, R. B. Franza, and D. L. Aronson, The effect of plasmin on prothrombin structure and activity, Fed. Proc. 35, 805 (1976).
111. B. H. Landis and J. W. Fenton, II, unpublished data.
112. M. P. Zabinski and J. W. Fenton, II, unpublished data.
113. R. L. Lundblad, H. S. Kingdon, and K. G. Mann, Thrombin, Methods in Enzymology, Proteolytic Enzymes (L. Lorand, ed.) Academic Press, New York, Vol. 15, Part B, pp. 156-176 (1976).
114. S. F. Mohammad, personal communication (1978).
115. J. Fareed, H. L. Messmore, and J. W. Fenton, II, unpublished data.
116. G. Glover and E. Shaw, The purification of thrombin and isolation of a peptide containing the active center histidine, J. Biol. Chem. 246, 4594-4601 (1971).
117. D. A. Walz and J. W. Fenton, II, unpublished data.
118. R. H. Landaburu and W. H. Seegers, The acetylation of thrombin, Can. J. Biochem. Physiol. 37, 1361-1366 (1959).
119. R. L. Lundblad and J. H. Harrison, The differential effect of tetranitromethane on the proteinase and esterase activity of bovine thrombin, Biochem. Biophys. Res. Commun. 45, 1344-1349 (1971).
120. L. C. Uhteg and R. L. Lundblad, The modification of tryptophan in bovine thrombin, Biochim. Biophys. Acta 491, 551-557 (1977).
121. M. Sokolovshy, J. F. Riordan, and B. L. Vallee, Tetranitromethane. A reagent for the nitration of tyrosyl residues in proteins, Biochemistry 5, 3582-3589 (1966).
122. S. A. Sonder and J. W. Fenton, II, unpublished data.
123. D. D. Cunningham, personal communication (1978).
124. T. Chase, Jr. and E. Shaw, Comparison of the esterase activities of trypsin, plasmin, and thrombin on guanidinobenzoate esters. Titration of the enzymes, Biochemistry 8, 2212-2224 (1969).
125. V. H. Donaldson, personal communication (1977).
126. J. J. Capone, personal communication (1977).
127. B. L. Reamer and J. S. Finlayson, unpublished data.
128. T. J. Ryan and J. W. Fenton, II, unpublished data.
129. B. W. Matthews, P. B. Sigler, R. Henderson, and D. M. Blow, Three-dimensional structure of tosyl-α-chymotrypsin, Nature 214, 652-656 (1967).
130. R. M. Stroud, M. Krieger, R. E. Koeppe, II, A. A. Kossiakoff, and J. L. Chambers, Structure-function relationships in the serine proteases, Proteases and Biological Control (E. Reich, D. B. Rifkin, and E. Shaw, eds.) Cold Spring Harbor Laboratory, New York, pp. 13-32 (1975).
131. K. Skaug and T. B. Christensen, The significance of the carbohydrate constituents of bovine thrombin for the clotting activity, Biochim. Biophys. Acta 230, 627-629 (1971).
132. K. A. Koehler, B. H. Landis, and J. W. Fenton, II, unpublished data.
133. R. S. Bauer and L. J. Berliner, unpublished data.
134. F. Markwardt, H. Landmann, and P. Walsmann, Comparative studies on the inhibition of trypsin, plasmin, and thrombin by derivatives of benzylamine and benzamidine, Eur. J. Biochem. 6, 502-506 (1968).
135. J. D. Geratz and R. R. Tidwell, The development of competitive reversible thrombin inhibitors, Chemistry and Biology of Thrombin (R. L. Lundblad, J. W. Fenton, II, and K. G. Mann, eds.) Ann Arbor Science Publishers, Michigan, pp. 179-196.
136. S. Okamoto, A. Hijikata, K. Ikezawa, K. Kinjo, R. Kikumoto, S. Tonomura, and Y. Tamao, New series of synthetic thrombin-inhibitors (Om-inhibitors) having extremely potent and selective action, Thromb. Res. 8, Suppl. 2, 77-82 (1976).
137. F. G. Prendergast, M. E. Nesheim, M. R. Downing, and K. G. Mann, Approaches to fluorescence studies with thrombin, Chemistry and Biology of Thrombin (R. L. Lundblad, J. W. Fenton, II, and K. G. Mann, eds.) Ann Arbor Science Publishers, Michigan, pp. 233-244 (1977).

138. J. D. Geratz, p-Amidinophenylpyruvic acid: a new highly effective inhibitor of enterokinase and trypsin, Arch. Biochem. Biophys. 118, 90-96 (1967).
139. F. J. Kezdy, L. Lorand, and K. D. Miller, Titration of active centers in thrombin solutions. Standardization of the enzyme, Biochemistry 4, 2302-2308 (1965)
140. L. Lorand and J. L. G. Nilsson, Molecular approach for designing inhibitors to enzymes involved in blood clotting, Drug Design (E. J. Ariensiens, ed.) Academi Press, New York, Vol. III, pp. 415-447 (1972).
141. G. E. Hein and C. Niemann, Steric course and specificity of -chymotrypsin-catalyzed reactions II, J. Am. Chem. Soc. 84, 4495-4503 (1962).
142. K. A. Koehler and S. Magnusson, The binding of proflavin to thrombin, Arch. Biochem. Biophys. 160, 175-184 (1974).
143. B. Conery and L. J. Berliner, unpublished data.
144. T-L. Chang, R. S. Bauer, and L. J. Berliner, unpublished data.
145. D. T. Elmore, The enzymic properties of thrombin and Factor Xa, Biochem. Soc. Trans. 1, 1191-1194 (1973).
146. W. H. Seegers, H. I. Hassouna, D. Hewett-Emmett, D. A. Walz, and T. J. Andary, Prothrombin and thrombin. Selected aspects of thrombin formation, properties, inhibition, and immunology, Semin. Thromb. Hemostasis 1, 211-283 (1975).
147. B. Blombäck, B. Hessel, D. Hogg, and G. Claesson, Substrate specificity of thrombin on proteins and synthetic substrates, Chemistry and Biology of Thrombin (R. L. Lundblad, J. W. Fenton, II, and K. G. Mann, eds.) Ann Arbor Science Publishers, Michigan, pp. 275-290 (1977).
148. P. Y. Chou and G. D. Fasman, Conformational parameters for amino acids in helical, β-sheet and random coil regions calculated from proteins, Biochemistry 13, 211-222 (1974).
149. R. A. Marlar, D. A. Walz, J. W. Fenton, II, and W. H. Seegers, The secondary structure requirements for thrombin susceptible bonds, Am. Chem. Soc., Div. Biol. Chem., 174th Natl. Mtg., Abst. 99 (1977).
150. B. Blombäck, B. Hessel, D. Hogg, and L. Therkildsen, A two-step fibrinogen-fibrin transition in blood coagulation, Nature 275, 501-505 (1978).
151. F. Markwardt, Hirudin as an inhibitor of thrombin, Methods in Enzymology, Proteolytic Enzymes (G. E. Perlmann and L. Lorand, eds.) Academic Press, New York, Vol. XIX, pp. 924-932 (1970).
152. H. Fritz and K. Krejci, Trypsin-plasmin inhibitors (Bdellins) from leeches, Methods in Enzymology, Proteolytic Enzymes (L. Lorand, ed.) Academic Press, New York, Vol. XLV, Part B, pp. 797-806 (1976).
153. P. C. Harpel and R. D. Rosenberg, α_2-Macroglobulin and antithrombin-heparin cofactor: modulators of hemostatic and inflammatory reactions, Prog. Hemostasis Thromb. 3, 145-189 (1976).
154. D. Bagdy, E. Barbas, L. Graf, T. E. Petersen, and S. Magnusson, Hirudin, Methods in Enzymology, Proteolytic Enzymes (L. Lorand, ed.) Academic Press, New York, Vol. XLV, Part B, pp. 669-678 (1976).
155. B. H. Landis, J. W. Fenton, II, and F. Markwardt, unpublished data.
156. T. C. Detwiler, personal communication (1976).
157. A. E. Davis, III and D. H. Bing, unpublished data.
158. B. H. Landis, S. A. Sonder, and J. W. Fenton, II, unpublished data.
159. M. A. Shuman, personal communication (1978).
160. T. C. Detwiler, personal communication (1978).
161. J. F. Perdue, personal communication (1978).
162. J. P. Quigley, personal communication (1978).
163. J. E. Folk and J. S. Finlayson, The ε-(γ-glutamyl)lysine crosslink and the catalytic role of transglutaminases, Adv. Protein Chem. 31, 1-133 (1977).
164. D. H. Carney and D. D. Cunningham, Role of specific cell surface receptors in thrombin-stimulated cell division, Cell 15, 1341-1349 (1978).
165. J. Koutts, P. N. Walsh, E. F. Plow, J. W. Fenton, II, B. N. Bouma, and T. S. Zimmerman, Active release of human platelet Factor VIII-related antigen by adenosine diphosphate, collagen, and thrombin, J. Clin. Invest. 62, 1255-1263 (1978).

166. S. Rittenhouse-Simmons and D. Deykin, The activation by Ca^{2+} of platelet phospholipase A. Effects of dibutyryl cyclic adenosine monophosphate and 8-(N,N-dimethylamino)octyl-3,4,5-trimethoxybenzoate, Biochim. Biophys. Acta 543, 409-422 (1978).
167. S. W. Tam and T. C. Detwiler, Binding of thrombin to human platelet plasma membranes, Biochim. Biophys. Acta 543, 194-201 (1978).
168. M. J. Weinstein and D. Deykin, Quantitative abnormality of an A α chain molecular weight form in the fibrinogen of cirrhotic patients, Brit. J. Haematol. 40, 617-730 (1978).

THE ROLE OF METAL IONS IN BLOOD COAGULATION

Bruce Furie and Barbara C. Furie
Hematology Division, Tufts-New England Medical Center
Tufts University School of Medicine, Boston, MA 02111

Calcium is a cofactor that is required in many physiologically important processes, including hemostasis. Metal ions participate in the intracellular metabolism of platelets, in events in plasma in which platelets play an active role, and in the enzymatic steps involved in blood coagulation. A summary of some of the reactions and features of the hemostatic mechanism which are of interest to this discussion is shown in Table I.

Table 1 Metal Ions and Hemostasis

1. Platelet aggregation is calcium-dependent
2. High calcium content of platelets; stored in dense granules
3. Calcium is released from platelets during platelet aggregation
4. Vitamin K-dependent blood coagulation proteins bind metal ions
5. Interaction of the vitamin K-dependent blood coagulation proteins and membrane surfaces is metal-dependent
6. γ-Carboxyglutamic acid, with unique metal binding properties, is present in the vitamin K-dependent blood coagulation proteins
7. Activity of factor XIIIa (fibrin stabilizing factor) is calcium-dependent
8. Early pathway of platelet prostaglandin synthesis is calcium-dependent
9. Structural transitions in the vitamin K-dependent proteins are induced by metal ions
10. Free calcium concentration in plasma is 1 mM

Current models of blood coagulation and platelet plug formation suggest the following description, with special emphasis of the role of calcium. As a response to tissue injury and abrasion of the vascular endothelium, platelets collect and adhere to the altered vascular surface. Platelets, containing high concentrations of calcium within their dense granules, undergo a series of reactions which can be observed biochemically and morphologically. Calcium is released into the local environment and these cells undergo calcium-dependent aggregation. The activation of the blood coagulation proteins leading to the formation of a fibrin clot also involves calcium. For instance, zymogen activation of the vitamin K-dependent proteins is metal-dependent. These proteins contain γ-carboxyglutamic acid and bind metal ions. Furthermore, the interaction of these proteins with platelet membrane surfaces requires metal ions. The generation of thrombin leads to the conversion of fibrinogen to fibrin. Activated factor XIII in the presence of calcium covalently cross-links fibrin to stabilize the fibrin clot. Our own studies have focused upon the metal binding properties of the vitamin K-dependent blood coagulation proteins, the functional role of metal ions in promoting zymogen activation, and the structural role of metal ions in stabilizing tertiary and quaternary structure of the blood coagulation proteins. In particular, the structure-function relationship of γ-carboxyglutamic acid in these proteins has been investigated. The results of these studies will be summarized and emphasized.

Like many other calcium-binding proteins, the vitamin K-dependent blood coagulation proteins have a weak affinity for calcium. This property, as well as the absence of spectroscopically interesting magnetic and electronic characteristics of calcium, has precluded detailed biophysical investigation of these and other calcium binding proteins. Approximately a decade ago, Williams (1) and Birnbaum, Gomez, and Darnall (2) independently suggested the use of lanthanide ions as probes of the metal binding sites of calcium binding proteins. Lanthanide ions have ionic radii similar to calcium. These ions, like calcium, have a preference for oxygen ligands and interact with these ligands electrostatically. However, they demonstrate several important differences. First, they are tripositive and, as such, interact more tightly with metal binding sites in proteins than do dipositive calcium ions. Second, lanthanide ions have spectral properties which may be exploited for study of their interaction with proteins. Some of these ions are paramagnetic or diamagnetic; others are fluorescent or have absorption transitions in the visible region; still others are available as radioactive isotopes. Exploiting these properties a number of laboratories have employed lanthanide ions in the study of calcium binding proteins as chemical shift and broadening reagents in nuclear magnetic resonance spectroscopy, as fluorescence probes for fluorescence spectroscopy, as heavy metal atom derivatives for X-ray crystallography, and for radiometric studies of metal-protein interactions, for example. We have used many of these properties to examine the metal binding properties of the vitamin K-dependent blood coagulation proteins, factor X and prothrombin.

Factor X and prothrombin, plasma proteins with a molecular weight of 56,000 and 70,000 respectively, are zymogens of the trypsin-like serine proteases, activated factor X and thrombin. These proteins, as well as factor IX and factor VII, require vitamin K during synthesis for complete expression of functional activity (3). These proteins are synthesized in an inactive precursor form; in the absence of vitamin K or in the presence of vitamin K antagonists, these precursors circulate in plasma as glycoproteins which lack the ability to participate in blood coagulation. Under normal conditions a vitamin K-dependent hepatic carboxylase is responsible for posttranslational modification of some of the glutamic acid residues near the N-terminus of the precursors to form γ-carboxyglutamic acid (Fig. 1).

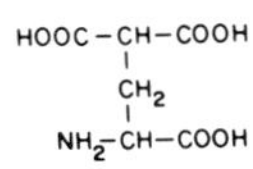

Fig. 1. γ-Carboxyglutamic Acid

This amino acid is found in the vitamin K-dependent blood coagulation proteins as well as other proteins. In the presence of metal ions, protein cofactors and membrane surfaces, these proteins may be converted enzymatically from an inactive zymogen to a serine protease.

Factor X and prothrombin have complex metal binding properties (for review, see (4)). Because of the relatively low affinity of these proteins for calcium, physical studies of the interaction of the vitamin K-dependent proteins and calcium have been difficult to interpret. However, trivalent lanthanide ions bind with greater affinity to these proteins than does calcium and facilitate the examination of the metal binding properties. Using lanthanide ions we have determined that bovine factor X contains two high affinity metal binding sites and many lower affinity metal binding sites (5). At least one of these sites is in close proximity of a tryptophan residue (5,6). Lanthanide ions, which compete directly with calcium for these sites, interact with these classes of sites with binding constants, K_D, of about 1 μM and 20 μM (5). The functional features of factor X differ in the presence of lanthanide ions compared to these features in the presence of calcium ions. Lanthanide ions cannot substitute for calcium in the metal-dependent activation of factor X by the coagulant protein from Russell's viper venom. However, they can facilitate metal-dependent protein complex formation of the venom protein and factor X.

Lanthanide ions have also been used to evaluate the metal binding properties of bovine prothrombin and derivatives associated with prothrombin activation. Like factor X, prothrombin has two high affinity metal binding sites and a larger number of lower affinity metal binding sites (7). Fragment 1, a proteolytic fragment of prothrombin representing the N-terminal one-third of prothrombin and containing the γ-carboxyglutamic acid residues, has metal-binding properties similar to prothrombin. Unlike the case for factor X, lanthanide ions can substitute for calcium in the metal-dependent activation of prothrombin by activated factor X in the presence of factor V and phospholipid vesicles. At optimal concentrations of Gd(III), for instance, the rates of thrombin generation are about 25% of that observed using calcium. Maximal rates of thrombin generation are seen employing 10 μM Gd(III) or 0.75 mM calcium. These studies have emphasized that lanthanide ions not only can substitute for calcium in the metal binding sites of this protein but can fulfill the functional role that calcium apparently plays.

But what is the relationship of γ-carboxyglutamic acid to bound metal ions? Indirectly, γ-carboxyglutamic acid has been implicated in metal binding. Observation that the precursor form of prothrombin which lacks γ-carboxyglutamic acid does not bind metal ions has suggested that the γ-carboxyglutamic acid residues of prothrombin are metal ligands (8,9). We have had the opportunity to examine the contribution that γ-carboxyglutamic acid makes to the binding of metal ions and to the tertiary structure of the protein.

The metal-binding properties of free γ-carboxyglutamic acid were examined using lanthanide ions as spectroscopic probes (10). By examining the effect of pH on the chemical shift of resonances of carbon nuclei in the natural abundance ^{13}C nuclear magnetic resonance spectrum, the pK_1 and pK_2 values of the γ-carboxyl groups of γ-carboxyglutamic acid were found to be 4.3 and 2.0. Thus, like aspartic acid and glutamic acid residues in proteins, γ-carboxyglutamic acid residues are completely ionized at physiologic pH. The interaction of the fluorescent lanthanide ion, Tb(III), and γ-carboxyglutamic acid was studied by measurement of the fluorescence enhancement of Tb(III) in the binary complex. At pH 6.5 this interaction is characterized by a K_D of 50 μM and a stoichiometry of 2 mol of γ-carboxyglutamic acid to 1 mol of Tb(III). The absolute distances between the bound metal ion and various carbon atoms in γ-carboxyglutamic acid were established using paramagnetic relaxation enhancement NMR techniques and paramagnetic Gd(III). Using a computer molecular modelling program, these distances were used to generate a geometry for the metal-γ-carboxyglutamic acid complex. This complex is shown in Fig. 2. Several important features of the interaction of γ-carboxyglutamic acid and metal ions were appreciated from this study. First, the metal ion is bound symmetrically by the two γ-carboxyl groups. Second, the oxygen ligands interact with the primary coordination sphere of the metal. Third and most importantly, the carboxyl groups of γ-carboxyglutamic acid interact with only half of the coordination sphere of the metal ion. The other half of the coordination sphere of the metal is available for interaction with other ligands. This conclusion thus explains why γ-carboxyglutamic acid binds metal ions with a 2:1 molar stoichiometry. Furthermore, it suggests that the primary structural role of γ-carboxyglutamic acid in proteins is to participate in reversible metal-dependent non-covalent electrostatic bridging.

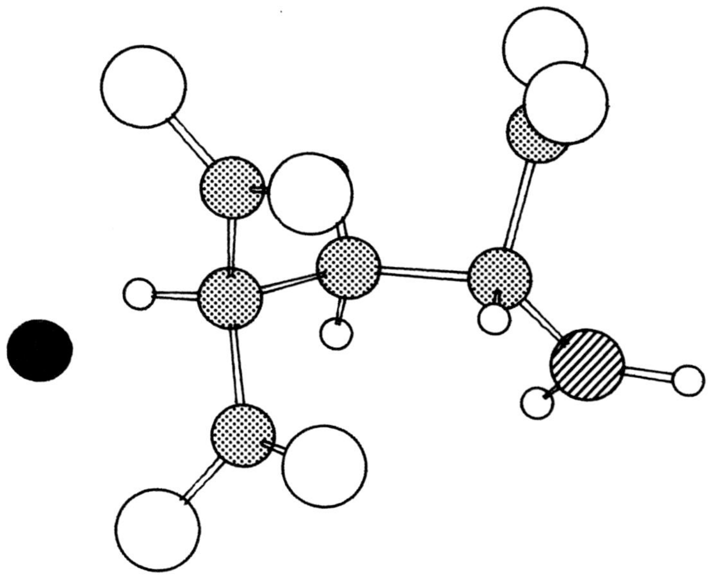

Fig. 2. Geometry of metal-γ-carboxyglutamic acid complex. Carbon (speckled), oxygen (white), metal (black), nitrogen (diagonal lines), hydrogens (small white).

This hypothesis was explored by evaluating the interaction of metal ions with a proteolytic fragment of prothrombin. Because prothrombin is too large to yield adequate natural abundance ^{13}C NMR spectra, a γ-carboxyglutamic acid-rich fragment of prothrombin was studied (11). This fragment, fragment (12-44), is a tryptic peptide of prothrombin. It contains eight γ-carboxyglutamic acid residues, a disulfide bond connecting cysteine 18 and cysteine 23, and has a molecular weight of 4100 (Fig. 3). This peptide has one high affinity metal binding site and multiple (4 to 6) lower affinity metal binding sites which bind lanthanide ions with a K_D of 0.4 μM and 12 μM respectively. Since γ-carboxyglutamic acid binds lanthanide ions with a K_D of 50 μM, it would appear that this high affinity metal binding site must involve more than one γ-carboxyglutamic acid residue. The ^{13}C NMR spectrum of fragment (12-44) at 67.88 MHz shows complete or partial resolution of the resonance of each carbon atom in the peptide. The proximity of bound paramagnetic lanthanide ions to individual carbon atoms was estimated by monitoring the perturbation of carbon resonances by these ions. These studies provide direct evidence that γ-carboxyglutamic acid is involved in metal liganding. Furthermore, the metal bound to the single high affinity metal binding site is located near the C_ε of the two arginine residues. The integrity of the high affinity site is dependent upon the presence of an intact disulfide bond connecting cysteine 18 and cysteine 23. If this disulfide bond is reduced and alkylated, only a single class of metal binding sites can be identified. These sites have a K_D of 10 μM. Also, the C_ε of the two arginine residues bear no special relationship to the bound metal ions. On the basis of these experiments we have concluded that the high affinity site is composed of two γ-carboxyglutamic acid residues. γ-Carboxyglutamic acid residues 15 and 26, located in close proximity of arginine 16 and arginine 25, may form this site. Construction of molecular models indicate that these residues are geometrically situated so that they can interact with a single metal ion. This site represents an intramolecular bridge interconnecting two regions of a polypeptide chain. The low affinity metal binding sites on the peptide are single γ-carboxyglutamic acid residues, as evidenced by the similarity of the K_D of lanthanide ions for the low affinity binding site and free γ-carboxyglutamic acid. These residues may be involved in the formation of metal-dependent intermolecular bridges between proteins or proteins and membranes. The nature of the metal ligand on the platelet membrane is not known, but the phosphate group of phosphotidylserine is likely involved when synthetic liposomes are employed. The intramolecular metal bridges participate in the stabilization of the tertiary structure of prothrombin. The intermolecular metal bridges participate in the macromolecular assembly of the complex of prothrombin, activated factor X, and membrane surfaces, i.e. the generation of quaternary structure. These conclusions can be seen within the context of observations of others. Nelsestuen (12) and Prendergast et al. (13) have indicated that the metal-dependent conformational change that prothrombin undergoes can be induced by a large variety of metal ions. However, the metal-dependent binding of prothrombin with membrane surfaces can be supported with only a limited number of metal ions, including calcium (14). These results emphasize that the two classes of metal binding sites on these proteins may be distinguished by their affinity and specificity for metal ions as well as by their functional role.

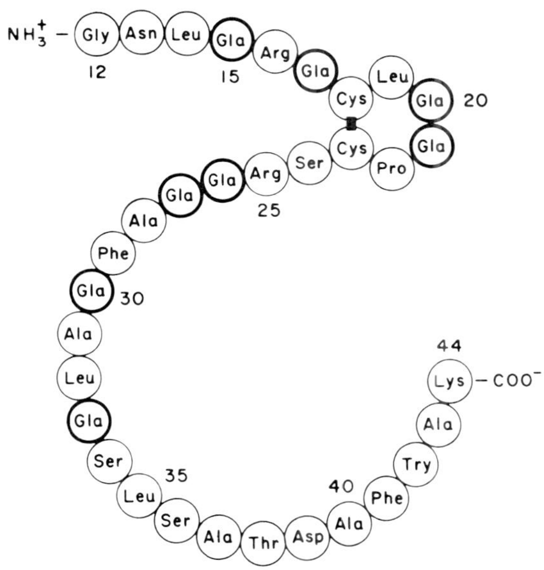

Fig. 3. Prothrombin fragment (12-44). This thirty-three residue peptide isolated from a proteolytic digest of prothrombin contains eight of the ten γ-carboxyglutamic acid (Gla) residues in prothrombin.

Such a view is consistent with other current experimental information. Fluorescence (12,13) and circular dichroism (15) studies provide a persuasive argument for metal-induced conformational changes in prothrombin. In addition, we have isolated a subpopulation of antibodies prepared against native prothrombin which is specific for the calcium-liganded conformation of prothrombin (16). This antibody binds to prothrombin only in the presence of calcium. Preliminary experiments suggest that this subpopulation is directed against antigenic determinants on both the fragment 1 and prethrombin 1 region of native prothrombin. Calcium thus induces a generalized alteration of the conformation of prothrombin. Using another antibody subpopulation specific for the γ-carboxyglutamic acid-rich region of prothrombin, we have identified the 12-44 region of prothrombin as a region which contains at least one antigenic determinant whose conformation is altered by the presence of calcium (17). These experiments emphasize the role of metal ions and γ-carboxyglutamic acid in determining protein conformation in the vitamin K-dependent proteins.

A fundamental question arises as to the role of calcium ions in the sequence of proteolytic reactions which are part of the coagulation pathways. The enzymes of the zymogens of blood coagulation are serine proteases. These enzymes share important structural and mechanistic features with other enzymes in the trypsin class. Unlike trypsin and related enzymes, however, these reactions proceed at a reasonable rate only in the presence of calcium. Calcium is not involved in enzyme catalysis. Rather, calcium is involved in the macromolecular assembly of the enzyme, substrate, and protein cofactors on a membrane surface.

As an example, prothrombin activation may be considered. In this reaction prothrombin is the substrate and activated factor X is the enzyme. Factor V, calcium and membrane surfaces are required for maximal rates of prothrombin activation. From recent data it would appear that activated factor X binds to specific receptor sites on the surface of activated platelets in the presence of calcium (18). This site is at least in part composed of factor V. The complex, which may be now considered as enzyme, can proteolytically cleave specific peptide bonds in the substrate, prothrombin (Fig. 4). Calcium thus functions in part to facilitate the reversible interaction of macromolecular surfaces containing metal ligands such as γ-carboxyglutamic acid.

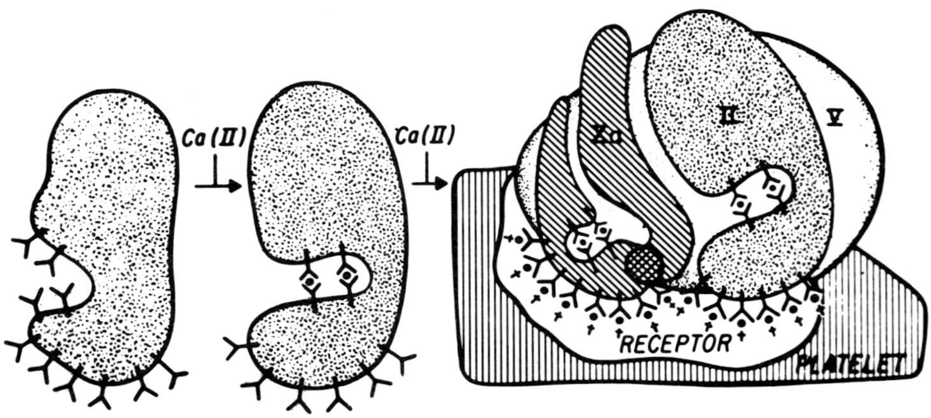

Fig. 4. Macromolecular assembly of the complex of activated factor X (Xa), factor V (V), and prothrombin (II) on the platelet receptor. Calcium (•) and γ-carboxyglutamic acid (Y) participate in intramolecular and intermolecular bridging.

This metal-dependent molecular assembly might serve two separate but related purposes in the regulation of hemostasis. On one hand, the formation of the blood clot and the reactions associated with this process must be localized in the blood to the area in which injury has occurred. By design, blood coagulation takes place on platelet surfaces and platelets have the unique property of adhering to the injured or disrupted vascular wall. Thus, calcium-dependent binding of the blood coagulation proteins to the platelet surfaces offers a mechanism to contain the clotting reactions to a specific locale and to minimize the amount of activated clotting proteins which float downstream from the site of vascular injury. Second, the extent of clot formation must in some way be proportional to the extent of injury. Mechanisms of control of the rate of each enzyme reaction and the extent to which each enzyme reaction proceeds must exist. At present it is not known how these reactions are regulated but it is possible that the protein cofactors (factor V or factor VIII) or calcium ions may play a role in modulation. These issues should be addressed and defined during the next phase of investigation of the role of metal ions in hemostasis.

ACKNOWLEDGEMENTS

The participation of Dr. Michael Blumenstein and our colleagues in our laboratory is gratefully acknowledged.

This work was supported by grants from the National Institutes of Health (HL-18834 and HL-21543) and the American Heart Association (76-996). Bruce Furie is an Established Investigator of the American Heart Association and its Massachusetts Affiliate. Barbara C. Furie is the recipient of a Research Career Development Award from the National Institutes of Health.

REFERENCES

(1) R. J. P. Williams, The biochemistry of sodium, potassium, magnesium, and calcium, Quart. Rev. Chem. Soc. London 24, 331 (1970).

(2) E. R. Birnbaum, J. E. Gomez, and D. W. Darnall, Rare Earth Metals as probes of electrostatic binding sites in proteins, J. Amer. Chem. Soc. 92, 5297-5288 (1970).

(3) J. Stenflo and J. W. Suttie, Vitamin K-dependent formation of γ-carboxyglutamic acid, Ann. Rev. Biochem. 46, 157-172 (1977).

(4) Y. Nemerson and B. Furie, Zymogens and cofactors of blood coagulation, Crit. Rev. Biochemistry. In press (1979).

(5) B. C. Furie and B. Furie, Interaction of lanthanide ions with bovine factor X and their use in the affinity chromatography of the venom coagulant protein of Vipera russelli, J. Biol. Chem. 250, 601-608 (1975).

(6) B. Furie and B. C. Furie, Spectral changes in bovine factor X associated with activation by the venom coagulant protein of Vipera russelli, J. Biol. Chem. 251, 6807-6814 (1976).

(7) B. C. Furie, K. G. Mann and B. Furie, Substitution of lanthanide ions for calcium ions in the activation of bovine prothrombin and the derivatives of prothrombin activation, J. Biol. Chem. 251, 3235-3241 (1976).

(8) J. Stenflo and P. O. Ganrot, Binding of Ca(II) to normal and dicoumarol-induced prothrombin, Biochem. Biophys. Res. Comm. 50, 98-104 (1973).

(9) G. L. Nelsestuen and J. W. Suttie, Mode of action of vitamin K. Calcium binding properties of bovine prothrombin, Biochemistry 11, 4961-4964 (1972).

(10) R. Sperling, B. C. Furie, M. Blumenstein, B. Keyt and B. Furie, Metal-binding properties of γ-carboxyglutamic acid: Implications for the vitamin K-dependent blood coagulation proteins, J. Biol. Chem. 253, 3898-3906 (1978).

(11) B. C. Furie, M. Blumenstein, and B. Furie, Structure of the metal binding sites of the vitamin K-dependent blood coagulation proteins, Fed. Proc. 37, 1292 (1978).

(12) G. L. Nelsestuen, Role of γ-carboxyglutamic acid. An unusual protein transition required for the calcium-dependent binding of prothrombin to phospholipid, J. Biol. Chem. 251, 5648-5656 (1976).

(13) F. G. Prendergast and K. G. Mann, Differentiation of metal ion-induced transitions of prothrombin fragment 1, J. Biol. Chem. 252, 840-850 (1977).

(14) G. L. Nelsestuen, M. Broderius, and G. Martin, Role of γ-carboxyglutamic acid. Cation specificity of prothrombin and factor X-phospholipid bindings. J. Biol. Chem. 251, 6886-6893 (1976).

(15) J. W. Bloom and K. G. Mann, Metal ion induced conformational transitions of prothrombin and prothrombin fragment 1, Biochemistry 17, 4430-4438 (1978).

(16) M. Tai, B. C. Furie and B. Furie, Conformation-specific antibodies as probes of the metal-dependent tertiary structure of bovine prothrombin, Fed. Proc. In press (1979).

(17) B. Furie, K. Provost, R. A. Blanchard, and B. C. Furie, Antibodies directed against a γ-carboxyglutamic acid-rich region of bovine prothrombin. Preparation, isolation, and characterization, J. Biol. Chem. 253. In press (1978).

(18) J. P. Miletich, C. M. Jackson, and P. W. Majerus, Properties of the factor Xa binding site on human platelets, J. Biol. Chem. 253, 6908-6916 (1978).

CONTACT ACTIVATION OF COAGULATION, FIBRINOLYSIS, AND KININ-FORMATION.

Allen P. Kaplan, M.D.
Professor of Medicine and Head
Division of Allergy, Rheumatology, and Clinical Immunology
The State University of New York at Stony Brook
Stony Brook, New York 11794

During the past decade, considerable progress has been made in understanding the mechanism by which the intrinsic coagulation and fibrinolytic pathways are activated and defining their relationship to the generation of the vasoactive peptide, bradykinin. In fact, the three proteins of the plasma kinin-forming system; namely, Hageman factor (Ratnoff and Rosenblum, 1958), prekallikrein (Wuepper, 1973A Weiss, et al, 1974; Saito et al, 1974) and high molecular weight (HMW) kininogen (Colman et al, 1975; Wuepper et al, 1975) have been shown to be the major factors required for contact activation of plasma. In this review I will present a detailed analysis of our present concept of the early events of these pathways. Emphasis will be placed upon the role of HMW-kininogen as a cofactor that is essential for surface dependent activation of coagulation and fibrinolysis and the molecular mechanisms by which this function is accomplished.

In Fig. 1 is shown the rate of activation of the intrinsic coagulation and fibrinolytic pathways in normal plasma compared to plasmas deficient in Hageman factor, HMW-kininogen, or prekallikrein. The normal plasma rapidly activates, the plasmas deficient in either Hageman factor or HMW-kininogen do not activate, while the prekallikrein deficient plasma has a diminished rate of activation which increases as the time of incubation with the surface is increased.

Interaction of Prekallikrein, Factor XI, and HMW-Kininogen in Plasma

It is clear that Hageman factor, prekallikrein, HMW-kininogen, factor XI, and plasminogen are intimately related functionally but they clearly represent different plasma proteins that are antigenically unrelated and are represented in the genome by distinct structural genes. However, reports suggesting that kallikrein can be purified as a complex with another plasma protein (Wendel et al 1972) and that prekallikrein appears to circulate in plasma as a complex (Nagasawa and Nakayasu, 1973), prompted the studies of Mandle, Jr. et al (1976) and Thompson et al (1977) in which prekallikrein and factor XI were each shown to circulate bound to HMW-kininogen.

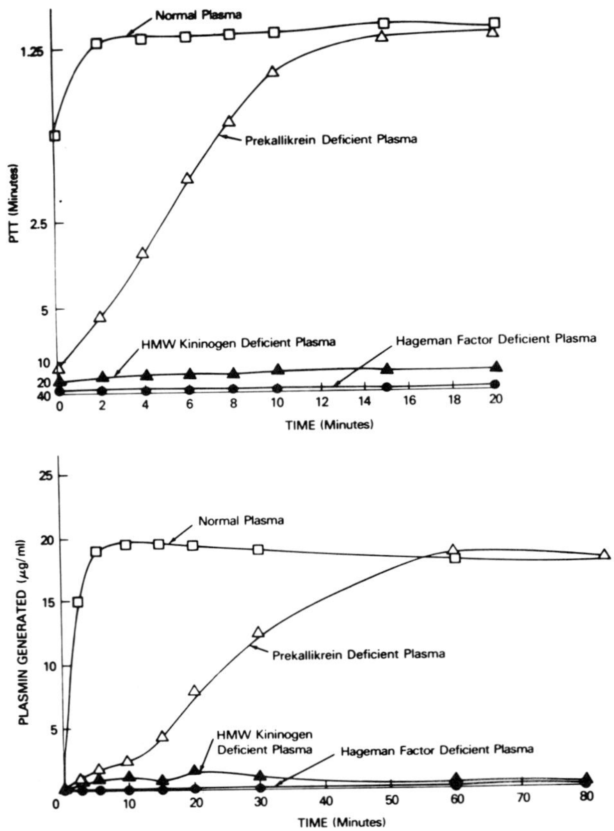

Fig. 1. Time course of activation of the Hageman factor-dependent coagulation and fibrinolytic pathways.

When normal human plasma was fractionated on Sephadex G-200, the apparent molecular weight of each of the above proteins could be determined. As shown in Fig. 2, factor XI was found at a molecular weight of 380,000, prekallikrein was found at 260,000, Hageman factor fractionated at 115,000, and plasminogen was located at 95,000. However when the molecular weights of purified factor XI and prekallikrein were assessed by gel filtration, values of 175,000 and 100,000 respectively were obtained, a discrepency of approximately 200,000. Purified Hageman factor and plasminogen fractionated at the same position as they did when whole plasma was assessed, and therefore did not appear to circulate as part of a complex. When

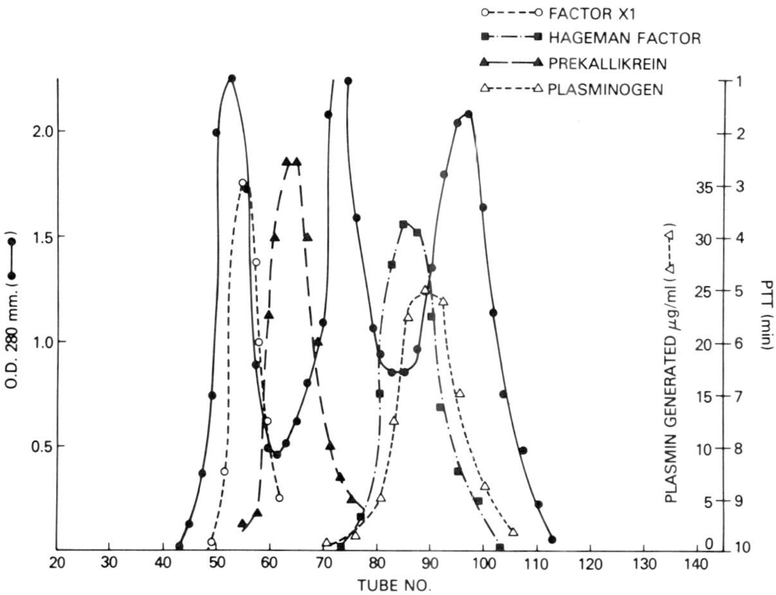

Fig. 2. Sephadex G-200 gel filtration of 4.0 ml of normal plasma indicating the relative position of the factor XI-HMW kininogen complex, the prekallikrein-HMW kininogen complex, Hageman factor, and plasminogen.

the molecular weight of prekallikrein and factor XI was determined in plasma that is deficient in HMW-kininogen, factor XI was found at 175,000 and prekallikrein was found at 100,000 suggesting that each protein normally circulates bound to HMW-kininogen. Reconstitution of HMW-kininogen deficient plasma with purified HMW-kininogen followed by fractionation by Sephadex G-200 gel filtration reproduced the chromatographic pattern of factor XI and prekallikrein in normal plasma (Mandle, Jr., et al, 1976; Thompson et al, 1977). In addition, direct binding of purified prekallikrein to HMW-kininogen (Mandle, Jr., et al, 1976) and direct binding of partially purified factor XI to HMW-kininogen (Thompson, et al, 1977) have been demonstrated. When a 10-fold excess of purified HMW-kininogen was incubated with partially purified factor XI for 10 minutes at 23°C and then fractionated on Sephadex G-200, the pattern shown in Fig. 3 was observed. The factor XI preparation had an apparent molecular weight of 175,000 (the contaminating IgG is seen at 160,000 purified HMW-kininogen was found at a molecular weight of 210,000 and the mixture of factor XI and HMW-kininogen yielded a peak of activity at 380,000 containing all of the factor XI and approximately 10 percent of the HMW-kininogen. Normal plasma contains approximately twice the concentration of HMW-kininogen as the sum of the factor XI and prekallikrein concentrations, thus complete binding of factor XI and prekallikrein results and the major peak of HMW-kininogen seen represents uncomplexed protein. No complex has been observed containing prekallikrein, factor XI, and HMW-kininogen as a single entity; prekallikrein and factor XI appears to circulate bound to different molecules of HMW-kininogen. Binding to HMW-kininogen also appears to be a specific property of the Hageman factor substrates and the complexes of prekallikrein-HMW-kininogen and factor XI-HMW-kininogen are each absorbed to surfaces where they they interact with surface bound Hageman factor. A schematic diagram showing the critical constituents bound to the surface is shown in Figure 4.

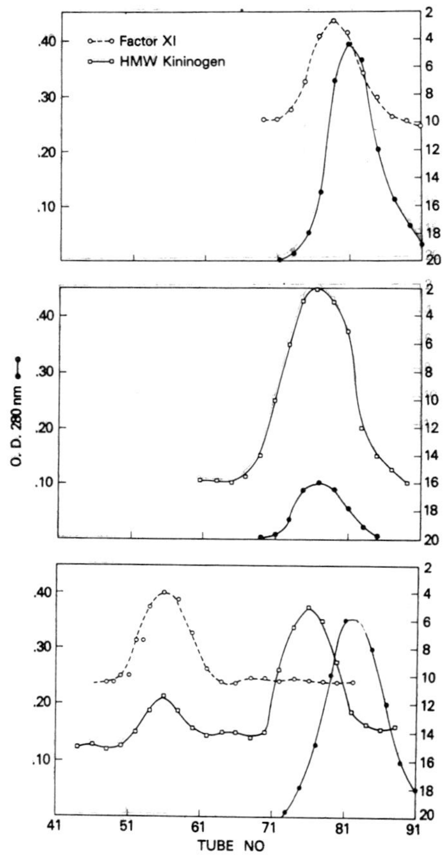

Fig. 3. Sephadex G-200 gel filtration of 2 ml of factor XI (5 units/ml) (upper panel), 2 ml of purified HMW kininogen (50 units/ml) (center panel) and a mixture of 2 ml factor XI plus 2 ml HMW kininogen (bottom panel). Buffer was added so that a total of 4.0 ml was applied to the column in each case.

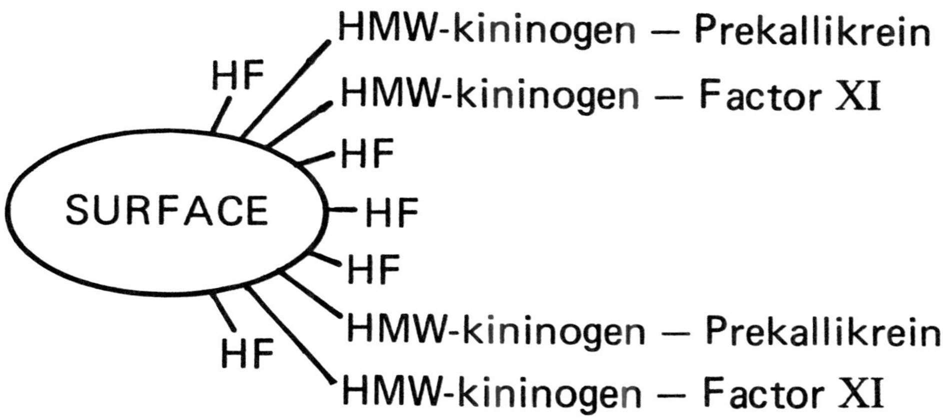

Fig. 4. Schematic diagram depicting the interaction of surface-bound Hageman factor with complexes of HMW kininogen and prekallikrein and complexes of HMW kininogen and factor XI.

Activation and Fragmentation of Hageman Factor: The Role of the Surface, HMW-Kininogen, and Prekallikrein.

The activation of Hageman factor, to be described herein, may occur by at least two different mechanisms. The first consists of a cleavage without obvious fragmentation in which the active enzyme consists of chains linked by disulfide bonds, and the second, a cleavage which liberates one or more active fragments. The discovery of the active fragments of Hageman factor by Kaplan and Austen (1970) provided the first evidence that activation could be performed enzymatically (Kaplan and Austen, 1971). The final product, a prealbumin fragment observed as two closely migrating bands upon alkaline disc gel electrophoresis, functioned as a potent prekallikrein activator but retained only 2 to 5 percent of the coagulant activity of the unfragmented Hageman factor. Subsequently, plasmin was shown to be capable of directly digesting Hageman factor to yield these fragments (Kaplan and Austen, 1971). Similar prealbumin activities described in the rabbit, (Wuepper et al, 1970) guinea pig (Trelcar and Movat,1970) and man (Movat et al 1971; Wuepper and Cochrane, 1971) were subsequently shown to be derived from Hageman factor (Cochrane and Wuepper 1971; Soltay et al 1972) and the ability of plasmin to activate and fragment Hageman factor was confirmed (Burrowes et al, 1975). Although not purified, an activated preparation of Hageman factor was also described whose molecular weight upon gel filtration (115,000) was identical to that of unactivated Hageman factor, yet it readily clotted Hageman factor deficient plasma in the absence of kaolin. This preparation was designated intact activated Hageman factor (Kaplan and Austen, 1971). In addition, at least two active fragments were described whose molecular weight was intermediate between that of the prealbumin fragments and the unfragmented active molecule. Thus by gel filtration, active species were detected at molecular weights of 115,000, 90,000, 60,000 and 40,000 (Kaplan et al, 1971), and each of the first three species could be converted to the 40,000 mol. wt. prealbumin fragment (Kaplan et al, 1971; Kaplan and Austen, 1971).

The discovery of prekallikrein deficient plasma lead to an examination of the ability of kallikrein to activate and fragment Hagman factor. Kallikrein was found to function in a similar manner to plasmin, however it was approximately 10 times as effective (Cochrane et al, 1973) and could act upon either surface bound or fluid phase Hageman factor. When Hageman factor was iodinated, digested, and examined by SDS gel electrophoresis, trypsin, plasmin, and kallikrein were found to yield similar patterns (Revak et al, 1974). The molecular weight of Hageman factor was 90,000 in unreduced gels and 80,000 after reduction; upon digestion it was converted to a 28,000 active fragment which corresponded to the stable prealbumin fragment previously described, and a 50,000 dalton fragment remained. Further digestion converted 50,000 dalton fragment to fragments of 40,000 and 10,000. However the formation of an active, unfragmented form of Hageman factor was not detected. The 50,000 dalton fragment was subsequently shown to be the portion of the molecule that binds to surfaces (Revak and Cochrane, 1976). In Fig. 5 is shown the pattern of ^{125}I-Hageman factor digestion upon incubation with 2 percent plasma kallikrein for 30 min at 37 C. The starting material, seen at 80,000 daltons was converted to 50,000 and 28,000 dalton fragments. In the insert is shown an alkaline disc gel electrophoresis of Hageman factor before (left) and after (center) digestion with plasma kallikrei When the digested product was incubated with kaolin, centrifuged, and the supernatant subjected to alkaline disc gel electrophoresis (right) only the active prealbumin fragments were seen. Bagdasarian and Colman investigated the cleavage of Hageman factor with kallikrein or plasmin (Bagdasarian et al, 1973) and observed that cleavage with kallikrein routinely generated the prealbumin fragments while plasmin digestion could yield a larger active fragment (Bagdasarian et al, 1972) which appeared to resist further digestion to the prealbumin fragments. This cleavage product may be identical to one of the intermediate sized active fragments described earlier, however the inability to further digest it to the prealbumin fragment has not yet been confirmed.

With the discovery of HMW kininogen deficiency, it became clear that a reciprocal mechanism in which activated Hageman factor converts prekallikrein to kallikrein, and kallikrein in turn activates the Hageman factor, was an over-simplification. For example, addition of activated Hageman factor to Hageman factor deficient plasma causes coagulation on the absence of kaolin by activation of factor XI. Addition of factor XIa to factor XI deficient plasma causes coagulation in the absence of kaolin by activation of factor IX. However addition of kallikrein to prekallikrein deficient plasma, in the absence of a surface, did not result in appreciable coagulation (Kaplan et al, 1974). Thus the surface appeared to be required for this function of kallikrein to be expressed. Furthermore, the addition of activated Hageman factor to HMW kininogen deficient plasma, even in the presence of a surface, did not significantly shorten its partial thromboplast: time (Meier et al, 1976; Liu et al, 1976). HMW kininogen therefore appeared to be required for the activation of Hageman factor and/or the expression of Hageman factor activity. When the role of HMW kininogen was further examined it was found to enhance both the function of activated Hageman factor and the formation of activated Hageman factor.

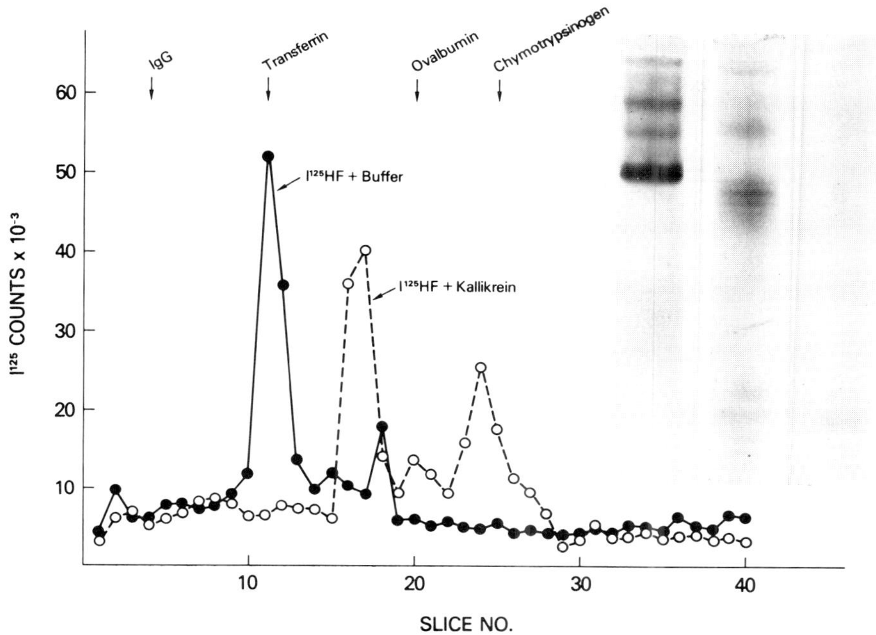

Fig. 5. SDS gel electrophoresis of ^{125}I Hageman factor before and after digestion with kallikrein. The gels were sliced, each sliced eluted, and the eluate counted. Conversion of ^{125}I Hageman factor seen at 80,000 daltons to 52,000 dalton and 28 dalton fragments was observed. In the insert is shown an alkaline disc gel electrophoresis of purified Hageman factor (left gel), Hageman factor that has been digested with kallikrein (center gel) and the supernatant obtained from kallikrein-digested Hageman factor after absorption with kaolin. The preparation demonstrates heterogeneity upon alkaline disc gel electrophoresis (left gel) and after digestion yields a series of bands at the center of the gel and prealbumin bands at the anode. After absorption with kaolin (right gel) only the prealbumin bands remain.

In Fig. 6 is shown the ability of HMW kininogen to augment the function of surface bound Hageman factor upon prekallikrein, factor XI, and the converstion of plasminogen to plasmin. For a fixed quantity of surface bound Hageman factor, the subsequent activation of each Hageman factor substrate appeared proportional to the quantity of HMW kininogen added (Meier et al, 1976; Griffin and Cochrane, 1976A;Griffin and Cochrane, 1976B; Meier et al, 1977_A). Such an experiment demonstrates the effect of HMW kininogen upon the system but does not distinguish an effect upon the function of activated Hageman factor from the formation of activated Hageman factor. However augmentation of the ability of Hageman factor fragments to convert prekallikrein to kallikrein in the absence of a surface has

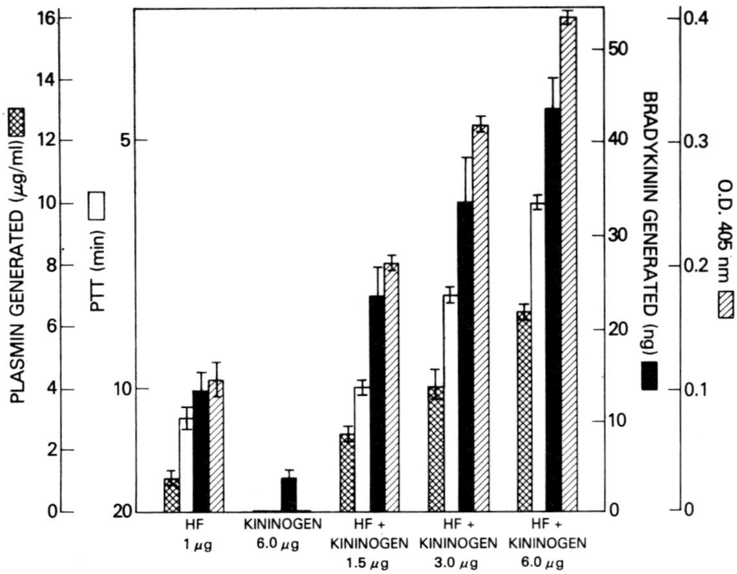

Fig. 6. The effect of increasing quantities of HMW kininogen upon the ability of Hageman factor to activate prekallikrein, factor XI, and generate plasminogen activating activity.

been reported (Liu et al, 1976; Meier et al, 1977 B Liu et al, 1977); in this case the Hageman factor utilized is already active thus the effect observed is upon its function. Furthermore, addition of Hageman factor fragments to HMW-kininogen deficient plasma failed to yield the predicted activation of either prekallikrein or factor XI and this abnormality was corrected upon reconstitution with HMW-kininogen (Liu et al, 1977). Limited trypsin treatment of surface-bound Hageman factor could also be utilized to achieve activation, and the enhancing effect of HMW kininogen upon the subsequent activation of prekallikrein or factor XI could then be observed (Griffin and Cochrane, 1976). In Fig. 7 is shown a dose response of the ability of HMW kininogen to augment the function surface-bound Hageman factor as assessed by prekallikrein activation. The reaction appeared stoichiometric in that the activity observed was proportional to the HMW kininogen input. There appeared to be an optimal concentration of HMW kininogen that could be used and excess HMW kininogen was inhibitory (Meier et al, 1977 A) The same profile has been reported for the effect of HMW kininogen upon the function of the Hageman factor fragments (Liu et al, 1977) however, the cause of this inhibition is not known. In order to perform these assays, the Hageman factor was first absorbed to the surface in the presence or absence of HMW kininogen, centrifuged, and the pellet was extensively washed. The pellet was then incubated with the Hageman factor substrates in order to assay for the presence of activated Hageman factor. Critical to the

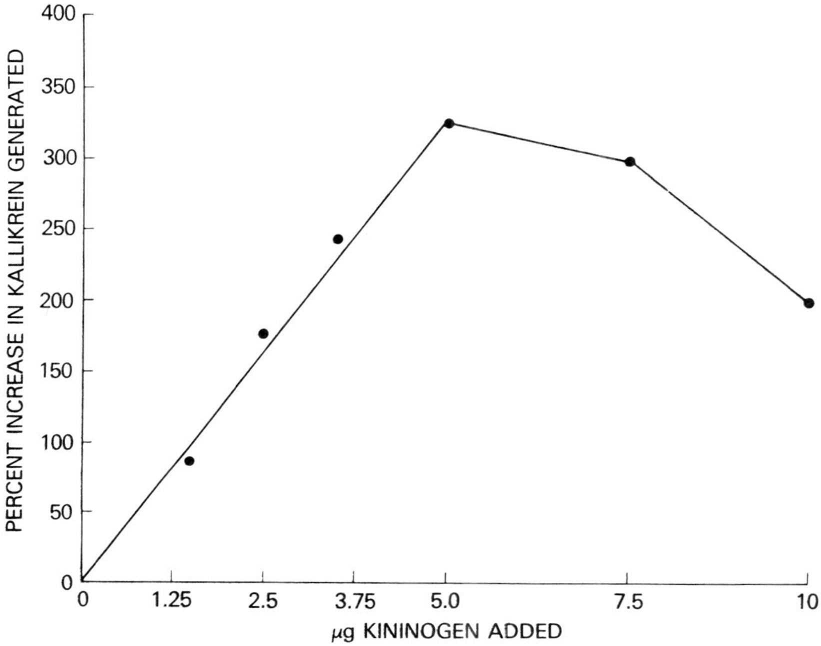

Fig. 7. Enhancement of the activity of surface-bound Hageman factor upon prekallikrein as a function of the HMW kininogen added.

interpretation of these experiments is a determination of whether HMW kininogen affects binding of Hageman factor to surfaces. When this was examined no effect was found (Meier et al, 1977_A) Furthermore any activated Hageman factor detected in the second step of the assay was firmly adsorbed to the surface suggesting that the molecular form of activated Hageman factor detected was not the prealbumin fragments since these fragments lack the binding site for the surface (Fig. 5).

Although these data demonstrate an effect of HMW kininogen upon the function of activated Hageman factor they do not preclude in effect upon the activation of Hageman factor. Griffin and Cochrane (1976) reported that the rate of cleavage of Hageman factor by kallikrein appeared to be enhanced by HMW kininogen suggesting an effect upon Hageman factor activation. Meier et al (1977_A)assessed this reaction functionally and demonstrated that the ability of kallikrein to activate Hageman factor was markedly augmented by HMW kininogen. Fig. 8 is a demonstration of the ability of kallikrein to activate Hageman factor as assessed in the same two-stage assay described above. Unactivated Hageman factor and kallikrein were adsorbed to the surface in the presence or absence of HMW kininogen. The mixture was centrifuged, the pellet was washed and the washed pellet then assayed for its ability to convert prekallikrein to kallikrein. Activation of Hageman factor during the initial incubation with kallikrein was observed only in the presence of HMW kininogen and the active moiety generated was bound to the surface. In Table I is shown the incorporation of ^{3}H-DFP

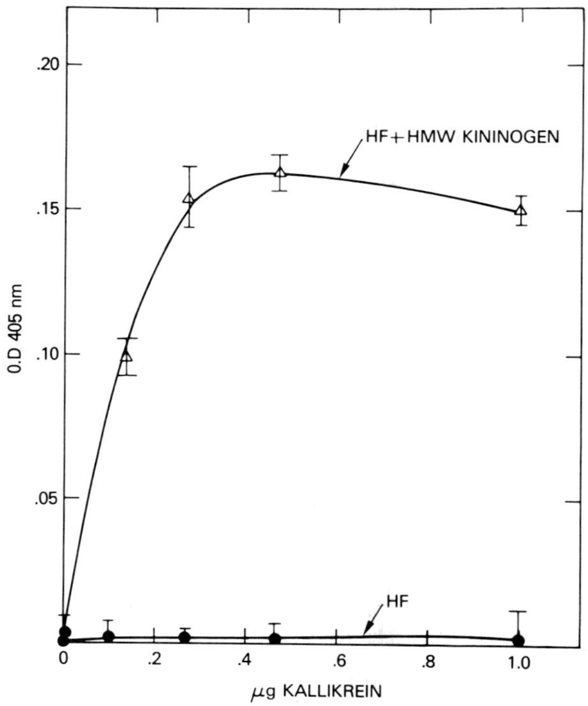

Fig. 8. Dose-response of the activation and function of bound Hageman factor by kallikrein in the presence and absence of HMW kininogen.

into the surface-bound reactants. Non-specific uptake of 7200 counts by the surface was observed. However incubation of the surface with Hageman factor alone or with Hageman factor plus HMW-kininogen did not yield a significant further uptake of radioactivity. There was no evident activation of the Hageman factor by the surface, and HMW kininogen did not activate the Hageman factor. However incubation with kallikrein did activate the Hageman factor as indicated by the additional incorporation of 6,000 counts (the kallikrein alone could only incorporate 500 counts). However the function of these additional sites would not be fully expressed in the absence of HMW kininogen. Incubation of surface-bound Hageman factor with kallikrein and HMW kininogen followed by incubation

TABLE I

Incorporation of ^{3}H DFP by Surface-Bound Hageman Factor, HMW kininogen, and Kallikrein

Proteins added to surface	Counts ^{3}H DFP
	cpm
---	7,240 ± 442
Hageman Factor	7,924 ± 438
HMW kininogen	7,635 ± 480
Hageman factor + HMW kininogen	8,081 ± 505
Kallikrein	8,426 ± 470
Kallikrein + HMW kininogen	8,269 ± 498
Kallikrein + Hageman factor	14,175 ± 770
Kallikrein + Hageman factor + HMW kininogen	34,395 ± 1,123
DFP-Kallikrein + Hageman factor + HMW kininogen	9,230 ± 521

with ^{3}H-DFP led to incorporation of an additional 34,000 counts. Thus HMW kininogen augmented the activation of Hageman factor by kallikrein when the presence of activated Hageman factor was assessed functionally (Figure 8), or when the formation of new active sites was determined. In the presence of HMW kininogen, the function of each of these sites could then be fully expressed. Figure 9 is a schematic diagram of this reciprocol interaction of surface-bound Hag-man factor and prekallikrein indicating that the reaction rate in each direction is augmented by HMW kininogen.

with ^{3}H-DFP led to incorporation of an additional 34,000 counts. Thus HMW kininogen augmented the activation of Hageman factor by kallikrein when the presence of activated Hageman factor was assessed functionally (Fig. 8), or when the formation of new active sites was determined. In the presence of HMW kininogen, the function of each of these sites could then be fully expressed. Fig. 9 is a schematic diagram of this reciprocal interaction of surface-bound Hageman factor and prekallikrein indicating that the reaction rate in each direction is augmented by HMW kininogen.

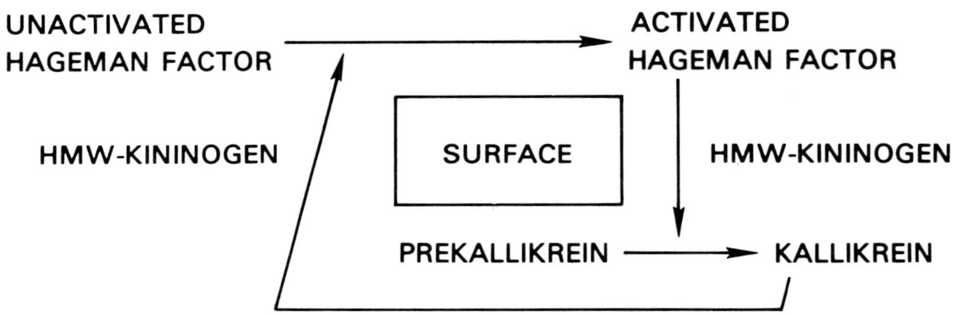

Fig. 9. Schematic diagram of the reciprocal activation of surface-bound Hageman factor and prekallikrein that is catalyzed by HMW kininogen.

It should be emphasized that the surface and the active site of kallikrein were required for this activation of Hageman factor (Meier et al, 1977A; Meier et al, 1977B) to proceed. Thus kallikrein did not correct prekallikrein deficient plasma in the absence of a surface (Weiss et al, 1974; Meier et al, 1977A) DFP-kallikrein did not correct prekallikrein deficient plasma in the presence of a surface (Meier et al, 1977B) and DFP-kallikrein would not activate purified surface-bound Hageman factor (Table I). The surface has been estimated to augment the rate of cleavage of Hageman factor by kallikrein bound by as much as 50-fold (Griffin, 1978 and, when activation of Hageman factor was examined by incorporation of ^{3}H-DFP, no activation of Hageman factor by the surface was observed in the absence of prekallikrein and HMW kininogen. Thus the surface appears to augment the rate of interaction of the reactants, and, in particular, render the Hageman factor a better substrate for plasma kallikrein. The ability of HMW kininogen to augment the function of activated Hageman factor has been estimated to be 3-4 fold while its effect upon the activation of Hageman factor yields a 40 fold enhancement (Meier et al, 1977_A). When combined with the surface, the rate is augmented 6000 fold. The major theoretical consideration that is not yet resolved is whether some combination of the surface, Hageman factor, prekallikrein and HMW kininogen generates an active site or whether trace quantities of one of the enzymes normally circulates in an active form. In the latter case, binding to the surface in the presence of HMW kininogen might augment the reaction rate sufficiently to initiate the cascade. It is possible that changes observed upon binding of Hageman factor to surfaces or ellagic acid (McMillin et al, 1974) may relate to the increased rate of cleavage of Hageman factor rather than the generation of a new active site in the Hageman factor.

The initial cleavage of human Hageman factor has been reported to occur within a disulfide bridge such that the product was the same size as the starting material (Revak et al, 1977; Revak et al, 1978). A second cleavage external to the disulfide bond liberated the 28,000 dalton fragment. This is shown diagrammatically in Figure 10. The initial cleavage, shown above, yields the intact, activated Hageman factor (HFa) in which a heavy chain that is attached to the surface is disulfide linked to a light chain. The cleavage shown below would serve to liberate the major portion of the light chain and/or the light chain attached to a small portion of the heavy chain to yield Hageman factor fragment (HFf) in the fluid phase. However the site of this latter cleavage is uncertain. For example, if cleavage were at the opposite side of the disulfide bond, a smaller HFf would be liberated and these two possible sites of cleavage have not been distinguished. In addition, we do not know whether formation of HFf is an alternative to formation of HFa (as shown) or whether cleavage within the disulfide bond occurs first to yield HFa followed by one or more additional cleavages to form HFf.

Alternative Mechanisms of Hageman Factor Activation

Since the major activator of Hageman factor is kallikrein, it is likely that one or more alternative enzymes account for the gradual activation of Hageman factor observed in prekallikrein deficient plasma. Both plasmin and factor XIa have been shown to be capable of activating and cleaving Hageman factor in the fluid phase (Kaplan and Austen, 1971; Cochrane et al, 1973; Revak, et al, 1974) and the ability of both of these enzymes to activate surface-bound Hageman factor has been investigated (Meier et al, 1977C; Griffin, 1978). At ratios of enzyme/ Hageman factor of 1:50, both plasmin and factor XIa activated Hageman factor as assessed by the subsequent ability of the surface bound Hageman factor to convert prekallikrein, to kallikrein. Plasmin was approximately one-tenth as effective an activator as kallikrein, and, in contrast to kallikrein, no augmentation by HMW kininogen was evident. When factor XIa was assayed, it was also about one-tenth as potent a Hageman factor activator as kallikrein, however Hageman factor activation, as assessed by the subsequent conversion of prekallikrein to kallikrein, was augmented 2-3 fold in the presence of HMW kininogen (HMW kininogen augmented the ability of kallikrein to activate Hageman factor 40-fold). When the effect of HMW kinogen upon the rate of cleavage of Hageman factor was assessed, no augmentation was seen when plasmin was used as the activator, however no significant effect was seen when factor XIa was the activator (Griffin, 1978). It is possible that the small functional augmentation seen when factor XIa is the activator represents an effect upon prekallikrein activation, which is utilized to assay for HFa. Nevertheless, it is clear that the major effect of HMW kininogen upon Hageman factor activation occurs when kallikrein is used as the activator. In all cases, the presence of the surface augmented the rate of cleavage of Hageman factor by each of the enzymes tested (Griffin, 1978).

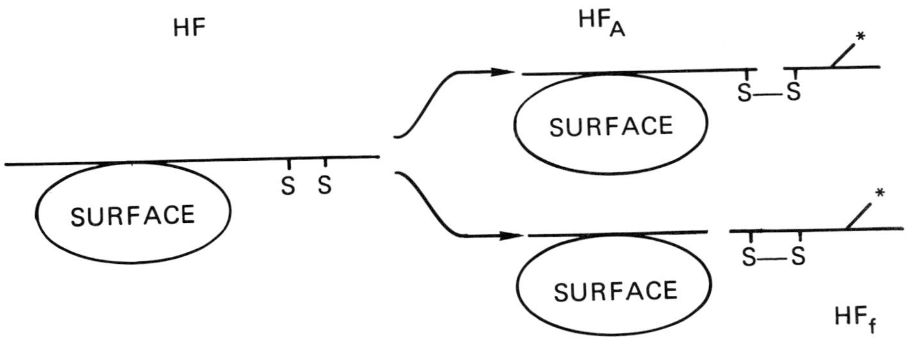

Fig. 10. Diagram illustrating the proposed cleavages of Hageman factor that can lead to activation. The initial cleavage shown above, is within a disulfide bond, to form HFa, while cleavage external to that disulfide bond shown below, liberates HFf from the surface. The asterisk (*) indicates the presence of an active site.

The main effect of HMW kininogen is to place the Hageman factor substrates on the surface in an optimal position for their subsequent interaction with Hageman factor (Mandle, Jr. et al, 1976; Thompson et al, 1977). In the absence of HMW kininogen, less prekallikrein or Factor XI are bound to the surface (Wiggins et al 1977) and neither activation of Hageman factor, nor activation of prekallikrein or Factor XI proceed at a normal rate. The augmentation of the rate of activation and cleavage of prekallikrein and factor XI by activated Hageman factor observed in the presence of HMW kininogen may therefore reflect an effect upon the Hageman factor substrates. However it is also possible that HMW kininogen directly augments the function of the active site of Hageman factor. Evidence to suggest this possibility is the observation that the rate of cleavage of acetyl-glycyl-lysyl-methyl ester by Hageman factor fragments is augmented by HMW kininogen (Liu et al, 1977).

PREKALLIKREIN

Purification and Properties of Human Prekallikrein

Human prekallikrein has been partially purified from plasma by fractionation on anion exchangers such as DEAE-cellulose (or Sephadex) or QAE-Sephadex. Under conditions of alkaline pH (8.0-8.5) at a conductivity of less than 1 mS, prekallikrein did not bind to these exchangers and was found in the effluent with the bulk of IgG. At this point prekallikrein was effectively separated from Hageman factor and HMW kininogen as well as plasma protease inhibitors. It is interesting to note that the prekallikrein-HMW kininogen complex was readily dissociated by a single passage over the ion exchanger. The other contaminating proteins identified after this first column step were β_2 glycoprotein I, factor XI, and the complement components Cl_q and properdin. Further purification of human prekallikrein utilized fractionation on SP Sephadex and Sephadex G 150 to yield a product that was contaminated with IgG and variable quantities of β_2 glycoprotein ^{125}I. However, fractionation in the absence of inhibitors lead to conversion of 25-35 percent of the material to kallikrein. Prekallikrein has been purified by Mandle and Kaplan (1977) utilizing each of the above steps followed by passage over a combined immunoadsorbent to IgG and β_2 glycoprotein I. Precautions taken to minimize conversion of prekallikrein to kallikrein included the addition of hexadimethine bromide (360 mg/ml) to the starting plasma, the addition of either 10 mM benzamidine or 10^{-4}M diisopropylfluorophosphate to all buffer systems, and use of plastic columns and test tubes. Estimates of the plasma concentration of prekallikrein range from 15-45 ug/ml and the final yield based upon these estimates was approximately 5-10 percent.

The molecular weights reported for human prekallikrein as assessed by gel filtration have ranged from 100,000 to 127,000. However, when purified prekallikrein was examined by SDS gel electrophoresis, two molecular variant were identified at 88,000 and 85,000 daltons respectively (Fig. 11) which have been designated prekallikreins I and II. Upon immunoelectrophoresis, in 1% agar at pH 8.3, prekallikrein migrated as a fast γ globulin and its isoelectric point was determined to be between 8.5 and 9.0 (peak value at 8.7) utilizing ampholytes that ranged from pH 7 to 10.

The Mechanism of Activation of Human Prekallikrein

Activation of human prekallikrein by HFa proceeds by limited proteolytic digestion. Each of the molecular forms of prekallikrein seen at 88,000 and 85,000 daltons is cleaved and upon reduction, a two-chain disulfide linked enzyme results. A heavy chain of 52,000 daltons is linked to a light chain of either 36,000 or 33,000 daltons corresponding to the two forms of the starting material. Fig. 12 shows a preparation of ^{125}I prekallikrein which was partially activated so that approximately 50 percent was converted to kallikrein. The mixture was then reduced, subjected to SDS gel electrophoresis, and an autoradiogram of the gel was made. One can readily visualize the undigested prekallikrein, the kallikrein heavy chain and the two kallikrein light chains. On the same figure is shown an identical experiment in which non-radiolabeled prekallikrein was activated, incubated with ^3H-DFP, reduced, and subjected to SDS gel electrophoresis and autoradiography. All of the ^3H-DFP was seen in the light chains indicating that this portion of the molecule contains the active site of kallikrein (Mandle and Kaplan, 1977). A time course of cleavage of 15 ug prekallikrein with 0.5 ug Hageman factor fragments as assessed after reduction and SDS gel electrophoresis is shown in Fig. 13. As the two forms of prekallikrein were cleaved, there was a gradual formation of the kallikrein heavy chain and the two light chains. The evolution of functional activity has been shown to parallel the percent conversion to the cleaved form. In the absence of reducing agents, the molecular weight of prekallikrein and kallikrein were the same, thus there was no evidence of release of any peptide during activation, and activation occurred by cleavage within a disulfide bridge. The difference in molecular weight of prekallikreins I and II (Fig. 11) was reflected in the light chains. The evidence that both bands represent prekallikrein included: 1) both were cleaved by Hageman factor

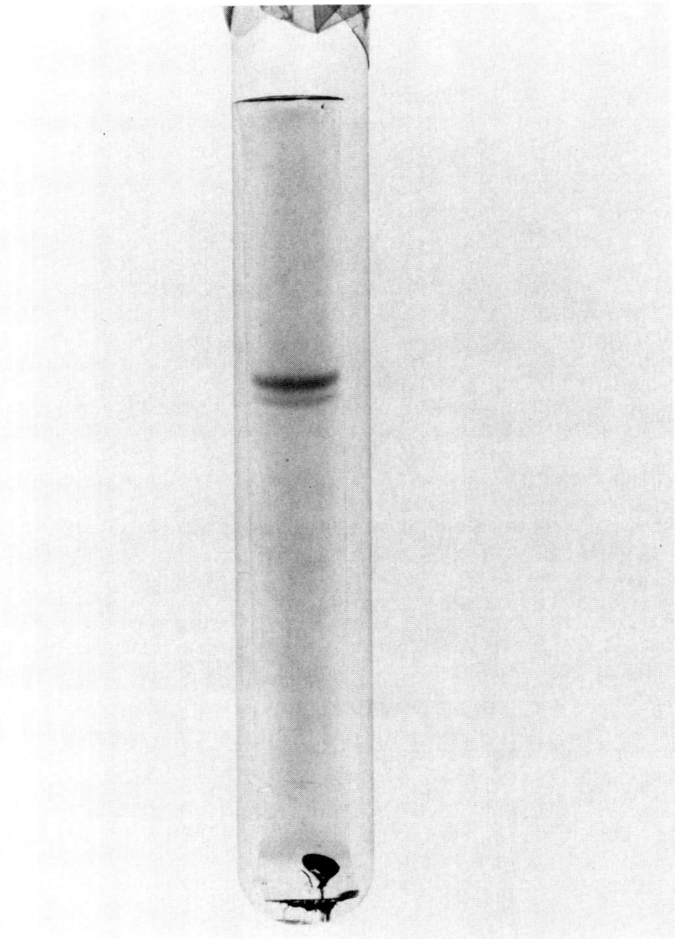

Fig. 11. SDS gel electrophoresis of 20 μg of reduced human prekallikrein.

fragments and yielded similar activation patterns, 2) they were not interconvertible upon activation by Hageman factor or incubation of prekallikrein with kallikrein, 3) they contained the same antigenic determinants, 4) DFP was incorporated into the light chains of each molecular form of the active enzymes and 5) neither band was seen when prekallikrein deficient plasma was fractionated.

Prekallikrein has been purified in other species and its mechanism of activation has been examined. Bovine prekallikrein (Nagasawa et al; 1968; Takahashi et al, 1972) was shown to be a single chain proenzyme that was digested by bovine Hageman factor to yield a two chain disulfide-linked enzyme in a fashion analagous to that seen in man. Rabbit prekallikrein was found to be a β globulin with a molecular weight of 90,000 daltons and an isoelectric point of 5.9 (Wuepper and

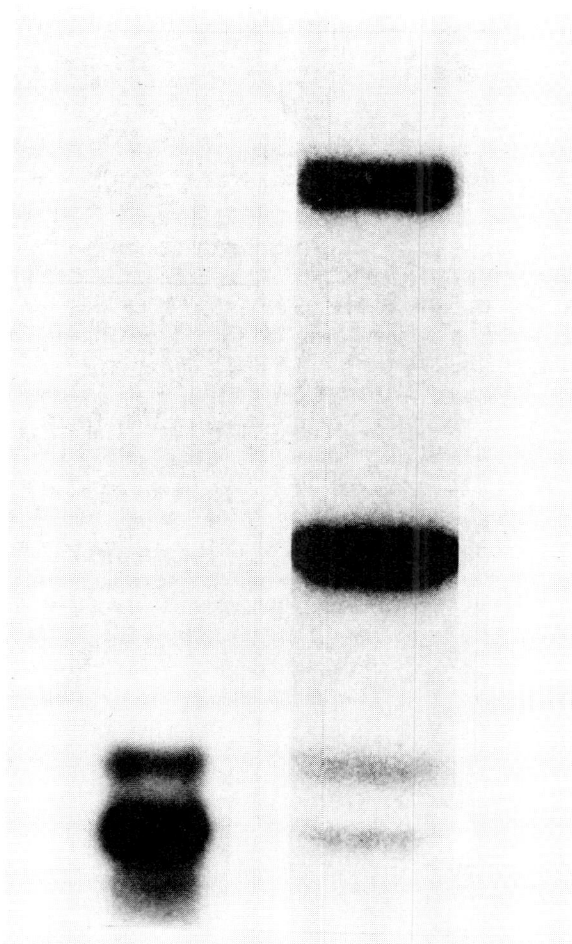

Fig. 12. Autoradiogram of a mixture of ^{125}I-labeled kallikrein and prekallikrein showing the prekallikrein, the kallikrein heavy chain and the two kallikrein light chains (right gel). The left gel is an autoradiogram of a reduced SDS-polyacrylamide gel electrophoresis of ^{3}H-DFP treated kallikrein showing incorporation of ^{3}H-DFP into both kallikrein light chains.

Cochrane, 1972_A). Upon conversion to kallikrein, not only was a kinin-generating enzyme formed but the kallikrein was found to shorten the PTT of rabbit plasma and human kallikrein behaved similarly (Wuepper and Cochrane, 1972_B). Thus the function of kallikrein as a coagulation factor can be detected in rabbit plasma. Addition of kallikrein to human plasma or to congenitally deficient plasmas (other than Fletcher trait) has no effect. When the mechanism of conversion of rabbit prekallikrein to kallikrein was examined, activation was associated with

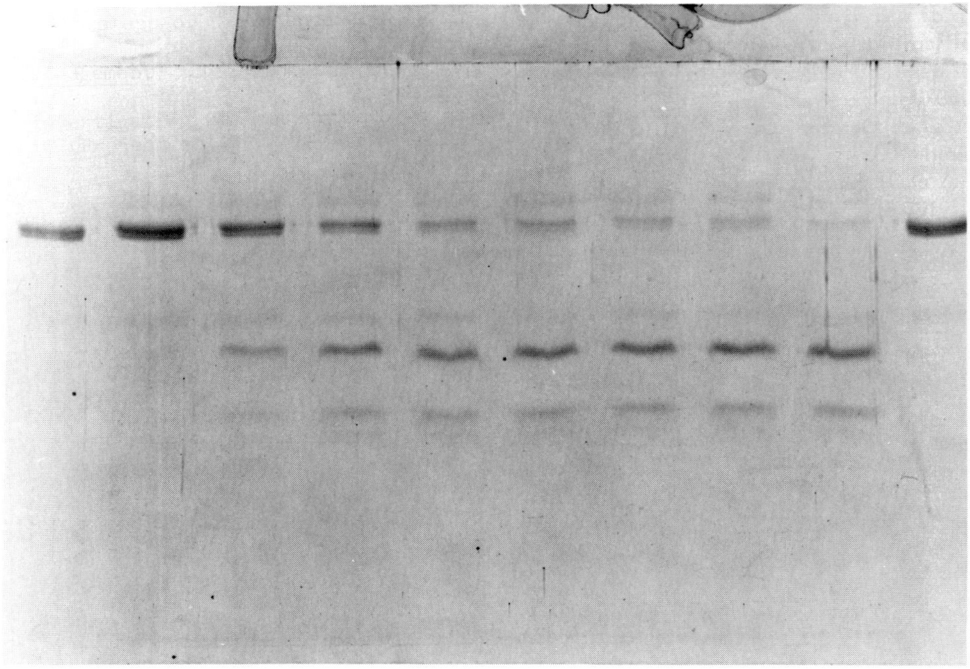

Fig. 13. Kinetics of prekallikrein activation by Hageman factor fragments. From left to right the gel contains the starting material followed by 0, 2, 5, 10, 15, 25, 40 and 60 min time-points after addition of Hageman factor. The final sample is a premixed control of SDS-buffer plus starting material and Hageman factor fragments incubated at 37 C for 60 min.

the loss of an 8,000 dalton peptide (Wuepper and Cochrane, 1972_A). However, when the mechanism was examined in greater detail, activation in the presence of trasylol yielded conversion to a two-chain disulfide-linked enzyme without any change in molecular weight (Johnson et al, 1976). Since trasylol inactivates kallikrein but not Hageman factor (Burrowes et al, 1975), it appeared that the peptide released was secondary to digestion of prekallikrein (or kallikrein) by the kallikrein produced. This phenomenon has been observed for human prekallikrein as shown in Fig. 14. Digestion of ^{125}I prekallikrein with 5 percent non-radiolabeled kallikrein followed by SDS gel electrophoresis and autoradiography resulted in the formation of a prekallikrein which was diminished in size by approximately 10,000 daltons (Mandle and Kaplan, 1977). The molecule remained as a single chain and no conversion to kallikrein was detected.

Purification and Characterization of Human HMW Kininogen.

Highly purified human HMW kininogen was prepared by Pierce and Guimaraes (Pierce and Guimaraes, 1974) who utilized chromatography on DEAE cellulose, elution from an anti-kininogen immunadsorbant with 6M guandine hydrochloride, followed by gel filtration. The resulting preparation of HMW kininogen had considerable size

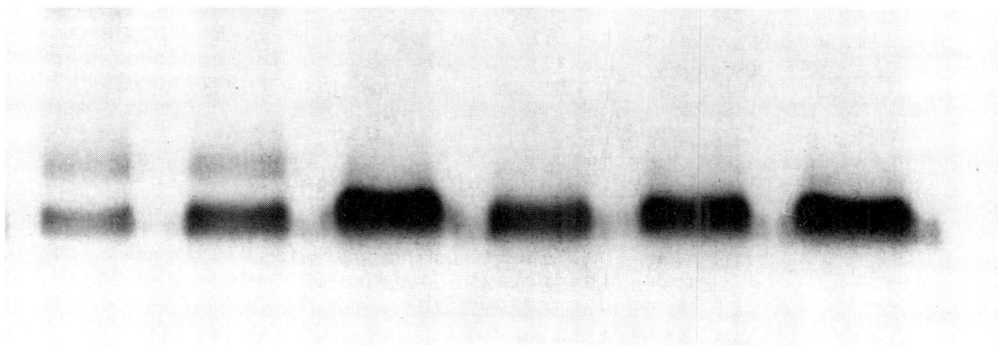

Fig. 14. Autoradiogram of ^{125}I labeled prekallikrein plus non-labeled kallikrein. The samples from left to right are: prekallikrein plus kallikrein plus 2000 units/ml Trasylol incubated for 0, 30, and 60 min: followed by prekallikrein plus kallikrein incubated for 0, 30 and 60 minutes without any Trasylol.

heterogeneity with peaks of activity at 200,000, 160,000 and 80,000 daltons. Each of these kininogens was readily cleaved by plasma kallikrein thus distinguishing them functionally from the bulk of low molecular weight kininogen, and each of these purified kininogens functioned as a coagulation factor and could correct HMW kininogen deficiency. The relative proportion of these three isolated forms were 4:6:1. It is not clear whether the smaller forms are enzymatically derived from the larger.

Habal et al (1974) and Habal and Movat (1974) purified human HMW kininogen utilizing QAE Sephadex, ammonium sulfate precipitation, SP Sephadex, and gel filtration. The product had a molecular weight of 210,000 upon Sephadex G200 gel filtration and an isoelectric point of 4.5 (Habal et al, 1975). Upon reduction and rechromatography on Sephadex G200, proteins of 70,000 and 50,000 daltons were obtained suggesting that the HMW kininogen had a two chain structure. Nagasawa and Nakayasu have isolated human HMW kininogen in the presence of benzamidine and DFP and reported finding only a single chain form of 120,000 daltons (Nagasawa and Nakayasa 1974). More recently, Thompson et al (1978) have utilized a modification of the procedure of Habal et al to purify human HMW kininogen. Plasma was collected in hexadimethrine bromide and was first fractionated on QAE Sephadex A-50 equilibrated in 10 mM Tris Cl pH 8.0 containing 0.15 M NaCl,

0.1 mM DFP and 20 mM benzamidine. The column was then washed with the same buffer containing 0.2M NaCl and the kininogen batch eluted with 0.45 mM NaCl. The kininogen was then precipitated with 50 percent saturated ammonium sulfate and fractionated on CM-sepharose followed by gel filtration. For concentration, pooled fractions were dialyzed against 0.1 ammonium bicarbonate, lyophilized, and redissolved in phosphate buffered saline.

The purified HMW kininogen had a molecular weight of 210,000 upon Sephadex G-200 gel filtration, an isoelectric point of 4.3, and a molecular weight of 120,000 when assessed by SDS gel electrophoresis. Over 90 percent of the material remained at 120,000 daltons after reduction indicating that the HMW kininogen isolated was a single chain. It therefore appears likely that two-chain forms of human or bovine HMW kininogen that have been isolated were partially cleaved during the purification.

Digestion of HMW Kininogen by Plasma Kallikrein.

When human HMW kininogen was digested by plasma kallikrein and examined by SDS gel electrophoresis, an apparent loss of approximately 15,000 daltons was seen. The peptides released, have not been isolated (other than bradykinin) however release of a fragment analagous to bovine fragment 1.2 has not been observed. When a time course of digestion of human HMW kininogen by plasma kallikrein was performed, the mixture reduced, and then examined by SDS gel electrophoresis, the pattern shown in Fig. 15 was seen. A heavy chain represented by two closely spaced bands at approximately 66,000 and 56,000 daltons, and a light chain seen at 37,000 daltons, were progressively formed as the starting HMW kininogen was cleaved. The reason for the heavy chain heterogeneity is not clear; it was present in the small amount of cleaved HMW kininogen in the starting material and conversion of the 66,000 dalton band to the 56,000 dalton band was not observed. When human HMW kininogen was cleaved by plasma kallikrein, there was no apparent loss in coagulant activity; furthermore, a combination of kallikrein cleavage, reduction and alkylation, and treatment with 6M quanidine hydrochloride did not inactivate it. Thus the individual chains could be isolated and tested for coagulant activity as shown in Fig. 16.

Antibody to HMW kininogen has been prepared and used to determine the distinguishing features of HMW kininogen and LMW kininogen. A sheep was immunized with kininogen and the sheep plasma adsorbed with Williams trait plasma to yield an antibody that reacts with both high and low molecular weight kininogens. When the sheep antiserum was adsorbed with Fitzgerald trait plasma (which has significant quantities of LMW kininogen) an antiserum that was monospecific for HMW kininogen resulted. When each of these antisera were reacted with normal plasma, the pattern shown in Fig. 17 was seen. Two arcs that fuse at one end are seen with the anti-kininogen serum indicating a reaction of partial antigenic identity (upper trough). When normal plasma was reacted against the anti-HMW kininogen serum placed in the lower trough, only the inner arc was seen. When this latter antiserum was then reacted with the isolated HMW kininogen heavy and light chains a precipitin was only obtained with the light chain. Thus the light chain appeared to possess the major antigenic determinants that distinguish HMW kininogen from LMW kininogen. Furthermore, the data demonstrated that the antigens they share were associated with the heavy chain as has been reported when the chains of bovine kininogens were compared (Kato et al, 1966 Komiya et al, 1974).

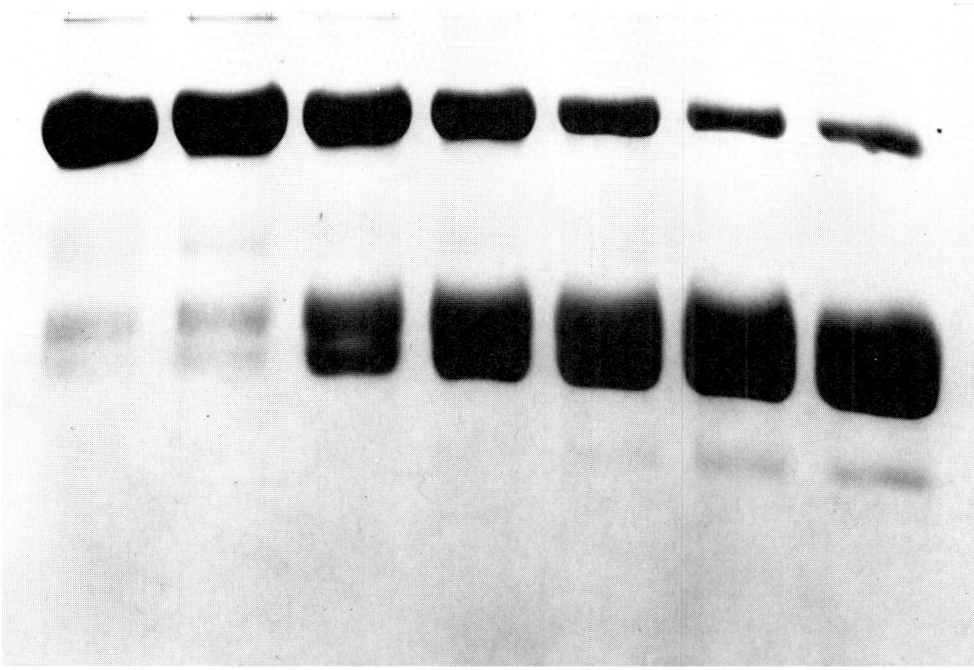

Fig. 15. Time course of interaction of 500 ug of HMW kininogen with 5 ug plasma kallikrein at 37°C. SDS polyacrylamide gel electrophoresis of 30 ug of reduced protein is shown after digestion for 0, 1, 5, 10, 20, 30 and 40 min. Two heavy chain bands at 66,000 and 56,000 daltons are seen as well as the light chain band at 37,000 daltons.

FACTOR XI

Purification and Properties.

Factor XI (Rosenthal et al; 1953) is a γ globulin of molecular weight 158,000 as assessed by SDS gel electrophoresis (Wuepper, 1972; Kaplan et al, 1974) and has an isoelectric point of 9.1 (Heck and Kaplan, 1974). It was first separated from Hageman factor by Schiffman et al (1960) who showed that it would not adhere to DEAE cellulose under dilute, alkaline conditions, while Hageman factor was completely bound. This initial step has been utilized in most purification procedures. Factor XI is thereby found in a fraction containing other γ globulins but it is free of virtually all the other plasma proteins. This is, however, the same fraction that contains prekallikrein and complete separation of these two proteins is difficult. The first direct demonstration that these two factors could be separated was reported by Harpel (1971), who incubated a mixture of both active enzymes with α_2 macroglobulin and fractionated the mixture by gel filtration. Kallikrein binds to this inhibitor while factor XIa does not, thus sephadex G-200 gel filtration of the mixture separated the kallikrein-α_2 macroglobulin complex from the factor XIa. The first chromatographic separation of kallikrein from factor XIa and prekallikrein from factor XI utilized a salt

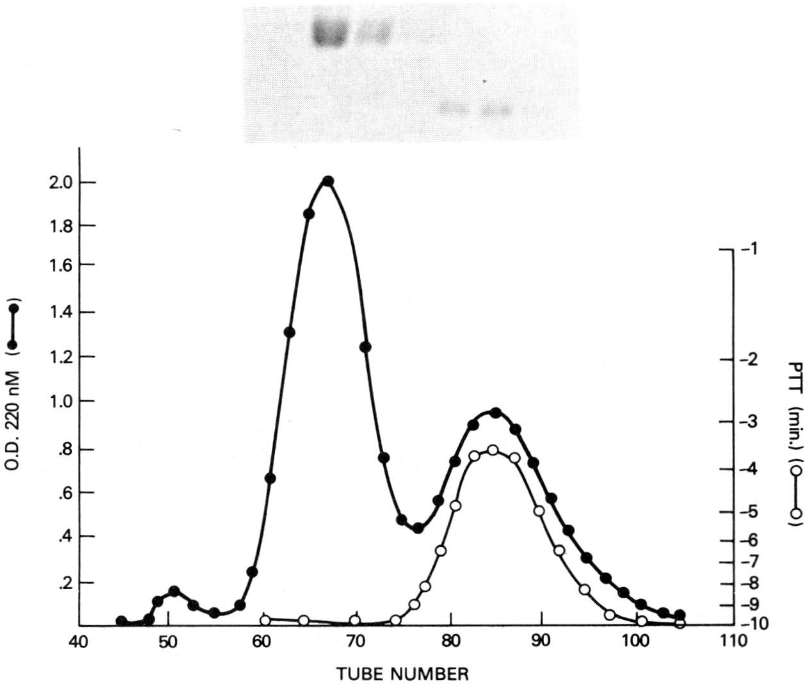

Fig. 16. Sephadex G-200 gel filtration of reduced, kinin-free HMW kininogen. The absorbance at 220 nm is shown as well as the ability of aliquots to correct the partial thromboplastin time of HMW kininogen deficient plasma. Above is shown the SDS-polyacrylamide gel electrophoretic pattern obtained after electrophoresis of 100 ul of tubes 60, 65, 70, and 75 (heavy chain) followed by electrophoresis of 100 ul of a 10-fold concentration of tubes 80, 85, and 90 (light chain).

gradient on SP sephadex (Kaplan et al, 197); prekallikrein was eluted first along the descending portion of the IgG peak at approximately 10-12 mS and factor XI eluted later at 18-20 mS. The factor XI preparation at this stage was still contaminated with prekallikrein, however over 90 percent of the IgG was removed. Fractionation on Sephadex G-200 yielded factor XI essentially free of prekallikre since the factor XI was eluted first at molecular weight 175,000 and prekallikrein eluted later at 100,000. This combination of three steps was also utilized by Saito et al (1973) to prepare highly purified factor XI however contamination with IgG and, at times, trace quantities of prekallikrein, remained.

Schiffman and Lee (1974) utilized a five-step procedure to prepare human factor XI of very high purity; however assessment by gel analysis was not reported and the percent contamination with residual IgG was not given. Wuepper (1972) utilized a separation by Pevikon block electrophoresis in which factor XI could be isolated such that it represented the major band seen upon SDS gel electrophoresis, and Heck and Kaplan (1974) removed residual IgG by passage over an anti IgG immunoadsorbant. The yield of factor XI obtained was approximately 6 percent

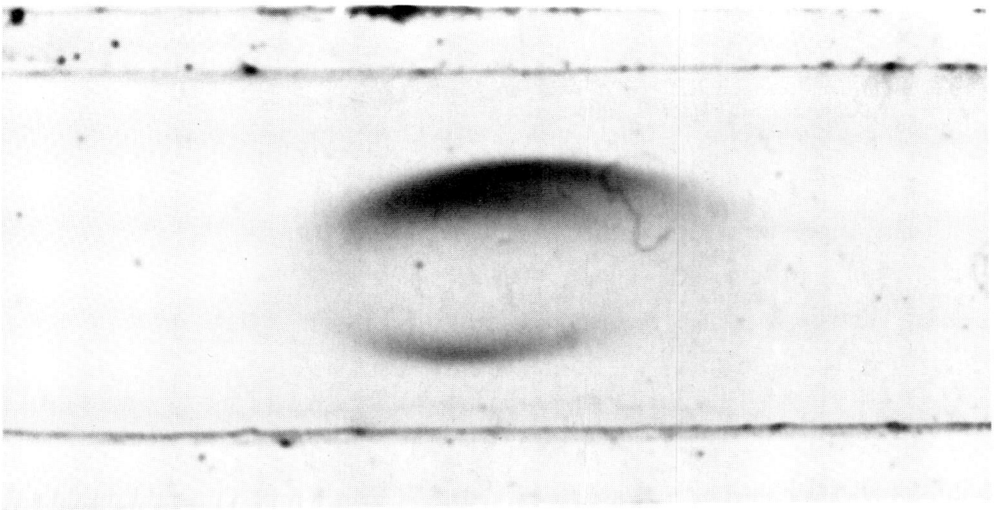

Fig. 17. Immunoelectrophoresis of normal plasma reacted against antibody to human kininogens (upper trough) and against antibody rendered specific for HMW kininogen (lower trough). A line of partial identity is seen.

Bouma and Griffin (1977) have reported a similar method for the isolation of Factor XI and by adding additional gradients on QAE sephadex and SP sephadex, eliminating the gel filtration step, and utilizing Conconavalin A sepharose to remove residual IgG, an increased yield resulted. Kurachi and Davie (1977) have also isolated human Factor XI and utilized its ability to bind to heparin sepharose and benzamidine sepharose to markedly simplify the isolation procedure.

Activation of Human Factor XI.

Purified preparations of human factor XI have a molecular weight of 155,000 to 160,000 upon SDS gel electrophoresis, however upon reduction, the molecular weight is 80,000 to 82,000 (Wuepper, 1972; Kaplan et al, 1974; Bouma and Griffin, 1977; Kurachi and Davie, 1977), and only a single band is seen. Thus it appears that factor XI is a two chain molecule and the two constituent chains are virtually the same size. A similar observation has been made when highly purified bovine factor XI was examined (Kaode et al, 1977) and, thus far, incorporation of high concentrations of benzamidine and DFP into the isolation procedure has not resulted in the formation of a single chain form of factor XI.

Clevage of human factor XI by trypsin (Wuepper 1972; Saito et al, 1973), Hageman factor fragments (Kaplan et al, 1974, Kaplan et al, 1976; Heck and Kaplan 1974) or surface bound activated Hageman factor (Bouma and Griffin, 1977) resulted in cleavage of the 80,000 daltons chains within a disulfide bridge. Thus in the absence of reduction, the molecular weight of factor XI and factor XIa were essentially the same. However, upon reduction, the two 80,000 chains of the starting material appeared to be cleaved to chains of 50,000 and 30,000. Factor XIa has been shown to be a serum protease (Kingdon et al, 1964) that can be inhibited by DFP. When factor XI was activated by Hageman factor, inactivated by ^{3}H-DFP, and reduced, ^{3}H-DFP was incorporated into the 30,000 dalton light chain (Bouma and Griffin, 1977). When binding of antithrombin III heparin by factor XIa was quantitated, two moles of antithrombin III appeared to be bound by each mole of factor XIa suggesting that there are two active sites in factor XIa, one for each light chain present (Kurachi and Davie, 1977).

Factor XI circulates as a complex with HMW kininogen (Thompson et al, 1977), the rate of conversion of factor XI to factor XIa is augmented by HMW kininogen (Shiffman and Lee 1975; Griffin and Cochrane 1976$_B$; Meier et al, 1977$_A$) and the rate of formation of activated Hageman factor (and factor XIa) are dependent upon prekallikrein. Yet prekallikrein circulates complexed to different HMW kininogen molecules than does factor XI thus a mechanism must exist in which Hageman factor that is activated by kallikrein can interact with the factor XI-HMW kininogen complex. This may require movement of either kallikrein or activated Hageman factor along the surface or release and readsorption of activated molecules at the surface-fluid phase interface. The ability of factor XIa-HMW kininogen to activate Hageman factor (Meier et al, 1977c) may, in part, account for the gradual correction of prekallikrein deficient plasma as the time of incubation with the surface is increased. The ability of factor XIa to completely correct the coagulation defect of Hageman factor, prekallikrein, or HMW kininogen deficient plasmas, and the normal rate of generation of plasmin and bradykinin upon activation of factor XI deficient plasma indicate that in a practical sense, activation of factor XIa represents the second step in the intrinsic coagulation pathway. It may, however, play an alternative role in the initial step when prekallikrein is absent.

THE ROLE OF THE EARLY STEPS OF THE INTRINSIC COAGULATION PATHWAY IN FIBRINOLYSIS.

Hageman factor dependent conversion of plasminogen to plasmin is readily demonstrable in whole plasma (Niewiarowski and Prow-Wartelle, 1959; Iatridis and Ferguson, 1962; McDonagh and Ferguson, 1970). Since prekallikrein and HMW kininogen are required for optimal activation and function of Hageman factor, they are also required for activation of the Hageman factor dependent fibrinolytic pathway. However, identification of the molecule or molecules that directly convert plasminogen to plasmin has been the subject of numerous investigations and the results have not been clear. Colman (1969) first reported that incubation of kallikrein with plasminogen leads to the generation of plasmin and the kinetics of the reaction appeared to be stoichiometric. Ogston et al (1969) demonstrated a cofactor required for Hageman factor dependent fibrinolysis that appeared to be distinguishable from kallikrein and factor XIa. However, it was clearly present in plasma fractions containing these factors. The assay for this protein was dependent upon reconstitution of glass-adsorbed plasma from which the fibrinolytic factor had been depleted. This "Hageman factor co-factor" had a molecular weight of 160,000 and it migrated with the γ globulins. Kaplan and Au (1972) subsequently demonstrated a Hageman factor-activatable plasma factor called plasminogen proactivator, which upon activation, was able to directly convert plasminogen to plasmin. These authors proposed that the plasminogen activator derived was responsible for the plasminogen-converting activity in kallikrein preparations. The demonstration of plasminogen proactivator activity in the γ globulin fraction of prekallikrein deficient plasma appeared to confirm their interpretation (Kaplan et al, 1973). However, Laake and Vennerod (1974) were unable to separate prekallikrein from plasminogen proactivator and concluded that kallikrein and plasminogen-activating activities are functions of the same molecule. When these authors examined the γ globulin effluent obtained from prekallikrein-deficient plasma, no plasminogen activator or proactivator activity was observed (Vennerod and Laake, 1976).

The successful purification of human prekallikrein has shed further light upon this question. First, when human prekallikrein was isolated in the presence of proteolytic inhibitors, the prekallikrein and plasminogen proactivator activates coincided and the two-banded pattern was shown to represent prekallikrein heterogeneity rather than two separate Hageman factor substrates (Mandle and Kaplan, 1977). Second, kallikrein was shown to cleave prekallikrein and decrease its molecular weight by 10,000 daltons; this difference in size corresponded to the previously reported difference in size between prekallikrein and plasminogen proactivator (Kaplan and Austen, 1972). Finally, fractionation of prekallikrein deficient plasma demonstrated that the plasminogen proactivator activity seen associated with prekallikrein was absent (Mandle and Kaplan, 1977). Hence the conclusion was reached that prekallikrein is a plasminogen proactivator and that the previous reported activity was a property of prekallikrein and/or the prekallikrein degradation product. However, plasminogen activating activity was again found in the γ globulin fraction of normal plasma (Mandle and Kaplan,1977B) which was not attributable to prekallikrein and this same activity was found in prekallikrein-deficient plasma. Further, fractionation of this material demonstrated that the activity was superimposed upon factor XI. In addition, two plasminogen proactivator peaks have been reported upon subsequent chromatography of the γ globulin fraction obtained from normal plasma (Kaplan et al, 1976) suggesting that factor XI may be a second proactivator. The observation that plasminogen activating activity does indeed reside in the γ globulin effluent of prekallikrein deficient plasma has been confirmed (Bouma and Griffin, 1978) however, these authors did not demonstrate that the activity was Hageman factor activatable and considered prekallikrein to be the only plasminogen proactivator. Clearly, the gradual conversion of plasminogen to plasmin observed in prekallikrein deficient plasma is secondary to a Hageman factor dependent enzyme that is not kallikrein. A recent report has presented evidence that activated Hageman factor itself, can also function as a plasminogen activator (Goldsmith et al, 1978) however when experiments are performed in which the fibrinolytic capacity of prekallikrein is assessed (i.e. Hageman factor fragments plus plasminogen) the contribution of HFf is less than 5 percent of the activity seen with kallikrein. Thus larger quantities of activated Hageman factor may be required for this effect to reach significant levels. It appears clear that prekallikrein is a plasminogen proactivator, factor XI may function as a second proactivator,and HFa and HFf may directly contribute to plasminogen activation.

The identity of the Hageman factor cofactor is not clear however the function these authors observed does not appear to be distinguishable from that of the known Hageman factor substrates. Glass adsorbed plasma, used in the assay for the Hageman factor cofactor has been shown to be depleted of prekallikrein (Wuepper, 1973_B) thus the kallikrein present in Hageman factor cofactor preparations may contribute to the fibrinolysis observed by its effect upon Hageman factor activation. Yet the molecular weight reported for this factor was quite different from kallikrein and the factor appeared to be separable from the bulk of kallikrein but not from factor XI (Ogston et al, 1969;Robyn, et al, 1972). The active factor was also inhibited by α_1 antitrypsin, a property it shares with factor XIa (Robyn et al, 1972). The molecular properties of this cofactor most closely resemble the activity we have observed with our factor XI preparation, thus it is possible that the activity being measured was a function of more than one protein.

Further studies in whole plasma are needed to distinguish the effect of kallikrein upon fibrinolysis via its ability to activate Hageman factor from its ability to convert plasminogen to plasmin. It is of interest that one estimate of the direct contribution of kallikrein to the conversion of plasminogen to plasmin was approximately 50 percent (Kluft, 1977) of the total Hageman factor dependent fibrinolytic activity present in plasma.

A summary of the known interactions leading to coagulation, fibrinolysis and kinin-formation is shown in Fig. 18.

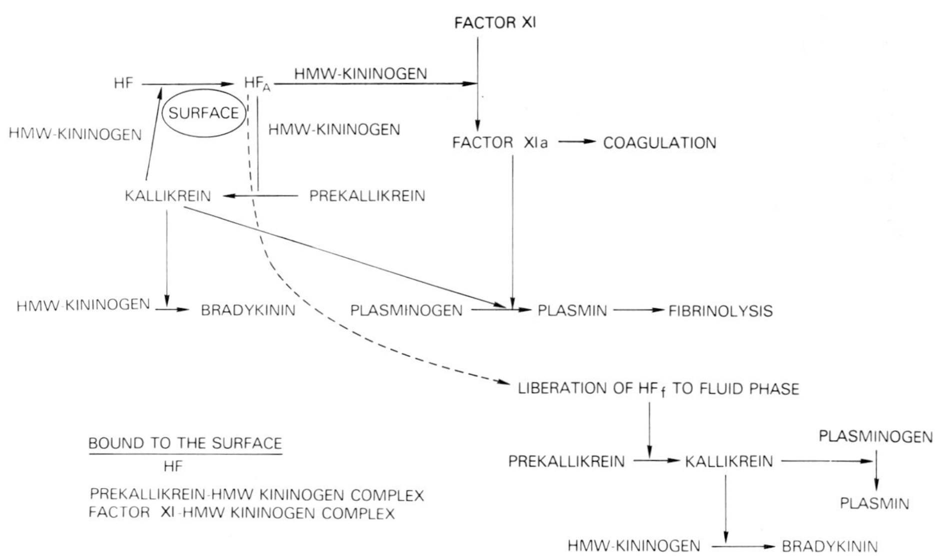

Fig. 18. Diagram of the known interactions leading to Hageman factor dependent coagulation, fibrinolysis and the generation of bradykinin.

Further studies in whole plasma are needed to distinguish the effect of kallikrein upon fibrinolysis via its ability to activate Hageman factor from its ability to convert plasminogen to plasmin. It is of interest that one estimate of the direct contribution of kallikrein to the conversion of plasminogen to plasmin was approximately 50 percent, (Kluft, 1977) of the total Hageman factor dependent fibrinolytic activity present in plasma.

A summary of the known interactions leading to coagulation, fibrinolysis and kinin-formation is shown in Figure 18.

REFERENCES

1. Bagdasarian, A., Talamo, R.C., and Colman, R.W., Isolation of high molecular weight activators of plasma prekallikrein. J. Biol. Chem. 248:3456-3463, 1972.

2. Bagdasarian, A., Lahiri, B., and Colman, R.W., Origin of the high molecular weight activator of prekallikrein, J. Biol. Chem. 248:7742-7747, 1973.

3. Bouma, B. N. and Griffin, J. H., Human blood coagulation factor XI: Purification, properties and mechanism of activation. J. Biol. Chem. 252:6432-6437, 1977.

4. Bouma, B. N., and Griffin, J. H., Deficiency of factor XII-dependent plasminogen proactivator in prekallikrein deficient plasma, J. Lab. Clin. Med. 91: 148-155, 1978.

5. Burrowes, C. E., Movat, H.Z., and Soltay, M. J., The kinin system of human plasma VI. The action of plasmin. Proc. Soc. Exp. Biol. Med. 135:959-966, 1975.

6. Cochrane, C.G., Revak, S.D., and Wuepper, K. D., Activation of Hageman factor in solid and fluid phases. J. Exp. Med., 138:1564-1583, 1973.

7. Colman, R.W., Activation of plasminogen by human plasma kallikrein. Biochem. Biophys. Res. Commun. 351:273-279, 1969.

8. Colman, R.W., Bagdasarian, A., Talamo, R.C., Scott, C.F., Seavey, M., Guimares, J.A., Pierce, J.V., and Kaplan, A.P., Williams Trait. Human kininogen deficiency with diminished levels of plasminogen proactivator and prekallikrein associated with abnormalities of the Hageman factor-dependent pathways. J. Clin. Invest. 56: 1650-1662, 1975.

9. Goldsmith, G.H., Saito, H., and Ratnoff, O.D., The activation of plasminogen by Hageman factor (factor XII) and Hageman factor fragments. J. Clin. Invest. 62: 54-60, 1978.

10. Griffin, J. H., Role of surface in surface-dependent activation of Hageman factor (Blood coagulation factor XII). Proc. Natl. Acad. Sci. 75: 1998-2002, 1978.

11. Griffin, J. H. and Cochrane, C.G., Involvement of high M.W. kininogen (HK) in surface dependent reactions of Hageman factor. Fed. Proc. 35: 692, 1976_A.

12. Griffin, J. H. and Cochrane, C.G., Mechanisms for the involvement of high molecular weight kininogen in surface-dependent reactions of Hageman factor. Proc. Nat. Acad. Sci., 8:2554-2558, 1976_B.

13. Habal, F.M. and Movat, H.Z., Some physico chemical and functional differences between low and high molecular weight kininogens of human plasma. In: The chemistry and biology of the kallikrein-kinin system in health and disease. John J. Pisano and K. Frank Austen, editors. Fogarty International Center Proceedings No . 27, U.S. Government Printing Office, Washington, D. C., pp. 129-131, 1974.

14. Habal, F.M., Movat, H.Z., and Burrowes, C.E., Isolation of two functionally different kininogens from human plasma - separation from proteinase inhibitors and interaction with plasma kallikrein. Biochem. Pharmacol. 23: 2291-2302, 1974.

15. Habal, F.M., Underdown, B.J., and Movat, H.Z., Further characterization of human plasma kininogens. Biochem. Pharm. 24:1241-1243, 1975.

16. Harpel, P.C., Separation of plasma thromboplastin antecedent from kallikrein by the plasma $_2$ macroglobulin, kallikrein inhibitor. J. Clin. Invest. 50:2084-2090, 1971.

17. Heck, L.W., and Kaplan, A.P., Substrates of human factor I. Isolation and characterization of PTA (Factor XI) and its inhibition by $_1$ antitrypsin J. Exp. Med. 140:1615 -1630 , 1974.

18. Iatridis, S.G. and Ferguson, J.H., Active Hageman factor. A plasma lysokinase of the human fibrinolytic system. J. Clin. Invest. 41:1277-1187, 1962.

19. Johnson, A.R., Ulevitch, R.J., and Ryan, K., Biochemical and biological properties of rabbit prekallikrein. Fed. Proc. 35:693., 1976.

20. Kaode, T., Hermodson, M.A., and Davie, E. W., Active site of bovine Hageman factor XI (plasma thromboplastin antecedent). Nature 266: 729-731, 1977.

21. Kaplan, A.P., and Austen, K.F., A prealbumin activator of prekallikrein. J. Immunol. 105:802-811, 1970.

22. Kaplan, A.P., and Austen, K.F., A prealbumin activator of prekallikrein II. Derivation of activators of prekallikrein from active Hageman factor by digestion with plasmin. J. Exp. Med. 133:672-712, 1971.

23. Kaplan, A.P., and Austen, K. F., The fibrinolytic pathway of human plasma. Isolation and characterization of the plasminogen proactivator. J. Exp. Med. 136: 1378-1393, 1972.

24. Kaplan, A.P., Goetzl, E.J., and Austen, K.F., The fibrinolytic pathway of human plasma II. Generation of chemotactic activity by activation of plasminogen proactivator. J. Clin. Invest. 52: 2591-2597, 1973.

25. Kaplan, A.P., Meier, H.W., and Mandle, Jr., R., The Hageman factor dependent pathways of coagulation, fibrinolysis, and kinin-generation. Seminars Thrombosis Haemostasis 3: 1-26, 1976.

26. Kaplan, A.P., Meier, H.S., Yecies, L.D., and Heck, L.W., Hageman factor and its substrates: the role of factor XI (PTA), prekallikrein, and plasminogen proactivator in coagulation, fibrinolysis and kinin-generation, In: Chemistry and biology of the kallikrein-kinin system in health and disease John J. Pisano and K. Frank Austen, editors. Fogarty Interantional Center Proceedings No. 27, U.S., Government Printing Office, Washington, D. C. pp. 237-254, 1974.

27. Kaplan, A.P., Spragge, J., and Austen, K.F., The bradykinin-forming system in man. In: Biochemistry of the acute allergic reaction. K.F. Austen and E.L. Becker, editors. Oxford, Blackwell Scientific Publications Ltd. pp. 279-298, 1971.

28. Kato, H., Han, Y.N., Iwanaga, S., Suzuke, T., and Komiya, M., Bovine plasma HMW and LMW kininogens. Structural differences between heavy and light chains derived from the kinin-free proteins. J. Biochem. 80:1299-1311, 1966.

29. Kurachi, K. and Davie, E. W., Activation of human factor XI (Plasma Thromboplastin Antecedent) by factor XIIa (Activated Hageman Factor). Biochem. 5831-5839, 1977.

30. Laake, K. and Vennerod, A.M., Factor Xii-induced fibrinolysis. Studies on the separation of prekallikrein, plasminogen proactivator, and factor XI in human plasma. Thromb. Res. 4:285-302, 1974.

31. Liu, C.Y., Bagdasarian, A., Meier, H., Scott, C.F., Pierce, J., Kaplan, A.P. and Colman, R.W. Potentiation of the action of Hageman factor fragments (HFf) by high molecular weight kininogen (HMW kng). Fed. Proc. 35:692, 1976.

32. Liu, C.Y., Scott, C.F., Bagdasarian, A., Pierce, J.V., Kaplan, A.P., and Colman, R.W., Potentiation of the function of Hageman factor fragments by high molecular weight kininogen. J. Clin. Invest. 60:7-17, 1977.

33. Mandle,Jr., R., Colman, R.W., and Kaplan, A.P., Identification of prekallikrein and HMW-kininogen as a circulating complex in human plasma. Proc. Natl. Acad. Sci. U.S.A. 73:4179-4183, 1976.

34. Mandle, Jr., R., and Kaplan, A.P., Hageman factor substrates. Human plasma prekallikrein: mechanism of activation by Hageman factor and participation in Hageman factor-dependent fibrinolysis. J. Biol. Chem. 252:6097-6104,1977.

35. McDonagh, K.S., and Ferguson, J.H., Studies on the participation of Hageman factor in fibrinolysis. Throm. et. Diath. Haemorrh. 24: 1-9, 1970.

36. McMillin, C.R., Saito, H., Ratnoff, O.D., and Walton, A.G., The secondary structure of human Hageman factor (Factor XII) and its alteration by activating agents. J. Clin. Invest. 54: 1312-1322, 1974.

37. Meier, H.S., Pierce, J.V., Colman, R.W., and Kaplan, A.P., Activation and function of human Hageman factor. The role of high molecular weight kininogen and prekallikrein. J. Clin. Invest. 60: 18-31, 1977_A.

38. Meier, H. L., Scott, C.F., Mandle, Jr., R., WEbster, M.E., Pierce, J.V., Colman, R.W., and Kaplan, A.P., Requirements for contact activation of human Hageman factor. Annals. N.Y. Acad. Sci. 283:93-103, 1977_B.

39. Meier, H.L., Thompson, R.E., and Kaplan, A.P., Activation of Hageman factor by factor XIa-HMW-kininogen. Throm. and Haemostasis 38:14, 1977_C.

40. Meier, H.L., Webster, M., Liu, C.Y., Colman, R.W., and Kaplan, A.P., Enhancement of surface dependent Hageman factor activation by high molecular weight kininogen. Fed. Proc. 35:692, 1976.

41. Movat, H.Z. Poon, M.C., and Tukeuchi, Y., The kinin system of human plasma I. Isolation of a low molecular weight activator of prekallikrein. Int. Arch. Allergy Appl. Immunol. 40:89-112, 1971.

42. Nagasawa, S. and Nakayasu, T., Human plasma prekallikrein as a protein complex. J. Biochem. 74: 401-403, 1973.

43. Nagasawa, S. and Nakayasa, T., Enzymatic and chemical cleavages of human kininogens. In: Chemistry and biology of the kallikrein-kinin system in health and disease. John J. Pisano and K. Frank Austen, editors. Fogarty International Proceedings No. 27, U.S. Government Printing Office, Washington, D.C., pp. 139-144, 1974.

44. Nagasawa, S., Takahashi, H., Koida, M., and Suzuki, T. Partial purification of bovine plasma kallikreinogen, its activation by the Hageman factor. Biochem. Biophys. Res. Commun. 32:644-649, 1968.

45. Biewiarowski, S. and Prow-Wartelle, O., Role du facteur contact (Facteur Hageman) dans la fibrinolyse. Throm. Diath. Haemorrhag. 3:593-603, 1959.

46. Ogston, D., Ogston, C.M., Ratnoff, O.D., and Forbes, C. O., Studies on a complex mechanism for the activation of plasminogen by kaolin and by chloroform the participation of Hageman factor and additional cofactors. J. Clin. Invest. 48: 1786-1801, 1969.

47. Pierce, J.V. and Guimaraes, J.A., Further characterization of highly purified human plasma kininogens. In: Chemistry and biology of the kallikrein-kinin system in health and disease. John J. Pisano and K. Frank Austen, editors. Fogarty International Center Proceedings No. 27 U.S. Government Printing Office, Washington, D.C. pp. 121-127, 1974.

48. Ratnoff, O.D. and Rosenblum, J.M., Role of Hageman factor in the initiation of clotting by glass: evidence that glass frees Hageman factor from inhibition. Am. J. Med. 25: 160-168, 1958.

49. Revak, S.D., Cochrane, C.G., Johnston, A., and Hugli, T., Structural changes accompanying enzymatic activation of Hageman factor. J. Clin. Invest. 54:619-627, 1974.

50. Revak, S.D. and Cochrane, C. G., The relationship of Structure and function in human Hageman factor. The association of enzymatic and binding activities with separate regions of the molecule, J. Clin. Invest. 57: 852-860, 1976.

51. Revak, S.D., Cochrane, C. G., Bouma,B.N., and Griffin, J.H., Surface and Fluid Phase Activities of Two Forms of Activated Hageman Factor Produced During Contact Activation of Plasma. J. Exp. Med. 147:719-229, 1978.

52. Revak, S.D., Cochrane, C.G., and Griffin, J.H., The binding and cleavage characteristics of human Hageman factor during contact activation. A comparison of normal plasma with plasmas deficient in factor XI, prekallikrein, or high molecular weight kininogen. J. Clin. Invest. 59: 1167-1175, 1977.

53. Robyn, J.C., Ogston, D., and Douglas, A.T. Further purification and properties of Hageman factor cofactor. Biochem. Biophys. Acta 271: 371-377, 1972.

54. Rosenthal, R.L., Dreskin, O.H. and Rosenthal, N., New hemophiliia-like disease caused by deficiency of a third plasma thromboplastin factor. Proc. Soc. Exp. Biol. Med. 82: 171-174, 1953.

55. Saito, H., Ratnoff, O.D., and Donaldson, V.H., Defective activation of clotting, fibrinolytic and permeability enhancing systems in human Fletcher trait plasma. Circ. Res. 34:641-651, 1974.

56. Saito, H., Ratnoff, O.D., Marshall, J.S. and Pensky, J., Partial purification of plasma thromboplastin antecedent (factor XI) and its activation by trypsin. J. Clin, Invest. 52:850-861, 1973.

57. Schiffman, S. and Lee, P. Preparation, characterization, activation of a highly purified factor XI. Evidence that a hitherto unrecognized plasma activity participates in the interaction of factors XI and XII. Brit. J. Haematol:27: 101-114, 1974.

58. Schiffman, S. and Lee, P. Partial purification and characterization of contact activation cofactor. J. Clin. Invest. 56:1082-1092, 1975.

59. Schiffman, S., Rapaport, S.I., Ware, A.O., and Mehl, J.W., Separation of plasma thromboplastin and antecedent (PTA) and Hageman factor (HF) from human plasma. Proc. Soc. Exp. Biol. Med. 105:453-455, 1960.

60. Soltay, M.J., Movat, H. Z. and Ozge-Anwar, A.H., The kinin system of human plasma V., The probable derivative of prekallikrein activator from activated Hageman factor. Proc. Soc. Exp. Biol. Med. 138:952-958, 1972.

61. Takahashi, H., Nagasawa, S., and Suzuki, T. Studies on prekallikrein of bovine plasma I. Purification and properties. J. Biochem. 71:471-483, 1972.

62. Thompson, R.E., Mandle, Jr., R., and Kaplan, A.P., Association of factor XI and high molecular weight kininogen in human plasma. J. Am. Invest. 60:1376-1380, 1977.

63. Thompson, R.E., Mandle, Jr., R., and Kaplan, A.P., Characterization of human high molecular weight kininogen. Procoagulant activity associated with the light chain of kinin-free high molecular weight kininogen. J. Exp. Med. 147:488-499, 1978.

64. Trloar, M.P. and Movat, H.Z., Isolation of two small molecular activators of the plasma kinin system in the guinea pig. Fed. Proc. 59:576, 1970.

65. Vennerod, A.M. and Laake, K., Prekallikrein and Plasminogen proactivator: Absence of plasminogen proactivator in Fletcher factor deficient plasma. Throm. Res. 8:519-522, 1976.

66. Weiss, A.S., Gallin, J.I., and Kaplan, A.P., Fletcher factor deficiency. Abnormalities of coagulation, fibrinolysis, chemotactic activity, and kinin generation attributable to absence of prekallikrein. J. Clin. Invest. 53:622-633, 1974.

67. Wendel, U., Vogt, W., and Seidel, G., Purification and some properties of a kininogenase from human plasma activated by surface contact. Hoppe Seylers Z. Physiol. Chem. 353: 1591-1606, 1972.

68. Wiggins, R.C., Bouma, B.N., Cochrane, C.G. and Griffin, J.H., Role of high molecular weight kininogen in surface-binding and activation of coagulation factor XI and prekallikrein. Proc. Natl. Acad. Sci. 77:4636-4640, 1977.

69. Wuepper, K.D., Biochemistry and biology of components of the plasma kinin-forming system. In: Inflammation: mechanism and control. I.H. Lepow and P.A. Ward, editors. New York, Academic Press, p. 93-117, 1972.

70. Wuepper, K.D., Prekallikrein deficiency in man. J. Exp. Med. 138: 1345-1355, 1973_A.

71. Wuepper, K. D. Prekallikrein-Hageman factor cofactor- Fletcher factor: are they identical? Clin. Res. 21:484, 1973_B.

72. Wuepper, K.D., and Cochrane, C.G., Isolation and mechanism of activation of components of the plasma kinin-forming system. In: the biochemistry of the acute allergic reactions - Second International Symposium. K.F. Austen and E.L. Becker, editors. Blackwell Scientific Publications Ltd., pp. 299-320, 1971

73. Wuepper, K.D. and Cochrane, C.G., Plasma prekallikrein: Isolation, characterization and mechanism of activation. J. Exp. Med. 135: 1-20, 1972_A.

74. Wuepper, K.D. and Cochrane, C.G., Effect of plasma kallikrein on coagulation in vitro. Proc. Soc. Exp. Biol. Med. 141:271-276, 1972_B.

75. Wuepper, K.D., Miller, D.R., and LaCombe, M.J., Flaujeac trait. Deficiency of human plasma kininogen. J. Clin. Invest. 56:1663-1672, 1975.

STRUCTURAL STUDIES OF THE VON WILLEBRAND PROTEIN

Daniel Deykin and Mark Weinstein
Boston Veterans Administration Medical Center

The thrust of the coagulation papers already presented today and of those to be given tomorrow demonstrates the change in coagulation research over the past fifty years. In 1928 the outlines of the coagulation sequences were dimly perceived. The complexity of clotting could hardly have been anticipated. In the twenty-five years between 1928 and 1953, research focussed primarily on the unraveling of the physiology of coagulation. Only within the last fifteen years have purified coagulation proteins other than fibrinogen been available. As today's papers have demonstrated, the present excitement in coagulation research derives from our expanding ability to relate structure to function.

Because of its enormous size and because of the lability of its clotting activity, Factor VIII has been one of the most difficult proteins to study. I should now like to present some of our recent work on the structure and function of Factor VIII carried out by my colleague, Dr. Mark Weinstein, in our laboratory at the Boston Veterans Administration Medical Center.

Factor VIII has two distinct properties. It shortens the abnormally prolonged clotting tests in patients with hemophilia or severe von Willebrand's disease. In addition, when certain Factor VII-enriched preparations are infused into patients with severe von Willebrand's disease, they shorten the patients' prolonged bleeding time. Although the *in vivo* attributes of Factor VIII define its biological activities, recent studies of the protein or proteins that are associated with Factor VIII activities have led to partial characterization of the proteins and also have led to several *in vitro* assays for both aspects of Factor VIII. Some of these properties and assays are summarized in Table 1.

The protein associated with the ability to shorten the bleeding time in patients with von Willebrand's disease is a large multimer with molecular weights between one to ten million. The multimer can be reduced to identical subunits with molecular weights of approximately 220,000. The multimer is readily isolated from plasma by gel filtration. When injected into rabbits, it elicits a precipitating antibody that facilitates identification of the von Willebrand-related protein by immunological techniques. The multimer and its subunits can be further identified by immuno- and SDS gel electrophoresis. Fortuitously, the von Willebrand protein potentiates the aggregation of platelets by the antibiotic, ristocetin, in a concentration dependent fashion that correlates with its biological properties.

TABLE 1 The Factor VIII Complex

PROTEIN	ACTIVITY	ASSAYS	MOLECULAR PROPERTIES
1. VIII RP:WF	SHORTENS BLEEDING TIME WHEN TRANS-FUSED INTO VON WILLEBRAND PATIENTS	a) BLEEDING TIME b) RISTOCETIN CO-FACTOR c) IMMUNOLOGICAL: PRODUCES PRE-CIPITATING HETEROLOGOUS Ab d) GEL ELECTRO-PHORESIS	2.2×10^5 mol. wt. SUBUNIT 10^6 to 10^7 mol. wt. MULTIMERS
2. VIII RP:C	SHORTENS CLOTTING TIMES IN PATIENTS WITH HEMOPHILIA AND SEVERE VON WILLEBRAND'S DISEASE	a) CLOTTING TESTS b) NEUTRALIZES HOMOLOGOUS HUMAN ANTI-BODY	1.5×10^5 mol. wt. (TENTATIVE)

Factor VIII preparations enriched with both clotting and von Willebrand activities are prepared by cryoprecipitation of plasma. The clotting activity is further purified in commercial concentrates. These concentrates, however, lack the abilit to correct the bleeding time in von Willebrand patients even though the concentrat contain large amounts of the von Willebrand-related protein identified by its anti genic properties. The purpose of our study was to examine the structural characteristics of the von Willebrand-related protein that could account for the functional differences betw-en cryoprecipitate and commercial concentrates of Factor V

We first isolated the von Willebrand-related protein from cryoprecipitate and from several samples of commercial concentrates by gel chromatography on A15m agarose, taking care to avoid proteolytic degradation of the multimers. The proteins in the void volume were examined by SDS gel electrophoresis on 1.5 per cent polyacryl amide - 0.5 per cent agarose gels, as shown in Fig. 1. The area within the bars contains the Willebrand protein multimers. The multimers in the cryoprecipitate increase in a uniform manner with a difference between the monomers consistent with an increment of two or three subunits per increment. By contrast the multime from the concentrates made by several manufacturers (a representative gel is shown appeared as doublets. Furthermore, the inter-multimer spacing appears heterogeneous. A second major difference between the multimers from the two sources is the average molecular weight of the multimer populations, best appreciated by comparing densitometry scans, as shown in Fig. 2. The peaks under the bars are the von Willebrand related protein multimers. Eighty-five per cent of the concentrate multimers lie between molecular weights of 1.4 to 5 million, but 75 per cent of the cryoprecipitate multimers lie aboe- a molecular weight of 5 million.

We have further examined the assembly of the multimers in each preparation by high resolution two-dimensional SDS gel chromatography. The proteins were first electrophoresed without reduction through 1.5 per cent polyacrylamide - 0.5 per cent agarose to separate multimers and then after reduction through 3 per cent polyacry amide - 0.5 per cent agarose to resolve the subunits of the multimers. The subuni of all the multimers in each preparation migrated identically, with apparent molec ular weights of 220,000.

Fig. 1. SDS gel electrophoresis of von Willebrand-related proteins

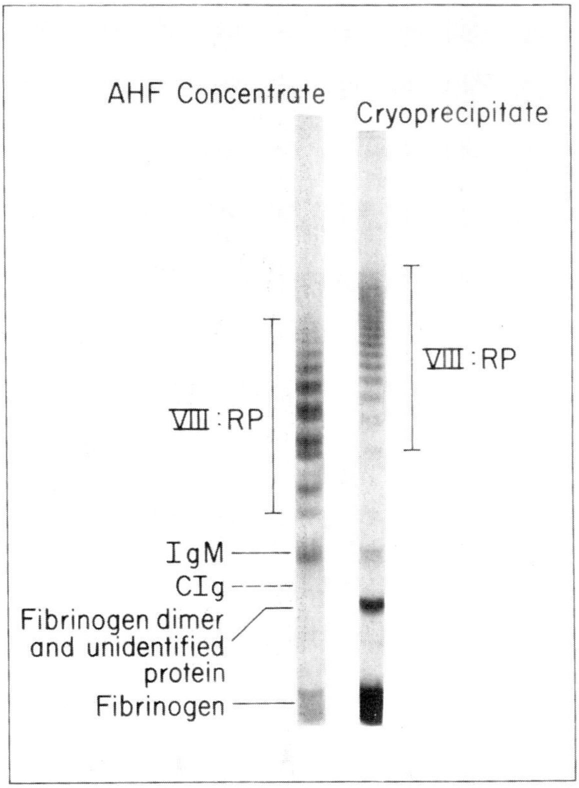

In parallel studies we confirmed the functional differences between the two preparations by measuring the ristocetin co-factor activities in each preparation. The cryoprecipitate was three times more potent per multimer subunit than the concentrate. Therefore, the biological differences between the two preparations lay not in their purity nor in their subunit content, but rather in the organization of the subunits into multimers of high molecular weight.

The technique of two-dimensional high resolution SDS gel electrophoresis we have developed provides a powerful additional method for examining the structure and function of the von Willebrand protein in both acquired and hereditary disorders affecting the Factor VIII complex.

Fig. 2. Densitometry scans of gels

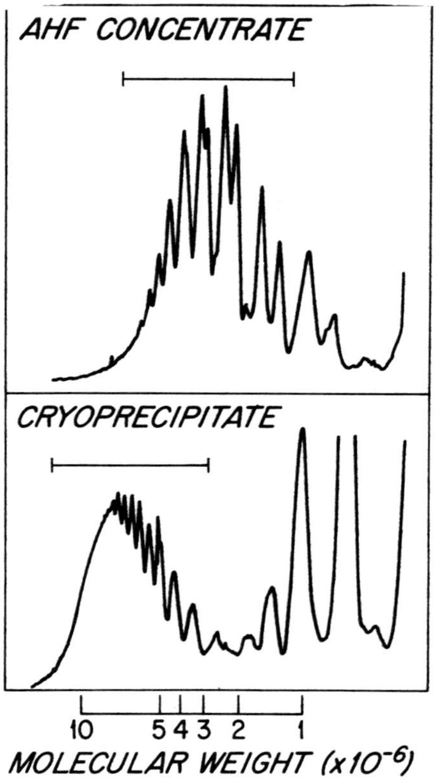

ACTIVATION MECHANISMS OF THE ALTERNATIVE COMPLEMENT PATHWAY AND AMPLIFICATION STEP*

Douglas T. Fearon+ and K. Frank Austen

Departments of Medicine, Harvard Medical School and Robert B. Brigham Division of the Affiliated Hospitals Center, Inc., Boston, Massachusetts.

ABSTRACT

Cleavage of C3 by the alternative complement pathway occurs in at least two distinct phases: continuous generation of C3b by low grade interaction of C3, B, D and P, and subsequent amplified cleavage of C3 by the interaction of C3b, B, D and P. Transition to C3b-dependent amplification is necessary to achieve substantial C3 cleavage and is normally prevented by C3bINA and β1H which limit formation and function of C3b,Bb. Activators of the alternative pathway provide sites that protect bound C3b and C3b,Bb from the actions of these regulatory proteins and permit C3b deposited by the low grade fluid phase reaction to assemble a membrane-associated amplification convertase which can deposit additional protected C3b. One biochemical characteristic of these privileged membrane sites is their lack of sialic acid, which is necessary for effective interaction between bound C3b and β1H. Sialic acid residues augment binding of β1H to favor competition with B, inactivation of C3b and decay-dissociation of C3b,Bb. The absence of this carbohydrate on the membrane in the environment of C3b results in low affinity binding of β1H, a circumstance that permits uptake of B to form the amplification convertase and impairs extrinsic decay of the C3-cleaving enzyme. This natural humoral host resistance reaction based on the relative content of sialic acid on target particles has a cellular counterpart in the capacity of human monocytes to engage in antibody-independent phagocytosis of sialic acid-deficient cells. Thus, the non-immune host may respond to such cells by dual humoral and cellular recognition mechanisms and this response may represent a primordial basis for protection against microbial invasion. The natural selective processes leading to the evolution of these systems may be based on the infrequent occurrence of sialic acid in microorganisms.

*Supported in part by grants AI-07722 and RR-05669 from the National Institutes of Health, and in part by a grant from the New England Peabody Home for Crippled Children.

+Dr Fearon is a recipient of a Research Career Development Award (K04 AI-00245) from the National Institutes of Health.

HISTORICAL PERSPECTIVES

In the early 1950's Pillemer and associates observed that inactivation of the third component of complement in human serum by incubation with zymosan, an insoluble polysaccharide-containing derivative of yeast cell walls, had characteristics of an enzymatic reaction (1). The reaction was temperature-dependent with an optimum at 37°C, required the presence of Mg^{2+} but not Ca^{2+}, involved a novel serum protein, properdin (P), which was felt to be distinct from immunoglobulin and apparently did not utilize the "classical" complement components, C1, C4 and C2. As removal of P from serum by adsorption to zymosan impaired certain bactericidal, virus-neutralizing and antibody-independent hemolytic activities of serum without affecting lysis of sensitized sheep erythrocytes, the original investigators considered the "properdin system" to represent a mechanism for complement activation that was distinct from the classical pathway. The apparent absence of a requirement for specific antibody for activation further suggested that the properdin system had an essential role in humoral natural immune reactions (1). However, the observations that preparations of properdin contained antibodies to zymosan, and that some consumption of C1 and C4 in serum did occur upon treatment with zymosan led to an alternative proposal that this reaction did not differ from the usual antibody-dependent activation of the classical complement pathway (2). This serious challenge to the concept of a distinct properdin system caused most immunologists to doubt its existence and as recently as 1968 a comprehensive review of the complement system did not refer to these early investigations of the alternative pathway (3).

During the period of 1968-1971 and coincident with the application of effective methods for the assay and purification of components of complement, independent observations in several laboratories reaffirmed the presence in serum of the properdin or alternative pathway of complement activation. Incubation of serum with lipopolysaccharide from gram negative bacilli caused consumption of C3-C9 with little utilization of C1, C4 and C2, findings which contrasted with the intense utilization of these classical pathway components when antigen-antibody complexes induce activation of C3 in serum (4). The C3-cleaving enzyme that was formed on lipopolysaccharide during incubation in serum was antigenically distinct from the classical C3 convertase, C4b,2a, as antiserum to C2 inhibited the latter enzyme but not the former (5). The earlier demonstration that highly purified P was not immunoglobulin or a known complement protein also supported the contention that the alternative pathway was comprised of plasma proteins other than C1, C4 and C2 (6). Immune complexes and aggregates of immunoglobulin that contained classes or fragments of antibody not capable of activating C1 were found to induce consumption of C3-C9 in serum (7, 8). The discovery of guinea pigs genetically deficient in C4 permitted experiments that demonstrated unequivocally C3 activation by lipopolysaccharide without involvement of the classical pathway (9). Finally, inactivation of C3-C9 by a protein of cobra venom (10) was shown to require the presence of a serum protein (11) subsequently identified as factor B of the original descriptions of the properdin pathway (12, 13). By 1971, the existence of the alternative pathway for activation of C3-C9 was no longer questioned. Since that time the six plasma proteins comprising this pathway have been identified (Fig. 1, Table 1) and the molecular basis has been delineated by which their interactions discriminate between activating and non-activating particle surfaces.

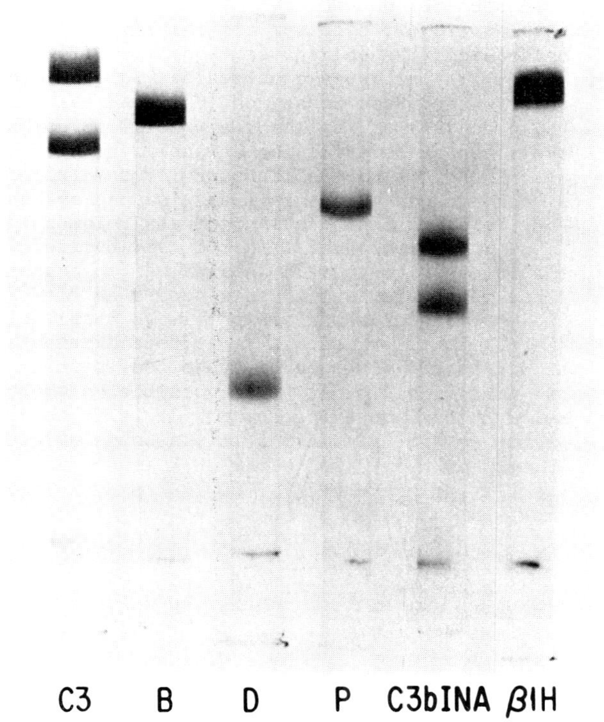

Fig. 1. Sodium dodecyl sulfate (SDS) - polyacrylamide gel electrophoresis cf purified, reduced proteins of the alternative complement pathway. [From (14).]

THE AMPLIFICATION C3 CONVERTASE

Although the amplification C3 convertase is not the first C3 convertase formed in the reaction sequence, it is essential for effective C3 cleavage by the alternative pathway; thus endogenous modulation of its formation and

TABLE 1 Proteins of the Alternative Pathway of Complement Activation

Protein	Average Plasma Concentration (μg/ml	Isoelectric Point	Polypeptide Chains	Apparent Molecular Weight of Polypeptide Chains	Cleavage Fragments
C3	1250	6.1 - 6.8	α (15, 16)	120,000	C3b, C3a, C3bi, C3c, C3d
			β	80,000	
Properdin	25	< 9.5	Four identical chains (17)	54,000	None
B	250	6.6 - 6.8	Single (18)	93,000	Bb, Ba
$\overline{D}$	2	7.2 - 7.5	Single (18)	23,500	None
C3b Inactivator	50	5.8 - 6.1	α (19, 20)	55,000	None
			β	42,000	
β1H	500	5.8 - 6.2	Single (21)	150,000	None

function determines whether the pathway responds to a particular microbial organism or mammalian cell. This critical concept of an amplification reaction evolved from the finding that interaction of C3b, B and $\overline{D}$ in the presence of Mg^{2+} resulted in the generation of C3 convertase activity concomitant with cleavage of B into fragments of 63,000 and 30,000 m.w., Bb and Ba, respectively (22). The positive feedback mechanism in which the product of C3 cleavage, C3b, participates in the formation of a C3 convertase was immediately recognized as the basis for the chronic hypercatabolism of C3 and B observed in a patient with an inherited deficiency of C3b inactivator (C3bINA)(23), and for the "spontaneous" cleavage of C3 and B in serum after immunochemical inhibition of C3bINA (24).

The amplification C3 convertase was recognized to be a labile bimolecular complex, C3b,Bb, when the enzyme was formed on sheep erythrocytes bearing C3b (25). Interaction of cell-bound C3b with B and $\overline{D}$ resulted in formation of cell-bound convertase sites which could be separated from unreacted B and $\overline{D}$ and quantitatively assayed by the extent of lysis of the erythrocytes upon the introduction of a source of C3-C9. The linear, stoichiometric relationship observed between the amount of cell-bound C3b and the number of C3b,Bb sites formed with B and $\overline{D}$ indicated that C3b was a constituent of the convertase. The first order, temperature-dependent decay of C3b,Bb sites on the cells secondary to release of Bb as inactive Bi demonstrated that Bb carried the C3-cleaving site which could be expressed only when the protein was bound to C3b. $\overline{D}$ (22, 26) functions in the amplification reaction to cleave B, releasing the Ba fragment and leaving Bb complexed to C3b. As this activity of $\overline{D}$ is irreversibly abolished by diisopropylphosphofluoridate (Dip-F)(27) the enzyme catalytic site contains a nucleophilic serine. However, $\overline{D}$ does not cleave isolated B and the requirement of this reaction for the simultaneous presence of C3b and Mg^{2+} suggests that the substrate or enzyme must be modified to permit proteolysis.

Evidence that C3b reversibly alters B was obtained when mixtures of purified C3b and B, with or without the stabilizing principles, P and C3 nephritic factor (C3NeF), were observed to generate C3 convertase activity (28-31). No $\overline{D}$ activity was detected in the reactants with an assay sensitive to 0.2 picogram $\overline{D}$/ml, and pretreatment of the proteins with 5mM Dip-F, a concentration sufficient to inactivate $\overline{D}$, failed to alter their capacity to generate C3 cleaving activity (30). This convertase has been isolated by sucrose density gradient ultracentrifugation in the presence of C3NeF (29) and by micro-disc electrophoresis (31) and shown to be a reversible bimolecular complex containing uncleaved B, i.e., C3b,B. Thus, binding of B to C3b induces a conformational alteration in B that can be detected by the partial expression of its C3-cleaving site and by cleavage-activation by $\overline{D}$ which allows full expression of the enzymatic site on Bb with release of the Ba fragment.

A requirement for Mg^{2+} in the activation of the alternative pathway by zymosan was recognized in the initial studies of this system (1) and the observation that formation of C3b,B was Mg^{2+}-dependent (22, 25, 31) localized the function of this cation to the complexing of these two proteins. The effect of Mg^{2+} on this reaction has been quantitatively assessed by measuring the uptake of ^{125}I-B by cell-bound C3b in the presence of increasing concentrations of Mg^{2+} (32) and calculating the affinity constants at equilibrium (Kassoc) by Scatchard analysis of the binding data. The association constant of ^{125}I-B for C3b increased in a dose-related manner with increasing concentrations of Mg^{2+}, ranging from $0.3 \times 10^6\ M^{-1}$ with 1.25 mM Mg^{2+} up to $3.0 \times 10^6\ M^{-1}$ in the presence of 15 mM Mg^{2+}. This Mg^{2+}-dependent ten-fold increment in the binding of

B to C3b would correspondingly enhance generation of C3b,Bb by $\bar{D}$ and may account for the observations that addition of this cation to human or guinea pig serum, which normally contain approximately 0.5 mM free Mg^{2+}, induced C3 cleavage by the alternative pathway in the absence of activating particles such as zymosan (33, 34).

In summary, the amplification C3 convertase is formed by a sequential reaction involving reversible complexing of B to C3b in the presence of Mg^{2+} to form C3b,B, and cleavage of the bound B by $\bar{D}$ to generate C3b,Bb, the labile convertase. The latter decays by dissociation of Bb which becomes functionally inactive Bi and the residual C3b and $\bar{D}$ which persist in their active states can regenerate the convertase with additional B (Fig. 2). These reactions are remarkably analogous to those occurring during formation, decay and regeneration of the classical pathway C3 convertase, C4b,2a. B and C2, which have similar amino acid compositions (35) and are synthesized by closely linked genes near the HLA complex of the human (36), bind reversibly to acceptor proteins, C3b and C4b, respectively, to permit expression of their enzymatic sites which have identical substrate specificities, C3 and C5, after cleavage-activation by enzymes of the serine esterase class, $\bar{D}$ and $C\bar{1}s$. C3b and C4b resemble one another not only in their capacities to bind to immune complexes and cell membranes, but also in their inactivation by the same plasma protein, C3bINA (37, 38), although different cofactors are required (21, 39, 40).

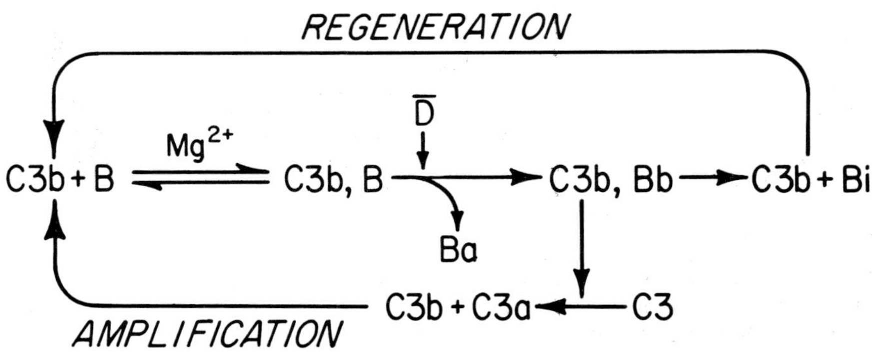

Fig. 2. The molecular reactions leading to formation, amplification, decay and regeneration of the C3b-dependent amplification C3 convertase.

STABILIZATION OF THE AMPLIFICATION CONVERTASE BY PROPERDIN

The lability of C3b,Bb, which spontaneously decays with a half-life of 4 min at 30°C, represents an intrinsic control that limits C3 cleavage by the amplification reaction of the alternative complement pathway. Two proteins have been shown to stabilize the amplification convertase, prolonging its half-life as much as ten-fold to augment its potential for activation of C3. The first of these, P, is a normal constituent of plasma, whereas the other, C3NeF, is an antibody which has been found only in some patients with membranoproliferative glomerulonephritis or with partial lipodystrophy.

P was defined initially as a factor in serum which bound to zymosan during incubation at 17°C, thereby rendering the adsorbed serum unable to generate C3-cleaving activity upon subsequent incubation with fresh zymosan at 37°C (1). The eluate of zymosan which had been incubated with serum at 17°C restored C3-cleaving activity to the adsorbed serum and the active principle was termed properdin. As incubation of zymosan with serum at 0°C or with purified P at any temperature did not result in binding of P, uptake of this principle by zymosan was presumed to be indirect and dependent on additional serum factors. Three groups of investigators independently found that P has an affinity for C3 and its cleavage fragments. Purified P bound to erythrocytes bearing C3b, but not to cells carrying C4b, in a temperature- and cation-independent reaction (41); P agglutinated erythrocyte-C3b intermediates (42); and P formed fluid phase complexes with C3, C3b and C3c (43). Therefore, the requirements for the binding of P in serum to zymosan reflect those conditions necessary for cleavage of C3 and adherence of C3b to the zymosan particles.

A functional consequence of this interaction of P and C3b is a decreased rate of decay-dissociation of Bb from C3b,Bb (41). Sheep erythrocytes bearing preformed C3b,Bb sites were incubated at 30°C in buffer alone or in the presence of increasing amounts of purified P and samples of cells were removed at timed intervals to assess the number of residual amplification convertase sites/cell. In the absence of P, cell-bound C3b,Bb decayed with a half-life of 4 min, whereas the presence of P retarded decay in dose-related manner, with the highest input of P extending the half-life to 30 min (Fig. 3). There was no detectable lag in the stabilizing effect of P, consistent with rapid binding of P to C3b,Bb sites, and decay was first order at all concentrations of P. This critical effect occurred whether P was introduced in the fluid phase or already bound to C3b on separate erythrocytes, indicating that P can transfer from C3b to C3b,Bb sites to effect stabilization of the recipient convertases (41). The presence of P during generation of C3b,Bb results in the detection of more convertase sites than occurs during interaction of cell-bound C3b, B and $\overline{D}$ alone; this effect is due to stabilization but was originally misinterpreted as being due to conversion of $\overline{D}$ from a non-active form of the protein termed D (44). Thus, one function of P in the alternative pathway is to augment C3 cleavage by the amplification convertase through binding to C3b and retarding decay-dissociation of Bb from that site.

THE AMPLIFICATION C5 CONVERTASE

The formation of a C5 convertase is essential for the generation of the C5b,6,7,8,9 cytolytic membrane insertion complex as well as for the elaboration of other biologic activities associated with these terminal components of complement. The C5-cleaving enzyme of the classical pathway is comprised of C4b,2a and C3b, the bimolecular complex carrying the enzymatic site for proteolysis of C5 and C3b apparently serving to present the

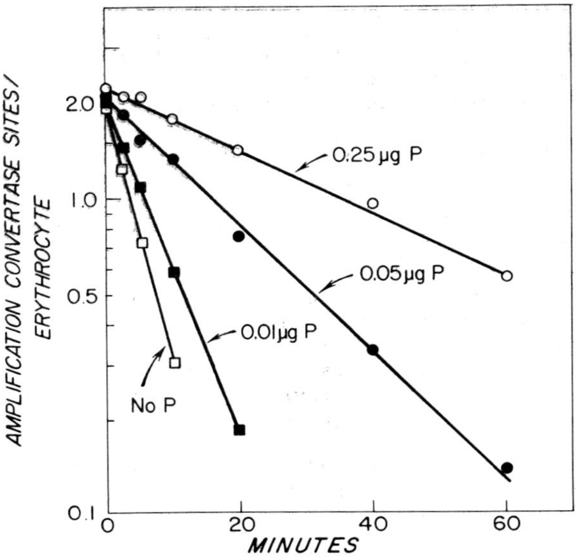

Fig. 3. Time course of decay at 30°C of C3b,Bb sites on sheep erythrocytes in buffer alone (□—□) or containing 0.01 µg P/ml (■—■), 0.05 µg P/ml (●—●), or 0.25 µg P/ml (O—O). [From (41).]

substrate in a manner that permits its cleavage (45, 46). Since the amplification C3 convertase already contains C3b as a subunit of the enzyme, a requirement for additional C3b to achieve C5-cleaving activity was not self-evident. However, the observation that sheep erythrocytes prepared with relatively limited amounts of C3b and bearing amplification C3 convertase sites were lysed by incubation with C3 and C5-C9 but not by C5-C9 alone, suggested that additional cell-bound C3b molecules are necessary for C5 convertase activity (25). Quantitative assessment of the different C3b requirements of the two convertases with ^{125}I-C3 revealed that 60 C3b molecules/erythrocyte sufficed for generation of amplification C3 convertase sites, whereas at least 200 C3b molecules/cell were necessary for C5 convertase activity (47). Cell-bound C3 convertase sites could be transformed into C5 convertase sites by interaction with C3 to increase the number of C3b molecules/cell without altering the content of C3b,Bb sites. These newly generated C5 convertases reverted to sites capable of cleaving only C3 when the additional cell-bound C3b was inactivated with C3bINA (47). The resistance to C3bINA of C3b forming the C3 convertase, C3b,Bb, as compared to the susceptibility of C3b necessary for C5 cleavage indicates that the former is protected by complexed Bb while the latter is exposed.

Although differing in their enzymatic capabilities, the two amplification convertases share a common proteolytic site which resides in the Bb fragment complexed to C3b. Both cell-bound convertases exhibit identical half-lives of 4 min at 30°C, and both decayed enzymes are regenerated to their original specificities upon the introduction of B in the presence of $\overline{D}$, indicating that the topographical relationships of membrane-associated C3b which determine C3 or C5 convertase activity are not disturbed by decay and regeneration of C3b,Bb sites (47). The inherent labilities of C3 and C5 convertase sites are overcome to the same extent by C3NeF which prolongs their half-lives to 40-60 min at 30°C without altering their substrate specificities (47). Thus, the composition of a cell-bound C5 convertase site is C3b,Bb with an additional, presumably adjacent C3b which permits interaction of C5 with the bimolecular complex in a manner analogous to the role of C3b in the classical pathway reaction of C4b,2a and C5.

ENDOGENOUS REGULATION OF THE AMPLIFICATION PHASE OF THE ALTERNATIVE COMPLEMENT PATHWAY

The positive feedback potential of the amplification C3 convertase requires stringent regulation to prevent inappropriate activation, and four mechanisms for regulation of the formation and function of this enzyme have been discerned: inactivation, which refers to the action of C3bINA and β1H on C3b; competition, which occurs between B and β1H for binding to C3b; intrinsic decay, which reflects the inherent lability of C3b,Bb; and extrinsic decay, which is mediated by the effect of β1H on the convertase.

The ability of C3b to form the amplification convertase is abolished by the proteolytic action of C3bINA in the presence of β1H which results in cleavage of the α polypeptide chain of C3b, to yield inactive C3bi. The participation in this reaction of β1H, which had been recognized previously only as a common contaminant of partially purified C3 (48), has been appreciated only recently, when this protein was isolated from plasma based on its capacity to increase the rate of inactivation of cell-bound C3b by C3bINA (21). It is thought that the binding of β1H to C3b (49) induces a reversible alteration in C3b to permit more effective interaction with C3bINA and the 30-fold increase in the association constant of C3b for C3bINA at 0°C in the presence of β1H (50) may reflect this presumed change. Furthermore, cleavage of C3b in the fluid phase by C3bINA apparently has an absolute requirement for the presence of β1H (20).

The capacity of β1H to bind to C3b (49, 51, 52) indicates that it may also regulate generation of the amplification convertase by impairing uptake of B by C3b. In equilibrium binding studies, β1H inhibited uptake of ^{125}I-B by C3b on sheep erythrocytes in a dose-related manner, with 50% inhibition occurring with a molar ratio of β1H/B of 0.3 (32). As these studies were performed in the presence of 5 mM Mg^{2+} to enhance detection of ^{125}I-B binding to C3b, competition by β1H, whose interaction with C3b is cation-independent, under physiologic conditions of 0.5 mM free Mg^{2+}, would be even more effective. Moreover, although serum contains approximately equimolar amounts of these two proteins, B is consumed during alternative pathway reactions while β1H remains intact, a circumstance that would increase the molar ratio of β1H/B and serve to dampen further generation of C3b,Bb.

Stabilization of the amplification convertase by P decreases the effectiveness of intrinsic decay-dissociation of C3b,Bb as a regulatory mechanism, thereby invoking the third function of β1H, that of extrinsic decay-dissociation of the convertases. Recognition of this activity of β1H occurred when a plasma protein was isolated as an inhibitor of the preformed,

P-stabilized amplification convertase (53) and shown to be β1H. Addition of β1H to sheep erythrocytes bearing P-stabilized C3b,Bb sites resulted in dose-dependent accelerated first order decay of convertase function. For example, 0.42 μg β1H/ml was sufficient to decrease the half-life of stabilized convertase sites from 60 min at 30°C to 4 min, the decay rate of unstabilized C3b,Bb sites (53). As the latter are also susceptible to accelerated decay by β1H, this effect of the control protein is directed at the convertase rather than at P. Loss of convertase function mediated by β1H is associated with loss of cell-bound ^{125}I-Bb, indicating that β1H functions to dissociate Bb from the C3b,Bb complex rather than to inhibit the enzymatic site, a mechanism that certainly reflects its higher affinity for C3b than B. Finally, release of Bb from C3b,Bb by β1H not only abolishes convertase activity, but also uncovers C3b for inactivation by C3bINA to prevent regeneration of C3b,Bb at that site (53).

INITIAL GENERATION OF C3b BY THE ALTERNATIVE COMPLEMENT PATHWAY

The description of the C3b-dependent amplification convertase permitted a focus on the alternative pathway reactions which led to generation of the initial C3b. Although an early study appeared to indicate that interaction of C3, B and $\overline{D}$ did not lead to C3 or B cleavage (22), a subsequent investigation with highly purified proteins yielded contrary results (54). The conclusion that C3, B and $\overline{D}$, each purified to homogeneity, interacted to form an initial C3 convertase was especially contingent upon excluding contaminating C3b in the C3. The C3 utilized in these studies was homogeneous and was devoid of C3b as assessed by immunoelectrophoresis and alkaline disc gel electrophoresis, the latter procedure being performed with ^{125}I-labeled protein to enhance the sensitivity of the analysis (54). Analytical isoelectric focusing in polyacrylamide gels of C3 revealed that eluates of gel slices having the capacity to interact with B and D corresponded to those containing C3 activity in a classical complement assay in which C3b is inactive. As these activities of C3 were isoelectric in the range of pH 6.3-6.7, and simultaneous analysis of C3b revealed it to be isoelectric at 5.3-5.8, any C3b that may have contaminated the C3 preparation would have been effectively separated. Further, pretreatment of the C3 with C3bINA did not alter its subsequent capacity to form an initial convertase with B and $\overline{D}$, whereas similar pretreatment of C3b diminished by 90% its capacity to interact with B and $\overline{D}$. Thus, C3 that was devoid of C3b by physicochemical and functional criteria could participate with B and $\overline{D}$ in initial generation of C3b (54). The additional finding that introduction of P into such reaction mixtures reduced by ten-fold the amounts of B or $\overline{D}$ necessary for initial cleavage of C3 indicates a role for P in this fluid phase reaction (28), and suggests that the apparent absolute requirement for P previously observed may have been a consequence of limited B or $\overline{D}$.

Although the manner in which C3, B and $\overline{D}$ interact to form an initial C3 convertase was not explicitly demonstrated (28, 54), it is postulated to be analogous to that of the C3b-dependent amplification reaction. Highly reversible binding of B to C3 is followed by cleavage of bound B with $\overline{D}$ to yield C3,Bb, a bimolecular complex containing uncleaved C3 that can act on free C3 to generate C3b. The enhancing effect of P is presumed to reflect stabilization of C3,Bb similar to its effect on C3b,Bb (41), and the capacity of P to form reversible fluid phase complexes with C3 in serum (43) supports this concept. The slower kinetics of this C3-dependent reaction and its requirement for higher concentrations of B and $\overline{D}$ as compared to the C3b-dependent amplification reaction would be consistent with a much lower association constant of C3 than C3b for B. The capacity of mixtures of C3,

B and $\overline{D}$ to generate initial C3b (54) has been confirmed (55), but direct analysis of the composition of the initial convertase is still lacking.

The inability of C3bINA to prevent mixtures of C3, B and $\overline{D}$ from advancing to amplified C3 cleavage (54) may have been the basis for the view that this mechanism for continuously generating small amounts of C3b did not operate in whole serum, and other protein factors were proposed to have a role in initial C3b generation and deposition on alternative pathway activating particles (56, 57). When β1H was recognized as the second essential control protein, it was possible for the first time to prepare a reaction mixture containing physiologic concentrations of purified C3, B, $\overline{D}$, P, C3bINA and β1H which engaged only in slow C3 cleavage and did not advance to amplification (14, 58). Thus, the alternative pathway, because of the normal presence of D, continuously generates small amounts of C3b which provide the potential for C3b-dependent amplification if regulation is impaired.

ACTIVATION OF THE ALTERNATIVE COMPLEMENT PATHWAY BY CIRCUMVENTION OF THE REGULATORY ACTIONS OF CONTROL PROTEINS

Because the alternative pathway has a mechanism for slow generation of C3b regardless of the presence of activating particles, attention was directed away from initial C3 cleavage to the effects of activators on the regulation of C3b-dependent amplification. These studies demonstrated that particulate activators provide sites that protect not only C3b deposited on their surfaces from inactivation by C3bINA and β1H but also the C3b,Bb convertases formed at those sites from decay-dissociation by β1H, resulting in surface-associated amplified C3 cleavage (14, 58, 59). The experiments defining this mode of alternative pathway activation utilized three types of activators that are diverse in their phylogenetic origins: zymosan, which was utilized in the discovery of this pathway (1); Gram negative bacteria, whose activating capacity reaffirmed the existence of the pathway (4), and rabbit erythrocytes (60), which indicated that the recognitive specificity of the pathway included mammalian cell membranes. As activation by each type of particle occurred by surface-dependent circumvention of the regulatory actions of C3bINA and β1H, this concept can be exemplified by the experiments dealing with a single activator, the rabbit erythrocyte.

It was demonstrated that rabbit erythrocytes, as compared to the reference non-activator, sheep erythrocytes, provided protection for bound C3b from the action of C3bINA and β1H (58). Each type of cell carried approximately the same number of C3b molecules, and the activity of C3b was assessed by its capacity to form the P-stabilized amplification convertase. As shown in Figure 4, a mixture of purified C3bINA and β1H at 1/100 their serum concentrations inactivated 86% of the C3b molecules on sheep erythrocytes after incubation for 45 min at 37°C, while only 19% of the C3b on rabbit erythrocytes were inactivated after 60 min. When whole human serum diluted 100-fold in ethylenediamine tetraacetate (EDTA) was used as the source of inactivating principles, comparable results were obtained after 60 min with 86% and 12% inactivation of C3b on sheep and rabbit erythrocytes, respectively. Thus, C3b molecules bound to this activator (58), as well as to zymosan (14) and *E. coli* (59), are relatively resistant to inactivation by C3bINA and β1H.

The susceptibility of the P-stabilized amplification convertase on rabbit and sheep erythrocytes to decay-dissociation by β1H was examined by comparing the dose-response effects of β1H on the decay rates of the cell-bound convertases (58). The half-life at 30°C of the unstabilized convertase sites on both

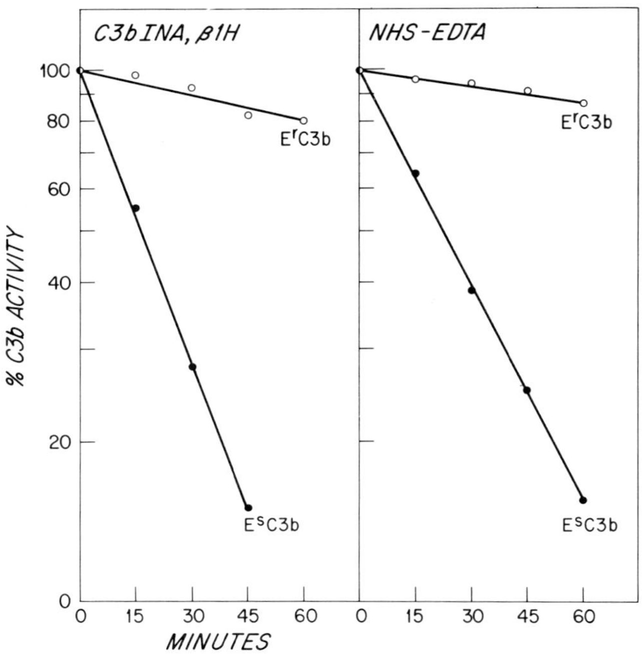

Fig. 4. Time course of inactivation of C3b bound to sheep (●—●) and rabbit erythrocytes (O—O) by C3bINA and β1H (left) and by diluted normal human serum (NHS-EDTA)(right). [Modified from (58).]

types of erythrocytes was 4 min and P effected similar degrees of stabilization, extending the half-lives to 28 and 29 min on the sheep and rabbit erythrocytes, respectively (Fig. 5). Thus the surface of an alternative pathway activator does not alter spontaneous decay-dissociation of Bb from C3b,Bb. However, P-stabilized convertase sites on rabbit erythrocytes were relatively resistant to extrinsic, β1H-mediated decay-dissociation. Whereas 0.22 μg β1H/ml reduced the half-life of the stabilized convertase on sheep erythrocytes to 11 min, 2.0 μg β1H/ml were required to effect a similar accelerated decay-dissociation of the convertase sites on rabbit erythrocytes. Thus, the surface of this activator (58), and that of zymosan (14) and E. coli (59), by offering a protected microenvironment for C3b, facilitates formation of bound amplification convertase which, in turn, is relatively resistant to the action of β1H; this convertase deposits additional C3b by cleavage of C3, thereby shifting the alternative pathway to its amplification phase.

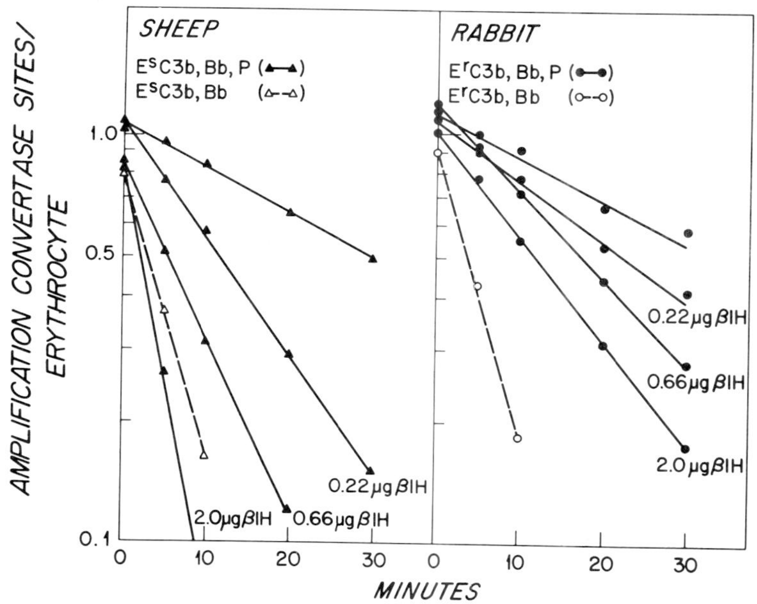

Fig. 5. Time course of decay of P-stabilized amplification convertase sites on sheep (▲—▲, left panel) and rabbit erythrocytes (●—●) alone and in the presence of increasing amounts of β1H. Decay of C3b,Bb sites in the absence of P and in buffer alone is indicated by the dashed lines. [From (58).]

That only six alternative pathway proteins are required for induction of rapid C3 cleavage by the activating particles was demonstrated with a mixture of C3, B, $\overline{D}$, P, C3bINA and β1H, each of which had been purified to homogeneity (Fig. 1). Incubation of these proteins at one-tenth their respective serum concentrations with zymosan (14) or rabbit (58) erythrocytes advanced their low grade fluid phase interaction to amplified C3 cleavage and deposited C3b on the activating particle; incubation of the protein mixture alone or with sheep erythrocytes resulted in no accelerated C3 cleavage. Deletion of either regulatory protein permitted C3 and B cleavage to occur in the absence of activating particles.

In summary, C3b molecules, which are slowly generated by the low grade fluid phase interaction of C3, B, $\overline{D}$ and P, primarily remain in the fluid phase because of rapid decay of their covalent binding sites, and only a few molecules may attach to bystander surfaces. C3b molecules in the fluid phase or bound to a non-activating surface are rapidly inactivated and amplification cannot occur. In contrast, C3b molecules bound to activators advance the reaction to surface-dependent amplified C3 cleavage by circumvention of the actions of the regulatory proteins, C3bINA and β1H. This view that the alternative pathway is comprised of only six proteins (14, 58) has recently been confirmed by studies in which a previously stated requirement for a postulated initiating factor (56, 57) was withdrawn (55).

ROLE OF MEMBRANE SIALIC ACID IN ACTIVATION OF THE ALTERNATIVE COMPLEMENT PATHWAY

Despite their different origins, zymosan, E. coli and rabbit erythroctes share a unifying characteristic of impairing the actions of C3bINA and β1H on bound C3b and C3b,Bb, and it seemed likely that there would be a biochemical characteristic common to all three surfaces. The realization that rabbit erythrocytes have less sialic acid than sheep erythrocytes (61) and that zymosan particles (62) and strains of E. coli lacking the K1 antigen comprised of coliminic acid (63) do not have sialic acid suggested that a relative paucity of this carbohydrate might be a critical common biochemical characteristic. The conversion of the sheep erythrocytes into activators of the alternative pathway in human serum by enzymatic removal of membrane sialic acid residues (51, 64) or chemical conversion to their heptulosonic acid derivative (64) established this concept.

The capacity of membrane sialic acid to modulate the effects of β1H on membrane-bound amplification convertase sites was examined (64) with sheep erythrocytes which had been prepared by removal of graded amounts of sialic acid with sialidase or by limited oxidation with periodate followed by reduction with borohydride to remove only the C8 and C9 hydroxylated carbon atoms from the exocyclic side chain of sialic acid. P-stabilized amplification convertase sites were formed on normal and on the modified sheep erythrocytes with purified proteins, and the amounts of β1H required to decay-dissociate the convertase sites were measured. With removal or modification of increasing amounts of erythrocyte sialic acid, there were corresponding requirements for increasing concentrations of β1H to effect decay of the P-stabilized C3b,Bb sites. In order to compare the effects of the two treatments of sheep erythrocyte membranes on β1H activity, the relative activities of β1H are plotted as a function of the percent of sialic acid removed or modified (Fig. 6). The dose response lines of the two treatments are superimposable, thereby indicating that chemical removal of the two terminal exocyclic carbons from membrane sialic acid impairs β1H interaction with cell-bound C3b,Bb to the same extent as removal of the entire sialic acid moiety. Therefore, secondary effects of the latter reaction, such as diminution of the membrane net negative charge or exposure of penultimate galactose residues are not responsible for the reduction in the capacity of β1H to dissociate Bb from C3b,Bb. Rather, sialic acid, with its side chain apparently being essential, appears to have a direct role in enhancing the interaction between cell-bound C3b and fluid phase β1H. Furthermore, this effect is critical as a 1% decrease in intact membrane sialic acid is associated with a 1% decrease in relative β1H activity (64)(Fig. 6).

These studies involving experimental manipulation of membrane sialic acid have been confirmed by examination of the effects of natural variations in membrane sialic acid (65). Mouse erythrocytes from 21 inbred strains were shown to have variable capacities for activation of the human alternative pathway. Activating capacity was inversely related to the membrane sialic acid content of erythrocytes from 20 individuals of the 4 strains that were examined. Linear regression analysis also demonstrated a significant inverse correlation between the alternative pathway activating capacity of erythrocytes from 4 strains and the concentration of β1H required for decay-dissociation of amplification convertase sites on the erythrocytes. Genetic studies extended these observations as erythrocytes from F_1 hybrids derived from strains with erythrocytes having high and low activating capacities demonstrated intermediate activating capacities and sialic acid

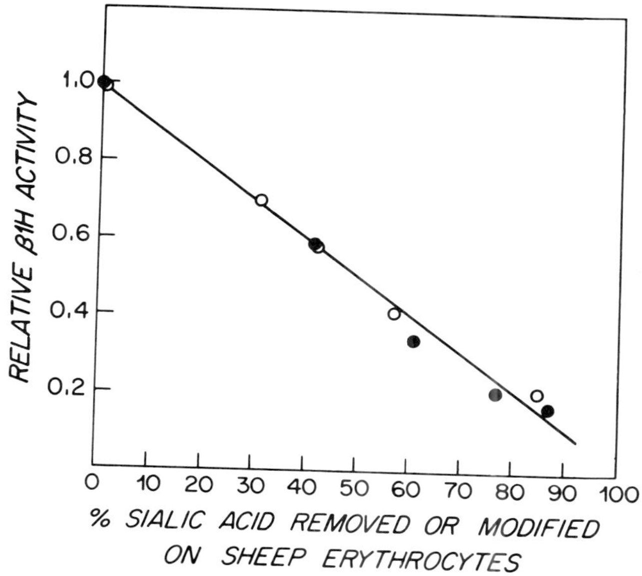

Fig. 6. Relationship between the percent sialic acid on sheep erythrocytes removed by sialidase (●) or modified by treatment with $NaIO_4$ and $NaBH_4$ (O) and the relative capacity of β1H to decay-dissociate P-stabilized C3b,Bb sites on the erythrocytes. [Modified from (64)].

content. Erythrocytes from mice of the backcross and F_2 generations exhibited distributions of activating capacity and sialic acid content that would be expected if these traits were controlled by codominant alleles of a single autosomal locus (65). Thus, a relative deficiency of sialic acid on a particle surface, whether experimentally induced or genetically determined, represents a critical biochemical characteristic of alternative pathway activators.

The molecular basis for the inverse relationship between sialic acid content of a membrane and the capacity of β1H to decay-dissociate amplification convertases on that membrane has been examined by analyzing uptake of β1H by C3b on modified erythrocyte membranes (32). Recent studies have shown decreased binding of β1H to rabbit as compared to sheep erythrocytes bearing C3b (51), and the applicability of Scatchard analysis to the binding of β1H to C3b on sheep erythrocytes (52). Therefore, the effect of sheep erythrocyte membrane sialic acid residues on the binding of B and β1H to membrane-associated C3b has been determined (32) with radiolabeled proteins and a technique for separating bound from free ligand by centrifugation of the erythrocytes through an oil/aqueous interphase. The affinity constants at equilibrium (Kassoc) and the effective number of C3b binding sites for B and β1H on the cells were calculated by Scatchard analysis of the binding data. Similar analyses were performed with C3b-bearing zymosan particles which represented an activator of the alternative pathway naturally lacking sialic acid (Table 2). The Kassoc for the interaction of B and β1H with C3b on normal sheep erythrocytes in the presence of 5 mM Mg^{2+} were $2.1 \times 10^6\ M^{-1}$ and $1 \times 10^7\ M^{-1}$, respectively, indicating an approximately five-fold greater affinity of β1H for the C3b binding sites which were present in approximately equal numbers for the two ligands and in the same range as estimated by the amount of ^{125}I-C3b/cell. The affinity of B for C3b on the sheep erythrocytes from which 80% of the sialic acid had been enzymatically removed or chemically modified and for C3b on the zymosan particles was relatively unchanged, and the number of effective binding sites again corresponded to the independent assessment of ^{125}I-C3b present. In contrast, the number of C3b binding sites having a Kassoc for β1H of approximately $10^7\ M^{-1}$ on the sialic acid-deficient erythrocytes or zymosan particles was only 1/5 to 1/6 the number interacting with B. The presence of additional C3b binding sites for β1H having an affinity so low that they were not revealed by Scatchard analysis because of the dominant effect of the high affinity C3b sites was determined in competitive binding studies measuring the capacity of β1H to inhibit uptake of B by C3b on the sialic acid-deficient surfaces. The Kassoc for the interaction of β1H with these C3b sites is approximately $4 \times 10^5\ M^{-1}$, an affinity that is between 10 and 100-fold less than that of the sialic acid-dependent high affinity C3b sites. Furthermore, the relative inefficiency of β1H in competing with B for binding to C3b on the sialic acid-deficient particles correlated with the decreased capacity of β1H to decay-dissociate Bb from C3b,Bb convertase sites on such particles (32). Thus, the content of sialic acid-containing glycoproteins and glycolipids in the microenvironment of bound C3b regulates its interaction with β1H. The presence of sialic acid augments binding of the regulatory protein to favor competition with B, inactivation of C3b and decay-dissociation of C3b,Bb, while the absence of sialic acid residues results in low affinity C3b binding of β1H, a circumstance that permits uptake of B to form the amplification convertase and impairs extrinsic decay of the C3 cleaving enzyme (Fig. 7). Although these investigations emphasize the capacity of the alternative pathway to recognize cell surfaces in the absence of an acquired immune response, the presence of some types of specific antibody to rabbit (66) and sheep (8) erythrocytes, pneumococci (67), virus infected cells (68, 69), and allotypic cellular antigens (70) has been shown to augment or even initiate activation of this pathway. Although the mechanism for these antibody-dependent effects is not known, these studies indicate the broad biological potential of the alternative pathway which includes acquired as well as natural immune reactions.

THE SYNERGISTIC INTERACTION OF THE ALTERNATIVE COMPLEMENT PATHWAY AND HUMAN MONOCYTES IN RECOGNITION OF SIALIC ACID-DEFICIENT SURFACES

As an effective natural immune response requires both humoral and cellular recognition of foreign organisms, a cellular counterpart to the alternative complement pathway was sought by examination of the capacity of human peripheral blood monocytes to engage in antibody-independent phagocytosis of activators of the alternative pathway. Monolayers of human monocytes directly ingested zymosan and rabbit and mouse erythrocytes in a synthetic medium devoid of serum proteins (71). The rank order of the percentage of monocytes that ingested erythrocytes from rabbits and C57BL/6 and CBA mice was the same as that for the percentage of lysis of these erythrocytes by the alternative pathway when C2-deficient human serum is used. Sheep and guinea pig erythrocytes, which do not activate the human alternative pathway, were not directly ingested by human monocytes. The capacity of human monocytes to ingest zymosan particles and rabbit erythrocytes was largely diminished when

TABLE 2 Analysis of Binding of ^{125}I-B and ^{125}I-β1H to C3b on Particle Surfaces Differing in their Sialic Acid Content

Particle	^{125}I-C3b/Particle	B		β1H	
		Kassoc (M^{-1})	C3b Sites/Particle	Kassoc (M^{-1})	C3b Sites/Particle
Sheep erythrocytes					
Unmodified	30,000	2.1×10^{6}	34,500	1.0×10^{7}	25,900
80% sialic acid removed	8,000	3.8×10^{6}	7,740	3.1×10^{7}	1,620
80% sialic acid modified	10,000	3.2×10^{6}	10,800	0.9×10^{7}	2,400
Zymosan	2,800	2.0×10^{6}	4,000	5.7×10^{7}	650

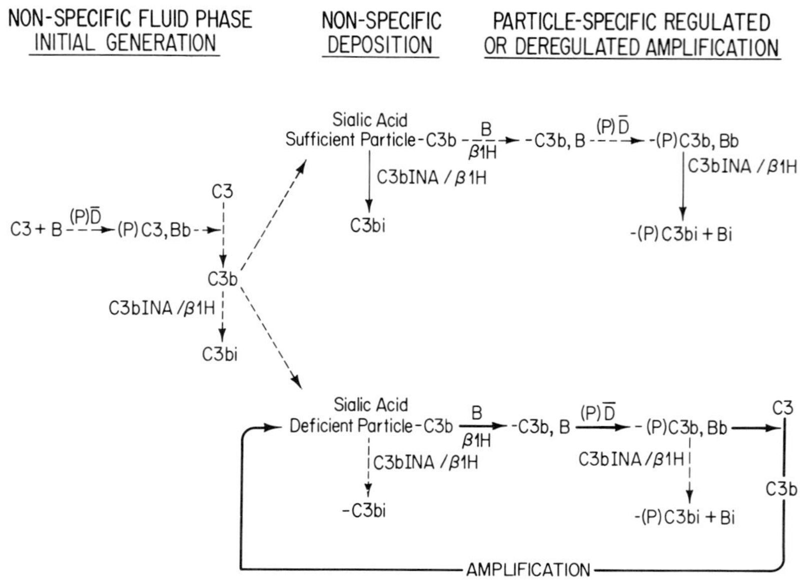

Fig. 7. Activation of the alternative complement pathway by a sialic acid-deficient particle. C3b is slowly generated in the fluid phase and may attach to bystander surfaces. Those molecules remaining unbound or on sialic acid-sufficient particles are rapidly inactivated by C3bINA/β1H, and exhibit higher affinities for β1H than for B. In contrast, C3b on sialic acid-deficient surfaces is relatively resistant to inactivation and binding of β1H is impaired, thereby permitting formation and function of the amplification convertase.

the monocytes were pretreated with quantities of affinity-purified trypsin which had no effect on monocyte Fc or C3b receptor function. This trypsin-sensitive mechanism of monocytes involved in ingestion of alternative pathway activating particles was regenerated over 48 hr during *in vitro* culture in a serum-free medium, a result compatible with the restoration of function of a membrane-associated protein. Thus, the human monocyte possesses a mechanism for the recognition of particulate activators of the alternative complement pathway in the absence of opsonizing factors such as IgG or C3b that had not previously been recognized as distinct (71).

Direct evidence was obtained that the monocyte phagocytic response is initiated by the same surface characteristics that enable a particle to activate the alternative complement pathway. Sheep erythrocytes, which do not ordinarily activate the human alternative pathway or initiate a direct monocyte phagocytic response were modified to exhibit both functions by deletion or alteration of membrane sialic acid residues (64, 72). Enzymatic removal of the sialic acid residues with sialidase or their conversion to the heptulosonic acid derivative by limited oxidation with periodate and reduction with borohydride had equivalent dose-response effects on the capacity of sheep erythrocytes to initiate directly the monocyte phagocytic response and to activate the alternative pathway. The trypsin-sensitive monocyte membrane protein(s) involved in ingestion of the natural activators, zymosan and rabbit erythrocytes, was also involved in recognition of the altered sheep erythrocytes. Fixation of C3b to the surface of the desialated sheep erythrocytes increased the number of monocytes ingesting the particles, revealing a synergistic interaction between the monocyte C3b receptor and the trypsin-sensitive receptor for activators of the alternative pathway. Since such particles would naturally become coated with C3b in vivo through activation of the alternative pathway, the synergistic interaction between these two monocyte receptors would normally be operative for phagocytosis. The capacity of the non-immune human host to respond to desialated particles by a dual humoral (64) and cellular (72) recognition mechanism may represent a primordial biochemical basis for protection against microbial assault.

C3 NEPHRITIC FACTOR: AN AUTOANTIBODY THAT ACTIVATES THE ALTERNATIVE COMPLEMENT PATHWAY

"Non-physiologic" activation of C3 by an alternative pathway occurs in some patients with membranoproliferative glomerulonephritis who exhibit marked depressions of C3 but relatively normal levels of C1, C4 and C2 in their sera (73). Addition of serum from these patients to normal serum induced C3 cleavage and this activity was ascribed to a principle termed C3 nephritic factor (C3NeF)(74). The action of C3NeF was dependent on the presence in normal serum of Mg^{2+} and B, but not Ca^{2+} or C4, indicating that cleavage of C3 was occurring by the alternative rather than the classical pathway (75, 76). A principle with similar characteristics was subsequently identified in the serum of most patients with partial lipodystrophy with or without glomerulonephritis (77).

Functional studies preceded physicochemical characterization of C3NeF as purification of the protein from contaminating IgG was hindered by its m.w. of 160,000 and γ electrophoretic mobility. A specific function for this protein in the alternative pathway was discovered when partially purified C3NeF extended the half-life of C3b,Bb sites on sheep erythrocytes from 4 min up to 45-60 min at 30°C (78). Stabilization of the fluid phase amplification convertase also occurs and this activity of C3NeF led to isolation by sucrose density gradient ultracentrifugation of a complex that contained equimolar amounts of C3b and Bb and possessed C3-cleaving activity (78). However, stabilization of the amplification C3 convertase alone could not account for the capacity of C3NeF to induce activation of the alternative pathway, as the normal protein, P, has a similar function and yet its presence in plasma does not induce amplified C3 cleavage. Appreciation of the essential role of β1H in extrinsic decay-dissociation of C3b,Bb led to an examination of the effect of C3NeF on this regulatory step (53). Dose-response studies indicated that the amount of β1H required to reduce the half-life of the C3NeF-stabilized convertase on sheep erythrocytes by 50% was 200-fold greater than that needed to achieve the same relative effect on the P-stabilized amplification convertase. The resistance of C3b,Bb(C3NeF) to extrinsic decay-dissociation was confirmed by the limited ability of β1H to dissociate ^{125}I-Bb from these convertase sites. Thus, C3NeF induces amplified C3 cleavage in serum by creating a stable amplification convertase that is resistant to the regulating action of β1H (53). Further, C3b in the stabilized convertase is protected from inactivation with C3bINA by the complexed Bb. This mechanism of alternative pathway activation is conceptually analogous to that of particulate activators of the alternative pathway, i.e., circumvention of the regulatory actions of control proteins.

In retrospect, the identity of C3NeF with a specific plasma protein had occurred relatively early, when partially purified C3NeF was found to be adsorbed by insolubilized rabbit anti-human IgG (79). Although entirely consistent with the molecular weight and charge of C3NeF, the conclusion that C3NeF is IgG was disputed. The purified protein was reported to lack antigenic identity with IgG in Ouchterlony analysis with the use of antisera specific for heavy and light chain determinants (80). These investigators further distinguished C3NeF from proteins of the immunoglobulin class by observing a composition for C3NeF of two disulfide-linked polypeptide chains of 85,000 m.w. (81), and stated that the protein was an activated form of "initiating factor", a postulated constituent of the alternative pathway (56, 57). However, the observations that C3NeF activity appeared to be trans- ported across the placenta (82), a characteristic of IgG and not of complement proteins, and that C3NeF activity in serum was heterogeneous in charge as assessed by isoelectric focusing were more consistent with C3NeF being an immunoglobulin (83). The capacities of insolubilized antisera (83) to kappa and lambda light chain determinants, as well as anti-Fc and anti-Fab antisera, to adsorb C3NeF activity from serum also reaffirmed the findings from the first study (79) of the antigenic reactivity of this protein.

Structural evidence of the identity of C3NeF with IgG was obtained when a method for its purification from contaminating non-specific IgG was developed (84). C3NeF was found to bind to erythrocyte intermediates bearing C3b,Bb and to dissociate upon decay of convertase function (81). Further, the interaction of partially purified C3NeF with C3, B and $\overline{D}$ in the fluid phase, followed by analytical sucrose density gradient ultracentrifugation, revealed that C3NeF activity had shifted from its usual 7S position to the 10S region (84). The apparent increase in m.w. of the principle was secondary to formation of a trimolecular complex containing equimolar amounts of C3NeF, C3b and Bb, indicating that C3NeF had been incorporated into the fluid phase convertase (84). C3NeF released from the 10S complex during spontaneous dissociation of Bb from C3b,Bb at 37°C exhibited no alteration in function, apparent m.w. or isoelectric point, but was free of contaminating non-specific IgG which had sedimented in the 7S region. As residual C3b and Bi could be removed by anion exchange chromatography, the affinity of C3NeF for C3b,Bb afforded a unique method for purification of the protein preparatory to analysis of its polypeptide chain composition. C3NeF was purified from the sera of three patients with membranoproliferative glomerulonephritis and of two patients with partial lipodystrophy by standard chromatography followed by the affinity method described above. Ninety-two to 98% of the purified preparations, radiolabeled with ^{125}I, bound to sheep erythrocytes bearing C3b,Bb; only 0.6 to 18% of ^{125}I-C3NeF was taken up by erythrocytes carrying C3b alone, and no binding to erythrocytes lacking complement proteins was observed (85). All preparations were adsorbed by insolubilized antiserum to IgG, but not by anti-α, μ or δ. Analysis of each ^{125}I-C3NeF preparation by polyacrylamide gel electrophoresis in the presence of SDS revealed apparent m.w.'s identical to non-specific human IgG, and reduction with dithiothreitol of each ^{125}I-C3NeF preparation yielded polypeptide chains of 54,000 and 23,500 m.w., which corresponded to the positions of the heavy and light chains of IgG (85). Thus, C3NeF is an autoantibody of the IgG class with specificity for C3b,Bb to which it binds, resulting in resistance of the complex to intrinsic and β1H-mediated extrinsic decay.

REFERENCES

1. L. Pillemer, L. Blum, I. H. Lepow, O. A. Ross, E. D. Todd, and A. C. Wardlaw, The properdin system and immunity: I. Demonstration and isolation of a new serum protein, properdin, and its role in immune phenomena, Science 120, 279 (1954).

2. R. A. Nelson, Jr., An alternative mechanism for the properdin system, J. Exp. Med. 108, 515 (1958).

3. H. J. Müller-Eberhard, Chemistry and reaction mechanisms of complement, Adv. Immunol. 8, 1 (1968).

4. H. Gewurz, H. S. Shin, and S. E. Mergenhagen, Interactions of the complement system with endotoxic lipopolysaccharide: Consumption of each of the six terminal complement components, J. Exp. Med. 128, 1049 (1968).

5. R. L. Marcus, H. S. Shin, and M. M. Mayer, An alternate complement pathway: C3-cleaving activity, not due to C4b,2a, on endotoxic lipopolysaccharide after treatment with guinea pig serum, Proc. Natl. Acad. Sci. USA 68, 1351 (1971).

6. J. Pensky, C. F. Hinz, Jr., E. W. Todd, R. R. Wedgwood, J. T. Boyer, and I. H. Lepow, Properties of highly purified human properdin, J. Immunol. 100, 142 (1968).

7. P. H. Schur and E. L. Becker, Pepsin digestion of rabbit and sheep antibodies: The effect on complement fixation, J. Exp. Med. 118, 891 (1963).

8. A. L. Sandberg and A. G. Osler, Dual pathways of complement interaction with guinea pig immunoglobulins, J. Immunol. 107, 1268 (1971).

9. M. M. Frank, J. May, T. Gaither, and L. Ellman, In vitro studies of complement function in sera of C4-deficient guinea pigs, J. Exp. Med. 134, 176 (1971).

10. R. A. Nelson, Jr., A new concept of immunosuppression in hypersensitivity reactions and in transplantation immunity, Survey Ophthalmol. 11, 498 (1966).

11. O. Götze and H. J. Müller-Eberhard, The C3-activator system: An alternate pathway of complement activation, J. Exp. Med. 134, Suppl. 90 (1971).

12. L. Pillemer, I. H. Lepow, and L. Blum, The requirement for a hydrazine-sensitive serum factor and heat-labile serum factors in the inactivation of human C3 by zymosan, J. Immunol. 71, 339 (1953).

13. I. Goodkofsky and I. H. Lepow, Functional relationship of factor B in the properdin system to C3 proactivator of human serum, J. Immunol. 107, 1200 (1971).

14. D. T. Fearon and K. F. Austen, Activation of the alternative complement pathway due to resistance of zymosan-bound amplification convertase to endogenous regulatory mechanisms, Proc. Natl. Acad. Sci. USA 74, 1683 (1977).

15. U. R. Nilsson, R. J. Mandle, Jr., and J. A. Mapes, Human C3 and C5: Subunit structure and modifications by trypsin and C42-C423, J. Immunol. 114, 815 (1975).

16. V. A. Bokisch, M. P. Dierich, and H. J. Müller-Eberhard, Third component of complement (C3): Structural properties in relation to functions, Proc. Natl. Acad. Sci. USA 72, 1989 (1975).

17. J. O. Minta and I. H. Lepow, Studies on the subunit structure of properdin, Immunochemistry 11, 361 (1974).

18. O. Götze, Proteases of the properdin system, in Cold Spring Harbor Symposium on Cell Proliferation: Proteases and Biological Control, Reich, E., Rifkin, D.B., and Shaw, E. eds., Cold Spring Harbor Laboratory, p. 255 (1975).

19. D. T. Fearon, Purification of C3b inactivator and demonstration of its two polypeptide chain structure, J. Immunol. 119, 1248 (1977).

20. M. K. Pangburn, R. D. Schreiber, and H. J. Müller-Eberhard, Human complement C3b inactivator: Isolation, characterization and demonstration of an absolute requirement for the serum protein β1H for cleavage of C3b and C4b in solution, J. Exp. Med. 146, 257 (1977).

21. K. Whaley and S. Ruddy, Modulation of the alternative complement pathway by β1H globulin, J. Exp. Med. 144, 1147 (1976).

22. H. J. Müller-Eberhard and O. Götze, C3 proactivator convertase and its mode of action, J. Exp. Med. 135, 1003 (1972).

23. C. A. Alper, F. S. Rosen, and P. J. Lachmann, Inactivator of the third component of complement as an inhibitor in the properdin pathway, Proc. Natl. Acad. Sci. USA 69, 2910 (1972).

24. P. A. E. Nicol and P. J. Lachmann, The alternate pathway of complement activation. The role of C3b and its inactivator (KAF), Immunology 24, 259 (1973).

25. D. T. Fearon, K. F. Austen, and S. Ruddy, Formation of a hemolytically active cellular intermediate by the interaction between properdin factors B and $\overline{D}$ and the activated third component of complement, J. Exp. Med. 138, 1305 (1973).

26. Hunsicker, L. G., S. Ruddy, and K. F. Austen, Alternate complement pathway: Factors involved in cobra venom factor (CoVF) activation of the third component of complement (C3), J. Immunol. 110, 128 (1973)

27. D. T. Fearon, K. F. Austen, and S. Ruddy, Properdin factor D: Characterization of its active site and isolation of the precursor form, J. Exp. Med. 139, 355 (1974).

28. D. T. Fearon and K. F. Austen, Properdin: Initiation of alternative complement pathway, Proc. Natl. Acad. Sci. USA 72, 3220 (1975).

29. M. R. Daha, D. T. Fearon, and K. F. Austen, Isolation of alternative pathway C3 convertase containing uncleaved B and formed in the presence of C3 nephritic factor (C3NeF), J. Immunol. 116, 568 (1976).

30. M. R. Daha, D. T. Fearon, and K. F. Austen, Formation in the presence of C3 nephritic factor (C3NeF) of an alternative pathway C3 convertase containing uncleaved B, Immunology 31, 789 (1976).

31. W. Vogt, W. Dames, G. Schmidt, and L. Dieminger, Complement activation by the properdin system: Formation of a stoichiometric C3 cleaving complex of properdin factor B with C3b, Immunochemistry 14, 201 (1977).

32. M. K. Kazatchkine, D. T. Fearon, and K. F. Austen, Human alternative complement pathway: Membrane-associated sialic acid regulates the competition between B and β1H for cell-bound C3b, J. Immunol., in press.

33. F. Lew, Y. Yukiyama, H. S. Waks, and A. G. Osler, Activation of the alternative (properdin) pathway by divalent cations, J. Immunol. 115, 884 (1975).

34. J. E. May, W. Rosse, and M. M. Frank, Paroxysmal nocturnal hemoglobinuria: Alternate complement pathway-mediated lysis induced by magnesium, New Engl. J. Med. 289, 705 (1973).

35. M. A. Kerr and R. R. Porter, The purification and properties of the second component of human complement, Biochem. J. 171, 99 (1978).

36. C. A. Alper, Inherited structural polymorphism in human C2: Evidence for genetic linkage between C2 and Bf, J. Exp. Med. 144, 1111 (1976).

37. N. Tamura and R.A. Nelson, Jr., Three naturally occurring inhibitors of complement in guinea pig and rabbit serum, J. Immunol. 99, 582 (1967).

38. N. R. Cooper, Isolation and analysis of the mechanism of action of an activator of C4b in human serum, J. Exp. Med. 141, 890 (1975).

39. S. Nagasawa and R. M. Stroud, Mechanism of action of the C3b inactivator: Requirement for a high molecular weight cofactor (C3b-C4bINA cofactor) and production of a new C3b derivative (C3b'), Immunochemistry 14, 749 (1977).

40. T. Fujita, I. Gigli, and V. Nussenzweig, Human C4-binding protein. II. Role in proteolysis of C4b by C3b inactivator, J. Exp. Med. 148, 1044 (1978).

41. D. T. Fearon and K. F. Austen, Properdin: Binding to C3b and stabilization of the C3b-dependent C3 convertase, J. Exp. Med. 142, 856 (1975).

42. R. D. Schreiber, R. G. Medicus, O. Götze, and H. J. Müller-Eberhard, Properdin and nephritic factor-dependent C3 convertases: Requirements of native C3 for enzyme formation and the function of bound C3b as properdin receptor, J. Exp. Med. 142, 760 (1975).

43. J. Chapitis and I. H. Lepow, Multiple sedimenting species of properdin in human serum and interaction of purified properdin with the third component of complement, J. Exp. Med. 143, 241 (1976).

44. D. T. Fearon, K. F. Austen, and S. Ruddy, Properdin factor D. II. Activation to $\overline{D}$ by properdin, J. Exp. Med. 140, 426 (1974).

45. H. S. Shin, R. J. Pickering, and M. M. Mayer, The fifth component of the guinea pig complement system. III. Dissociation and transfer of C5b, and the probable site of C56 fixation, J. Immunol. 106, 480 (1971).

46. N. R. Cooper and H. J. Müller-Eberhard, The reaction mechanism of human C5 in immune hemolysis, J. Exp. Med. 132, 775 (1970).

47. M. R. Daha, D. T. Fearon, and K. F. Austen, C3 requirements for formation of alternative pathway C5 convertase, J. Immunol. 117, 630 (1976).

48. U. R. Nilsson and H. J. Müller-Eberhard, Isolation of β1F-globulin from human serum and its characterization as the fifth component of complement, J. Exp. Med. 122, 277 (1965).

49. K. Whaley and S. Ruddy, Modulation of C3b hemolytic activity by a plasma protein distinct from C3b inactivator, Science 193, 1011 (1976).

50. M. K. Pangburn, R. D. Schreiber, and H. J. Müller-Eberhard, Molecular interactions of the control proteins, C3b inactivator and β1H, with various complement intermediates, J. Immunol. 120, 1791 (1978).

51. M. K. Pangburn and H. J. Müller-Eberhard, Complement C3 convertase: Cell surface restriction of β1H control and generation of restriction on neuraminidase-treated cells, Proc. Natl. Acad. Sci. USA 75, 2416 (1978).

52. D. H. Conrad, J. R. Carlo, and S. Ruddy, Interaction of β1H with cell-bound C3b: Quantitative analysis of binding and influence of alternative pathway components on binding, J. Exp. Med. 147, 1792 (1978).

53. J. M. Weiler, M. R. Daha, K. F. Austen, and D. T. Fearon, Control of the amplification convertase of complement by the plasma protein β1H, Proc. Natl. Acad. Sci. USA 73, 3268 (1976).

54. D. T. Fearon and K. F. Austen, Initiation of C3 cleavage in the alternative complement pathway, J. Immunol. 115, 1357 (1975).

55. R. D. Schreiber, M. K. Pangburn, P. H. LeSavre, and H. J. Muller-Eberhard, Initiation of the alternative pathway of complement: Recognition of activators by bound C3b and assembly of the entire pathway from six isolated proteins, Proc. Natl. Acad. Sci. USA 75, 3948 (1978).

56. R. D. Schreiber, O. Götze, and H. J. Müller-Eberhard, Alternative pathway of complement: Demonstration and characterization of initiating factor and its properdin-independent function, J. Exp. Med. 144, 1062 (1976).

57. R. G. Medicus, R. D. Schreiber, O. Götze, and H. J. Müller-Eberhard, A molecular concept of the properdin pathway, Proc. Natl. Acad. Sci. USA 73, 612 (1976).

58. D. T. Fearon and K. F. Austen, Activation of the alternative complement pathway with rabbit erythrocytes by circumvention of the regulatory action of endogenous control proteins, J. Exp. Med. 146, 22 (1977).

59. D. T. Fearon, Activation of the alternative complement pathway by Escherichia coli: Resistance of bound C3b to inactivation by C3bINA and β1H, J. Immunol. 120, 1772 (1978).

60. T. A. E. Platts-Mills and K. Ishizaka, Activation of the alternate pathway of human complement by rabbit cells, J. Immunol. 113, 348 (1974).

61. D. Aminoff, W. C. Bell, J. Fulton, and N. Ingebrightsen, Effect of sialidase on the viability of erythrocytes in circulation, Amer. J. Hematol. 1, 419 (1976).

62. H. J. Phaff, Cell wall of yeasts, Ann. Rev. Microbial. 17, 15 (1963).

63. G. T. Barry, Colominic acid, a polymer of N-acetylneuraminic acid, J. Exp. Med. 107, 507 (1958).

64. D. T. Fearon, Regulation by membrane sialic acid of β1H-dependent decay-dissociation of amplification C3 convertase of the alternative complement pathway, Proc. Natl. Acad. Sci. USA 75, 1971 (1978).

65. U. E. Nydegger, D. T. Fearon, and K. F. Austen, Regulation by an autosomal locus of the inverse relationship between sialic acid content and the capacity of mouse erythrocytes to activate the human alternative complement pathway, Proc. Natl. Acad. Sci. USA, in press.

66. R. B. Polhill, S. L. Newman, K. M. Pruitt, and R. B. Johnson, Jr., Kinetic assessment of alternative complement pathway in a hemolytic system. II. Influence of antibody on alternative pathway activator, J. Immunol. 121, 371 (1978).

67. J. A. Winklestein and H. S. Shin, The role of immunoglobulin in the interaction of pneumococci and the properdin pathway: Evidence for its specificity and lack of requirement for the Fc portion of the molecule, J. Immunol. 112, 1635 (1974).

68. L. H. Perrin, B. S. Joseph, N. R. Cooper, and M. B. A. Oldstone, Mechanism of injury of virus-infected cells by anti-viral antibody and complement: Participation of IgG, $F(ab')_2$, and the alternative complement pathway, J. Exp. Med. 143, 1027 (1976).

69. A. Ehrhst, Separate pathways of complement activation by measles virus cytotoxic antibodies: Subclass analysis and capacity of Fab molecules to activate complement via the alternative pathway, J. Immunol. 121, 1206 (1978).

70. S. Ferrone, N. R. Cooper, M. A. Pellegrino, and R. A. Reisfeld, Activation of human complement by human lymphoid cells sensitized with histocompatibility alloantisera, Proc. Natl. Acad. Sci. USA 70, 3665 (1973).

71. J. K. Czop, D. T. Fearon, and K. F. Austen, Opsonin-independent phagocytosis of activators of the alternative complement pathway by human monocytes, J. Immunol. 120, 1132 (1978).

72. J. K. Czop, D. T. Fearon, and K. F. Austen, Membrane sialic acid on target particles modulates their phagocytosis by a trypsin-sensitive mechanism on human monocytes, Proc. Natl. Acad. Sci. USA 75, 3831 (1978).

73. H. Gewurz, R. J. Pickering, S. E. Mergenhagen, and R. A. Good, The complement profile in acute glomerulonephritis, systemic lupus erythematosus and hypocomplementemic chronic glomerulonephritis, Int. Arch. Allergy 34, 556 (1968).

74. R. E. Spitzer, E. H. Vallota, J. Forristal, E. Sudora, A. Stitzel, N. C. Davis, and C. D. West, Serum C3 lytic system in patients with glomerulonephritis, Science 164, 436 (1969).

75. E. H. Vallota, J. Forristal, R. E. Spitzer, N. C. Davis, and C. D. West, Characteristics of a non-complement dependent C3 reactive complex formed from factors in nephritic serum and normal serum, J. Exp. Med. 131, 1306 (1970).

76. E. H. Ruley, J. Forristal, N. C. Davis, C. Andres, and C. D. West, Hypocomplementemia of membranoproliferative nephritis: Dependence of the nephritic factor reaction on properdin factor B, J. Clin. Invest. 52, 896 (1973).

77. J. G. P. Sissons, R. G. West, J. Fallows, D. G. Williams, B. J. Boucher, N. Amos, and D. K. Peters, The complement abnormalities of lipodystrophy, New Engl. J. Med. 297, 461 (1976).

78. M. R. Daha, D. T. Fearon, and K. F. Austen, C3 nephritic factor (C3NeF): Stabilization of fluid phase and cell-bound alternative pathway convertase, J. Immunol. 116, 1 (1976).

79. R. A. Thompson, C3 inactivating factor in the serum of a patient with chronic hypocomplementemic proliferative glomerulonephritis, Immunology 22, 147 (1972).

80. E. H. Vallota, O. Götze, H. H. Spiegelberg, J. Forristal, C. D. West, and H. J. Müller-Eberhard, A serum factor in chronic hypocomplementemic nephritis distinct from immunoglobulin and activating the alternative pathway of complement, J. Exp. Med. 139, 1249 (1974).

81. R. E. Schreiber, O. Götze, and H. J. Müller-Eberhard, Nephritic factor: Its structure and function and relationship to initiating factor of the alternative pathway, Scand. J. Immunol. 5, 705 (1976).

82. A. E. Davis, III, M. A. Arnaout, C. A. Alper, and F. S. Rosen, Transfer of C3 nephritic factor from mother to fetus, New Engl. J. Med. 297, 144 (1977).

83. A. E. Davis, III, J. B. Ziegler, E. W. Gelfand, F. S. Rosen, and C. A. Alper, Heterogeneity of nephritic factor and its identification as an immunoglobulin, Proc. Natl. Acad. Sci. USA 74, 3980 (1977).

84. M. R. Daha, K. F. Austen, and D. T. Fearon, The incorporation of C3 nephritic factor (C3NeF) into a stabilized C3 convertase, C3b,Bb(C3NeF), and its release after decay of convertase function, J. Immunol. 119, 812 (1977).

85. M. R. Daha, K. F. Austen, and D. T. Fearon, Heterogeneity, polypeptide chain composition and antigenic reactivity of C3 nephritic factor, J. Immunol. 120, 1389 (1978).

COMPLEMENT ANAPHYLATOXINS AS PLASMA MEDIATORS, SPASMOGENS AND CHEMOTAXINS

Tony E. Hugli
Department of Molecular Immunology, Scripps Clinic and Research Foundation, La Jolla, California 92122

I. INTRODUCTION

As interest in the functional aspects of the blood complement system has increased in intensity during the past twenty-five years, our understanding of the structures of complement components has also grown, particularly in the last decade. Müller-Eberhard's laboratory has been the undisputed leader in elaborating the molecular nature of human complement components. Recently Reid and Porter's (1,2) elegant chemical descriptions of human C1q and Tack, Prahl and colleagues' (3,4,5) work with human C3, C4 and C5 have provided detailed biochemical definition of these pivotal complement factors.

The complement system is a multifunctional complex of proteins that serves an integral role in the primary defense mechanisms of higher organisms. Complement products participate in numerous major systemic processes, mediated via diverse cellular responses including immune adherence, enhanced phagocytosis, cytolysis, chemotaxis, chemokinesis, aggregation and specific release phenomena. Additionally, immune surveillance and inflammation are vital defense mechanisms that use and depend on complement in maintaining a state of physiologic normalcy. Imbalances of body chemistry, as in certain hypersensitivity conditions, may reflect deleterious manifestations of this same complement system. Unfortunately, some devices of medical science's advanced technology may stimulate complement activation artificially, causing secondary pathologic complications of major consequence, such as the side effects from nylon fiber filtration leukapheresis (6,7) or from renal dialysis in patients with acute kidney failure. Contact activation of the complement cascade can occur from interaction with the cellophane-like surfaces of commercial dialysis membranes (8), and the associated leukopenia (9) and pulmonary dysfunction (10) may be related to formation of a complement-derived chemotactic factor. Although this leukopenia is transient and reversible, serious clinical ramifications may accrue from recurrent massive activation of complement during sequential dialysis treatment of patients or by repeated filtration leukapheresis of normal donors. Evaluation of all the complement products and their importance in maintaining integrity and balance *in vivo* constitutes a new horizon in clinical research and will become the focus for future investigation of this complex humoral system.

Basically three groups of proteins constitute the entire complement system. These are the activator components of the cascade (C1, C2, C4, properdin, Factors B and D), the functional components that participate directly in expression of activity (C3, C4, C5, C6, C7, C8 and C9), and the inhibitory or control components (C1 Inh, C3b INA, C1q Inh, S protein, SCPB)*. These combined complement proteins account for more than 4% of all serum proteins or more than 10% of all serum proteins exclusive of albumin. So, by sheer bulk alone the complement proteins form an impressive assemblage of novel structures.

The low molecular weight activation fragments of C3 and C5, called anaphylatoxins, constitute our main research interest. These fragments are the pharmacologically active factors, C3a and C5a. Both are spasmogens, i.e., release mast cell histamine and contract smooth muscle, and in addition C5a is a potent chemotactic factor. This report addresses the current status of our structure-function studies with the serum polypeptides and delves into the physiologic behavior of these humoral factors.

II. HISTORICAL PERSPECTIVE

The desire to commemorate 1920 as the beginning of Dr. E.J. Cohn's leadership in plasma protein research and 1953 as the founding of the Protein Foundation, stimulated this Symposium. The premise of using these dates as milestones around which to build my presentation seemed particularly fitting and novel on this occasion. Unfortunately, I could not cite a single article published in either year that contained an appropriate mention of the anaphylatoxins. Nevertheless, well before 1920 a plasma-derived principle had been identified as an anaphylatoxin (Friedberger 11, 12),or as a serotoxin (Bordet 13),because of its functional behavior.

The name anaphylatoxin reflects this active principle's often lethal physiologic effect (e.g. anaphylactic-like shock) when it is injected into experimental animals. Unknown at the time were the facts that: a) the serum principle originated from activated complement, b) only the "classical" or C5a anaphylatoxin was involved, c) the apparent anaphylactic shock phenomenon may actually have been respiratory collapse partially mediated by liberated histamine, d) and individual species manifest different intensities of responsiveness depending on the relative efficacy of their internal serum control mechanisms. Despite these limitations, the pre-1920 era was an exciting period of discovery in which the anaphylatoxin gradually emerged as an identifiable serum factor with dramatic physiologic consequences (Bordet (13)). Nearly one decade of research was required to establish that the origins of this toxic principle was in the "activated serum" and not just a by-product of the activators used to generate anaphylatoxin.

Originally the additives used in generating anaphylatoxin in serum had contained immunoglobulins and were themselves suspect as providers of the toxic activity. However, a wide variety of substances were later found to produce anaphylactic activity in animal sera, including antigen-antibody complexes, precipitated immunoglobulin, kaolin, barium sulfate, agar, starch and inulin. Eventually, Nathan (14), in attempting to isolate a single causative factor, found that blood contained the true source of the toxin. Discovery of a toxic humoral factor came at a time when Dale strongly advocated the cellular theory of anaphylaxis (15,16), which had already gained wide acceptance. Dale theorized that cellular liberation of potent mediators such as histamine could account for the anaphylactic phenomenon. Friedberger's opposing claim of a genuinely humoral toxic principle (12) became known as the humoral theory of anaphylaxis that Nathan (14) subsequently supported. This debate prompted the inception of valuable studies into the nature of this humoral factor and stimulated the second era of anaphylatoxin research.

*Terminology for complement components conforms to the recommendations of the World Health Organization Committee on Complement Nomenclature (Bull. W.H.O. 39, 939 (1968)). Abbreviations used are: C1 Inh, C1 inhibitor; C3b INA, C3b inactivator; C1q Inh, inhibitor; S protein, inhibits cellular binding of the C5b-7 complex; and SCPB, serum carboxypeptidase

Between 1920 and the early 1950s, investigation in the field of protein chemistry reached a zenith in America and established it as a permanent and indispensible discipline of research. Although blood proteins became a major focus for the protein chemists, anaphylatoxins did not draw much attention, and little progress was made in understanding the chemical or physical nature of the humoral "shock" factors. However, the relatively few, important advances of that time led to a unifying theory of anaphylaxis. This new theory, espoused by Rocha e Silva (17, 18), embodies the influences of both cellular and humoral mediators into a general scheme for explaining anaphylaxis. Most significant to this work were the experiments of Hahn and Oberdorf (19), who showed that antihistamines can block anaphylatoxin induced shock, and the observation by Rocha e Silva and Aronson (20) that anaphylatoxin in activated rat plasma can release histamine from isolated guinea pig lung. These physiologic studies solidly confirmed the ability of anaphylatoxins to excite cellular mediator release. Hahn and Oberdorf's demonstration that antihistamines can attenuate the action of anaphylatoxin suggested a role for humoral factors in systemic processes such as hypersensitivity and surveillance mechanisms like inflammation.

The greatest growth in our understanding of the structural and functional properties of the anaphylatoxins postdates 1950, as is apparent in the historical outline of anaphylatoxin research presented in Table 1. Although progress has steadily accelerated in recent years, the foundations on which we as current researchers build clearly emanate from the efforts of our predecessors.

III. BIOLOGICAL BEHAVIOR OF THE ANAPHYLATOXINS

The biological behavior of the anaphylatoxins, as demonstrated in numerous *in vitro* bioassays, seems quite distinct from their true biological function *in vivo*, for the later processes are intertwined in a massive network of concurrent reactions. Therefore, the specific function or significance of a lone cellular mediator is as difficult to assign as appraising the contribution of a single instrument in a symphony orchestra. Similarly, if just one apparently insignificant instrument is eliminated an entire performance may nonetheless suffer. This may be exactly the dilemma we face when deleting a single mediator from a complex system as a means of detecting the associated physiologic function. Because certain defense mechanisms in higher organisms seem to operate with safeguards such as duplication of function or alternative pathways of protection, the researcher is challenged with the problem of how best to define the functional importance of a factor that may be supported by other endogenous backup systems. Actually, only when one understands the chemical nature of the factor, its mode of activation, and the appropriate control mechanisms is an accurate interpretation of the factor's physiologic significance possible. However, crude *in vivo* tests of biological function are often the first step toward characterizing such factors and these may include blocking or stimulating formation of the factors, introduction of an excess of the active factors or of a suitable analog, or manipulating mechanisms that control or inactivate the factors. Although this discussion is limited to describing the behavior of anaphylatoxins that relates to their potential function *in vivo*, the stage is now set for obtaining unequivocal proof as to the roles C3a and C5a play in maintaining health and, on occasion, their involvement in pathophysiologic mechanisms.

In Vitro Functions

Purified C3a and C5a readily induce responses from isolated smooth muscle preparations, that is, they contract ileal, bronchial, tracheal, uterine, colonic and cardiac muscle strips. To be sure, the responsiveness of various muscle types differ, perhaps in proportion to the relative content of tissue mast cells. In general, the order of tissue sensitivity is ileum > uterus > trachea > atrium in guinea pig tissue, although in the rat the level and order of sensitivity are quite different. The

TABLE 1 Important Events in the History of the Anaphylatoxins

1910	First description of a factor in "activated" serum causing an anaphylactoid-like shock syndrome: Friedberger (11).
1911-13	Evidence that the active factor was serum derived and not a product of the activators: Bordet (13) and Nathan (14).
1950	Demonstration that the action of "classical" anaphylatoxin (C5a) is blocked by antihistamines: Hahn and Oberdorf (19).
1952	Tissue histamine release is induced by anaphylatoxin (C5a). Support for the histamine shock theory: Rocha e Silva and Aronson (20).
1959	Anaphylatoxinogens are components of the blood complement system: Osler, et al. (21).
1967	Discovery of an anaphylatoxin derived from guinea pig C5: Jensen (22).
	Discovery of an anaphylatoxin derived from human C3: Dias da Silva et al. (23).
1968	Evidence that there are two distinct human anaphylatoxins: Cochrane and Müller-Eberhard (24).
	Identification of serum carboxypeptidase (SCPB) as an enzyme that controls spasmogenic activity of C3a and C5a: Lepow et al. (26) and Bokisch (27).
1971	Preliminary characterization of C3a obtained from purified human C3: Budzko et al. (28).
1973	Demonstration of both active C3a and C5a in C-activated human serum: Vallota and Müller-Eberhard (29).
1975	The complete chemical structure of human C3a is reported: Hugli (30).
1976	Description of human C5a as glycopolypeptide: Fernandez and Hugli (31).
1977	Discovery of novel synthetic peptides that mimic the biological activity of C3a: Hugli and Erickson (32).
1978	Initial chemical evidence that C3a and C5a share a common genetic ancestry: Fernandez and Hugli (33).
	Demonstration that both C5a and $C5a_{des\ Arg}$ stimulate neutrophil migration. Proof that C3a is inactive as a chemotaxin: Fernandez et al. (34).
	Primary structure of the human C5a polypeptide is reported: Fernandez and Hugli (35).
	Preliminary characterization of a neutrophil receptor for human C5a: Chenoweth and Hugli (36).

order of sensitivity in experimental animals appears to be guinea pig>rabbit>rat for responsiveness of ileal tissues to applied anaphylatoxin. Furthermore, animals with the greatest susceptibility to anaphylatoxin-induced shock have tissues that seem to be particularly responsive to these factors. Several types of muscle react to anaphylatoxins, and each may reflect responses induced by a separate group of mediators. For instance, histamine may be primarily responsible for the smooth muscle contractions elicited by C3a or C5a in digestive and respiratory tissues, whereas uterine tissue may contract as a result of serotonin or neuromotor mediator release. Conceivably, anaphylatoxins could act directly on muscle tissue; however, on histamine-sensitive tissue, H-1 type histamine antagonists effectively block the action. Cardiac muscle appears to represent yet another situation, possibly involving anaphylatoxin's release of mediators that stimulate neuromuscular reflex action.

Tissues stimulated by the anaphylatoxins share a common and characteristic feature manifested as tissue desensitization. Smooth muscle can be selectively desensitized by either anaphylatoxin, a condition known as tachyphylaxis. Although C3a preparations from humans and other animals are mutually cross-tachyphylactic, C3a shows no tachyphylaxis (desensitization) toward C5a, or vice versa. These results suggest to us that each anaphylatoxin has its own receptor population on the cellular target.

Cellular responses to the anaphylatoxins have recently taken on new meaning with the realization that a wider variety of circulating cell types respond to these factors than was previously appreciated. Responsive cell types include neutrophils, macrophages, eosinophils, basophils and platelets. The mast cell undergoes a selective release reaction and remains the best characterized of the target tissue cells responsive to C3a and C5a stimulation. Table 2 contains a summary of these cellular responses and a compilation of the effects directly associated with the action of anaphylatoxins.

TABLE 2 Cellular activities of the serum anaphylatoxins

Cell Type	C3a	C5a	Specific Effects
Mast cells	+	+	Vasoamine release
	+	+	degranulation
Polymorphonuclear leukocytes	-	+	chemotaxis
	±	±	enzyme release
	?	+	enhanced phagocytosis
	-	+	aggregation
Basophils	-	+	chemotaxis
	+	+	histamine release
	+	+	degranulation
Eosinophils	-	+	chemotaxis
Platelets	+	?	serotonin release
	+	?	aggregation
Peripheral macrophages	-	+	enhanced migration
Alveolar macrophages	-	+	enhanced migration
Lymphocytes	+	?	cytolytic

Responsiveness of a single cell type to the anaphylatoxins might be viewed as relatively insignificant, but the recognized interplay that occurs between the variety of cell types affected and their cooperation to evoke systemic responses are of major concern. Systemic processes such as hypersensitivity and inflammation evolve from a concert of mediator-elicited cellular reactions as outlined in Fig. 1. The proposed role of the anaphylatoxins has been purposefully emphasized in the scheme displayed in this figure. Beneficial or not, these processes originate from direct interactions between plasma components and cellular elements in the blood. Anaphylatoxins represent only one of three categories of endogenous humoral polypeptides reported to mediate such cellular functions; the other two include the kinins and the fibrinopeptides.

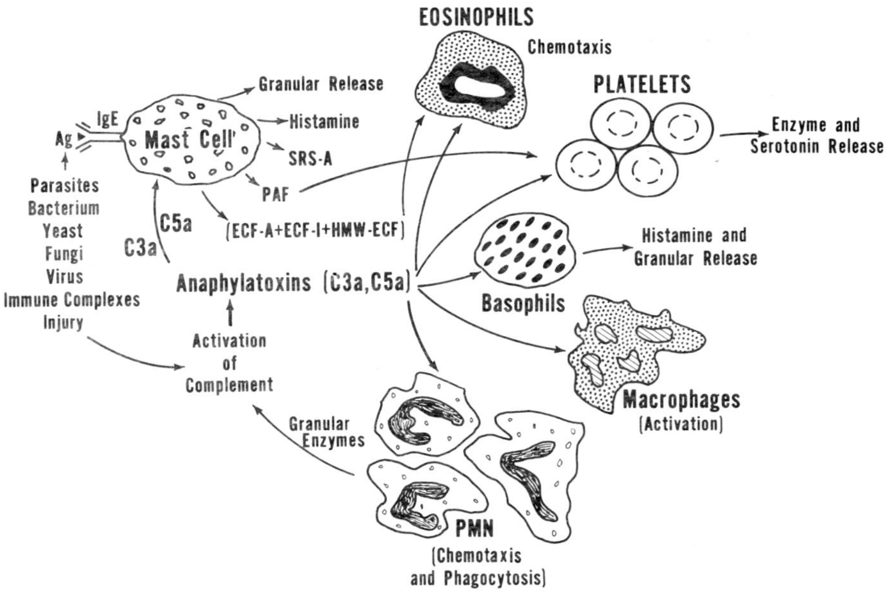

Figure 1. Mediators serve to communicate changes in the environment to the cells and in that capacity the anaphylatoxins stimulate the proposed cellular responses shown above. A possible mechanism for anaphylatoxin involvement in hypersensitivity reactions can be portrayed by focusing on their well-known ability for releasing histamine from tissue mast cells. A variety of additional mediators are presumably released from the stimulated mast cell and these factors in turn excite cellular components in the blood, particularly eosinophils. Anaphylatoxins also act directly on a number of circulatory cell types that play a prominent role in host defense mechanisms. Thereby both C3a and C5a may prove intimately associated with major systemic processes such as inflammation.

In Vivo Functions

A summary of the wide variety of *in vivo* functions stimulated by the anaphylatoxins emphasizes the potential impact of these potent factors on tissue or systemic reactions during acute injury or insult (See Table 3). The fact that complement activation must precede the involvement of C3a or C5a clearly establishes these factors primarily as protective and pathophysiologic rather than preventive in their function.

TABLE 3 Effects of the anaphylatoxins as measured *In Vivo*

Description of Procedure	Quantity of C3a	Quantity of C5a	Anaphylatoxin Source	Effects
Intravenous injection in guinea pigs	NA	10 - 20µg (1.2 - 2.4 nmoles)	rat porcine	Lethal shock
in guinea pigs	NA	5 - 10 µg (0.6 - 1.2 nmoles)	rat guinea pig	Respiratory distress Circulatory hypertension
Kidney perfusion in porcine kidney	—	C-activated serum	porcine	Resistance to blood flow (vasoconstriction)
Topical application to exposed rabbit omentum	10^{-8} - 10^{-9}moles	ND	human	Arteriolar constriction Pressure changes Hemostasis, local
Intradermal injection in guinea pigs	10^{-10} - 10^{-12}moles	10^{-13} - 10^{-14}moles	human porcine	Wheal (enhanced vascular permeability, 20-100mm^2)
in human	10^{-10} - 10^{-12}moles	10^{-13} - 10^{-14}moles	human	Flare (mast cell vasoamine release, 75 to 1200mm^2)
Skin-mounted chambers (chemotaxis)				
on human skin	NA	diluted serum	human	Attraction of neutrophils
on rabbit skin	NA	1.2 - 6.0 x 10^{-7}M	human	

NA, not active
ND, not determined

Although lethal shock is the most dramatic manifestation of C5a action, less extreme local responses such as histamine release and vascular changes are believed more important in man because an efficient control mechanism abrogates broader systemic effects. Unlike animal sera, complement-activated human serum contains little if any spasmogenically active C5a because of the regulating enzyme known as serum carboxypeptidase B (SCPB, EC 3.4.12.7). Since the spasmogenic activity of C3a and C5a is dependent on the presence of an essential C-terminal arginyl residue, simple removal of this arginine by SCPB efficiently controls this activity and leads to the formation of $C3a_{des\ Arg}$ and $C5a_{des\ Arg}$, respectively. Presumably it is a structural feature that distinguishes human from other animal C5a molecules, for residual spasmogenic activity is expressed in the complement-activated sera of most animals. The only function that is known to be associated with the des Arg forms of either anaphylatoxin is the induction of polymorphonuclear leukocyte (PMN) migration by the $C5a_{des\ Arg}$ molecule. It is this separation of spasmogenic and chemotactic activities that infers a unique duality of function for C5a.

Chemotaxis

Shin et al. (25) first described C5 as a chemotaxinogen in 1968, and since that time C5 activation peptides have been recognized for their potent chemotactic properties directed toward leukocytes. One year later, Jensen et al. (37) further described the properties of the guinea pig C5a, and Ward and Newman (38) reported that human C5 serves as a chemotaxinogen with the active factor being generated in this case by trypsinization. Recently, Ward and his colleagues proved that chemotactic factor formation can be initiated by plasmin (39) or lysosomal granular enzymes of neutrophils (40), and they have demonstrated that a chemotactic factor inactivator (CFI) can be isolated from normal human serum (41). Although its nature has yet to be established, CFI appears to be either a protease of limited action or a specific inhibitor of insufficient quantity to abrogate C5a-related chemotactic activity in normal sera. The role of CFI may ultimately be understood through examination of disease states associated with elevated levels of CFI such as certain inflammatory (sarcoidosis and hepatic cirrhosis), infectious (lepromatous leprosy) and neoplastic (Hodgkin's) diseases (42). Although it is generally agree that the predominant chemotactic factors generated in plasma are derived from complement components, the origin and chemical form of these active factors are still somewhat controversial. Currently, there is strong evidence that the major humoral factors are all C5-derived, but other minor factors may indeed originate from C3 and other plasma proteins. The C3-derived factors must, however, arise from a structural region distinct from the C3a portion of the parent molecule. C5-derived fragments may indeed exist in forms other than those most extensively characterized i.e., C5a and $C5a_{des\ Arg}$. In fact, a recent report describes a C5-derived factor that selectively attracts tumor cells (Walker carcinosarcoma cells), but differs physically and chemically from the classical anaphylatoxin molecule (43). In view of the above description, we shall define chemotactic factors for the purpose of this discussion as those humoral factors that attract human PMN.

Chemically pure human C3a and C5a have now been carefully examined for chemotactic behavior. While C3a is inactive, C5a stimulates cellular migration over a range of 0.04 to 1.7 x 10^{-8}M in the Boyden chamber assay (34) (Table 4). The spasmogenically inactive form of C5a ($C5a_{des\ Arg}$) has also proven to be chemotactically active, but only in the presence of added serum proteins. At higher concentrations, these humoral chemotactic factors elicit cellular responses that rise and then fall to a nominal level implying that the cells are being desensitized or are otherwise rendered unresponsive. Much like the response obtained with isolated PMN _in vitro_, when _in vivo_ conditions are simulated by allowing cells to migrate into chambers attached to an abraded skin surface, PMN are attracted by C5a or $C5a_{des\ Arg}$. Desensitization apparently also occurs _in vivo_ for when levels of the C5a or $C5a_{des\ Arg}$ in the chambers are elevated, no cells were attracted.

TABLE 4 Quantitative estimates of human C5a and $C5a_{des\ Arg}$ Interactions with Polymorphonuclear Leukocytes

Measurement	C5a	$C5a_{des\ Arg}$
1. Chemotaxis	ED_{50} Values (M)	
Boyden chamber method	0.9×10^{-9}	2.0×10^{-8}
Agarose method	1.0×10^{-9}	6.3×10^{-8}
Skin window technique (rabbit PMN)	1.7×10^{-7}	3.3×10^{-7}
II. PMN Receptor Affinity		
Cellular uptake	$3\text{-}7 \times 10^{-9}$	not determined
III. Lysosomal Enzyme Release		
β-glucuronidase	3.0×10^{-9}	no effect
	Sites per cell	
IV. Receptor sites on PMN	$1\text{-}3 \times 10^{5}$	not determined

The amount of chemoattractants necessary to stimulate migration of the PMN is about the same in the Boyden and in the "under agarose" assay of Chenoweth et al. (44) in terms of comparative ED_{50} values for C5a and $C5a_{des\ Arg}$ (See Table 4). Therefore, the two techniques are equally useful for quantitating humoral chemotactic factors. However, the agarose method may be more advantageous since cellular morphology of the PMN reflects the extent of stimulation and the shape of the migratory pattern may provide valuable information concerning the physical nature (e.g. the size) of the stimulant applied.

Evidence that C5a stimulates movement of the PMN after some direct physical interaction with cellular receptors was recently obtained by using human PMN and ^{125}I-labeled C5a (36). In these studies, saturation was taken as an indication that specific uptake had occurred (Fig. 2A). Furthermore, the uptake was rapid, and little if any of the labeled factor was released from the cells over a 90 min. period indicating either that the affinity of the factor-receptor interaction was very high or that the factor had been internalized (Fig. 2B). An apparent half-saturation value for human C5a was $3\text{-}7 \times 10^{-9}$M. The ED_{50} values for ^{125}I-C5a cellular binding were 3.3 nM to 5.3nM and compared favorably with the ED_{50} values estimated from assays of chemotactic activity (Table 4). The apparent PMN receptor affinity (i.e. ^{125}I-$C5a_{des\ Arg}$ uptake) for $C5a_{des\ Arg}$ was less than for C5a differing perhaps by more than two logs. This conclusion is derived from the fact that a 100-fold molar excess of ^{125}I-$C5a_{des\ Arg}$ was less than 60% as effective as C5a for inhibiting ^{125}I-C5a uptake by the PMN.

Quantitative activity values were obtained for C5a in a pure form and extrapolated back to the serum levels assuming total complement conversion of C5, these two values agree to within a factor of 2. Measurement of chemotactic activity in EACA*-protected human serum activated by

*EACA, epsilon-aminocaproic acid is a competitive inhibitor of the serum carboxypeptidase (SCPB), used during serum activation to prevent degradation of the anaphylatoxins.

Figure 2A. Uptake of ^{125}I-C5a by human PMNs was measured as a function of the ligand concentration of 1.4×10^7 cells/ml, binding of labeled human C5a was saturable at a concentration of 2.5×10^{-7} g/ml of polypeptide. Uptake was specific and was inhibited by unlabeled C5a indicating that the active factor bound to a select population of surface receptors.

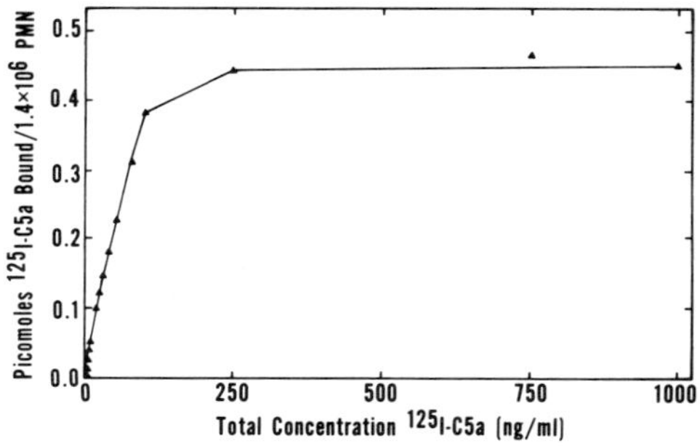

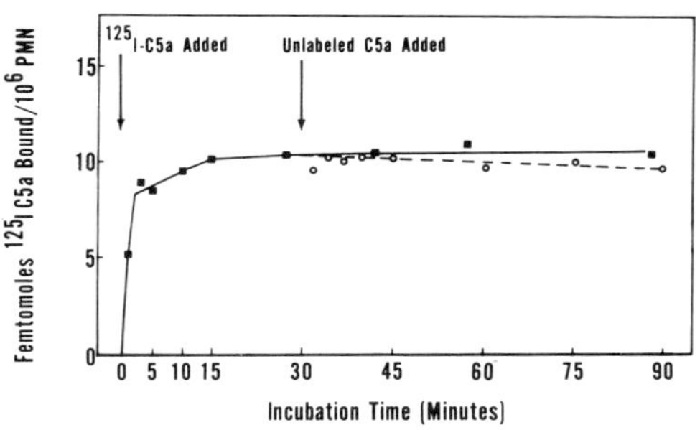

Figure 2B. Rate of cellular ^{125}I-C5a uptake by PMNs.

A final concentration of 2 ng/ml (0.24 nM) ^{125}I-C5a was added to 10^9 PMNs and the quantity of cell-bound ligand was determined. At 30 minutes (see arrow) a 1000-fold excess of unlabeled C5a was added and the off rate of ^{125}I-C5a was measured. O, ^{125}I-C5a bound in the presence of 1000-fold excess of unlabeled C5a.

zymosan also yields a value consistent with that predicted from C5 conversion alone. Unfortunately, neither approach resolves the question of whether other humoral chemotactic factors exist and have sufficient activity to be considered functionally important. Perhaps a better attempt at answering this question is the recent experiments with specific antibody raised to the human C5a molecule (45). Activated human serum (ZAS) can be rendered free of measurable chemotactic activity by adding immunospecific C5a antibody. As Fig. 3 illustrates, the specific antibody neutralized all activity, which confirms our hypothesis that only C5a or C5a-related humoral factors represent major chemotactic activity in activated plasma or serum.

Physiologic and Clinical Importance

Present knowledge is just beginning to reveal the variety of physiologic responses influenced by the anaphylatoxins. Two categories of responses that might be expected to occur are those related to effects induced by the spasmogenic activity of C3a and C5a and those that exist as a manifestation of C5a-dependent granulocyte chemotaxis. Perhaps the most difficult functions to perceive and define are the roles of these factors under normal conditions, that is, when the factors participate in what is believed to be their usual defense roles of supporting the inflammatory process and the consequent promotion of healing. Various clinical conditions resulting from complement component deficiencies, inhibitor deficiencies, or hyperactivation of complement imply a direct involvement of the anaphylatoxin, and have recently been brought into sharper focus by a number of studies concerned exclusively with the nature and extent of anaphylatoxin action in man. Thus far, there is no unifying statement about how these factors act systemically, but from

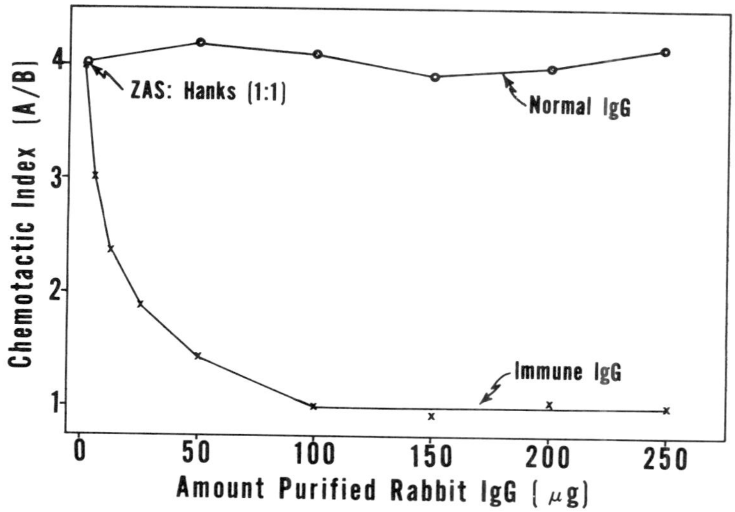

Figure 3. Zymogen activated human serum (ZAS) serves as a convenient source of complement-derived chemoattractant. When purified rabbit IgG is added to the ZAS no effect is observed on the ability to induce PMN migration. However, addition of rabbit anti-human C5a immunoglobulin totally neutralizes the chemotactic activity of ZAS indicating that the major chemoattractant in complement-activated serum is related antigenically to C5a. Chemotaxis was estimated using 2.5×10^{-5} human PMN in the modified "chemotaxis under agarose" procedure (44).

the various isolated cases and the preliminary results, it seems clear that multiple biological effects might be attributed to the presence of anaphylatoxins. A brief outline of known and suspected physiologic activities of the anaphylatoxins is presented.

Complement component deficiencies are inborn disorders that provide valuable data related to the pathophysiology of a defined molecular defect. Case reports of separate individuals exhibiting early component deficiency (e.g. C1r, C2 or C3) indicate a depressed or delayed ability to generate chemotactic activity (46) One C3-deficient individual, described as only partially deficient and having approximately 50% the normal C3 level, is not subject to recurrent infections and shows no clinical abnormalities other than depressed chemotaxis (47). However, total C3 deficiency in a young girl led to a marked reduction of her host defense mechanisms (48). Another C3 deficient individual, who experiences hypercatabolism of C3, maintains plasma C3 levels only 4 to 8% of normal, displays an enhanced susceptibility to infection and reportedly has expressed urticaria under stress (49). The latter effect may be directly related to the rapid formation of C3a anaphylatoxins during excessive C3 turnover. This individual's serum is also depressed in chemotaxin formation, as is predictable for anyone deficient in the early complement components, including C3, if the defect adversely affects conversion of C5. Miller and co-workers (50,51) described a familial clinical syndrome that presents as a plasma-associated defect of both leukocyte phagocytosis and chemotaxis resulting in dysfunction of the individual's inflammatory response. The clinical manifestation is an enhanced susceptibility to recurrent infection by gram-negative bacteria. The defect, in this patient does not appear to be a quantitative deficiency but rather a dysfunction of the C5, perhaps chemical in nature somehow preventing the selective cleavage of C5 into C5a and C5b. Serum from this individual was reconstituted in its phagocytosis-enhancing ability by the addition of normal purified C5 (51).

Mechanisms controlling the spasmogenic and chemotactic properties of the anaphylatoxins are known to constitute separate processes. C3a and C5a spasmogenic activities are short-lived in plasma if it contains a normal level of the SCPB. A recently identified patient with a SCPB deficiency suffered clinical effects outwardly characterized as idiopathic angioedema. This patient had a plasma SCPB level only 20% of normal (52) and is the only individual presently known who is deficient in the particular enzyme that controls the spasmogenic action of the anaphylatoxins. The causal relationship between the individual's clinical status and the SCPB deficiency is not yet established, and there is no firm evidence that defective control of the anaphylatoxins is responsible for the patient's recurrent angioedema. Only circumstantial evidence indicates that the enzymatic defect permits enhanced expression of C3a and C5a,factors that are usually under the rigorous control of the inhibitor. What is presently established is that the patient suffers from a genetic defect, presumably an enzyme deficiency and not a dysfunction.

A separate mechanism appears to exist for controlling the chemotaxins, the previously mentioned inactivator CFI may influence expression of humoral chemotactic activity. The nature of CFI is uncertain; however, its activity in normal individuals and certain disease states varies significantly. The serum level of CFI is reported to be depressed in individuals with a Pi ZZ phenotype for α-anti trypsin deficiency (53). Excessive levels of CFI are found in the sera of individuals experiencing certain inflammatory, infectious and neoplastic diseases (36), but interpretation is limited until more is known of the CFI mechanism. It does appear that a major CFI interaction in vivo is with the C5a des Arg form of the anaphylatoxin molecule and that in normal plasma the inactivator exhibits a very limited capacity for control. This means either that CFI is not an enzyme or that it is inhibited from acting by yet another component in normal plasma.

Finally, when the humoral chemotactic factor is repeatedly infused, it seems to initiate severe clinical conditions such as a pronounced transient neutropenia observed in rabbits only seconds after the introduction of C5a-related chemotactic factor (8). As early as 1969, Kaplow and Goffinet reported profound neutropenia in patients during the early phase of hemodialysis, and later neutrophils were detected in the pulmonary bed during hemodialysis (54). Craddock and co-workers (7,9) have since associated complement activation with the complication of neutrophil sequestration in the lung, presumably related to the effect of C5a ($C5a_{des\ Arg}$) on granulocytes (PMN) increasing their adherence and enhancing their tendency to aggregate (55). Although pulmonary calcification is a known complication of chronic kidney failure, recent studies suggest that patients on long-term hemodialysis have an increased frequency of this complication. Taken together these studies implicate humoral chemotactic factors in mediating the cellular induction of pulmonary calcification. Therapeutic dialysis serves to enhance this process, a newly found potential effect, albeit deleterious, of the anaphylatoxins in pathophysiology. Another clinical procedure that may involve C5a-induced aberrant leukocyte behavior is the practice of neutrophil transfusion in humans with leukemia. A technique used for harvesting the leukocytes, called filtration leukapheresis (FL), selectively separates leukocytes from other plasma cells by differential adherence of the neutrophils to nylon wool filters. This process induces preferential degranulation of the leukocytes leading to complement activation in the donor (56). Adverse side effects that are associated with FL (without the concurrent elevation of serum histamine) include transient neutropenia, hypotension, urticaria, and lower abdominal cramping in female donors (57,58) indicating that the spasmogenic form of C5a is not involved. Although transfusion of these harvested leukocytes may be a useful form of hematologic support in severely neutropenic patients, it is now evident that cells obtained by FL are functionally defective. Avoidance of complement activation during collection may result in the isolation of fully functional leukocytes. Therapeutic use of such "non-activated" granulocytes might alleviate the usually severe side effects thereby enhancing the potential value of this clinical treatment.

We seem to be just at the threshold of assigning major functional roles to the anaphylatoxins in mediating essential host surveillance mechanisms such as phagocytosis and cellular migration. Possibly, the transient effects of anaphylatoxins such as their actions on smooth muscle and vascular permeability are more important functions than previously recognized and become detrimental only when the rigorous control mechanisms fail to limit their action to localized sites. Ultimately, it seems that nature's inherent defense mechanisms must be respected and maintained under proper control if clinical techniques such as hemodialysis, granulocyte transfusion, and possibly even tissue transplantion are to be employed without adverse side effects.

IV. CHEMICAL STRUCTURE OF THE ANAPHYLATOXINS

Since the complete chemical structure of an anaphylatoxin was first reported less than four years ago, human C3a and C5a, have been characterized chemically and numerous shared features observed. However, it is not so much the similarities as the subtle differences responsible for the individual functions of each that now draws our attention. Chemical structural analyses of the two human anaphylatoxins indicate that they are genetically related and the acquired functional differences may result from amino acid replacements occurring near the C-terminal arginine. Since the arginyl residue is essential for all spasmogenic activity, knowing the C-terminal sequence proved instructive for interpreting functional differences between C3a and C5a. Structural analyses of anaphylatoxins obtained from various animal sources have contributed greatly to our present knowledge by indicating trends in the conservation of specific features that correlate with the functional expression of the molecule.

Distribution, formation and control

Anaphylatoxins certainly are not restricted to the blood of mammals alone. Among members of the animal kingdom, the hemolytic complement system is found in all vertebrates, although that of non-mammals occurs in a somewhat more primative form (59). Quantitative levels of the anaphylatoxinogens seem to vary little among the species of higher mammals studied to date, except in certain murine strains that are markedly deficient in the component C5 (60,61). In man, the potential serum levels of the anaphylatoxin are between 40 and 90 μg/ml C3a ($0.45-1.0 \times 10^{-5}$M) and 3.3 to 9.3 μg/ml C5a ($3.0 - 8.5 \times 10^{-7}$M); however, these values should be viewed in terms of the biological activities these factors engender even in the nanomolar range (see Table 3).

Anaphylatoxin formation by complement proteases represents one of the most selective enzymatic scissions to be produced by any of the plasma proteases. The C3 or C5 convertases are not known to cleave any plasma protein substrate other than the complement components for which they are specific. In the human C3 molecule the larger alpha chain (110,000 m.w.) is cleaved between residue positions 77 and 78, and the smaller beta chain (75,000 m.w.) remains undisturbed. C3a may be released by either the C3 convertase (C4b, 2a complex) of the classical pathway or by the C3 convertase (C3b, Bb complex) of the alternative pathway depending on the mode of activation. However, functional essentiality of the C-terminal arginyl residue in C3a dictates that cleavage by either of these serum enzymes must occur at exactly the same site. The alpha chain of human C5 is cleaved in a very similar manner between residue positions 74 and 75. C5 is activated by the corresponding C5 convertases of the classical (C4b, 2a, 3b complex) and the alternative (C3b, Bb complex) pathways. A major difference between the C3 and C5 convertase systems is that C3 enzymes can function adequately in the fluid phase, whereas the C5 convertase acts almost exclusively from a surface attachment position. Furthermore, the rate and extent of anaphylatoxin formation is controlled by two simple mechanisms, one is the inherent lability of the self-associated enzyme complexes, and the other is the relatively low substrate turnover rate for the various convertases, particularly for the C5 convertase.

Once formed the anaphylatoxin is under the rigorous control of SCPB. Human SCPB is a large protein of 280,000 m.w. composed of four subunits. Levels of SCPB activity vary slightly among animal sources with pig and rat having considerably higher levels and cow and rabbit lower levels than man. Presumably no other protease in serum acts on the anaphylatoxins, because after long-term contact of the purified factors with whole serum, only arginine can be detected in the digest and both $C3a_{des\ Arg}$ and $C5a_{des\ Arg}$ have been isolated in good yields from complement-activated serum. Therefore, the catabolic end-products of anaphylatoxins in blood are believed to be $C3a_{des\ Arg}$ and $C5a_{des\ Arg}$. Interestingly, the specificity of SCPB is directed more toward C-lysl groups than to arginine, nonetheless, normal levels of SCPB in serum are sufficient to render either human anaphylatoxin spasmogenically harmless in 3 to 6 seconds. Understandably, C3a is inactivated more rapidly than C5a, presumably because the C-terminal dipeptide sequence is Ala-Arg in C3a and Gly-Arg in C5a, and it is well known that a penultimate alanyl residue is kinetically preferred to a glycyl residue for digestion by pancreatic carboxypeptidase B (62). SCPB is a metallo-enzyme, much like pancreatic carboxypeptidase, and contains Zn^{++} as the metal ion co-factor. Substitution of Co^{++} for Zn^{++} in the pancreatic carboxypeptidase only increases the turnover number for hippuryl-L-arginine by two-fold (63), while cobalt activation of SCPB appears much more pronounced and increases activity by nearly six-fold (64). Since SCPB removes C-terminal arginine from bradykinin much more slowly than from the anaphylatoxins, the predominant physiological role of this enzyme must be to keep the spasmogen activity of C3a and C5a in check rather than to control the kinins as has previously been suggested.

Characteristics

In addition to low molecular weight, the anaphylatoxins have several other distinguishing features that set them apart from any other factor in plasma. These molecules are perhaps the most cationic polypeptides of their size range to be found in plasma, particularly the human C3a molecule, with its pI of about 9.5, which is comparable to that of the lysine-rich histones. The isoelectric pH condition for human C5a is approximately pH 8.6, as judged by its failure to migrate significantly during electrophoresis on cellulose acetate strips at that pH. Although C5a contains a sizeable oligosaccharide unit in contrast to other mammalian C5a molecules, the net charge of both human and porcine C5a, for instance, are surprisingly similar. In addition, both C3a and C5a are remarkably heat-stable structures that resist functional inactivation up to 80°C and become denatured only slowly at 100°C. For example, after boiling for 15 minutes, human C3a loses only half of its biological activity, but C5a seems to be thermally inactivated somewhat more rapidly. However, the functional loss induced by heating is irreversible for both factors.

Insensitivity to acidic or alkaline conditions is another feature indicating the unique stability of the anaphylatoxins. Neither structure is functionally affected by extremes of pH from 1 to 13 at 4°C; although sizeable conformational effects can be detected by circular dichroism (CD) as the pH varies. These effects are entirely reversible, and in fact, the structural integrity of anaphylatoxins is a self-determined and reversible characteristic of these molecules. Their conformations may be dramatically altered by a variety of treatments other than heating, resulting in partial or total loss of function, but when the denaturant is removed, both structure and function are restored. Reversible folding of denaturated C3a or C5a occurs rapidly and is believed to be enhanced by reformation of helical regions estimated to involve the particpation of 40 to 45% of the total residues in each structure. The shapes of the CD spectra for C3a and C5a suggest that a major portion of the polypeptide chain assumes an alpha helical arrangement (65,66). Reductive scission of the three disulfide bonds found in each polypeptide produces major changes in the CD spectra indicating these disulfide linkages tend to reinforce and stabilize the existing helical structure. In view of the combination of helical structure and multiple internal disulfide bonds, the folded molecule apparently assumes a very compact form.

Chemical Nature

Since we reported the complete amino acid sequence of human C3a (23) in 1975, structures of human C5a and two other C3a molecules, each purified from animal sources, have been elucidated giving us a unique investigative opportunity. By comparing the sequences of these molecules, we have begun to unravel the many mysteries of these special structures. A summary of the accummulated sequence data is presented in Fig. 4, where each sequence is compared to human C3a as the reference primary structure. Such a comparison graphically illustrates features common to both C3a and C5a, and the sizeable number of identities substantiate their genetic relatedness. For instance, 17 of a total of 78 positions are identical in all four structures examined, given that the alignments shown were arbitrarily assigned. Of these numerous identities, many must represent residues that contribute in some essential way to either the structure and/or function of the anaphylatoxins thus explaining their immutability. This contention seems especially true of specific residues known to participate actively in the secondary folding of the molecule, as in the case of half-cystine residues that form an ordered array of intrachain disulfide linkages. Conservation of the six half-cystine positions strongly implicates these residues as integral elements for maintaining structural integrity of the native anaphylatoxin molecules. Presently, reasons for other identities are less clear, and their involvement can not be explained without further information concerning the three dimensional conformations of both C3a and C5a. However, the rigorous conservation of a glycyl residue, as at position 25 or 44, suggests that the polypeptide backbone is forced into a sharp turn that accomodates only a glycyl residue, which characteristically lacks a bulky side chain. It is known the polypeptide chain must fold back upon itself in the regions of sequence that contain the conserved glycines, because disulfide linkages between nearby half-cystines dictate such a turn. Note the location of the two glycyl residues in the diagrammatic model of C5a that is portrayed in Fig. 5. Arrangement of the disulfide bonds are not yet assigned in either C3a or C5a, however it is known that three bonds interconnect all six half-cystines.

Six of the 17 conserved residues possess hydrophobic side chains and may be relatively resistant to substitution, because their side chains may constitute an internal hydrophobic domain as previously illustrated for many globular proteins (67). Yet, residues that assume a surface disposition in water-soluble globular protein are more often replaced without affecting molecular function than are their internalized counterparts (68). This empirical rule is particularly true for the anaphylatoxins, since only three polar arginine residues, one already known to be functionally essential, are conserved in the four structures thus far determined.

Chemical features also distinguish the three C3a molecules from one another. Human and porcine C3a differ at 24 residue positions, and all but 6 of these differences are genetically conservative replacements. Human and rat C3a differ at 26 sites and the rat molecule is composed of 78 instead of the 77 residues that consitute the human and porcine C3a polypeptide chains. The increased length of rat C3a results from insertion of an aspartyl residue between assigned positions 16 and 17 in the reference human molecule. Significantly, the sequence adjacent to the essential C-terminal arginine, positions 73 to 77, has remained homologous in all three structures. An oligopeptide, Leu-Gly-Leu-Ala-Arg, was synthesized that mimics the common C-terminal portion of C3a and this fragment alone exhibits all the activities of an anaphylatoxin (See section V), presumably explaining why this region of C3a has been so rigorously conserved among species.

In human C5a only 28 of the 74 residues share identities with corresponding positions in the

```
                                1                                          10
I.    Human C3a       NH2-SER-VAL-GLN-LEU-THR-GLU-LYS-ARG-MET-ASN-LYS-VAL-GLY-LYS-TYR-PRO-( )-LYS-GLU-LEU-
II.   Porcine C3a         —— —— —— —— MET —— —— —— —— —— —— LEU —— GLN —— SER-( ) —— —— ——
III.  Rat C3a             —— —— —— —— MET —— ARG —— —— ASP —— ALA —— GLN —— THR-ASP —— GLY ——
                                        1                                  10
IV.   Human C5a                   NH2-THR —— GLN-LYS —— ILE-GLU-GLU-ILE-ALA-ALA —— —— LYS-HIS-SER-VAL-VAL-

                          20                                     30
I.                        ARG-LYS-CYS-CYS-GLU-ASP-GLY-MET-ARG-GLN-ASN-PRO-MET-ARG-PHE-SER-CYS-GLN-ARG-ARG-
II.                       —— ARG —— —— —— HIS —— —— —— ASN —— —— —— LYS —— —— —— —— —— ——
III.                      —— —— —— —— —— —— —— —— —— ASP-ILE —— —— LYS-TYR —— —— —— —— ——
                                                                     30
IV.                       LYS —— —— —— TYR —— —— ALA-CYS-VAL —— ASN-ASP-GLU-( )-THR —— GLU-GLN ——

                          40                                     50
I.                        THR-ARG-PHE-ILE-SER-LEU-GLY-GLU-ALA-CYS-LYS-LYS-VAL-PHE-LEU-ASP-CYS-CYS-ASN-TYR-
II.                       ALA-GLN —— —— HIS-GLN —— ASN —— —— VAL —— ALA —— —— ASN —— —— GLU ——
III.                      ALA —— LEU —— THR-GLN —— —— SER —— —— LEU-ALA —— MET —— —— —— —— ——
                                  40                                     50
IV.                       ALA-ALA-ARG —— —— —— —— PRO-ARG —— ILE —— ALA —— THR-GLU —— —— VAL-VAL-

                          60                                     70                                  77
I.                        ILE-THR-GLU-LEU-ARG-ARG-GLN-HIS-ALA-ARG-ALA-SER-HIS-(      )-LEU-GLY-LEU-ALA-ARG-CO2H
II.                       —— ALA-LYS —— —— GLN —— —— SER —— ASN-LYS-PRO-(      ) —— —— —— —— ——
III.                      —— —— LYS —— —— GLU —— —— ARG —— ASP-HIS-VAL-(      ) —— —— —— —— ——
                                  60                                           70                74
IV.                       ALA-SER-GLN —— —— (          ) —— ASN-ILE —— —— LYS-ASP-MET-GLN —— GLY ——
                                                            |
                                                          (CHO)
```

Figure 4. Comparison of the primary structures of human, porcine and rat C3a with human C5a.

Open spaces indicate identity with the human C3a sequence. Rat C3a contains an extra aspartic acid residue located between positions 16 and 17 of the reference human sequence. Alignment of the human C5a structure requires an indentation of two residues at the NH_2-terminus and several gaps to maximize the homology. Note that 17 positions were identical in all four sequences with a particularly unique feature being that six half-cystine positions were conserved. The single oligosaccharide unit of C5a is attached to Asn 64 as indicated. The amino acid sequence of rat C3a was recently reported, being a molecule that shares 65% homology with human C3a (J.W. Jacobs, et al., Purification, Characterization, and Amino Acid Sequence of Rat Anaphylatoxin (C3a). Biochemistry 17, 5031 (1978).

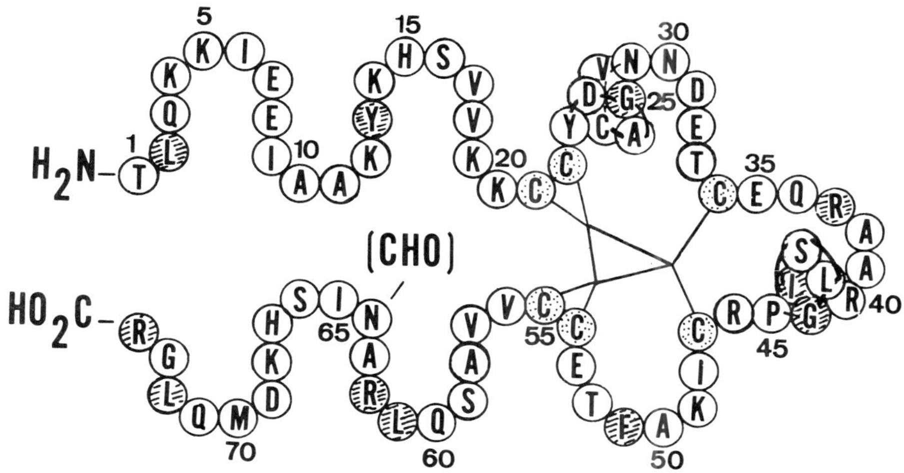

Figure 5. A schematic representation of the human C5a molecule was designed to illustrate several features of the secondary structure. Portions of the NH_2- and COOH terminal regions are believed to assume alpha helical conformation. The exact disulfide bonding arrangement is unknown, but it is certain that three distinct loops are formed of the polypeptide backbone. Conservation of glycyl residues at positions 25 and 44 suggest structural constraints may exist that will not permit the presence of a bulky side chain. Shaded residue positions identify the 17 locations that are conserved between all C3a and C5a molecules whose structures are known. Amino acids are designated by the one-letter abbreviation proposed by Dayhoff (Atlas of Protein Sequence and Structure Suppl. I, Vol 5, 5-10 (1973)).

human C3a sequence, and indentions, deletions and insertions are all manipulations required to maximize the degree of similarity between these two polypeptide chains. Three marked differences are evident between the C3a and C5a structures: 1) The odd number of seven half-cystine residues in C5a compared to six in C3a with no role yet assigned to the unpaired half-cystine. 2) The chemical deviation in sequence near the essential C-terminal arginine in C3a and C5a that is largely responsible for the characteristic individuality of the two molecules' expression of spasmogenic activity; 3) The most obvious difference is the presence of a large oligosaccharide, a complex carbohydrate of approximately 3,000 daltons with 3 to 4 mannose, 2 galactose, 3-4 glucosamine, and 3 sialic acid residues, attached to the side chain of an asparaginyl at position 64 in human C5a (see Fig. 5).

V. APPROACHES TO STRUCTURE-FUNCTION RELATIONSHIPS

The C-terminal arginyl residue of C3a is essential for all known functional activities of the molecule, and the enzymatic removal of this residue abrogates all such activity (27). Recently, the similar dependence of C5a was demonstrated in that a C-terminal arginyl residue is also essential for the expression of spasmogenic activity by human C5a (29). However, the unique ability of C5a to induce PMN migration is only reduced, not abrogated, by removing the C-terminal residue (34). These few facts serve as a basis for our examination of the C-terminal regions of both

C3a and C5a as possible active centers of the anaphylatoxins. Both molecules must maintain their native conformations to express maximal activity; any disruption of this native form causes major losses in activity. Reduced and carboxymethylated derivatives of intact C3a or C5a are less than 5% as active as their respective native forms. These alkylated derivatives, while nearly inactive, each retain residual alpha helical structure, implying that scission of disulfide bridges alone seriously affects the functional capabilities of the polypeptides. Unfolding induced by a combination of either guanidium chloride or urea and a reducing agent such as mercaptoethanol, seems to convert the polypeptides to a random state, as judged by CD measurements, yet both activity and the original conformations are recovered when the denaturants are removed. Such reversibility is not remarkable for structural polypeptides with highly ordered structures, but the unusual quality is that these molecules are but fragments of much larger proteins that are themselves readily and irreversibly denatured.

Relationships in Structure, Genetics and Evolution

Limited evidence now suggests that the C3a and C5a molecules may share highly similar conformations. Much of the linear structure is folded in an alpha helical arrangement, as interpreted from CD spectra, and the six common half-cystines are believed to be paired identically and to form three intrachain disulfide linkages. Given these assumptions, and the homologous positions held by 36% of the residues in human C3a and C5a, one might predict that the native folded polypeptides assume very similar forms.

Structural studies have quite firmly established the genetic relationship between C3a and C5a, undoubtedly arising from their apparently common ancestry. Interestingly, the anaphylatoxinogens C3 and C5 do not seem to be genetically linked in higher mammals, nor is there convincing evidence that even their cellular sites of synthesis are shared (69). This incongruence presumably reflects the dilemma of interpreting a genetic process long after gene duplication has occurred. Fortunately, the structural data provide more telling evidence regarding the divergence of anaphylatoxin molecules than do purely genetic approaches. For example, crude analysis using the limited assemblage of chemical structures presently available places the event of gene duplication at or before the reptilian era, as illustrated in Fig 6. From such computations, a working hypothesis should develop eventually that will delineate the evolution of the entire complement system.

Synthetic C3a Peptides

In the two years since selected peptides that mimic C3a function were first synthesized much has been learned regarding specific structural requirements of these anaphylatoxin analogs and their relationships to intact C3a. Originally, an octapeptide, Ala-Ser-His-Leu-Gly-Leu-Ala-Arg or C3a 70-77,* which corresponds exactly to the C-terminal sequence of human C3a, was examined and proved to express the same activities as the native molecule (32), although the synthetic octapeptide is only 1-2% as potent as intact C3a. The most dramatic statement that can be made concerning synthetic C3a 70-77 is that the "active site" of C3a is most certainly represented by this limited portion of the primary C3a structure. From the synthesis of additional model C3a peptides we now know that both activity and specificity of the parent molecule are localized in and controlled by a very short C-terminal portion of the polypeptide chain.

We have directed a series of studies toward establishing the effect of peptide length on biological activity (71). Our results indicate that each active peptide can cause contraction of guinea

---

* C3a 70-77 is an abbreviation used for identifying the synthetic oligopeptides as analogs of C3a or C5a structure. The numbers identify portions of the natural sequence that are being duplicated in the synthetic fragment.

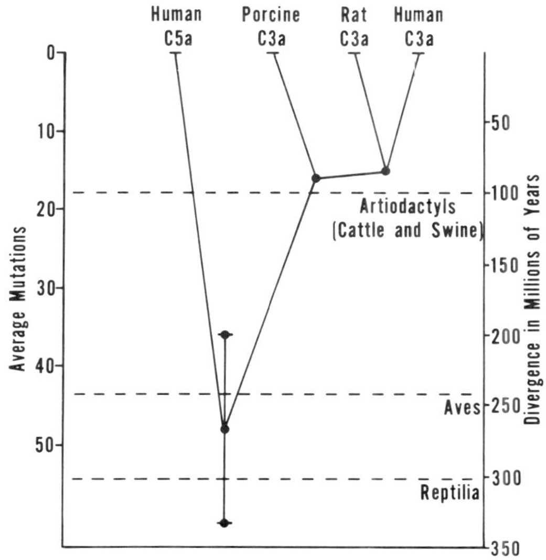

Figure 6. A phylogentic tree was constructed according to the methods described by Fitch and Margoliash (70). Construction of protein difference matrices used in developing the diagram shown above were produced employing the minimal mutational difference (MMD) method. Further estimates of the C3a/C5a gene duplication event range between 200 million years using the amino acid difference method to 335 million years using the random evolutionary hits (REH) methodology.

pig ileal or uterine muscles, induce release of vasoamines from rat mast cells, and increase vascular permeability when injected into either human or guinea pig skin. However, routine evaluations of peptide activity involve observing only the contraction of guinea pig ileal strips and enhanced vascular permeability in guinea pig or human skin as indicators of their functional capability. Relative capacities for inducing smooth muscle contraction of several C3a analog peptides that are from 4 to 13 residues in length are summarized in Fig. 7A. The 13 residue peptide (C3a 65-77) is no more active than the octapeptide C3a 70-77; therefore, elongation apparently contributes little information to that stored in the shorter C-terminal octapeptide. Shortening the synthetic oligopeptide to below 8 residues, however, leads to an immediately measurable reduction in activity. The heptapeptide (C3a 71-77) is only slightly less active, whereas the hexapeptide (C3a 72-77) is approximately 50% less active, than the octapeptide. Activity diminishes further in the pentapeptide (C3a 73-77) as in the tetrapeptide (C3a 74-77), which is 100-fold less active than the pentapeptide. The tripeptide's (C3a 75-77) activity is not detectable. Hence although a major break in the activity curve occurs at the 4 to 5 residue level, even the tetra-and pentapeptide forms of synthetic C3a can desensitize the smooth muscle so that it does not respond to native C3a, proving that both selectivity and specificity remain intact. Skin sensitivity to the injected peptides parallels the smooth muscle response; however, the difference in activity between the pentapeptide and the tetrapeptide appears to be less *in vivo* than is observed *in vitro* (Fig. 7B).

Modification of the synthetic C3a peptides has provided additional information concerning the structural requirements of the "active site" portion of C3a. For instance, when the free carboxyl group of the C-terminal arginine is converted to an amide or a methyl ester, activity is

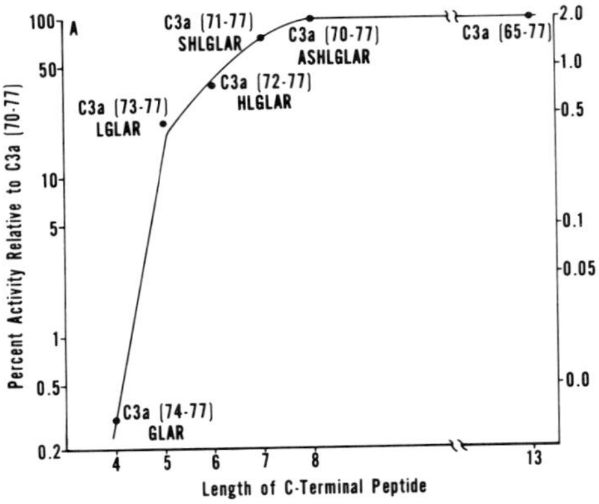

Figure 7A. Relative activities of synthetic C3a peptides of various lengths are shown. The biological assay employed here was the contractile response of a guinea pig ileal strip. Octapeptide C3a 70-77, ASHLGLAR, was approximately 300-fold more active than was the tetrapeptide C3a 74-77 with the peptapeptide (C3a 73-77), hexapeptide (C3a 72-77) and heptapeptide (C3a 71-77) each exhibiting only slightly less activity than the octapeptide for eliciting a contraction of the ileum. All peptides shown were capable of desensitizing the muscle to native C3a proving a specificity of the interaction.

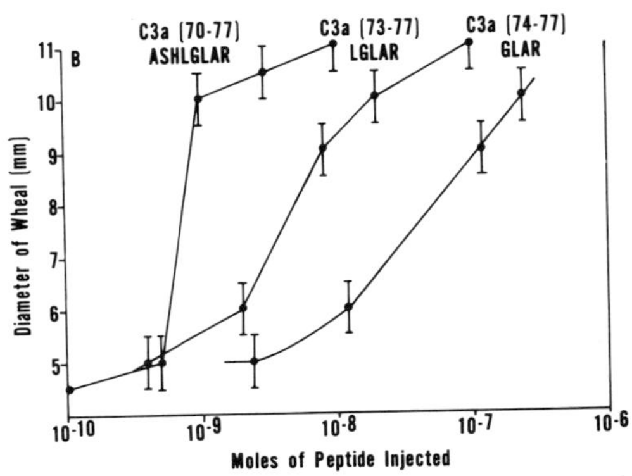

Figure 7B. An estimate of the biological activity of synthetic C3a peptides *in vivo* is obtained by intradermal injection. Development of a wheal and erythema at the site of injection signifies induced vascular changes and histamine release. Dose dependence of the synthetic peptides for producing a visible wheal indicate relative activities are consistent with the in vitro responses on the isolated ileum. The cutaneous response to octapeptide is approximately 2 percent of that observed for the native C3a on a mole per mole basis.

markedly reduced. Attachment of a glycyl residue to the C-terminal carboxyl group of the synthetic peptides reduces activity considerably; that is, C3a 70-77 is 100-fold more active than C3a 70-77 glycine (32). These results suggest that the carboxyl group of the terminal arginine is somehow directly involved in C3a function. Substitution of the C-terminal arginine with another basic residue such as lysine eliminates all activity of the synthetic peptides which seems to indicate that the positively charged guanidino group is essential; consequently, not just any formal positively charged side chain can act as a viable replacement.

The amino-terminal end of the synthetic C3a peptides proved much less sensitive to modification than the carboxyl end. N-acetylation of either the pentapeptide or the octapeptide had little effect on their respective activities, and substitution in the octapeptide (i.e. Ala-Ala-Ala-Leu-Gly-Leu-Ala Arg) of Ser 71 or His 72 with an alanyl residue did not alter overt biological activity. Since the positions corresponding to 70, 71 and 72 in human C3a are occupied by dissimilar residues in rat and porcine C3a, it is not surprising that replacement at these residue positions had little effect on the function of the resultant synthetic peptides. The core of the C3a active site unquestionably seems to be the C-terminal region represented by Leu-Gly-Leu-Ala-Arg, a sequence that has remained unchanged in all C3a structures studied to date.

Synthetic C5a peptides

Unlike the C3a studies, C5a synthetic peptides used as an approach toward elucidating C5a structure-function relationships have not provided results that are easily interpretable. First, the synthetic C-terminal pentapeptide analog of C5a, C5a 70-74, exhibits neither spasmogenic nor chemotactic activity at molar levels 1000-fold higher than correspond to maximal activity levels for the native factor. These results alone illustrate the extent of the dissimilarity between receptor interactions for C3a and C5a, since a 100-fold molar excess of the C3a peptapeptide is spasminogenically active. Second, the two anaphylatoxins are known to interact with individual populations of receptors, but we must now conclude that each factor pursues a unique mode for this interaction. The fact that $C5a_{des\ Arg}$ retains activity as a chemotaxin proves that the C-terminal arginine of C5a is less influential in exciting cellular migration than for promoting spasmogenic activity. However, the third difference from the prior model, was the surprising total absence of any spasmogenic activity exhibited by the synthetic C-terminal peptide of C5a (C5a 70-74). Fourth, the synthetic pentapeptide also fails to desensitize smooth muscle toward native C5a, further evidence of its inability to interact adequately with the C5a receptor.

Since N-formylated peptides have been shown to possess potent chemotactic abilities (72), we formylated the synthetic C5a pentapeptide (N-f-Met-Gln-Leu-Gly-Arg) and re-examined its biological properties. The formylated synthetic peptide remained inactive as a spasmogen, but exhibited chemotactic activity for human neutrophils ($ED_{50} = 3.2 \times 10^{-4}M$) and induced β-glucuronidase release from cytochalasin-B treated neutrophils ($ED_{50} = 3.3 \times 10^{-4}M$). Removal of the C-terminal arginine to produce N-f-Met-Gln-Leu-Gly yielded a tetrapeptide that was surprisingly even more active than the parent pentapeptide (chemotaxis $ED_{50} = 3.3 \times 10^{-5}M$ and enzyme release $ED50 = 5.1 \times 10^{-5}M$). However, in further studies of specificity, the formylated C5a fragments seemed to interact only with receptors specific for N-formylmethionyl peptides and not for C5a (73). In summary then, our studies with synthetic C5a peptides show that their behavior is quite different from that of the C3a analogs. Unlike C3a, C5a does not seem to have a short sequence at the C-terminus with sufficient structural information to trigger a cellular response.

Several other novel features of the human C5a molecule also demand further examination. For instance, what role does the rather bulky oligosaccharide group play in C5a function? Neither C3a nor animal C5a molecules contain significant carbohydrate, yet animal C5a seems to function as well as does human C5a. What is the reason for the odd half-cystine that is disulfide linked to a free cysteine in C5a obtained from human plasma (74)? Purified C5a can be freed of this covalently attached cysteine by reduction and air oxidation, but the product thus obtained is equally as active as the original material. Although the synthetic pentapeptide Met-Gln-Leu-Gly-Arg is inactive as a chemotaxin, enzymatic removal of these same five residues from native C5a entirely destroys its chemotactic activity (45). Therefore, the C-terminal primary structure of C5a as in C3a, must play a significant role in the expression of biological activity, but the latter picture is obviously more complicated and will obviously require further interpretation.

VI. CONCLUSION

In essence, current advances in anaphylatoxin chemistry have ushered in a new era of investigation for this aspect of plasma protein research. Human mediators derived from plasma components promise to play a major role in host defense mechanisms, although the exact import of such factors as C3a and C5a are yet to be accurately and specifically defined. Major advances in our understanding of the chemical nature of these complement fragments has permitted the active site of C3a to be localized to the C-terminal pentapeptide (LGLAR) and recent work implies a similar functional role for the C-terminal region of C5a. Duality of function by C5a, acting both as a spasmogen and a chemotaxin, points up the wide diversity of biological actions mediated by the serum anaphylatoxins. As more detail is accummulated concerning interactions between C3a or C5a and a variety of target cells, it becomes clear that highly specific receptors exist on responsive cells and that physical binding precedes mediator-induced release or other stimulated cellular activities. Cellular recruitment by chemotaxins is undoubtedly a means of enhancing the organism's systemic responsiveness to foreign invaders and as such represents a possible amplification mechanism for cellular sequestration. Amplification may occur, as the feedback loop for PMNs in Fig. 1 suggests, when stimulated cells release proteases capable of converting complement components to release anaphylatoxins and hence generate additional chemotaxin. These hypotheses form the basis for future studies that will ultimately answer lingering questions concerning the rightful role of anaphylatoxins in normal physiological events.

ACKNOWLEDGEMENTS

The author wishes to thank Mrs. Phyllis Minick and Mrs. Andrea Rothman for their able editorial assistance. I also wish to recognize the assistance of Miss Holly Wimer in preparing the final manuscript. The author is supported by Grant HL 20220 from the U.S. Public Health Service and by Program Project Grant HL 16411, both grants are awards from the National Heart and Lung Institute. Pub. # 1671

REFERENCES

1. Reid, K.B.M, Isolation, by partial pepsin digestion, of the three collagen-like regions present in subcomponent C1q of the first component, Biochem. J. 155, 5 (1976).

2. Reid, K.B.M. and Porter, R.R., Subunit composition and structure of subcomponent C1q of the first component of human complement, Biochem. J. 155, 19 (1976).

3. Tack, B.F. and Prahl, J.W., Third component of human complement: Purification from plasma and physicochemical characterization, Biochemistry 15, 4513 (1976).

4. Bolotin, C., Morris, S., Tack, B. and Prahl, J.W., Purification and structural analysis of the fourth component of human complement, Biochemistry 16 2008 (1976).

5. Tack, B.F., Morris, S.C. and Prahl, J.W., The purification and physicochemical characterization of human C5, Fed. Amer. Soc. Exp. Biol. 35, 494 (Abst. 1594) (1976).

6. Fehr, J., Complement as a mediator of granulocyte adherence and margination: Studies based on the acute neutropenia of filtration leukapheresis. In T.J. Greenwalt and G.A. Jamieson, (eds). The Granulocyte: Function and Clinical Utilization. Liss, New York, p 243,1977.

7. Nusbacher, J., Rosenfeld, S.I., Mac Pherson, J.L., Thiem, P.A. and Leddy, J. P., Nylon Fiber Leukapheresis: Associated complement component changes and granulocyteopenia, Blood, 51 359 (1978).

8. Craddock, P., Fehr, J., Dalmasso, A., Brigham, K. and Jacob, H., Hemodialysis leukopenia: Pulmonary vascular leukostasis resulting from complement activation by dialyzer cellophane membranes, J. Clin, Invest. 59, 879 (1977).

9. O'Flaherty, J.T., Showell, H. and Ward, P.A., Neutropenia induced by systemic infusion of chemotactic factors, J. Immunol. 118, 1586 (1977).

10. Craddock, P., Fehr, J., Brigham, K., Kronenberg, R. and Jacob, H., Complement and leukocyte mediated pulmonary dysfunction in hemodialysis, New Engl. J. Med. 296, 769 (1977).

11. Friedberger, E., Weitere Untersuchungen uber Einweissanaphylaxie. IV. Mitteilung, Z. ImmununForsch 4, 636 (1910).

12. Friedberger, E., Die Anaphylaxie mit besonderer Berucksichtigung ihrer Bedeutung für Infektion und Immunität Dtsch. Med. Wsch. 37, 481 (1911)

13. Bordet, J., Le Mecanisme de L' anaphylaxie, C.R. Soc. Biol., Paris 74, 225 (1913).

14. Nathan, E., Ueber Anaphylatoxin bildung durch Agar Z. Immun Forsch 17, 478 (1913).

15. Dale, H.H., The anaphylactic reaction of plain muscle in the guinea pig. J. Pharmacol Exp. Ther. 4, 167 (1913).

16. Dale, H.H., Croonian lecture: The biological significance of anaphylaxis, Proc. Roy. Soc. (B) 91, 126 (1920).

17. Rocha e Silva, M., Concerning the mechanisms of anaphylaxis and allergy, Brit. med. J., i, 779 (1952).

18. Rocha e Silva, M., Aronson, M., and Bier, O.G., Histamine release by anaphylatoxin Nature, 168, 465 (1951).

19. Hahn, F. and Oberdorf. A., Anti histaminica and anaphylaktoide reaktionen, Z. Immun Forsch. 107, 528 (1950).

20. Rocha e Silva, M. and Aronson, M., Histamine release from the perfused lung of the guinea pig by serotoxin (anaphylatoxin). Exp. Path. 33, 577 (1952).

21. Osler, A.G., Randall, H.G., Hill, B.M. and Ovary, Z., Studies on the mechanisms of hypersensitivity phenomena III. The participation of complement in thr formation of anaphylatoxin, J. Exp. Med. 110, 311 (1959).

22. Jensen, J.A., Anaphylatoxin in its relation to the complement system, Science 155, 1122 (1967).

23. Dias da Silva, W., Eisele, J.W. and Lepow, I.H., Complement as a mediator of inflammation. III Purification of the activity with anaphyatoxin properties generated by interaction of the first four components of complement and its identification as a cleavage product of C'3, J. Exp. Med. 126, 1027 (1967).

24. Cochrane, C.G. and Müller-Eberhard, H.J., The derivation of two distinct anaphylatoxin activities from the third and fifth components of human complement, J. Exp. Med. 127, 371 (1968).

25. Shin, H.S., Snyderman, R., Friedman, E., Mellors, A. and Mayer, M.M., Chemotactic and anaphylatoxic fragment cleaved from the fifth component of guinea pig complement, Science 162, 361 (1968).

26. Lepow, I.H., Dias da Silva, W. and Patrick, R.A., Biologically active cleavage products of components of complement. In Cellular and Humoral Mechanisms in Anaphylaxis and Allergy, H. Movat (eds), S. Karger, Basel p. 237 (1969).

27. Bokisch, V.A., Müller-Eberhard, H.J. and Cochrane, C.G., Isolation of fragment (C3a) of the third component of human complement containing anaphylatoxin and chemotactic activity and description of an anaphylatoxin inactivator of human serum, J. Exp. Med.129, 1109 (1969).

28. Budzko, D.B., Bokisch, V.A. and Müller-Eberhard, H.J., A fragment of the third component of human complement with anaphylatoxin activity. Biochemistry 10, 1166 (1971).

29. Vallota, E.H. and Müller-Eberhard, H.J., Formation of C3a and C5a anaphylatoxins in whole human serum after inhibition of the anaphylatoxin inactivator, J. Exp. Med. 137, 1109 (1973).

30. Hugli, T.E., Human anaphylatoxin (C3a) from the third component of complement, J. Biol. Chem. 250, 8293 (1975).

31. Fernandez, H.N. and Hugli, T.E., Partial characterization of human C5a anaphylatoxin, I. Chemical description of the carbohydrate and polypeptide portion of human C5a, J. Immunol. 117, 1688 (1976).

32. Hugli, T.E. and Erickson, B.W., Synthetic peptides with the biological activities and specificity of human C3a anaphylatoxin. Proc. Natl. Acad. Sci. USA 74, 1826 (1977).

33. Fernandez, H.N. and Hugli, T.E., Chemical evidence for common genetic ancestry of complement components C3 and C5 J. Biol. Chem. 252, 1826 (1977).

34. Fernandez, H.N., Henson, P.M., Otani, A. and Hugli, T.E., Chemotactic response to human C3a and C5a anaphylatoxins. I. Evaluation of C3a and C5a leukotaxis in vitro and under simulated in vivo conditions, J. Immunol. 120, 109 (1978).

35. Fernandez, H.N. and Hugli, T.E., Primary structural analysis of the polypeptide portion of human C5a, J. Biol. Chem. 253, 6955 (1978).

36. Chenoweth, D.E. and Hugli, T.E., Demonstration of specific C5a receptor on intact human polymorphonuclear leukocytes, Proc. Natl. Acad. Sci. USA 75, 3943 (1978).

37. Jensen, J.A., Snyderman, R. and Mergenhagen, S.E., Chemotactic activity of guinea pig C'5-anaphylatoxin. In Cellular and Humoral Mechanisms in Anaphylaxis and Allergy, H.Z. Movat (eds). Karger, Basel p 265 (1969).

38. Ward, P.A. and Newman, L.J. A neutrophil chemotactic factor from human C5. J. Immunol. 102, 93 (1969).

39. Ward, P.A., A plasmin-split fragment of C'3 as a new chemotactic factor, J. Exp. Med. 126, 189 (1967).

40. Ward, P.A. and Hill, J.H., C5 chemotactic fragments produced by an enzyme in lysosomal granules of neutrophils, J. Immunol. 104, 535 (1970).

41. Berenberg, J.L. and Ward, P.A., The chemotactic factor inactivator in normal human serum, J. Clin. Invest. 52, 1200 (1973).

42. Ward, P.A., Kreutzer, D.L., Jones, M.L. and Brozna, J.P., Biology of the chemotactic factor inactivator, In Clinical Aspects of the Complement System, W. Opferkuch, K. Rother and D.R. Schultz (eds), Georg Thieme-Pub., Stuttgart, p 145 (1978).

43. Romualdez, A.G. Jr. and Ward, P.A., A unique complement derived chemotactic factor for tumor cells, Proc. Natl. Acad. Sci. USA, 72, 4128 (1975).

44. Chenoweth, D.E., Rowe, J.G. and Hugli, T.E., A modified method for chemotaxis under agarose, J. Immunol. Methods (1978) in press.

45. Chenoweth, D.E. and Hugli, T.E., Chemotactic response to human C3a and C5a anaphylatoxins. II. Assessment by a modified chemotaxis under agarose method, J. Immunol. in press.

46. Snyderman, R. and Meadows, L., Chemotaxis and the complement system: Methodology to quantify a biological activity of complement in humans. In Clinical aspects of the complement system, W. Opferkuch, K. Rother, and D.R. Schultz, (eds), Georg Thieme Pubs., Stuttgart, p 42 (1978).

47. Alper, C.A., Propp, R.P., Klemperer, M.R., and Rosen, F.S., Inherited deficiency of the third component of human complement (C3). J. Clin. Invest. 48, 553 (1969).

48. Ballow, M., Shira, J.E., Harden, L., Yang, S.Y. and Day, N.B., Complete absence of the third component of complement in man, J. Clin. Invest. 56, 703 (1975).

49. Alper, C.A., Abramson, N., Johnston, R.B., Jandl, J.H. and Rosen, F.S., Increased susceptibility to infection associated with abnormalities of complement-mediated functions and of the third component of complement (C3). New Engl. J. Med. 282, 349 (1970).

50. Miller, M.E., Seals, J., Kaye, R., A Familial plasma-associated defect of phagocytosis a new cause of recurrent bacterial infections. Lancet 2, 60 (1968).

51. Miller, M.E. and Nilsson, U.R., A familial deficiency of the phagocytosis-enhancing activity of serum related to a dysfunction of the fifth component complement (C5). New Engl. J. Med. 282, 354, (1970).

52. Mathews, K., Personal Communication.

53. Ward, P.A. and Talamo, R.C., Deficiency of the chemotactic factor inactivator in human serum with α1-antitrypsin deficiency, J. Clin. Invest. 52, 516 (1973).

54. Kaplow, L.S. and Goffinet, J.A., Profound neutropenia during the early phase of hemodialysis JAMA, 203, 1135 (1968).

55. O'Flaherty, J.T., Craddock, P.R. and Jacob, H.S., Effect of intravascular complement activation on granulocyte adhesiveness and distribution, Blood, 51, 731 (1978).

56. Wright, D.G. and Gallin, J.I., A functional differentiation of human neutrophil granules: Generation of C5a by a specific (secondary) granule product and inactivation of C5a by azurophil (primary granule products), J. Immunol. 119, 1068 (1977).

57. Schiffer, C.A., Aisner, J., Betts, S.W. and Wiernik, P., Clinical experience with transfusion of granulocytes obtained by continuous flow filtration leukapheresis, Am. J. Med. 58, 373 (1975).

58. Hammerschmidt, D.E., Craddock, P.R., McCullough, J., Kronenberg, R.S., Dalmasso, A.P. and Jacob, H.S., Complement activation and pulmonary leukostasis during nylon fiber filtration leukapheresis, Blood 51, 721 (1978).

59. Ballow, M., Phylogenetics and ontogenetics of the complement systems. In Comprehensive Immunology 2, Good, R.A. and Day, S.B. (Series eds). Biological Amplification Systems in Immunology, N.K. Day and R.A. Good, (eds), Plenum Med. Book Co., New York, p 183 (1977).

60. Nilsson, U.R. and Müller-Eberhard, H.J., Efficiency of the fifth component of complement in mice with an inherited complement defect, J. Exp. Med. 125, 1 (1967).

61. Cinader, B., Dubiski, S. and Wardlaw, A.C., Distribution, inheritance and properties of an antigen, MUBI, and its relation to hemolytic complement, J. Exp. Med. 120, 897 (1964).

62. Folk, J.E. and Gladner, J.A., Carboxypeptidase B: I. Purification of the zymogen and specificity of the enzyme, J. Biol. Chem. 231, 379 (1958).

63. Folk, J.E., Carboxypeptidase B. In The Enzymes, P.D. Boyer, (eds), Academic Press, New York, Vol. III, p 57 (1971).

64. Erdös, E.G., Sloane, E.M. and Wohler, I.M., Carboxypeptidase in blood and other fluids. I. Properties, distribution, and partial purification of the enzyme, Biochem. Pharm. 13, 893 (1964).

65. Hugli, T.E., Morgan, W.T. and Müller-Eberhard, H.J., Circular dichroism of C3a anaphylatoxin, J. Biol. Chem. 250, 1479 (1975).

66. Morgan, W.T., Vallota, E.H. and Müller-Eberhard, H.J., Circular dichroism of C5a anaphylatoxin of porcine complement, Biochem. Biophys. Res. Commun. 57, 572 (1974).

67. Epstein, D.J., Non-randomness of amino acid changes in the evolution of homologous proteins, Nature 215, 355 (1967).

68. Perutz, M.F., Kendrew, J.C. and Watson, H.C., Structure and function of hemoglobin. II. Some relations between polypeptide chain configuration and amino acid sequence, J. Mol. Biol. 13, 669 (1965).

69. Colten, H.R., Biosynthesis of complement, In Advances in Immunology, F.J. Dixon and H.G. Kunkel, (eds), Academic Press, New York, vol. 22, p 67 (1976).

70. Fitch, W.M. and Margoliash, E., Construction of phylogenetic tree, Science 155, 279 (1967).

71. Caporale, L.H., Erickson, B.W. and Hugli, T.E., Synthetic oligopeptides from human C3a anaphylatoxin that mediate the inflammatory response. In Peptides - Proceedings of the Fifth American Peptide Symposium, M. Goodman, and J. Meienhofer (eds), John Wiley & Co. New York, p 225 (1977).

72. Schiffman, E., Corcoran, B.A. and Wahl, S.M., N-Formylmethionyl peptides as chemoattractants for leukocytes, Proc, Nat. Acad. Sci. USA 72, 1059 (1975).

73. Chenoweth, D.E., Erickson, B.W. and Hugli, T.E., Human C5a-related synthetic peptides as neutrophil chemotactic factors, Biochem. Biophys. Res. Commun. (1978), in press.

74. Fernandez, H.N., Blockage of an unpaired sulfhydryl group by cysteine in human C5a anaphylatoxin, Proc. Fed. Am. Soc. Exp. Biol. 37, 1495 (Abst. 1237) (1978).

ACTIVATION MECHANISM OF THE CLASSICAL PATHWAY OF COMPLEMENT

Rodney R. Porter
Department of Biochemistry, Oxford University,
South Parks Road, Oxford OX1 3QU, England

As the earlier speakers have discussed, complement is perhaps the most complex of the several activation systems in blood and its special role is the elimination of foreign substances from the body. Activation of the complement system may be due to interaction of an antibody in the blood with an antigen as in the classical pathway of activation, or there may be direct activation by the foreign cells or particles as in the alternative pathway (1). The initial steps in the latter are still not entirely clear, but in the classical pathway it has been established that, following aggregation of the antibody by reaction with antigen, the first component of complement (C1), a complex of 3 proteins (C1q, C1r and C1s), binds to the Fc part of the antibody. In so doing it is converted to an active protease which in turn activates the second (C2) and fourth component (C4). The activated components $C\overline{4}$ and $C\overline{2}$ form a complex enzyme, C3 convertase, which activates C3. This in turn associates with $C\overline{42}$ to give $C\overline{423}$ which is a C5 convertase and activates C5. This is the last proteolytic step in the pathway and C5 associates with C6, C7, C8 and C9 to form a lytic complex which causes lysis of cells, apparently non enzymically.

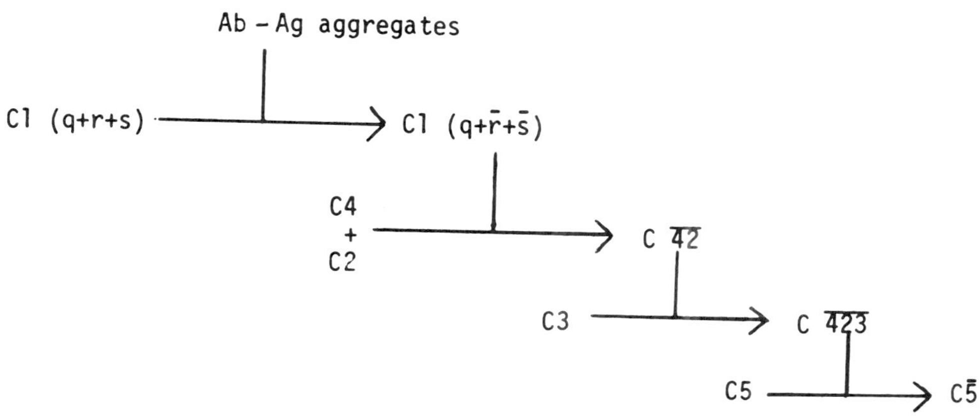

Fig. 1 Activation of the classical pathway by antibody-antigen (Ab-Ag) aggregates.

I wish to discuss the assembly and activation of the early components which occurs as shown in Fig. 1.

The nature of the antigen appears to be unimportant and binding and activation of the first component occurs whether the antibody is present as an aggregate with a soluble antigen or is bound on to a cell surface. It was uncertain however if a cell surface could play any role in subsequent activation steps as lysis of the cells at the final stage of complement activation clearly occurs at the cell membrane.

Binding and activation of complement by aggregated and cell bound antibody

A quantitative study has been made therefore of the relative effectiveness of aggregated and cell bound antibody in activating the early components (2). Rabbit IgG antiovalbumin precipitated with ovalbumin has been compared with rabbit IgG anti sheep red cell bound on to red cells. When the units of total complement destroyed in human serum by addition of antibody in either form was measured, aggregated and cell bound antibody behaved in a quantitatively similar manner. Destruction of added C4 by the bound $C\overline{1}$ was 50%-100% more, per given weight of antibody, for cell bound than aggreated antibody but this may be due only to the greater accessibility of antibody when spread on a cell surface rather than in aggregates. Similarly, when Clq and Cls binding per 1,000 molecules of antibody was measured using radioimmune assay the number of molecules bound was about 50% higher for cell bound than aggregated antibody. As expected, 2 Cls moles were bound per molecule of Clq as the active Cl complex has been shown to be formed from association of one Clr_2-Cls_2 tetrameric complex per molecules of Clq, the Clr_2-Cls_2 complex being dependent on the presence of Ca^{++}. Thus in agreement with previous work the binding and activation of Cl is likely to be a function only of the aggregated antibody however it is present in the serum.

When C4 binding was measured, 10-15 times more C4 molecules bound per 1,000 molecul of antibody to cell surface antibody than to antibody aggregates, suggesting that much of the C4 must be bound on the cell membrane. This was not unexpected as the binding of $C\overline{4}$ to the red cell surface had been reported earlier (3), but as total complement consumption per given weight of antibody is similar in both cases it suggested that most of the $C\overline{4}$ bound to the cell surface could not be effective in the lytic system. The only function of $C\overline{4}$ known, in the complement sequence, is in the formation of the complex enzyme, C3 convertase, $C\overline{42}$ with $C\overline{2}$. The formation of this enzyme was estimated therefore by measuring the rate of destruction of C3 by antibody antigen $C\overline{1}$ complexes when increasing amounts of $C\overline{4}$ were bound in the presence of excess C2. Figure 2 shows that maximal C3 convertase activity is reached when about 5%-10% of the total C4 is bound on the red cells and 50% of the total on aggregates, i.e. 50% of the $C\overline{4}$ bound is ineffective in the complement sequence with antibody aggregates and 95% with cell bound antibody giving 1.5 - 2 fold higher convertase activity per 1,000 molecules of antibody similar to the efficiency as measured by total complement consumption. This suggested that only half of the $C\overline{4}$ bound to antibody and probably none of the C4 on the cell surface could form the convertase. C4 activated by $C\overline{1}$ in solution has no haemolytic activity and rapid binding to antibody appears to be necessary to preserve activity. If so, with constant antibody and C4, effective C4 binding as measured by C3 convertase activity would be expected to be proportional to the $C\overline{1}$ on the antibody as a greater number of adjacent antibody binding sites would be available with increasing $C\overline{1}$ present. This proved to be correct (Fig. 3).

The antibody-C4 binding site could be on either the Fc or Fab portion or perhaps indirectly through the $C\overline{1}$ bound to the Fc part of the antibody. An attempt was made to measure this directly by splitting antibody aggregates, with $C\overline{1}$ and $C\overline{4}$ attached, with enzymes to give Fab and Fc fragments. However, conditions have not been found where this can be done without substantial splitting of the complement

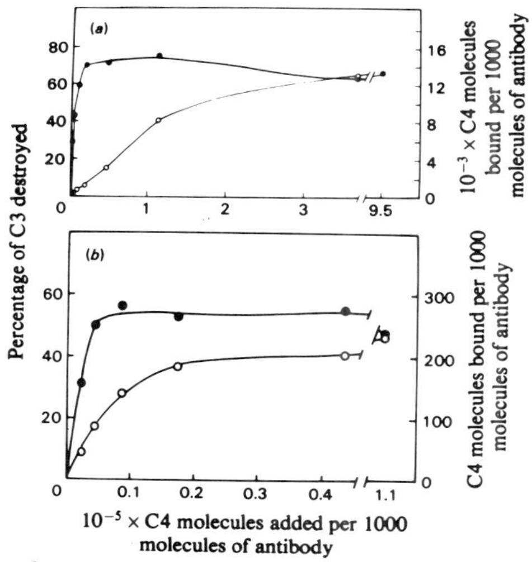

Fig. 2 *Comparison of the binding of C4 with the development of C3 convertase activity on antibody-coated erythrocytes (a) and on ovalbumin–anti-ovalbumin aggregates (b)* Samples of either 10^7 sensitized cells carrying 1.3×10^{12} IgG and 4.3×10^{11} $C\bar{1}s$ molecules or aggregates containing 14×10^{12} IgG and 11×10^{11} $C\bar{1}s$ molecules were incubated with various amounts of C4 for 30 min at 30°C. Samples were removed to measure bound C4 by specific radioimmunoassay. After a washing and addition of 5000 units of C2 for 15 min at 30°C to develop the C3 convertase ($C\bar{4}\bar{2}$), the samples were washed and incubated with 13 units of C3 for 30 min at 30°C. Finally, the cells or aggregates were separated by centrifugation and the residual C3 activity in the supernatant was determined by haemolytic assay. The percentage of C3 destroyed (●) and of C4 bound (○) is plotted versus the amount of C4 added to the samples.

components as well as of the antibody. An indirect approach was made of comparing C4 binding to antibody aggregates formed from interaction of antigen with either whole antibody or with 4:1 ratio of $(Fab')_2$ fragments and whole antibody. When the $C\bar{1}$ bound was the same in both cases, C4 binding was also the same and as the Fc was only 1/5th the amount in the mixed aggregates it is most probable that C4 binds to the Fab part of the antibody. Other experiments showed that the C4 bound increases with the amount of antibody present when C1 was kept constant and hence indirect binding to antibody through $C\bar{1}$ bound to the Fc portion is unlikely. Though no evidence is available it would be expected that if the C4 binds to the Fab portion of the antibody it is likely to be to the first constant domain, i.e. the C terminal halves of the light chain and Fd section of the heavy chain.

With earlier data, a picture can be build up of the assembly of the early complement components on the aggregated antibody (Fig. 4). It has been shown in several ways that Clq binds to the C_H2 comain, perhaps most directly by the demonstration that the $(Facb)_2$ fragment after precipitation with antigen will bind and activate C1 while $(Fab')_2$ will not and the only difference between the fragments is the presence of the C_H2 domain in $(Facb)_2$ and its absence in $(Fab')_2$ (4,5). Binding

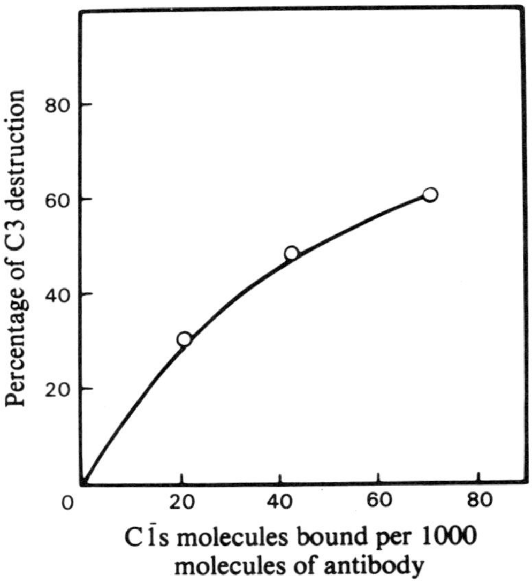

Fig. 3 *Development of C3 convertase activity by ovalbumin–anti-ovalbumin aggregates carrying increasing amounts of C$\bar{1}$ (measured as C$\bar{1}$s) but constant amounts of C4*

Samples of antibody aggregates (1.4μg of IgG) carrying increasing amounts of C$\bar{1}$ and constant amount of C4 (105 C4 molecules per 1000 IgG molecules) were incubated with 1 × 10^4 units of C2 for 15min at 30°C to generate C3 convertase activity (C$\overline{42}$). After a washing and incubation for 30min at 30°C with 5.4 units of C3, residual C3 in the supernatant was haemolytically titred.

is through the heads of the C1q molecules (6) and as, in excess C1q, 1 C1q molecule binds per 3-5 antibody molecules, cross-linking by the hexameric C1q to several antibody molecules is probable (2). Reid and colleagues (7) have shown that the collagenous tails of C1q (isolated after peptic digestion of C1q) will inhibit the binding of the C1r$_2$-C1s$_2$ tetramer to the C1q attached to antibody and hence it is probable that the tetramer is binding to C1q through the collagenous stems. The attachment and activation of C1 is efficient (95% or higher in excess antibody) in contrast to the activation and binding of C4 where only 5%-10% appears to take part in forming C3 convertase with cell bound antibody and 50% with aggregates (2). It is suggested as indicated in the diagram that this difference arises because C1 is bound first and then activated, while C4 (and presumably C2) are activated by the bound C$\bar{1}$ and then bind subsequently. Activated C$\bar{4}$ loses haemolytic activity rapidly possibly by reaction with the C4 binding protein and C3 INA (8) but is relatively stable when bound and hence the lower efficiency compared to C1 activation. C$\bar{2}$ is unstable in solution and when bound but the structural basis for the instability is not yet clear. It is suggested that some C$\bar{4}$ and C$\bar{2}$ molecules, seperately or as complex (as a complex has been shown to exist in solution) (9), diffuse after activation and bind on to the first constant domain of the adjacent antibody molecules, as an active C3 convertase complex,

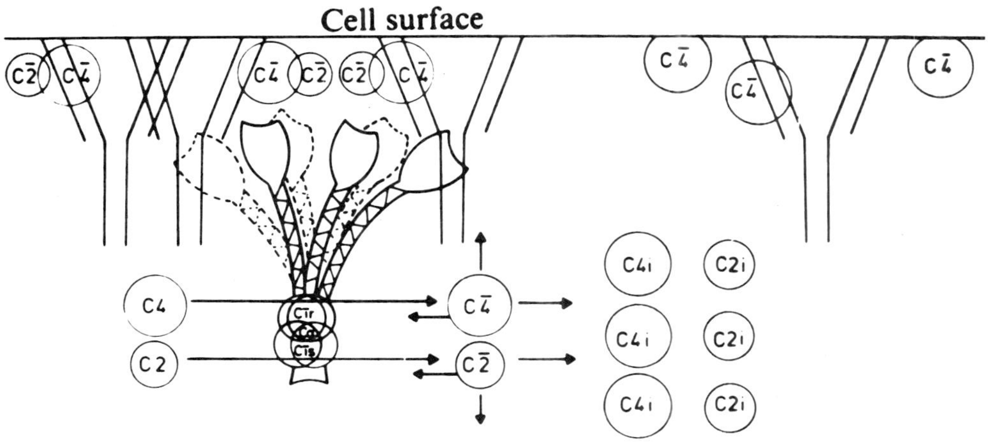

Fig. 4 Suggested assembly of the early components of the classical pathway of complement on antibody bound to a cell surface. The heads of the C1q molecule bind to the C_H2 domain of the antibody and the $C1r_2$–Ca^{2+}–C1s complex to the collagenous tails of C1q through C1r. The activated $C\bar{1}s$ formed splits C4 and C2. Most $C\bar{4}$ and $C\bar{2}$ is inactivated in the serum but some $C\bar{4}$ binds either to the Fab part of the antibody or to the cell surface. $C\bar{2}$ binds to adjacent $C\bar{4}$ molecules and forms C3 convertase, but is inactivated before reaching more distant $C\bar{4}$ molecules which are ineffective in the haemolytic sequence.

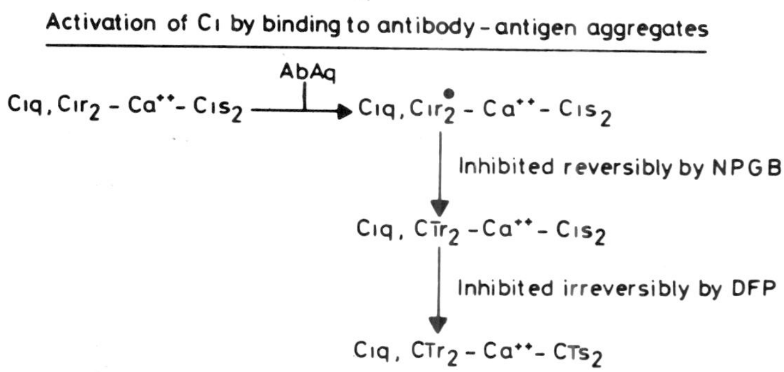

Fig. 5 When the tetrameric complex $C1r_2$–Ca^{2+}–$C1s_2$ interacts with C1q bound to aggregated antibody, the conformation of C1r is changed, exposing a proteolytic site ($C1r^{\bullet}$). It is this site in the unsplit peptide chain which catalyses the hydrolysis of a peptide bond and the conversion of $C1r^{\bullet}$ to $C\bar{1}r$. $C\bar{1}r$ activates C1s to $C\bar{1}s$. The active site of $C1r^{\bullet}$ is distinguished from that of $C\bar{1}r$ in that it reacts reversibly not irreversibly with nitrophenyl guanidine benzoate (NPGB) and it is not inhibited by diisopropyl phosphate fluoridate (DFP).

as shown. No measure has been made of the $\overline{C2}$ bound on to antibody aggregates and this will be difficult due to its lability but this may be overcome in part by prior treatment of the C2 with weak iodine solution (10).

It appears that a very complex intermolecular assembly of complement components may be formed on the aggregated antibody. It is probable that $\overline{C3}$ molecules may also be added to the bound $\overline{C42}$ complex to form the C5 convertase $\overline{C423}$ (11). The advantage of keeping the $\overline{C1}$, $\overline{C42}$ and $\overline{C423}$ proteases bound to the aggregated antibody could lie in the necessity to maintain them concentrated when surrounded by plasma containing about Ig/100 ml of different proteolytic inhibitors (12). Only by localisation is the temporary excess of protease over inhibitor achieved and this is essential for the continued sequential activation up to formation of $\overline{C5}$ which then interacts with the later components to form the lytic complex $\overline{C56789}$.

Activation of C1

Another related problem is the activation mechanism of C1 after binding to aggregated antibody. In $\overline{C1}$, C1q appears to be unchanged but C1r and C1s become serine esterase type proteases. The original 83,000 molecular weight single peptide chain present in both enzymes is split into an activation peptide of 56,000 molecular weight joined by a disulphide bond to the catalytic peptide containing the active site of 27,000 molecular weight (13). $\overline{C1s}$ will hydrolyse C4 and C2 in solution but $\overline{C1r}$ will not. $\overline{C1s}$ will not catalyse the activation of C1s in solution but $\overline{C1r}$ will (14). Hence it is probable that $\overline{C1r}$ activates C4 and C2, but it has not been clear as to how C1r is activated. Incubation of C1r with $\overline{C1r}$ (or with $\overline{C1s}$) does not cause activation in solution and hence simple autoactivation seems improbable (15). With the C1q, C1r and C1s complex bound to the antibody aggregates however autoactivation of C1r may occur. The position is complex as when C1r is added to antibody-C1q C1r binds firmly but is not activated (15). If C1s and Ca^{++} are present, C1s binds forming the tetrameric $C1r_2$-$C1s_2$ complex and C1r is activated. C1s can have no proteolytic role as it can be replaced either by $\overline{C1s}$ or by $\overline{C1s}$ which has been inactivated by two sequential treatments with 10 mM iPrP-F at 37°. C1s is an essential part of the activating complex not in a proteolytic role but presumably in a structural role. Autoactivation of C1r by $\overline{C1r}$ is still however improbable as if aggregated antibody C1q, C1r and C1s are mixed in optimum ratios in the presence of 10 mM iPr_2P-F, activation occurs of C1r but not of C1s (15). $\overline{C1r}$ is inactivated by iPr_2P-F under these conditions and the failure to activate C1s is due presumably to inactivation of $\overline{C1r}$ as it is formed. As activation of C1r is not inhibited, it suggests that when bound as well as when in solution C1r is not activated by $\overline{C1r}$. The only inhibitor found which will prevent the activation of C1r when bound in the C1 complex to antibody is nitrophenyl quanifinobenzoate (NPGB) which is effective at 1 mM in the activation mixture. This site directed reagent will inhibit $\overline{C1r}$ and $\overline{C1s}$ in solution irreversibly. However, if the antibody antigen-C1 complex formed in the presence of NPGB is spun down, washed and resuspended at 37^oC C1r and C1s are rapidly activated. That is, the inhibition is reversible. This suggests, as does the previous evidence, that the catalytic site responsible for C1r activation cannot be $\overline{C1r}$ which reacts irreversibly with NPGB.

As illustrated in Fig. 5, it is suggested that when the antibody antigen C1 complex forms, C1r undergoes a conformational change in such a way that a catalytic site is exposed in the unsplit peptide chain and is designated C1r˙ (15). This site is distinguished from the $\overline{C1r}$ active site in that it reacts much more slowly or not at all with iPr_2Pr-F and that while both react with NPGB, C1r˙ reacts with it reversibly and $\overline{C1r}$ irreversibly. That the peptide chain is unsplit when NPGB reacts in the complex is readily shown by acrylamide gel electrophoresis. C1r˙ is responsible for the hydrolysis of C1r (or C1r˙) to $\overline{C1r}$ and $\overline{C1r}$ activates C1s. Conclusive evidence for the existence of the postulated intermediary C1r˙ would be possible if an inhibitor reacting with it irreversibly could be found and the reaction product isolated and the catalytic site identified. No such irreversible inhibitor has been found so far and hence the postulated scheme can only be claimed to be a plausible explanation of the experimental results obtained.

The experiments described in this and in the previous section do suggest however that some of the complex assembly and activation mechanisms of the complement system can be unravelled by current techniques of protein and enzyme chemistry. No adequate explanations have yet been offered for the behaviour of the complex enzymes such as C3 convertase, C$\overline{42}$ and C5 convertase C$\overline{423}$ where the catalytically active site is believed to be in the C$\overline{2}$ component, but the specificity is apparently controlled by the associated proteins. Physical methods will be necessary to determine the steric arrangement of these multicomponent complexes and to relate their structure to their specific catalytic activity and it is not yet clear whether presently available methods are adequate to serve this difficult problem.

REFERENCES

1. Porter, R.R. in Defense and Recognition, 2nd Edition, Ed. E.S. Lennox, Butterworth, London (1979).
2. Goers, J.G. & Porter, R.R. Biochem. J. 175, 675 (1978).
3. Müller-Eberhard, H.J. & Lepow, I.H. J. Exp. Med. 121, 819 (1965).
4. Connel, G.E. & Porter, R.R. Biochem. J. 124, 53P (1971).
5. Colomb, M. & Porter, R.R. Biochem. J. 145, 177 (1975).
6. Knobel, N.R., Heusser, C., Rodrick, M.L. & Isliker, H. J. Immunol. 112, 2094 (1974).
7. Reid, K.B.M., Sim, R.B. & Faiers, A.P. Biochem. J. 161, 247 (1977).
8. Fujita, T., Gigli, I. & Nussenzweig, V. J. Exp. Med. 148, 1044 (1978).
9. Müller-Eberhard, H.J., Polley, M.E. & Calcott, M.A. J. Exp. Med. 125, 359 (1967).
10. Polley, M.E. & Müller-Eberhard, H.J. J. Exp. Med. 126, 1013 (1967).
11. Cooper, W.R. & Müller-Eberhard, H.J. J. Exp. Med. 132, 775 (1970).
12. Heimburger, N. in Bayer Symposium V. Protease Inhibitors (Ed. Fritz, H., Teshe, H., Green, L.J. & T heit, E.) Springer Verlag: New York (1974).
13. Sim, R.B., Porter, R.R., Reid, K.B.M. & Gigli, I. Biochem. J. 163, 219 (1977).
14. Gigli, I., Porter, R.R. & Sim, R.B. Biochem. J. 157, 541 (1976).
15. Dodds, A.W., Sim, R.B., Porter, R.R., Kerr, M.A. Biochem. J. 175, 383 (1978).

PLASMINOGEN AND PLASMIN
KINETICS OF ACTIVATION OF HUMAN PLASMINOGEN

Kenneth C. Robbins
Michael Reese Research Foundation, Chicago, IL., and
Departments of Medicine and Pathology,
Pritzker School of Medicine, University of Chicago,
Chicago, IL.

INTRODUCTION

It is the purpose of this manuscript to review recent knowledge on the biochemistry of the plasma components of the human fibrinolytic system. Plasminogen, a zymogen, of molecular weight $\sim$ 84,000, is found in plasma in a concentration of approximately 20 mg%. It can be activated to the proteolytic enzyme plasmin, of molecular weight $\sim$ 76,000, by substances called plasminogen activators which are found in plasma, the vascular endothelial cells, tissues and in bacterial culture filtrates. The zymogen to enzyme conversion involves the cleavage first of a specific Arg_{560}-Val peptide bond by the activator followed by the plasmic cleavage of a specific Lys_{77}-Lys peptide bond. Our studies on the kinetics of activation of plasminogen by specific activator species, in both isolated systems and in whole plasma, has permitted us to develop appropriate methodology to identify variant plasminogen molecules with low functional activities.

HUMAN PLASMINOGEN AND PLASMIN, AND PLASMIN-DERIVED HEAVY(A) AND LIGHT(B) CHAINS

The methods currently being used to prepare human plasminogen by affinity chromatography methods, the methods for preparing plasmin with highly purified preparations of both streptokinase and urokinase, and the properties of the zymogen and enzyme, have been described in recent reviews (1-5).

Native (Glu-forms) and partially-degraded (Lys-forms) plasminogens, and their respective affinity chromatography forms (1 and 2) have been isolated in a highly purified state. The native Glu-forms have molecular weights of $\sim$ 84,000, sedimentation coefficients between 5.0S and 5.7S, and isoelectric points between 6.0 and 6.6 (four isoelectric forms). The partially-degraded Lys-forms have molecular weights of $\sim$ 82,000, sedimentation coefficients between 4.2S and 4.8S, and isoelectric points between 6.6 and 8.5 (five isoelectric forms). The extinction coefficients of these proteins is between 16.8 and 17.0. The primary structure of human plasminogen has been determined; the zymogen contains 790 amino acid residues (6,7).

Plasmin, and its affinity chromatography forms (1 and 2), prepared in purified systems, are Lys_{78}-forms. The enzyme has a molecular weight of ∿ 76,000, sedimentation coefficients between 3.9S and 4.3S, and isoelectric points between 7.2 and 8.5 (two, to three, isoelectric forms). The extinction coefficient of this protein is between 16.8 and 17.0. A Glu_1-form of plasmin has been described which has the same molecular weight as Glu-plasminogen.

Plasmin is a two-chain molecule, with a heavy(A) chain (NH_2-terminus) and a light(B) chain (COOH-terminus), connected by apparently two interchain disulfide bonds. Glu_1-plasmin has a larger heavy(A) chain (Glu-, 560 residues) whereas Lys_{78}-plasmin has a smaller heavy(A) chain (Lys-, 483 residues). The Lys_{78}-heavy(A) chain has a molecular weight of ∿ 50,000, with an isoelectric point of 4.9 (reduced and carboxymethylated; one isoelectric form). It has both lysine-binding sites (for L-substituted-lysine Sepharose) and fibrin-binding sites. The Val_{561}-light(B) chain (Val-, 230 residues) is the same in both plasmin forms. The molecular weight of the light(B) chain is ∿ 26,000, with isoelectric points between 5.8 and 6.0 (reduced and carboxymethylated; three isoelectric forms).

Plasmin is a serine protease with trypsin-like specificity cleaving proteins and peptides at arginyl- and lysyl- peptide bonds, and basic amino acid esters and amides. An International Standard for human plasmin has been established (8). The specific activity of both the pure zymogen (after activation), and the enzyme, is about 30 I.U. per mg of protein.

MECHANISM OF ACTIVATION OF HUMAN PLASMINOGEN TO PLASMIN BY LOW ACTIVATOR CONCENTRATIONS

The molecular mechanism of activation of native human Glu-plasminogen, a single chain protein, to plasmin, a two chain protein, by either streptokinase (a bacterial protein) or urokinase (a human urinary protein), at low activator concentrations (1000 mol of zymogen : 1 mol of activator), involves the sequential cleavage of two major specific peptide bonds (1-5) (Fig. 1). These peptide bonds are Arg_{560}-Val (bond 1) and Lys_{77}-Lys (bond 2) which are cleaved at different rates, and differently under different conditions of activation. The single essential specific bond-cleaving event which takes place in the zymogen to enzyme conversion is the hydrolysis of the Arg_{560}-Val peptide bond. An enzyme species, Glu_1-plasmin, is formed when this peptide bond is cleaved. In isolated purified systems, in the presence of plasmin inhibitors, e.g. antithrombin III (plus heparin), α_1-antitrypsin, Trasylol (the basic bovine trypsin-kallikrein inhibitor), the pancreatic trypsin inhibitor-Kunitz, streptomyces leupeptin (Ac-L-Leu-L-Leu-L-Argal), the only bond-cleaving event which takes place is at the Arg_{560}-Val peptide bond (bond 1) producing the enzyme species Glu_1-plasmin. In the absence of plasmin inhibitors, the Lys_{77}-Lys peptide bond (bond 2) is cleaved producing the enzyme species Lys_{78}-plasmin; this bond-cleaving event is the result of plasmic cleavage, and not activator cleavage. The rates of cleavage of the two specific peptide bonds (1 and 2) are influenced by both lysine and ε-aminocaproic acid. The physiological form of plasmin formed in plasma has not as yet been determined.

EQUIMOLAR COMPLEXES OF HUMAN PLASMINOGEN AND PLASMIN

Both human plasminogen and plasmin form equimolar, or stoichiometric, complexes with streptokinase (1-5,9-11). This is a very specific reaction occurring with both crude and highly purified preparations of either plasminogen or plasmin, and native streptokinase, or large fragments of streptokinase. The binding-site

Fig. 1 Mechanism of activation of human plasminogen

Two bond-cleaving events[a]

(a) Purified system (low activator concentration)

$$\text{Glu-plasminogen} \xrightarrow{(1)} \text{Glu-plasmin} \xrightarrow{(2)} \text{Lys-plasmin}$$

$$\text{Glu-plasminogen} \xrightarrow{(2)} \text{Lys-plasminogen} \xrightarrow{(1)} \text{Lys-plasmin}$$

(b) Purified system + inhibitors (low activator concentration)

$$\text{Glu-plasminogen} \xrightarrow{(1)} \text{Glu-plasmin}$$

(c) Purified system (equimolar streptokinase concentration)

$$\text{Glu-plasminogen}\cdot\text{streptokinase} \longrightarrow \text{Glu-plasminogen}^{*}\cdot\text{streptokinase} \xrightarrow{(1)}$$

$$\text{Glu-plasmin}\cdot\text{streptokinase} \xrightarrow{(2)} \text{Lys-plasmin}\cdot\text{streptokinase}$$

[a] (1) Arg_{560}-Val; (2) Lys_{77}-Lys.

for streptokinase is found in the light(B) chain portion of the zymogen and enzyme (12). Streptokinase has a high degree of species specificity (13); the human and cat zymogens are the only mammalian zymogens which are readily activated in vitro by streptokinase (14). The molecular reactions between human plasminogen and streptokinase have been described (1-5,9-11,14,15). The equimolar human plasminogen (plasmin)•streptokinase complex, frequently called bovine plasminogen activator, appears to be an activator of all mammalian species of plasminogen.

A series of physical and chemical transformations takes place when the equimolar human plasminogen•streptokinase activator complex is formed. The first reaction, which is time dependent, is the formation of an intact complex in which plasminogen is transformed into a zymogen with an active site (plasminogen*) (16,17) without any apparent peptide bond cleavages in the zymogen, or in the streptokinase. Native Glu-plasminogen has no active site, but one forms during its interaction with streptokinase; a Lys-plasminogen* form has been prepared in the absence of streptokinase from the partially-degraded Lys-form (18). Glu-plasminogen* is then converted in the complex to Glu_1-plasmin and then to Lys_{78}-plasmin by plasmic cleavage (14). Also, in the complex, streptokinase is specifically cleaved, continuously, by limited proteolysis to give a series of high molecular components with the peptide fragments probably still bound to the complex (10,11,14,15,19-21). The large streptokinase fragments have been named SK1, or SK_c (∿40,000), SK2 or SK_f (∿36,000), SK3 (∿36,000) and SK4 (∿26,000); other high molecular weight streptokinase fragments have also been described: SK_b, SK_d, and SK_e. The rate of fragmentation of streptokinase is influenced by temperature and ε-aminocaproic acid. Streptokinase fragments SK2 and SK4 have been isolated and characterized (10); only fragment SK2 behaves like native streptokinase in the activation of human plasminogen.

THE FUNCTIONALLY-ACTIVE HUMAN PLASMIN-DERIVED LIGHT(B) CHAIN AND ITS STREPTOKINASE COMPLEX

A functionally-active human plasmin-derived light(B) chain and a functionally-active human plasmin-derived light(B) chain•streptokinase complex have been isolated and characterized (12). Limited reduction of human Lys-plasmin, to cleave the two interchain disulfide bonds, followed by specific affinity chromatography methods on L-lysine-substituted Sepharose, will permit the separation of the functionally-active light(B) chain, and its equimolar streptokinase complex, from the heavy(A) chain which is adsorbed to the affinity column. Only the isolated, functionally-active light(B) chain will form with streptokinase a stoichiometric activator complex (12,18) which will activate all mammalian plasminogens. The plasmin active site is located on the light(B) chain portion of the molecule (22) which is also the activator active site in the light(B) chain•streptokinase complex (12). The light(B) chain•streptokinase complex, both formed and preformed, has low proteolytic activity, less than 10% of the activity of the human plasmin•streptokinase complex (12). In this complex, streptokinase is transformed only to fragments SK1 and SK2 (23).

EFFICIENCY OF ACTIVATION OF HUMAN PLASMINOGEN BY THE EQUIMOLAR COMPLEXES OF STREPTOKINASE WITH HUMAN PLASMINOGEN, PLASMIN AND THE PLASMIN-DERIVED LIGHT(B) CHAIN

The equimolar activator complexes of streptokinase with various activated forms of human plasminogen (plasminogen*, plasmin and plasmin-derived light(B) chain) have been found to vary in their activator activities on bovine plasminogen (11,18,21,24). Fragmentation of streptokinase in the complexes leads to substantially lower activator activities.

Recent studies dealing with kinetics of activation of human plasminogen have made it possible to order the efficiency of plasminogen activators using kinetic constants (23, unpublished data). The second-order rate constant, or catalytic efficiency, for each activator species has been determined in coupled assays with synthetic substrates. Activation rates for the human plasminogen substrate with the streptokinase activator species were measured both at pH 6.0 and 30° with N^{α}-Cbz-L-lysine-p-nitrophenyl ester (23), and at pH 7.4 and 37° with H-D-valine-L-leucine-L-lysine-p-nitroanilide (unpublished data), with comparable results. The relative activator efficiencies, or second-order rate constants, of the various streptokinase complexes, all with intact streptokinase, and the urokinase activator species, at pH 7.4 and 37°, with human Glu-plasminogen as the substrate, are summarized in Table 1. In this series of highly purified

TABLE 1 Relative activities of activator species

Activator species	Relative activity[b]
1) Streptokinase[a]	
Light(B) chain·streptokinase	4.3
Glu-plasminogen·streptokinase	1.9
Streptokinase	1.7
Lys-plasmin·streptokinase	1.0
2) Urokinase	
High molecular weight	1.3
Low molecular weight	0.6

[a] Streptokinase complexes with intact SK.
[b] Kinetic analysis - catalytic efficiency, or second-order rate constants, of activator; values relative to Lys-plasmin·streptokinase

activator species, the plasmin-derived light(B) chain·streptokinase complex is the activator with the highest catalytic efficiency. The catalytic efficiency of the urokinase activator species is similar to the zymogen·- and enzyme·-streptokinase complexes but several-fold lower than the light(B) chain·streptokinase complex. In these studies, it was found that the Lys-plasminogen substrate is activated more rapidly (higher catalytic rate constants) than the Glu-plasminogen substrate by the streptokinase activator species.

PHYSIOLOGICAL ACTIVATION OF HUMAN PLASMA PLASMINOGEN BY STREPTOKINASE AND UROKINASE ACTIVATOR SPECIES: BASIC CONSIDERATIONS

The use of various streptokinase and urokinase activator species (see Table 1) in thrombolytic therapy, requires an understanding of the kinetic mechanisms of plasminogen activation in a physiological environment. For example, during the infusion of streptokinase into a human subject, several different concurrent types of biochemical reactions take place. Firstly, the streptokinase could react with circulating antibodies to streptokinase resulting in antigen-antibody complexes which may, or may not, have activator activity; these immune complexes are probably removed physiologically and could stimulate further antibody formation to streptokinase. Secondly, streptokinase will bind to circulating Glu-plasminogen to form the equimolar activator species. Since complexes do not form instantaneously with every molecule of plasminogen in the circulation, the formed activator species will activate a variable amount of plasminogen to plasmin. The plasmin will bind quickly either to streptokinase to form an activator complex, or to the primary α_2-plasmin inhibitor to form a plasmin-α_2-plasmin inhibitor complex (25). Thirdly, even with high doses of streptokinase, it is difficult to complex all the plasminogen in the circulation, and free streptokinase is rapidly removed from the circulation (biological half-life of less than 30 min) (26). At any fixed time, in the circulation, one can find immune complexes of streptokinase, inhibitor complexes of plasmin, streptokinase•-plasminogen and streptokinase•plasmin activator complexes, and some free streptokinase. There does not appear to be any natural inhibitor to the streptokinase activator complexes (unpublished data).

When equimolar streptokinase activator complexes (with plasminogen, plasmin, or light(B) chain) are infused into a human subject, a different set of biochemical reactions take place. Firstly, immune complexes of these activators with antibodies to streptokinase are probably formed which could behave differently from the streptokinase immune complexes and may be active activator complexes, and when removed from the circulation could also further stimulate antibody formation to streptokinase. Secondly, plasminogen is converted to plasmin, and the enzyme is complexed to the α_2-plasmin inhibitor to form a circulating inactive complex. These activator complexes have biological half-lifes of from 4 to 12 hours in an experimental dog model (unpublished data) and remain in the circulation much longer than uncomplexed streptokinase.

When urokinase is infused into a human subject, a third set of biochemical reactions take place. Firstly, complexes of urokinase are formed with circulating urokinase inhibitors, not antibodies, which will remove the activator from the circulation. Secondly, this activator species will, like the other activator species, convert plasminogen to plasmin which will form complexes with the α_2-plasmin inhibitor. The biological half-life of this activator species is under 30 min (26). All highly purified activator species will activate plasminogen to plasmin in a plasma milieu but the rates of activation will vary and will depend upon a variety of factors, including type and concentration of activator species.

KINETICS OF ACTIVATION OF HUMAN PLASMINOGEN

a) Isolated Systems

Studies on the kinetics of activation of highly purified human Glu- and Lys-plasminogen by various activator species (e.g. streptokinase and urokinase) allowed us to determine the apparent Michaelis constants and catalytic rate constants for the activator species (23, unpublished data). As a result of these steady-state kinetic studies, we propose that all plasminogen activators have a serine protease-like active center and they bind to plasminogen at a common region in the vicinity of the susceptible Arg_{560}-Val peptide bond to form an active activator complex. This enzyme now interacts with a second molecule of plasminogen, which is activated to plasmin. The activator enzyme species is always an activator•plasminogen complex whether transitory, with urokinase, or stable, with streptokinase. Also plasminogen activators vary in their catalytic efficiencies, or second-order rate constants. The low apparent Michaelis constants indicate a minimum of four pairs of interacting side chains for each plasminogen•activator-plasminogen complex. The high catalytic rate constants indicate that the specific Arg_{560}-Val peptide bond which is cleaved is uniquely labile in the presence of activator.

b) Human Plasma

Methodology has been developed for studying rates of activation of plasminogen with various activator species in whole human plasma (unpublished data). These studies are influenced by antibodies and inhibitors to the activators, and α_2-plasmin inhibitor which is the major plasmin inhibitor in plasma (25). Systems have been developed which permit us to measure the rate, or initial velocity, of plasmin generation in whole human plasma using synthetic substrates. The initial velocity of plasmin generation from plasminogen in the plasma milieu is at least 50-fold lower than in purified systems. For example, with streptokinase levels between 1×10^{-8} M ($\sim$ 40 units) and 1×10^{-7} M ($\sim$ 400 units), with 1 ml plasma (2.4×10^{-6} M plasminogen), plasmin generation is very rapid, in the presence of specific plasmin synthetic substrates. Plasma samples have been found which show an $\sim$ 2-fold slower plasmin generation rate. The steady-state kinetic parameters of activation of the plasminogens isolated from these plasma samples, with streptokinase, gave 3- to 10-fold higher apparent Michaelis constants, but normal catalytic rate constants. Other activator species gave over 200-fold higher apparent Michaelis constants, but also with normal catalytic rate constants, indicating a primary defect in the binding of the activator to the zymogen. This unusual, or different, class of zymogens can be called "variant" plasminogens.

REFERENCES

(1) K. C. Robbins, and L. Summaria, Human plasminogen and plasmin, In Methods Enzymol. (G. E. Perlmann and L. Lorand, Eds.), Vol. 19, pp. 184-199, Academic Press, New York, 1970.

(2) K. C. Robbins and L. Summaria, Plasminogen and plasmin, In Methods Enzymol. (L. Lorand, Ed.) Vol. 45, pp. 257-273, Academic Press, New York, 1976.

(3) K. C. Robbins, The biochemistry of plasminogen and plasmin, In Haemostasis: Biochemistry, Physiology and Pathology (D. Ogston and R. Bennett, Eds.), pp. 208-220, John Wiley and Sons, London, 1977.

(4) K. C. Robbins, Plasmin, In Handbook of Experimental Pharmacology, Vol. 46, Fibrinolytics and Antifibrinolytics (F. Markwardt, Ed.), pp. 317-336, Springer-Verlag, Berlin, 1978.

(5) K. C. Robbins, The human fibrinolytic system: Regulation and control, Mol. Cell. Biochem. 20, 149-157 (1978).

(6) L. Sottrup-Jensen, H. Claeys, M. Zajdel, T. E. Petersen and S. Magnusson, The primary structure of human plasminogen: Isolation of two lysine-binding fragments and one "mini"-plasminogen (M.W. 38,000) by elastase-catalyzed specific limited proteolysis, In Progress in chemical fibrinolysis and thrombolysis (J. F. Davidson, M. Samama, and P. Desnoyers, Eds.), Vol. 3, pp. 191-209, Raven Press, New York, 1978.

(7) B. Wiman, Biochemistry of the plasminogen to plasmin conversion, In Fibrinolysis: Current fundamental and clinical concepts, (P. J. Gaffney and S. Balkuv-Ulutin, Eds.), pp. 47-60, Academic Press, London, 1978.

(8) T. B. L. Kirkwood, P. J. Campbell, and P. J. Gaffney, A standard for human plasmin, Thromb. Diath. Haemorrh. 34, 20-31 (1975).

(9) F. B. Taylor, Jr., and R. H. Tomar, Streptokinase, In Methods Enzymol. (G. E. Perlmann and L. Lorand, Eds.), Vol. 19, pp. 807-821, Academic Press, New York, 1970.

(10) F. J. Castellino, J. M. Sodetz, W. J. Brockway, G. E. Siefring, Jr., Streptokinase, In Methods Enzymol. (L. Lorand, Ed.), Vol. 45, pp. 244-257, Academic Press, New York, 1976.

(11) K. C. Robbins and G. Markus, The interaction of human plasminogen with streptokinase, in Fibrinolysis: Current fundamental and clinical concepts (P. J. Gaffney and S. Balkuv-Ulutin, Eds.), pp. 61-75, Academic Press, London, 1978.

(12) L. Summaria and K. C. Robbins, Isolation of a human plasmin-derived, functionally active, light(B) chain capable of forming with streptokinase an equimolar light(B) chain-streptokinase complex with plasminogen activator activity, J. Biol. Chem. 251, 5810-5813 (1976).

(13) R. J. Wulf, and E. T. Mertz, Plasminogen VIII: Species specificity of streptokinase, Canad. J. Biochem. 47, 927-931 (1969).

(14) L. Summaria, L. Arzadon, P. Bernabe, and K. C. Robbins, The interaction of streptokinase with human, cat, dog, and rabbit plasminogens. The fragmentation of streptokinase in the equimolar plasminogen-streptokinase complexes, J. Biol. Chem. 249, 4760-4769 (1974).

(15) S. P. Bajaj and F. J. Castellino, Activation of human plasminogen by equimolar levels of streptokinase, J. Biol. Chem. 252, 492-498 (1977).

(16) D. K. McClintock and P. H. Bell, The mechanism of activation of human plasminogen by streptokinase, Biochem. Biophys. Res. Commun. 43, 694-702 (1971).

(17) K. N. N. Reddy and G. Markus, Mechanism of activation of human plasminogen by streptokinase. Presence of active center in streptokinase-plasminogen complex, J. Biol. Chem. 247, 1683-1694 (1972).

(18) R. C. Wohl, L. Arzadon, L. Summaria, and K. C. Robbins, Comparison of the esterase and human plasminogen activator activities of various activated forms of human plasminogen and their equimolar streptokinase complexes, J. Biol. Chem. 252, 1141-1147 (1977).

(19) L. Summaria, K. C. Robbins and G. H. Barlow, Dissociation of the equimolar human plasmin-streptokinase complex. Partial characterization of the isolated plasmin and streptokinase moieties, J. Biol. Chem. 246, 2136-2142 (1971).

(20) D. K. McClintock, M. E. Englert, C. Dziobkowski, E. H. Snedeker, P. H. Bell, Two distinct pathways of the streptokinase-mediated activation of highly purified human plasminogen, Biochemistry 13, 5334-5344 (1974).

(21) G. Markus, J. L. Evers and G. H. Hobika, Activator activities of the transient forms of the human plasminogen-streptokinase complex during its proteolytic conversion to the stable activator complex, J. Biol. Chem. 251, 6495-6504 (1976).

(22) W. R. Groskopf, B. Hsieh, L. Summaria and K. C. Robbins, Studies on the active center of human plasmin. The serine and histidine residues, J. Biol. Chem. 244, 359-365 (1969).

(23) R. C. Wohl, L. Summaria, L. Arzadon and K. C. Robbins, Steady state kinetics of activation of human and bovine plasminogens by streptokinase and its equimolar complexes with various activated forms of human plasminogen, J. Biol. Chem. 253, 1402-1407 (1978).

(24) G. Markus, J. L. Evers, and G. H. Hobika, Comparison of some properties of native (Glu) and modified (Lys) human plasminogen, J. Biol. Chem. 253, 733-739 (1978).

(25) D. Collen and B. Wiman, Physiological inhibitors of fibrinolysis, In Fibrinolysis: Current fundamental and clinical concepts (P. J. Gaffney and S. Balkuv-Ulutin, Eds.) pp. 17-26, Academic Press, London, 1978.

(26) W. R. Bell, Thrombolytic therapy: A comparison between urokinase and streptokinase, Semin. Thromb. Hemostas. 2, 1-13 (1975).

ACKNOWLEDGEMENT

The studies cited from our laboratory were supported in part by United States Public Health Service Grant HL04366 from the National Heart, Lung and Blood Institute

ASPECTS OF THE STRUCTURE AND ACTIVATION OF HUMAN PLASMINOGEN

Francis J. Castellino
Department of Chemistry, The University of Notre Dame, Notre Dame, Indiana 46556

Plasminogen is the inactive plasma protein precursor of the proteolytic enzyme, plasmin. The exact role of plasmin is not completely understood; but plasmin is known to function in several diverse pathways. Plasmin is certainly operative in the fibrinolytic system, digesting both the fibrin clot, and its precursor molecule, fibrinogen into soluble peptides (1). Additionally, plasmin may also exert controls on coagulation, other than strict involvement in fibrinolysis. For example, plasmin is known to possess proteolytic activity toward factor XIIa (activated Hageman Factor) (2). By virtue of its action on factor XIIa, plasmin can divert the function of factor XIIa from its role of initiation of the intrinsic blood coagulation pathway, into generation of kinins - an activity possessed by the plasminolysis products of factor XIIa (2). In addition to the above, plasmin may play a role in the complement system, since plasmin has been reported to be capable of activation of $C1_s$ (3), inhibition of C1 inactivator (4) and release of chemotactic substances from C_3 (5).

Research in the area of fibrinolysis was greatly advanced in 1970 when Deutsch and Mertz (6) published an affinity chromatographic method, utilizing Sepharose-lysine, for purification at plasminogen from whole plasma, in a single step. Subsequently, our laboratory reported (7) isolation of two plasminogen variants from plasma, utilizing a modification of the Deutsch and Mertz method, essentially as shown in Fig. 1.

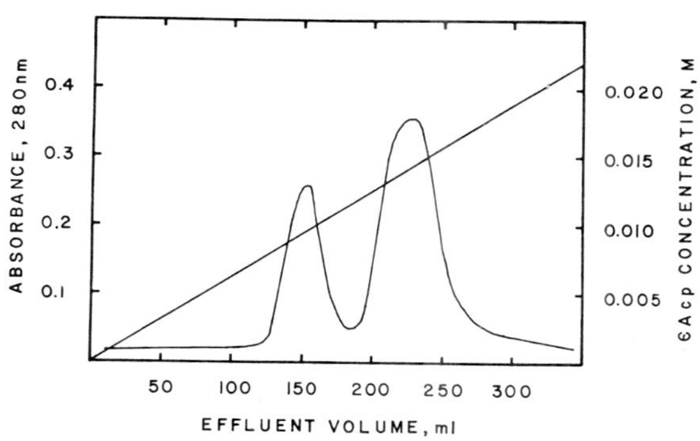

Fig. 1. Elution of human plasminogen variants by affinity chromatography.

Here, whole plasma was passed over a column of Sepharose-lysine, and the column washed free of weakly adsorbed proteins. At this point a linear gradient of ε-amino caproic acid (ε-ACA) was used to elute the two distinct fractions, as noted in Fig. 1, in a total yield > 90%. We have studied the chemical nature of the two plasminogen variants and have shown that their amino terminal sequences (8), molecular weights (9), propensity for activation into plasmin (9) and immunochemical cross-reactivities (10) are virtually the same. Additionally, metabolic studies on the two forms indicated that they are independently synthesized, independently degraded, and non-interconvertible in the plasma (10). The major differences in the two forms are their charge characteristics (9), affinity for ε-amino caproic acid (9) and their carbohydrate structures (8). This latter point is of considerable importance. We have recently completely sequenced the carbohydrate of the two human plasminogen variants. The sequences obtained are:

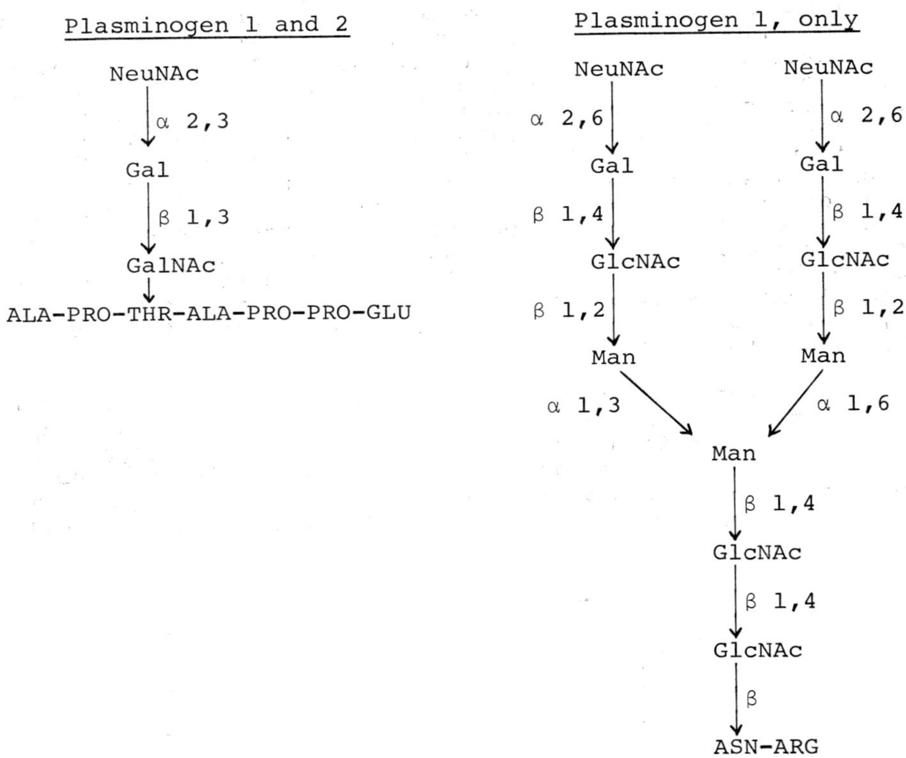

Both human plasminogen variant 1 (first peak eluted in Fig. 1) and variant 2 (second peak eluted in Fig. 1) contain the trisaccharide sequence sialic acid (NeuNAc)→galactose (Gal)→N-acetyl galactosamine (GalNAc) bound to threonine of the indicated sequence. In addition, plasminogen variant 1, only, contains the indicated branched carbohydrate sequence, above. Thus, there is an extra site of glycosylation in variant 1, compared to variant 2. This results in variant

1 containing considerable greater quantities of carbohydrate than variant 2, an observation which we previously reported (8). This appears to be the major structural difference in the two forms of human plasminogen. Electrophoretically distinct subforms of each plasminogen variant have been found (9,11), some of which arise as a result of partial desialyation of the parent variant (12). Complete removal of sialic acid from each plasminogen results in absolution of the charge differences between the plasminogen variants, without affecting their affinity chromatographic resolution (12). This suggests that the charge differences are not related to the differences in ε-amino caproic acid binding for the 2 plasminogen forms.

The ligand utilized for the affinity chromatographic separation of the plasminogen forms, L-lysine, represents one of a series of α,ω-amino acids which possess antifibrinolytic properties (13). These amino acids also affect the structure and activation properties of plasminogen. Before further examination of this topic, however, it is important to review the important structural features of plasminogen and plasmin. The latent activation intermediates and products of native human plasminogen can be represented as:

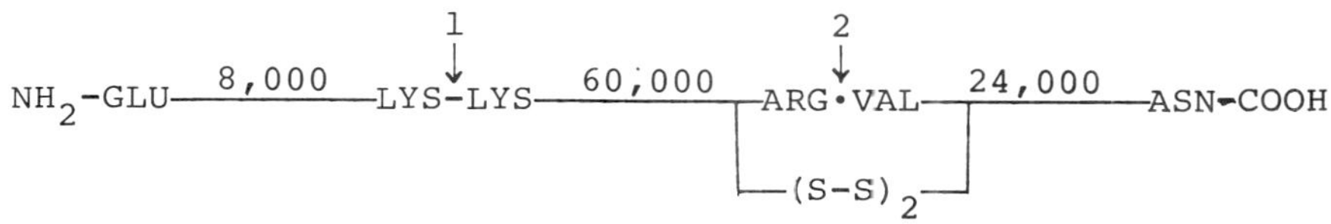

Native circulating plasminogen (GLU-Pg) possesses a molecular weight of 89,000-92,000 (14,15) and is a single chain protein, containing *ca.*, 20 disulfide bonds (16) - two of which are shown. GLU-Pg readily loses an amino terminal activation peptide (GLU-P), by cleavage at bond 1, above, forming LYS-plasminogen (LYS-Pg), of molecular weight 81,000-85,000 (15). The major catalyst for this bond cleavage is plasmin (15,17,18). The final plasmin formed upon activation of either GLU-Pg, or LYS-Pg, is LYS-plasmin (LYS-Pm), and results from cleavage of bonds 1 and 2, above. LYS-Pm is a two chain structure, linked by two disulfide bonds (19,20). It possesses a heavy chain, of molecular weight approximately 58,000-63,000 (15), containing all plasminogen carbohydrate (21), and an active site containing light chain (22), of molecular weight 23,000-26,000. The ε-amino caproic acid binding site(s) are also found in the plasmin heavy chain (23,24). Another plasmin GLU-plasmin (GLU-Pm), of molecular weight 89,000-92,000 (15), has been isolated and results from exclusive cleavage of bond 2, above, by the activator (15,17, 18,25). This form of plasmin is very unstable and is rapidly degraded to LYS-Pm, upon bond 1 cleavage by plasmin (15,17,18).

Each of these plasminogen and plasmin molecules interact with certain amino acids, such as lysine and ε-amino caproic acid in an extremely interesting and important manner. It has been shown that ε-amino caproic acid significantly alters the $S^{0}_{20,w}$ value of several species of plasminogen (7,26,27). We have studied, over the past several years, the effect of ε-amino caproic acid and its analogues on human plasminogen and plasmin conformation. Table 1 summarizes some of our findings.

TABLE 1 The Effect of ε-Amino Caproic Acid (ε-ACA) on the $S^{o}_{20,w}$ Values of Plasminogen and Plasmin[a]

Species	$S^{o}_{20,w}$ Native	$S^{o}_{20,w}$ Native + ε-ACA
GLU-Pg	5.73 S	4.80 S
LYS-Pg	4.75 S	4.65 S
GLU-Pm	5.68 S	4.83 S
LYS-Pm	4.80 S	4.82 S

[a]See reference 27 for experimental details.

Clearly, at ε-ACA levels which saturate its effect on the system, molecules which possess the activation peptide, *e.g.* GLU-Pg and GLU-Pm undergo a dramatic ligand-induced conformational alteration. On the other hand, molecules which do not possess the activation peptide, *e.g.* LYS-Pg and LYS-Pm, although fully capable of binding ε-ACA (27-29), do not undergo a significant conformational alteration as a result of this interaction. Interestingly, LYS-Pg and LYS-Pm, in the presence or absence of ε-ACA appear to possess a gross conformation similar to GLU-Pg or GLU-Pm, bound to ε-ACA (27).

Table 2 extends this data to measurement of the effect of analogues of ε-ACA on the overall conformation of human GLU-Pg, as monitored by the $S^{o}_{20,w}$ (30), change in intrinsic fluorescence (ΔF) (30) and alteration in rotational relaxation time (ρ_h) of GLU-Pg (31) in the presence and absence of the ligands.

TABLE 2 The Effect of Various ε-ACA Analogues on Human GLU-Pg Conformation

Ligand	$S^{o}_{20,w}$	ΔF (%)	ρ_h (nsec)
None	5.79 S	—	262
Gly,3-APr	5.72 S	0	259
4-ABt	4.90 S	7.2	157
5-APn	4.86 S	7.0	156
ε-ACA	4.87 S	7.0	156
7-AHp	4.85 S	7.1	155
8-AOt	4.88 S	7.0	160
t-AMCHA	4.79 S	11.5	160
L-lysine	4.80 S	7.0	159

Glycine (Gly) and 3-amino propionic acid (3-APr) do not appear to alter the conformation of GLU-Pg. However, as the number of carbon atoms between the COO^- and NH_3^+ is progressively altered from 4, in 4-amino butyric acid (4-ABt) through 8, in 8-amino octanoic acid, a dramatic decrease in the $S^{o}_{20,w}$ and ρ_h of GLU-Pg is noted, along with a corresponding increase in the intrinsic fluorescence of the protein. Interposition of a cyclohexane ring between the COO^-

and NH_3^+ groups, e.g., trans-aminomethylcyclohexane-1-carboxylic acid (t-AMCHA) also allows the conformational alteration in GLU-Pg to occur, and placement of an NH_3^+ in a position α to the COO^- (in L-lysine), does not alter its ability to induce the conformational alteration in human GLU-Pg. Considering the 3 conformational parameters in Table 2, it appears that upon interaction of human GLU-Pg with certain α,ω-amino acids, a conformational alteration occurs in GLU-Pg to a more extended and internally more flexible molecule. Additionally, there is likely an alteration in environment of a tyrptophan residue(s) as a result of this conformational alteration, as seen from the increase in ΔF of GLU-Pg, upon interaction with certain of these ligands. On the other hand, LYS-Pg, when bound to ε-ACA like molecules does not show significant alterations in the above parameters.

Since the magnitude of the conformation alteration induced by these agents is so large, any of the parameters of Table 2 can be titrated with these agents, such that their relative effeciencies in producing these alterations can be evaluated. Figure 2 shows the data obtained when the $S^o_{20,w}$ of human GLU-Pg is titrated with t-AMCHA (●), ε-ACA (■), and L-lysine (▲) (30):

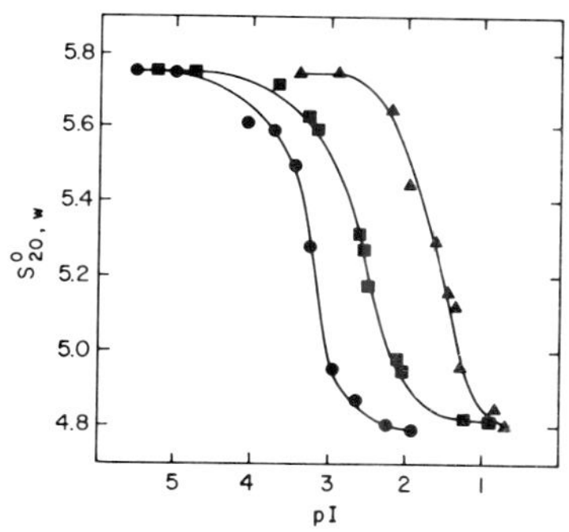

Fig. 2. The effect of various concentrations of amino acid, plotted as the negative logarithm of ligand concentration (pI), on the $S^o_{20,w}$ of human GLU-Pg.

As can be readily seen from the data, t-AMCHA appears to be more effective than ε-ACA, which, in turn, is more effective than L-lysine in altering the GLU-Pg conformation. Figure 3 shows similar data for the titration of the change in GLU-Pg intrinsic fluorescence (ΔF) with these same three ligands (30):

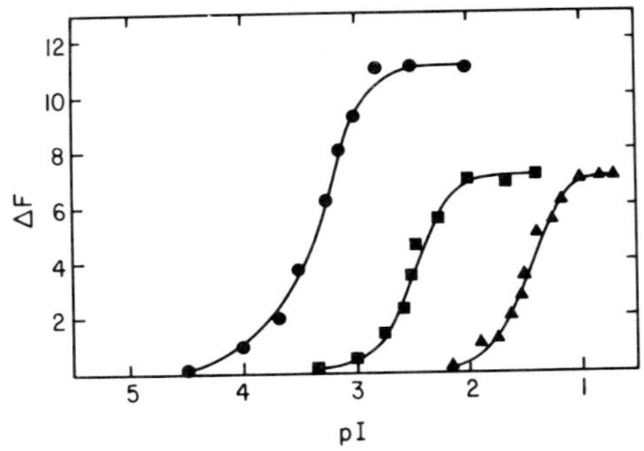

Fig. 3. The effect of various concentrations of amino acid on the ΔF of human GLU-Pg.

A similar trend is noted here, as was observed in Fig. 2. As a quantitative measure of the efficacy of the ligands employed for examination of the conformational alteration in human GLU-Pg, we have calculated the concentration of each amino acid required to produce one-half of the conformational alteration in GLU-Pg (30). The data are listed in Table 3.

TABLE 3 The Concentration of α,ω-Amino Acids Required to Produce One-Half of the Conformational Alteration (K 0.5) in Human GLU-Pg

	$K_{0.5}$ (mM)		
Ligand	$s^{o}_{20,w}$	ΔF	ρ_h
4-ABt	20.7	19.2	—
5-APn	4.9	4.0	—
ε-ACA	2.4	3.0	2.5
7-AHp	17.4	16.9	—
8-AOt	32.5	33.0	—
t-AMCHA	0.6	0.5	0.4
L-lysine	26.0	25.1	27.2

In scanning the columns, it appears as though the efficiency of these ligands increase as one proceeds stepwise from 4-ABt to ε-ACA. Upon further increase of the chain length separating the COO^- and NH_3^+ groups, in 7-AHp and 8-AOt, the efficacy of these agents again show decreases. The ligand, t-AMCHA, is the most effective of the ligands examined; whereas, cis-AMCHA does not induce alteration of GLU-Pg conformation, suggesting that steric considerations in the ligand are important to their effectiveness. L-lysine is much less effective than ε-ACA, suggesting that interposition of an α-NH_3^+ is deleterious to the ability of these agents to alter the conformation of GLU-Pg. Further inspection of Table 3, for t-AMCHA, ε-ACA, and L-lysine, indicates that the same $K_{0.5}$ is obtained for each amino acid upon titration of any conformational property. This shows that these 3 different conformational monitors are in fact reflections of the same ligand-induced conformational change in GLU-Pg.

Since these agents cause such dramatic changes in the structure of GLU-Pg and GLU-Pm, it is of considerable importance to ask how this is reflected in the activation properties of plasminogen. One important plasminogen activator is the proteolytic activator, urokinase (32). This particular activator has been purified from urine (33), and from cultured embryonic human kidney cells (33). Our laboratory has intensively studied the mechanism of activation of human plasminogen by urokinase and has published the following mechanism of activation (15):

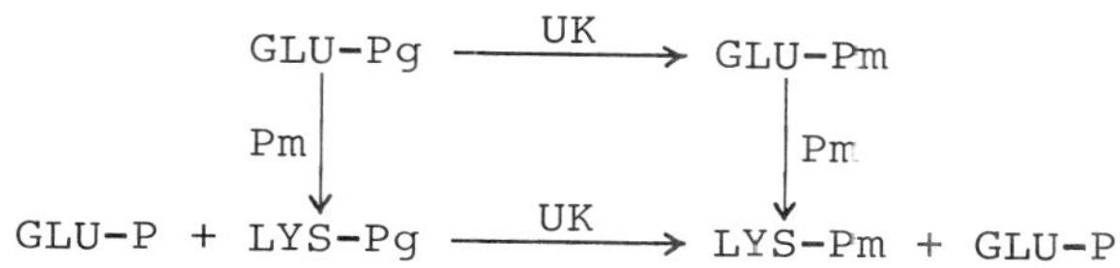

Here, the initial molecules of plasmin formed are GLU-Pm, as a result of the urokinase (UK)-catalyzed cleavage of bond 2 in GLU-Pg. GLU-Pm is not a stable species and is autocatalytically converted to LYS-Pm, by cleavage of the activation peptide (GLU-P) from the amino terminus of the GLU-Pm heavy chain. LYS-Pm and, quite possibly, GLU-Pm also catalyze ready removal of the same activation peptide from the amino terminus of remaining GLU-Pg molecules, yielding LYS-Pg, which is activated to LYS-Pm by UK. The actual pathway of LYS-Pm formation greatly depends upon environmental conditions, such as the amount of UK present (15) and the presence or absence of ε-ACA-like compounds (*vide infra*), and is not readily predictable.

It has been previously demonstrated that the activation rate of GLU-Pg to LYS-Pm is greatly accelerated by the presence of ε-ACA or *L*-lysine (34). On the other hand, the conversion of LYS-Pg to LYS-Pm is unaffected by the presence of ε-ACA (34). Therefore, it was of interest to us to examine the effect of a representative compound of the ε-ACA class, *L*-lysine, on the individual steps of the activation of GLU-Pg to LYS-Pm; *i.e.*, GLU-Pg → GLU-Pm; GLU-Pm → LYS-Pm; GLU-Pg → LYS-Pg (30). Figure 4 shows the effect of *L*-lysine on the conversion of GLU-Pg to GLU-Pm.

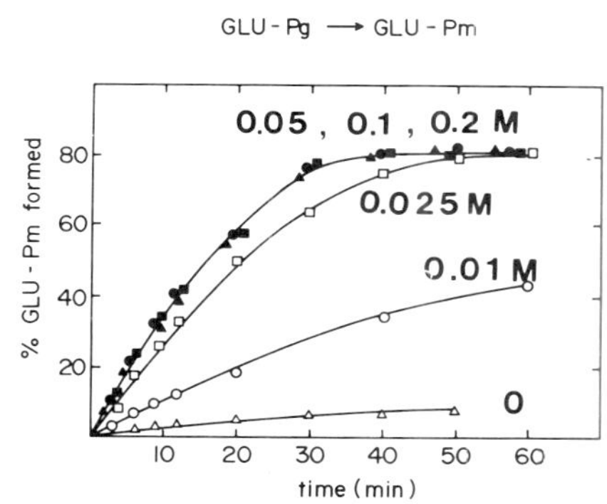

Fig. 4. The effect of *L*-lysine on the conversion of GLU-Pg to GLU-Pm by UK. The concentration terms on the individual curves represent the amount of *L*-lysine present.

As can be seen from Fig. 4, very slow conversion is noted in the absence of L-lysine. However, the rate of conversion of GLU-Pg to GLU-Pm is greatly accelerated as the concentration of L-lysine is increased from O(△) 0.01 M(O), 0.025 M(□), 0.05 M(●). No further rate increases are noted upon further increase in L-lysine concentration to 0.1 M(■), and 0.2 M(▲). Figure 5

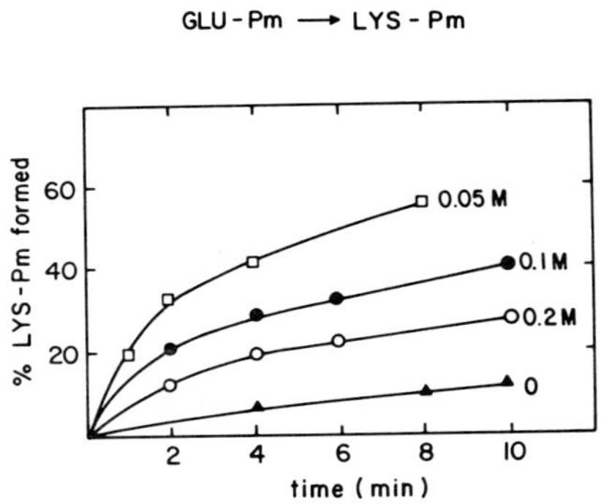

Fig. 5. The effect of L-lysine on the conversion of GLU-Pm to LYS-Pm, by plasmin.

shows the effect of L-lysine on the conversion of GLU-Pm to LYS-Pm by plasmin. In this case, the rate of conversion increases as the concentration of L-lysine increases to 0.05 M. Further addition of L-lysine serves to inhibit the reaction under study. This inhibition effect of L-lysine was not evident in the GLU-Pg to GLU-Pm conversion (Fig. 4). Figure 6

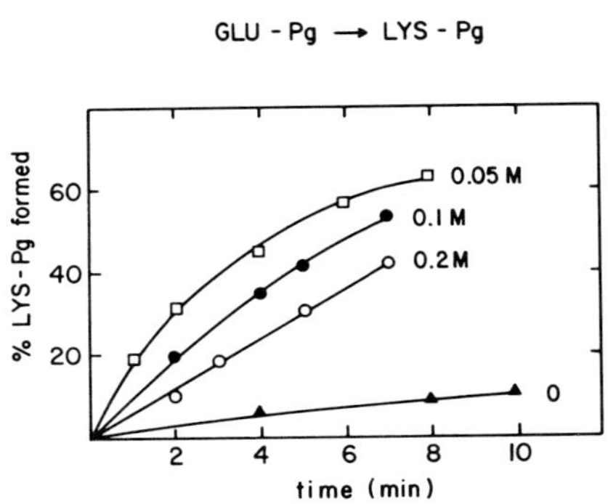

Fig. 6. The effect of L-lysine on the conversion of GLU-Pg to LYS-Pg, by plasmin.

shows the effect of L-lysine on the conversion of GLU-Pg to LYS-Pg, as catalyzed by plasmin. Again, the stimulating effect is maximal at 0.05 M L-lysine, after which an inhibition is again observed.

From these considerations, it is clear that compounds such as L-lysine may not only accelerate the activation of GLU-Pg, but may also affect the pathway of conversion of GLU-Pg to LYS-Pm, *i.e.*, may affect the proportion of GLU-Pg which is activated to LYS-Pm through LYS-Pg, or GLU-Pm (30). The data presented in Fig. 7 confirms these observations.

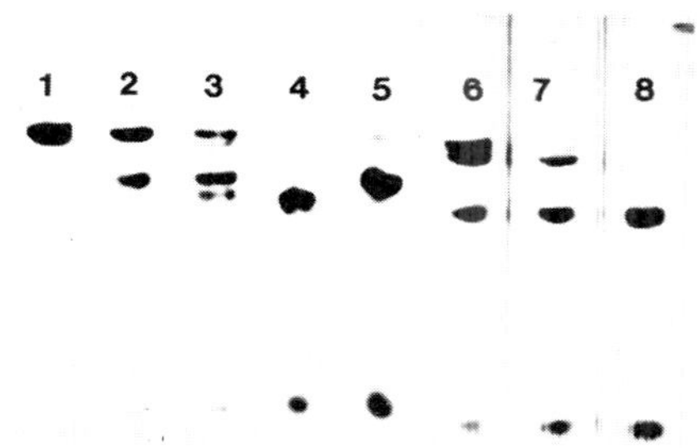

Fig. 7. Reduced sodium dodecyl sulfate gels depicting the activation of human GLU-Pg, by UK, in the presence and absence of L-Lysine.

The first 4 gels depict the time course of activation of GLU-Pg to LYS-Pm in the absence of L-lysine. The first gel is GLU-Pg and the fourth gel represents the heavy (Hb) and light (L) chains of LYS-Pm and gel 5 represents the heavy (Ha) and light (L) chains of GLU-Pm. Gels 2 and 3 are intermediate time points of the activation. In gel 2, at approximately 40% of activation, the only plasmin formed is GLU-Pm, as indicated by the presence of the GLU-Pm heavy (Ha) and light (L) chains. In gel 3, at approximately 70% of activation, still the predominant plasmin is GLU-Pm. Some LYS-Pm is formed here. Essentially all of the plasminogen remaining is GLU-Pg. At complete activation (gel 4) all plasmin is LYS-Pm. Therefore, in the absence of L-lysine, the predominant activation pathway is GLU-Pg → GLU-Pm → LYS-Pm. On the other hand, gels 6 and 7 represent incomplete activation mixtures of human GLU-Pg, performed in the presence of 0.05 M L-lysine. At 30% activation (gel 6), only LYS-Pm is obtained, and essentially 50% of the remaining plasminogen is LYS-Pg, precluding GLU-Pm formation from this fraction of plasminogen. At 70% activation (gel 7), all plasmin is LYS-Pm and all remaining plasminogen is LYS-Pg. Gel 8 represents the complete activation in the presence of 0.05 M L-lysine, and shows that LYS-Pm is again the most stable product. Thus, in the presence of L-lysine, it appears as though the predominant activation pathway is GLU-Pg → LYS-Pg → LYS-Pm. However, the activation mechanism which we proposed (above) can readily accommodate these effects.

Another interesting activator of human plasminogen is streptokinase. Streptokinase (SK) is a protein of molecular weight approximately 45,000 (35,36) isolated as a catabolic by-product of β-hemolytic streptococcus. The most interesting facet of the SK-induced activation of plasminogen is the fact that SK is not a protease. Thus, the question of how this non-proteolytic activator accomplishes cleavage of the peptide bond in plasminogen, to yield plasmin, has been the subject of intensive study. Studies from several different laboratories (37-41) have shown that there are two important steps in the activation of plasminogen by SK. The first step involves formation of the proteolytic species which actually activates plasminogen. The events which occur in the formation of plasminogen activator are generally agreed upon and are depicted as

$$\text{HPg} + \text{SK} \rightleftharpoons \text{SK}\cdot\text{HPg} \longrightarrow \text{SK}\cdot\text{HPg}' \longrightarrow \text{SK}^{*}\cdot\text{HPm}$$

$$\text{SK} + \text{HPm} \longrightarrow \text{SK}^{*}\cdot\text{HPm}$$

Here, human plasminogen (HPg) and SK bind in a 1:1 stoichiometry (SK•HPg). As a result of this interaction, an alteration occurs, producing an active proteolytic site in the complex (SK•HPg') (40). We have definitively shown this active site to be located in the plasminogen moiety of the complex (42). This particular complex, however, is unstable and is rapidly altered to a complex of streptokinase, which has now also lost a small peptide (36) and plasmin (SK*•HPm). Although plasmin, alone, will not activate plasminogen, the SK*•HPm (37-41), and likely SK•HPg' complexes (40,41,43) are potent activators of plasminogen. The above scheme also shows that SK*•HPm can also form from SK + human plasmin. Our laboratory has isolated and identified all of the above complexes (41).

We have further studied events which occur in the formation of plasminogen activator, in terms of the reactions of GLU-Pg, LYS-Pg, GLU-Pm, LYS-Pm, SK and SK*, within the activator complex (44). Figure 8 shows our scheme on the interconversions which occur.

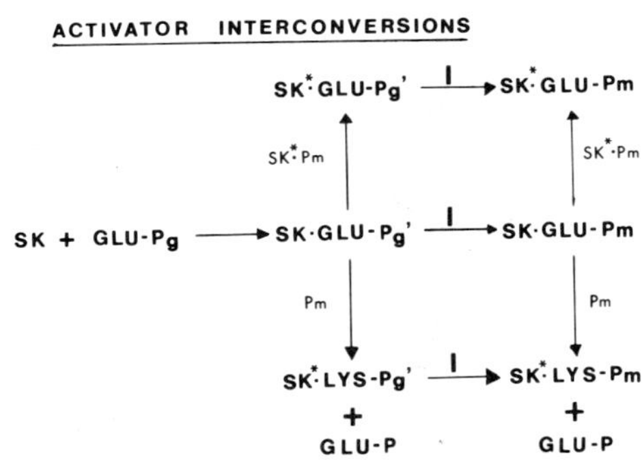

Fig. 8. Interconversions of the various streptokinase complexes with plasminogen and plasmin.

In this scheme (44), SK and human GLU-Pg ultimately form the SK•GLU-Pg' complex. In an intramolecular (I) step, the complex SK•GLU-Pm is formed. In the presence of small amounts of plasmin (Pm) or SK*•Pm, the SK moiety in the original SK•GLU-Pm complex, will lose an amino terminal peptide, and become SK*. Additionally, only Pm is capable of conversion of GLU-Pg' to LYS-Pg' within the complex. Either of these two complexes, SK*•GLU-Pg' or SK*•LYS-Pg', can form SK*•GLU-Pm or SK*•LYS-Pm, respectively in an intramolecular conversion. These latter two complexes can also form from SK•GLU-Pm, by action of SK*•Pm or Pm as shown in the scheme. The ultimate final activator complex is SK*•LYS-Pm, formed by any combination of steps shown in the scheme above.

The final step in plasminogen activation by streptokinase involves free plasmin generation by catalytic levels of plasminogen activator (SK*•LYS-Pm). The first, most widely favored mechanism (45,46) involves the enzymatic conversion of HPg to HPm by the activator complex, i.e.,

$$\text{HPg} \xrightarrow{\text{SK}^{*}\cdot\text{LYS-Pm}} \text{HPm}$$

Another, more indirect route, of plasmin formation has been recently postulated by Kosow (47). This is represented as:

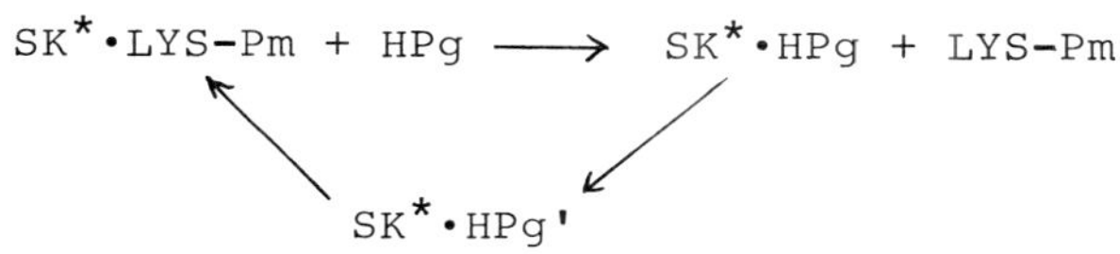

Here, it is believed that free plasminogen (HPg) displaces LYS-Pm from the SK*•LYS-Pm complex, yielding LYS-Pm. The SK*•HPg complex concomitantly formed then recyles to SK*•LYS-Pm, through SK*•HPg', in the manner postulated above. The SK*•LYS-Pm then continues the cycle.

Recent data from our laboratory are not in accord with the view of the Kosow mechanism. Table 4 shows some critical data in this regard (48).

TABLE 4. Transfer of SK* from SK*•HPm to Plasminogen and Plasmin

Incubation Time	% Label Recovered in SK*•HPm
0	91
15	87
30	91
control	91

Here, we incubated a catalytic level of SK*•^{125}I-HPm with a 1000-fold excess of unlabeled HPg. After 15 minutes of incubation, all HPg was converted to HPm, but essentially all of the label was recovered in the SK*•HPm complex. Lengthening the incubation time to 30 minutes did not alter the findings. Thus, it is evident that SK* is not transferred from the activator complex to other HPg or

HPm molecules, precluding the indirect activation mechanism of Kosow (47). We favor the mechanism suggesting that SK*•HPm is an enzyme for the conversion of plasminogen to plasmin.

REFERENCES

(1) S. V. Pizzo, M. L. Schwartz, R. L. Hill, and P. A. McKee, The effect of plasmin on the subunit structure of human fibrinogen, J. Biol. Chem. 247, 636 (1972).

(2) A. P. Kaplan, and K. F. Austen, A prealbumin activator of prekallikrein. II. Derivation of activators of prekallikrein from active Hageman factor by digestion with plasmin, J. Exp. Med. 133, 696 (1971).

(3) O. D. Ratnoff, and G. B. Naff, The conversion of $C1_s$ to C1 esterase by plasmin and trypsin, J. Exp. Med. 125, 337 (1967).

(4) P. C. Harpel, C1 inactivator inhibition by plasmin, J. Clin. Invest. 49, 568 (1970).

(5) P. A. Ward, A plasmin-split fragment of C3 as a new chemotactic factor, J. Exp. Med. 126, 189 (1967).

(6) D. Deutsch, and E. F. Mertz, Plasminogen: Purification from human plasma by affinity chromatography, Science 170, 1095 (1970).

(7) W. J. Brockway, and F. J. Castellino, Measurement of the binding of antifibrinolytic amino acids to various plasminogens, Arch. Biochem. Biophys. 151, 194 (1972).

(8) F. J. Castellino, G. E. Siefring, J. M. Sodetz, and R. K. Bretthauer, Amino terminal amino acid sequences and carbohydrate of the two major forms of rabbit plasminogen, Biochem. Biophys. Res. Comm. 53, 845 (1973).

(9) J. M. Sodetz, W. J. Brockway, and F. J. Castellino, Multiplicity of rabbit plasminogen. Physical characterization, Biochemistry 11, 4451 (1972).

(10) G. E. Siefring, and F. J. Castellino, Metabolic turnover studies of the two major forms of rat and rabbit plasminogen, J. Biol. Chem. 249, 1434 (1974).

(11) L. Summaria, F. Spitz, L. Arzadon, I. Boreisha, and K. C. Robbins, Isolation and characterization of the affinity chromatography forms of human glu- and lys-plasminogens and plasmins, J. Biol. Chem. 251, 3693 (1976).

(12) G. E. Siefring, and F. J. Castellino, The role of sialic acid in the determination of distinct properties of the isozymes of rabbit plasminogen, J. Biol. Chem. 249, 7742 (1974).

(13) S. Okamoto, S. Oshiba, H. Mihara, and U. Okomoto, Synthetic inhibitors of fibrinolysis: *in vitro* and *in vivo* mode of action, *Ann. N.Y. Acad. Sci.* 146, 414 (1968).

(14) E. E. Rickli, and P. A. Cuendert, Isolation of a plasmin - free human plasminogen with N-terminal glutamic acid, *Biochim. Biophys. Acta* 250, 447 (1971).

(15) B. N. Violand, and F. J. Castellino, Mechanism of the urokinase - catalyzed activation of human plasminogen, *J. Biol. Chem.* 251, 3906 (1976).

(16) K. C. Robbins, J. G. Boreisha, L. Arzadon, L. Summaria, and G. Barlow, Physical and chemical properties of the NH_2-terminal glutamic acid and lysine forms of human plasminogen and their derived plasmins with an NH_2-terminal lysine heavy (A) chain, *J. Biol. Chem.* 250, 4044 (1975).

(17) J. M. Sodetz, W. J. Brockway, K. G. Mann, and F. J. Castellino, The mechanism of activation of rabbit plasminogen by urokinase. Lack of a preactivation peptide, *Biochem. Biophys. Res. Comm.* 60, 729 (1974).

(18) J. M. Sodetz, and F. J. Castellino, Mechanism of the activation of rabbit plasminogen by urokinase, *J. Biol. Chem.* 250, 3041 (1975).

(19) K. C. Robbins, L. Summaria, B. Hsieh, and R. I. Shaw, The peptide chains of human plasmin. Mechanism of activation of human plasminogen to plasmin, *J. Biol. Chem.* 242, 4279 (1967).

(20) L. Sottrup-Jensen, H. Claeys, M. Zajdel, T. E. Petersen, and S. Magnusson, The primary structure of human plasminogen: Isolation of two lysine-binding fragments and one mini-plasminogen by elastase-catalyzed-specific limited proteolysis, *Prog. Chem. Fibrinolysis and Thrombolysis* 3, 191 (1978).

(21) M. L. Hayes, R. K. Bretthauer, and F. J. Castellino, Carbohydrate compositions of the rabbit plasminogen isozymes, *Arch. Biochem. Biophys.* 171, 651 (1975).

(22) W. R. Groskopf, B. Hsieh, L. Summaria, and K. C. Robbins, Studies on the active center of human plasmin: The serine and histidine residues, *J. Biol. Chem.* 244, 359 (1969).

(23) E. E. Rickli, and W. I. Otavsky, A new method of isolation and some properties of the heavy chain of human plasmin, *Eur. J. Biochem.* 59, 441 (1975).

(24) M. Gonzalez-Gronow, and F. J. Castellino, Purification and properties of the glu- and lys-human plasmin heavy chains, *J. Biol. Chem.* 252, 2175 (1977).

(25) L. Summaria, L. Arzadon, P. Bernabe, and K. C. Robbins, The activation of plasminogen to plasmin by urokinase in the presence of the plasmin inhibitor trasylol, *J. Biol. Chem.* 250, 3988 (1975).

(26) Alkjaersig, N., The purification and properties of human plasminogen, Biochem. J. 93, 171 (1964).

(27) B. N. Violand, J. M. Sodetz, and F. J. Castellino, The effect of ε-amino caproic acid on the gross conformation of plasminogen and plasmin, Arch. Biochem. Biophys. 170, 300 (1975).

(28) G. E. Siefring, and F. J. Castellino, De novo biosynthesis of plasminogen in the anephric rat, J. App. Physiol. 38, 114 (1975).

(29) G. Markus, J. L. Evers, and G. H. Hobika, Comparison of some properties of native (glu) and modified (lys) human plasminogen, J. Biol. Chem. 253, 733 (1978).

(30) B. N. Violand, and F. J. Castellino, The effect of α,ω-amino acids on human plasminogen structure and activation, J. Biol. Chem. 253, 5395 (1978).

(31) F. J. Castellino, W. J. Brockway, J. K. Thomas, H.-t. Liao, and A. B. Rawitch, Rotational diffusion analysis of the conformational alterations produced in plasminogen by certain antifibrinolytic amino acids, Biochemistry 12, 2787 (1973).

(32) N. O. Kjeldgoard, and J. Pluog, Urokinase, an activator of plasminogen from human urine, Biochim. Biophys. Acta 24, 289 (1957).

(33) G. H. Barlow, Urinary and kidney cell plasminogen activator, Methods in Enzymol. XLV, 239 (1976).

(34) H. Claeys, and J. Vermylen, Physiochemical and proenzyme properties of NH_2-terminal glutamic acid and NH_2-terminal lysine human plasminogen, Biochim. Biophys. Acta 342, 351 (1974).

(35) F. B. Taylor, and J. Botts, Purification and characterization of streptokinase with studies of streptokinase activation of plasminogen, Biochemistry 7, 232 (1968).

(36) W. J. Brockway, and F. J. Castellino, A characterization of native streptokinase and altered streptokinase isolated from a human plasminogen activator complex, Biochemistry 13, 2063 (1974).

(37) B. C. W. Hummel, F. F. Buck, and E. C. DeRenzo, Interaction of streptokinase with human plasminogen. III Plasmin and activator activities in reaction mixtures of streptokinase and human plasminogen and human plasmin of various molar ratios, J. Biol. Chem. 241, 3474 (1966).

(38) C.-M. Ling, L. Summaria, and K. C. Robbins, Isolation and characterization of bovine plasminogen activator from a human plasminogen-streptokinase mixture, J. Biol. Chem. 242, 1419 (1967).

(39) D. K. McClintock and P. H. Bell, The mechanism of activation of human plasminogen by streptokinase, Biochem. Biophys. Res. Comm. 43, 694 (1971).

(40) K. N. N. Reddy, and G. Markus, Mechanism of activation of human plasminogen by streptokinase. Presence of an active center in the streptokinase-plasminogen complex, J. Biol. Chem. 247, 1683 (1972).

(41) L. A. Schick, and F. J. Castellino, Interaction of streptokinase and rabbit plasminogen, Biochemistry 12, 4315 (1973).

(42) L. A. Schick, and F. J. Castellino, Direct evidence for the formation of an active site in the plasminogen moiety of the streptokinase-human plasminogen activator complex, Biochem. Biophys. Res. Comm. 57, 47 (1974).

(43) G. Markus, and W. C. Werkheiser, The interaction of streptokinase with plasminogen. I. Functional properties of the activated enzymes, J. Biol. Chem. 239, 2637 (1964).

(44) S. P. Bajaj, and F. J. Castellino, Activation of human plasminogen by equimolar levels of streptokinase, J. Biol. Chem. 252, 492 (1977).

(45) L. Summaria, C.-M. Ling, W. R. Groskopf, and K. C. Robbins, The active site of bovine plasminogen activator. Interaction of streptokinase with human plasminogen and plasmin, J. Biol. Chem. 243, 144 (1968).

(46) F. F. Buck, B. C. W. Hummel, and E. C. DeRenzo, Interaction of streptokinase and human plasminogen. V. Studies on the nature and mechanism of formation of the enzymatic site of the activator complex, J. Biol. Chem. 243, 3648 (1968).

(47) D. P. Kosow, Kinetic mechanism of the activation of human plasminogen by streptokinase, Biochemistry 14, 4459 (1975).

(48) M. Gonzalez-Gronow, and F. J. Castellino, The mechanism of activation of human plasminogen by the activator complex, streptokinase plasmin, J. Biol. Chem. 253, 1090 (1978).

THE FORMATION OF PLASMINOGEN ACTIVATOR DURING VIRAL TRANSFORMATION OF CHICK EMBRYO FIBROBLASTS

Dr. Myung-Hee Park, Dr. William H. Berg and
Dr. John M. Buchanan
Department of Biology
Massachusetts Institute of Technology
Cambridge, Massachusetts 02139

ABSTRACT

The production of plasminogen activator is one of the pleiotypic responses of the cell to transformation by tumor viruses. It is a catalyst for the conversion of serum plasminogen to plasmin which is the principal component of the fibrinolytic system. Since the transformation phenotype can be produced and maintained in the absence of plasminogen, plasminogen activator may play some other important role in cellular transformation.

With the discovery that the primary transforming agent produced in cells transformed with Rous sarcoma virus is a 60,000 dalton protein with protein kinase activity, we are looking for one of the several putative physiological substrates of its action. By use of ^{3}H-labeled diisopropylfluorophosphate (DFP), a specific inhibitor of the so-called "serine" proteases or esterases, we have identified a readily labeled 100,000 dalton component of normal resting and growing chick plasma membranes that is lost upon infection with the non-defective (nd) Rous sarcoma virus but not with the transformation-defective (td) virus. We have also found in transformed cells one species of plasminogen activator (M_r 37,000) in the plasma membrane and three species (M_r 70,000, 50,000 and 37,000) exported into the harvest fluid. The 50,000 dalton enzyme is readily labeled with ^{3}H-DFP. We are currently developing peptide maps of the 100,000 dalton component of membranes of normal cells and the 50,000 dalton plasminogen activator of the harvest fluid of transformed cells in order to establish a precursor-product relationship. The purpose of these experiments is to establish one site of the action of the sarc protein kinase activity in the transformed cell.

INTRODUCTION

Several experimental approaches have been taken to identify cell surface proteins that may be involved in the transformation of fibroblasts by tumorigenic viruses (1). Specifically, changes have been observed in the composition of cell proteins labeled with ^{35}S-SO_4 or methionine, ^{125}I or ^{131}I, ^{14}C or ^{3}H-carbohydrate derivatives, or by fluorescent dyes. Although consistent patterns of labeled proteins have been obtained in a comparison of the cell surface proteins of normal and Rous sarcoma virus-infected chick embryo fibroblasts, none of these investigations has been able to establish any one of these components as a primary agent of the transformation process.

For these reasons we initiated a new approach for the identification of sarcoma specific proteins in which we have compared by use of an in vitro translation system the radioactive products translated from RNA derived from non-defective (nd) Prague B Rous sarcoma virus and its transformation defective (td) counterpart. Proteins of three sizes, approximately of 60,000, 25,000 and 18,000 daltons, have been recognized, which are present in the SDS polyacrylamide electropherograms of radioactive proteins produced from the nd RNA but not from the td RNA (2,3). These proteins are not precipitated by antisera of the structural proteins of the Rous sarcoma virus (2). Comparable experiments have been reported by Beemon and Hunter (4) and by Erikson and his colleagues (5). Erikson has prepared antibodies to the 60,000 dalton protein (6) and demonstrated that the latter is capable of catalyzing the phosphorylation of its own IgG antibody (7), and thus has protein kinase activity. However, it is recognized that the antibody is only a fortuitous substrate of the kinase activity. The physiological substrates remain to be identified.

The characteristics of RSV-transformed as compared to normal chick embryo fibroblasts are: increased transport of glucose, ions and uridine, increase in rate of cell growth and cell density, decreased requirement for serum, production of surface ruffles together with reorganization of basic cell membrane structures, and finally production of proteases, including a plasminogen activator, that is inhibited by diisopropylfluorophosphate (DFP). This reagent reacts covalently with a reactive serine residue of several proteases and esterases.

This special property of DFP has enabled us to devise a unique approach to the identification of a possible precursor in normal cells to a characteristic product of transformation in the membrane and harvest fluid of RSV-infected chick embryo fibroblasts. We have been operating on the premise that the 60,000 dalton sarcoma (or sarc) protein kinase exerts a pleiotypic effect on a number of structural proteins of normal cells causing them to assume functions or activities characteristic of the transformed phenotype.

The production and secretion of a protease, a plasminogen activator, is a particularly characteristic feature of transformed cells. Christman and Acs (8) have purified to homogeneity a plasminogen activator of 50,000 daltons consisting of at least one subunit of 25,000 daltons from the harvest fluid of SV-40 transformed hamster cells. Rifkin et al. (9) have isolated a species of 48,000 daltons from human melanoma cells. Finally, Unkeless et al. (10) and Quigley (11) have isolated from plasma membranes and harvest fluids of RSV-transformed chick embryo fibroblasts a 39,000 dalton species, which is readily labeled with 70 μM DFP and which upon reduction yields a subunit of approximately 28,000 daltons. The chick cell plasminogen activator is found both intra and extracellularly in cultures of chick embryo fibroblasts infected with wild type Rous sarcoma virus. As far as is known, plasminogen found in plasma or serum is its only known substrate. However, the transformation of cells does occur in the absence of plasminogen. Therefore, plasmin is not necessary for the production or maintenance of the transformation phenotype. These latter experiments reported nearly three years ago from our laboratory (12) indicated that plasminogen activator may have another cellular substrate that is more directly associated with transformation.

The data to be presented in the following experimental section will document the conclusion that (1) a DFP-reactive protein of approximately 100,000 daltons is present in the membranes of normal chick embryo fibroblasts and is lost upon infection with the non-defective Rous sarcoma virus. In addition to a plasminogen activator in the plasma membranes of transformed chick cells, at least three species of enzyme have been isolated from harvest fluids. Of the three activities ranging in molecular weight from 70,000, 50,000 and 37,000, the second is particularly sensitive to labeling with ^{3}H-DFP.

The use of DFP to label components of plasma membranes of normal cells that are putative precursors of DFP-sensitive proteases of the harvest fluid and membranes of transformed cells is a new approach to a study of cell surface changes occurring during transformation. It makes use of a chemical property of a putative precursor in normal cells, i.e., its capacity to react with DFP, as a means of its identification and of establishing a relationship to a significant product of transformation, namely, a plasminogen activator.

MATERIALS AND METHODS

Fibrinolytic Assay

Highly purified fibrinogen, which was a generous gift of Dr. David Waugh, contained sufficient plasminogen to serve as substrate for plasminogen activator far in excess of that required for the enzyme concentrations present in concentrated protein solutions of harvest fluids of transformed cells.

Fibrin plates were prepared by mixing 1 mg/ml of fibrinogen in 0.1 M Tris-HCl, pH 8, with an equal volume of 1.5% agar in 0.1 M Tris-HCl, pH 8. The temperature of the mixture was kept close to 40°C. Purified thrombin was added at a concentration of 1 NIH unit/ml, and 5 ml of the resulting mixture were rapidly poured into 60 mm falcon plates. When the fibrin clots solidified, a hole 0.35 cm in diameter was made. Ten µl of test sample were added to the well and incubated at 37°C for 24 hr. The diameter of the cleared ring in the fibrin field was measured to estimate the fibrinolytic activity and is roughly proportional to the log of the concentration of the enzyme (13). The standards of different dilutions of urokinase approximate this relationship particularly at the higher concentrations of enzyme (Table 1, experiment 7). This method is not particularly sensitive in estimating plasminogen activator activity, but it is useful in locating activity in a large number of analytical samples.

Tissue Culture

Primary chick embryo fibroblasts were grown in medium 199 containing 10% calf serum (Colorado Serum Company). Secondary chick embryo fibroblasts were used as such or infected with Prague B -Rous sarcoma virus (PRB-RSV), with Schmidt-Ruppin RSV, subgroup A or D (SRA and SRD, respectively), or with the transformation-defective (td) Prague B RSV. The medium was changed daily with Dulbecco's modified Eagle's medium (DME) containing tryptose phosphate broth, calf serum and chicken serum in the following percentages, respectively; 2-1-1 or 5-3-1. Cultures infected with the non-defective viruses were well transformed after 4 or 5 days.

Preparation and Labeling of Proteins of Membranes and Harvest Fluids of Normal and Transformed Fibroblasts

Crude preparations of plasma membranes were obtained by the method of Unkeless et al. (10). Serum-free harvest fluids were prepared according to the method described by Unkeless et al. (10) with minor modifications, namely that the media were clarified of virus and were not acidified to pH 3.5 before addition of ammonium sulfate for concentration of proteins. Cells and virus of the harvest fluids were removed by centrifugation at 10,000 rpm for 10 min, followed by centrifugation at 10,000 rpm for 5-6 hr in a small Sorvall GSA rotor. The cleared harvest fluid was kept frozen at -20°C until ready for use. The proteins of the harvest fluid were precipitated by the slow addition of ammonium sulfate to a final concentration of 70 g/100 ml. The precipitate was centrifuged at 11,000 rpm for

Table 1 Fibrinolysis Assay of Plasminogen Activator Activity of Membranes and Harvest Fluids of Normal and Transformed Chick Embryo Fibroblasts

Experiment	System Tested	Diameter of Cleared Ring (cm)
1	normal CEF membrane	0.35
	SRD-CEF membrane	0.75
2	normal CEF harvest fluid	0.35
	SRD-CEF harvest fluid	0.8
	SRD-CEF harvest fluid + 1 mM DFP	0.7
3	70K protein of SRD-CEF harvest fluid	0.75
	70K protein + 0.1 mM DFP	0.75
	70K protein + 1 mM DFP	0.68
4	37K protein of SRD-CEF harvest fluid	0.85
	37K protein + 0.1 mM DFP	0.85
	37K protein + 1 mM DFP	0.75
5	urokinase (10 units)	3.6
	urokinase + 1 mM DFP	1.2
6	SRD-CEF harvest fluid	0.8
	10^{-1} dilution of SRD-CEF harvest fluid	0.65
	10^{-2} dilution of SRD-CEF harvest fluid	0.4
7	urokinase (10 units)	3.6
	urokinase (1 unit)	2.6
	urokinase (0.1 unit)	1.8
	urokinase (0.01 unit)	0.9
	control (no urokinase)	0.35

Fibrinolytic activities were measured on plasminogen containing fibrin plates. The diameter of cleared ring after incubation for 24 hr at 37°C is reported without substraction of that of the initial well. The diameter of 0.35 cm represents zero activity. Abbreviations: CEF, chick embryo fibroblasts, SRD-CEF, CEF infected with nd Schmidt-Ruppin Rous sarcoma virus, subgroup D.

---

15 min in a Sorvall GSA rotor and resuspended in a minimum volume of the desired buffer and then dialyzed against the same buffer to remove excess salt. A 100-fold concentration of proteins was achieved by this procedure.

In order to label the proteins of the plasma membrane with ^{3}H-DFP the membrane pellet was resuspended in TD buffer (0.14 M NaCl, 0.005 M KCl, 0.024 M Tris-HCl and 0.0004 M Na_2HPO_4, pH 7.4) to a protein concentration of 10 mg/ml. ^{3}H-DFP was added at a concentration of 10 to 50 μM, and the membrane suspension was incubated at 37°C for 2 to 24 hr. The labeled membrane was then sedimented by centrifugation and washed once with TD buffer to free the sample of unreacted ^{3}H-DFP.

The washed membrane pellet was dissolved in sample buffer containing 1% SDS and prepared for electrophoresis on a 5-15% gradient SDS-polyacrylamide gel as described by Laemmli (14). The sample was incubated either with or without 2-mercaptoethanol for one min at 100°. For the detection of the ^{3}H-DFP labeled bands, the gel was subjected to fluorography as described by Laskey and Mills (15).

The concentrated proteins of the harvest fluid were reacted with 10 to 50 μM ^{3}H-DFP in TD buffer for 2 to 3 hr at 37°C. Free ^{3}H-DFP was removed by dialysis first against TD buffer and then against distilled water. The resulting labeled harvest fluid concentrate was lyophilized and redissolved in sample buffer for SDS polyacrylamide gel electrophoresis.

Chromatography on a Sephadex G 200 Column

The ammonium sulfate precipitate of cleared harvest fluid was resuspended in the minimum volume of column buffer (0.1 M Tris-HCl, pH 8.1, 0.5 M NaCl), dialyzed against the column buffer, and then applied on a Sephadex G 200 column (2.5 x 55 cm).

RESULTS

DFP-Labeled Proteins of Membranes of Normal and Viral-Infected Chick Embryo Fibroblasts

As shown in Fig. 1 we have compared the capacity of ^{3}H-DFP to combine covalently with proteins of the membranes of normal cells, both growing and resting, and of cells infected with the transformation-defective (td) and non-defective (nd) Rous sarcoma virus. After SDS-polyacrylamide gel electrophoresis and subsequent fluorography we were able to identify one strongly DFP-labeled band in the electropherogram of proteins derived from plasma membranes of normal growing or resting chick fibroblasts. The protein migrated to a position corresponding to a size of 100,000 daltons. The labeled membrane protein of 100,000 daltons was missing from cells transformed with Prague B non-defective Rous sarcoma virus (channels, A,F,K, Fig. 1). The presence of the band in the electropherograms of proteins of cells infected with the transformation-defective (td) Rous sarcoma virus is evidence that the loss of the band is a result of transformation rather than of viral infection alone (channels B,G,L, Fig. 1). The same relative intensity of bands was obtained whether the membrane proteins were incubated with 50 μM ^{3}H-DFP for either 1.5 hr at 37°C (K,L), for 3 hr at 37° (A-D) or for 24 hr at room temperature (F-I). In channels E and J, ^{35}S-methionine-labeled translation products of nd Rous sarcoma virus RNA are shown to calibrate the sizes of proteins measured in this experiment.

On the basis of previous information (10,11) one might have expected to detect an increase of DFP-labeled components in the membrane of transformed cells attributable to plasminogen activator. Although several minor bands of DFP-labeled proteins smaller than 100,000 daltons were evident in the electropherograms of proteins of normal and transformed cells, the pattern of these bands was approximately the same in both instances. Therefore, as judged by the intensity of labeling of a component with ^{3}H-DFP, we could not detect a product in the membranes of transformed cells comparable to the loss of the DFP-sensitive, 100,000 dalton protein of normal cells.

Production of Proteases (Plasminogen Activators) by Cells Transformed by Rous Sarcoma Viruses

Membrane Proteases: As evident from previous reports (10,11) and from our data,

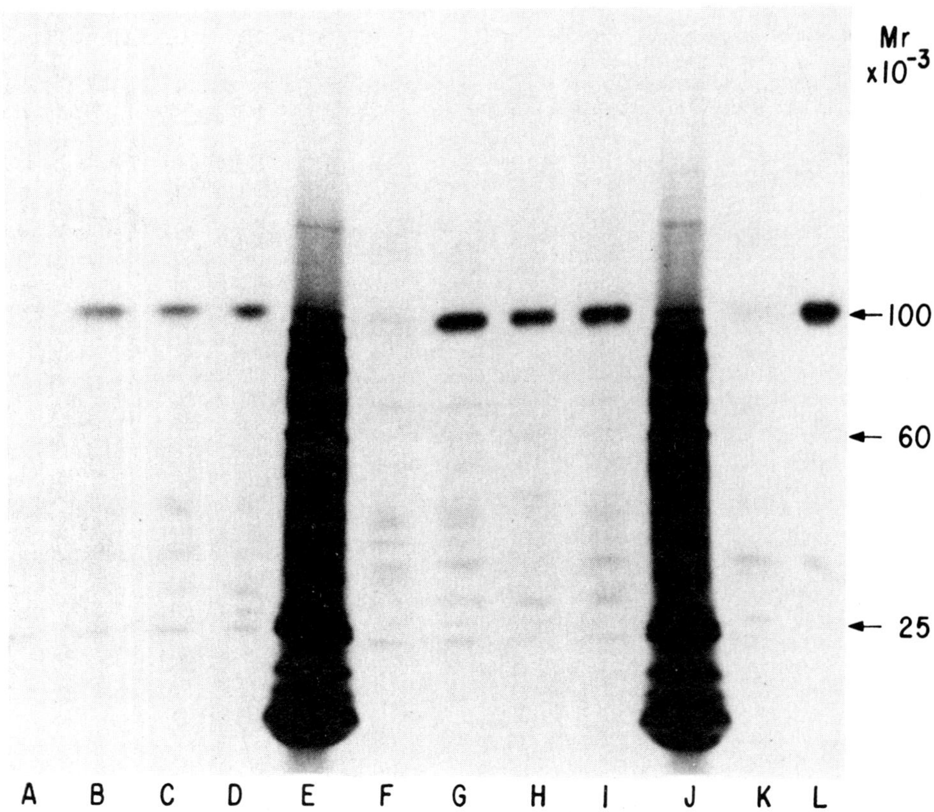

Fig. 1. ^{3}H-DFP Labeling of Membranes

Fig. 1. A-D; membranes were labeled with 50 µM ^{14}C-DFP for 3 hours at 37°C. A, nd-PrB-RSV CEF; B, td-PrB-RSV CEF; C, normal growing CEF; D, normal resting CEF. F-I; membranes were labeled with 50 µM of ^{3}H-DFP for 24 hour at room temperature. F, nd-PrB-RSV CEF; G, td-PrB-RSV CEF; H, normal growing CEF; I, normal resting CEF. K-L; membranes were labeled with 50 µM of ^{3}H-DFP for 1.5 hour at 37°C. K, nd-PrB-RSV CEF; L, td-PrB-RSV CEF. E-J; cell-free translation of nd-PrB-RSV mRNA in the presence of ^{35}S-methionine for calibration of membrane protein bands. All gels were run under reducing conditions.

(Table 1, experiment 1) plasma membranes of transformed chick embryo fibroblasts have a high level of fibrinolytic activity when added to plasminogen-containing plates, whereas membranes of normal fibroblasts have little or no plasminogen activator activity. In order to characterize this activity we dissolved the membranes of both normal and transformed cells (SRA-CEF) in sample buffer containing 1% SDS and subjected the proteins to electrophoresis on an SDS-containing polyacrylamide gel column. The samples had not been reduced with mercaptoethanol in order to retain proteolytic activity. The gel columns were sliced into 3 mm sections, and the plasminogen activator activity of each section measured by the assay described in Materials and Methods. One species of plasminogen activator activity was identified with a molecular weight of approximately 37,000 (Fig. 2).

Since the ^{3}H-DFP labeled proteins were analyzed on reducing gels and enzyme activity on non-reducing gels, the location of a putative ^{3}H-labeled component representing this protease activity would not necessarily reside in the 37,000 dalton area of the electropherogram.

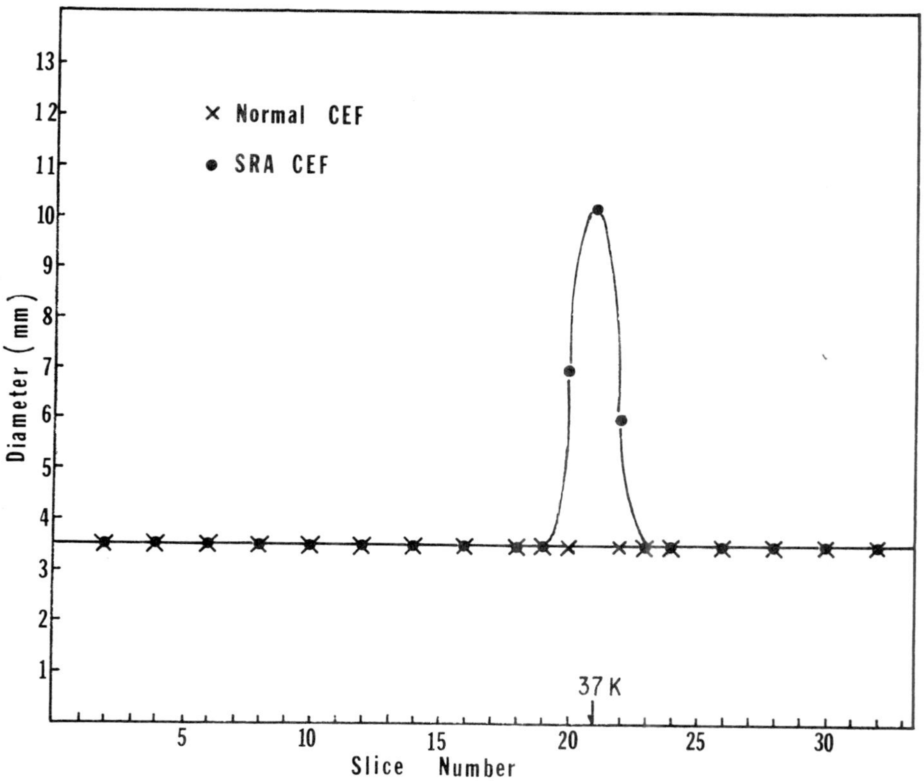

Fig. 2. Electrophoresis of Fibrinolytic Activity of Membranes on SDS-Polyacrylamide Gel

Fig. 2. Membranes of normal CEF and SRA-CEF were electrophoresed on SDS-polyacrylamide gels. Each gel was sliced into sections of 3 mm thickness. The fibrinolytic activity of each slice was tested on plasminogen-containing fibrin plates.

Closed Circle (●), SRA-RSV CEF membranes;
Cross (X), normal CEF membranes

Esterase Activities of Membranes: Although DFP is generally viewed as a protease inhibitor, it has a relatively broad specificity for both proteases and esterases with serine at the active site. In fact many of the so-called serine proteases exhibit esterase activity.

Normal cells have been reported to contain a membrane-bound acetylcholine esterase of approximately 100,000 daltons, which with a serine at its active site is readily inhibited and labeled covalently with ^{3}H-DFP (16). In collaboration with Dr. Su-Ray Lee we have measured the acetylcholine esterase activity (17) of normal and transformed membranes that had been extracted with the non-denaturing detergent NP_{40}. The amount of acetylcholine esterase activity was exceedingly low in either sample, and within the experimental error there was no difference in the activities of either the normal or transformed membrane preparation. It therefore seems unlikely that the 100,000 dalton component of the membrane of normal cells is acetylcholine esterase. There is in fact no evidence as yet that it possesses any enzymatic activity, but may instead be a zymogen, or the precursor of an active protease or esterase present in the membranes or, more likely, exported into the harvest fluid of transformed cells.

Proteolytic Enzymes Released into Harvest Fluid of Transformed Cells

Separation on a Sephadex G 200 Column: Since a highly DFP-sensitive plasminogen activator could not be located in the membranes of RSV-transformed cells (Fig. 1), we have examined the harvest fluids of normal and transformed cells to identify proteolytic activities (Table 1, experiment 2). As indicated in the Methods and Materials section, the proteins were concentrated by use of ammonium sulfate precipitation.

In a preliminary experiment the concentrated proteins from the harvest fluids of Prague B RSV-transformed cells were applied to a Sephadex G 200 column and eluted with column buffer (see Methods and Materials). Five peaks of proteolytic activity could be distinguished (Fig. 3). These same five activities could be separated and distinguished regardless of whether the harvest fluid was maintained near neutrality during ammonium sulfate precipitation or whether it was acidified to pH 3.5 as prescribed in the procedure of Unkeless et al. (10).

This experiment then revealed that there is more than one form of proteolytic activity released into the harvest fluid of transformed cells. Since these activities were not evident when plasminogen-free fibrinogen was used to prepare the fibrin plates, we assume that they are specific for plasminogen activation or that plasminogen via plasmin serves as an amplifying system for detecting low levels of proteolytic activities that may have more than one cellular substrate.

Separation on SDS-Polyacrylamide Gel Columns: As another approach to the separation and study of the proteolytic activities produced and exported by transformed cells, the concentrated proteins of the harvest fluid were dissolved in sample buffer containing 1% SDS and were subjected to electrophoresis on SDS-polyacrylamide gel columns with omission of the reducing agent 2-mercaptoethanol. The gel was sliced into sections 3 mm thick, and the activity of each slice was tested on plasminogen-containing fibrin plates. Since preparation of samples for electrophoresis requires heating them at 100° in SDS, only those resistant enzymes are detected.

As shown in Fig. 4 three bands with plasminogen activator activity were detected in the harvest fluid of transformed cells, whereas none was evident in harvest fluids of normal cells. The three bands traveled on the polyacrylamide gels with apparent molecular weights of 70,000, 50,000 and 37,000. The 37,000 dalton protein exhibited the highest activity and the 50,000 dalton protein the lowest.

The above experiment was then repeated with the modification that the proteins of the concentrated harvest fluid were first reacted for 2 hr at 37° with 10 μM ^{3}H-DFP. After electrophoresis, half of each slice was tested for fibrinolytic activity; the other half was measured for its radioactivity. As shown in Fig. 5 a 50,000 dalton protein was heavily labeled with 10 μM DFP, whereas activities at 70,000 and 37,000 reacted only slightly at this concentration of inhibitor.

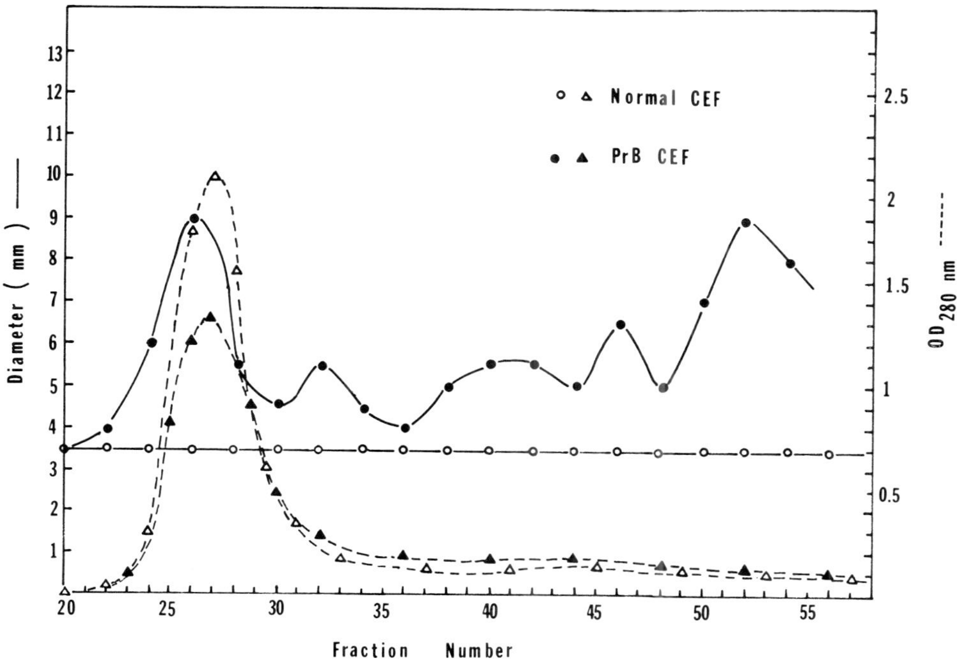

Fig. 3. Separation of Fibrinolytic Activities of Harvest Fluid on a Sephadex G-200 Column

Fig. 3. Harvest fluids of normal CEF and PrB-RSV CEF were fractionated on a Sephadex G-200 column (2.5 cm diameter x 55 cm length). 4.5-ml fractions were collected. Fibrinolytic activity of each fraction was tested on plasminogen-containing fibrin plates. Closed circles (●), fibrinolytic activity of PrB-RSV CEF harvest fluid; open circles (O), fibrinolytic activity of normal CEF harvest fluid; closed triangle (▲), optical density of PrB-RSV CEF harvest fluid; open triangle (Δ), optical density of normal CEF harvest fluid.

In view of the residual activity in the 50,000 dalton region of the electropherogram it is possible either that all of this plasminogen activator species was not labeled under the conditions of our experiment or that other forms of this size are present that are more resistant to inactivation by the inhibitor.

In order to test further the sensitivity of the 70,000 and 37,000 dalton species to inhibition with unlabeled DFP, bands containing these activities were excised from gel columns for incubation with DFP at higher concentrations, namely 0.1 and 1 mM. Only at 1 mM DFP was there a decrease in activity. Since our method of assay reflects changes in enzyme activity with a low sensitivity, we have calibrated the extent of ring development in the fibrin field as a function of the concentration of the untreated harvest fluid. As may be seen in Table 1, a tenfold decrease in concentration of harvest fluid reduces the ring diameter from 8 to 6.5 mm (Table 1, experiment 6). Hence the reduction of ring diameter of 1 mm by samples of the 70,000 and 37,000 dalton proteolytic activities may represent considerable inhibition (Table 1, experiments 3 and 4). Further experi-

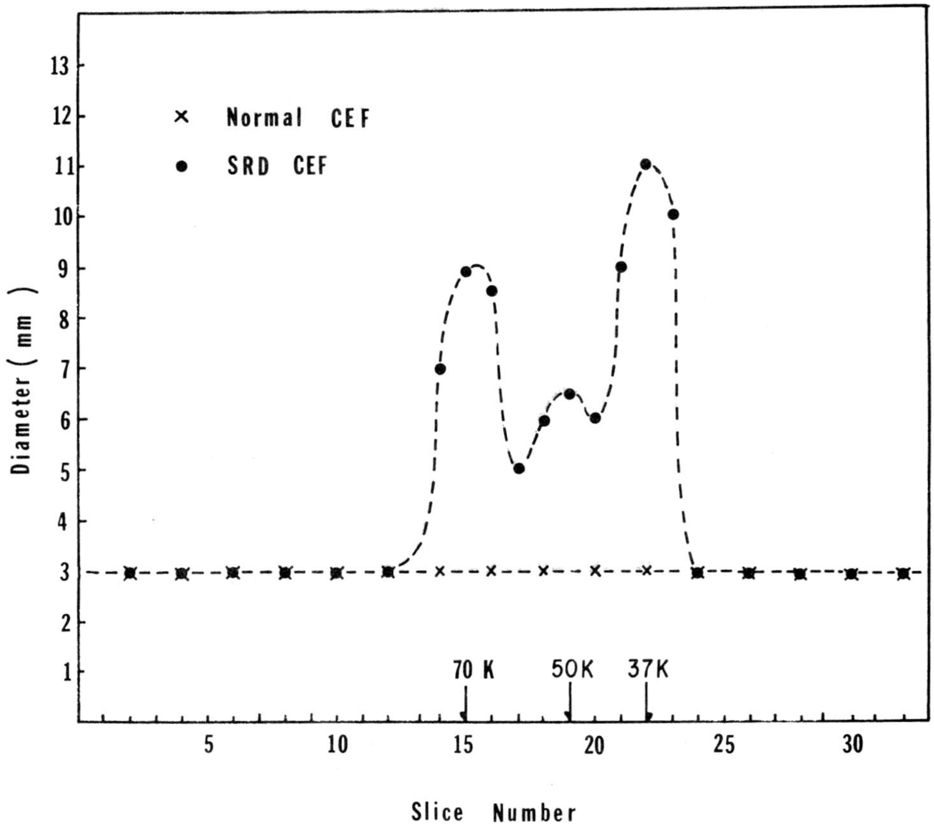

Fig. 4. Electrophoresis of Fibrinolytic Activity of Harvest Fluid on SDS-Polyacrylamide Gels

Fig. 4. Proteins of harvest fluids of normal CEF and SRD-RSV CEF were electrophoresed on SDS-polyacrylamide gels. The gel was sliced into 3 mm sections and the fibrinolytic activity of each slice was tested on plasminogen-containing fibrin plates.

Closed Circle (●), SRD-RSV CEF harvest fluid;
Cross (X), normal CEF harvest fluid

---

ments are required with a more sensitive assay system to establish this point quantitatively. When 10 units of urokinase were reacted with 1 mM DFP, less than 1% of the activity remained (Table 1, cf experiments 5 and 7).

DISCUSSION

The RNA of Rous sarcoma virus (RSV) is believed to contain a gene, termed the sarcoma or sarc gene, that is responsible for the cellular transformation of infected fibroblasts in culture and the induction of sarcomas in animals. Deletion or transformation-defective (td) mutants that lack this gene can infect

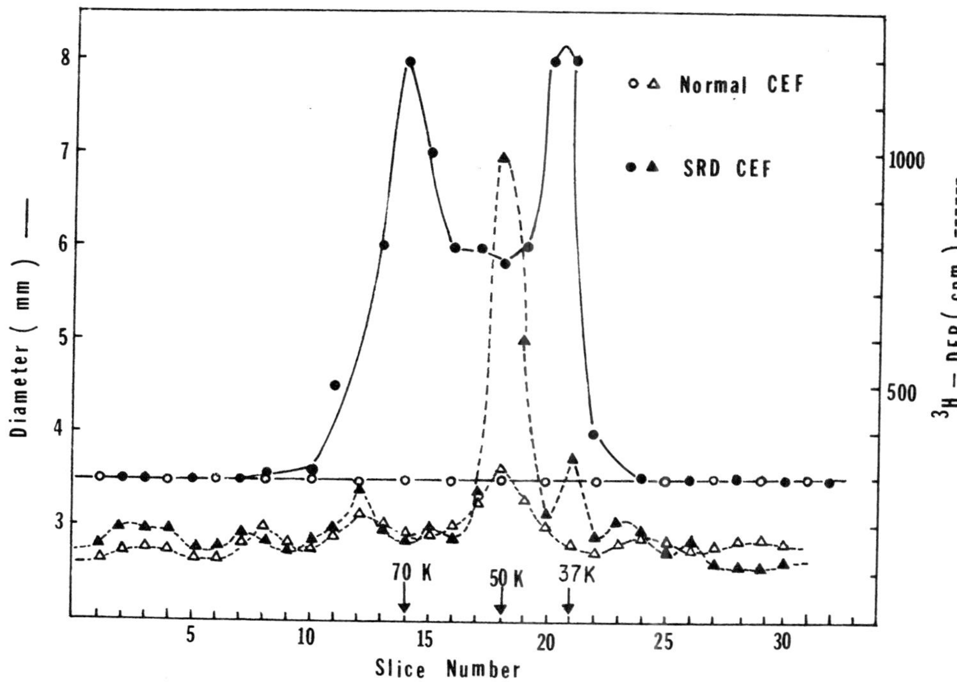

Fig. 5. Fibrinolytic Activities of ^{3}H-DFP-Labeled Harvest Fluid

Fig. 5. The details are the same as in Fig. 4 except that concentrated harvest fluids were labeled with ^{3}H-DFP (10 μM) for 2 hours at 37°C. Half of each slice was tested for fibrinolytic activity. The other half was used to measure radioactivity.

Closed Circle (●), fibrinolytic activity of SRD-RSV CEF harvest fluid;

Open Circle (O), fibrinolytic activity of normal CEF harvest fluid;

Closed Triangle (▲), ^{3}H-DFP-labeling of SRD-RSV harvest fluid;

Open Triangle (Δ), ^{3}H-DFP-labeling of normal CEF harvest fluid.

---

cells and can replicate at the normal rate but are not capable of generating the transformed phenotype (18,19). The existence of temperature-sensitive mutants of RSV for cellular transformation, which map in the sarc gene region, suggests that a protein coded for by this gene is specifically involved in cellular transformation (20). Oligonucleotide mapping studies of RNA from transforming RSV and deletion mutants have estimated the size of the sarc gene to be 10-15% of the 38 S viral RNA (21,22). Recent electron microscope analyses of heteroduplexes between viral RNA and cDNA have estimated that the sarc gene may comprise 20% of the 38 S genome, enough information to code for a 65,000 dalton protein (23).

Recent investigations from this (3) and other laboratories (5) have identified a 60,000 dalton protein as being a translation product of this sarc gene. Smaller translation products of 25,000 and 18,000 (2-4) with structures corresponding to that of the larger sarc protein have also been described. Collett and Erikson have isolated the 60,000-dalton protein from RSV-transformed chick cells and have shown that the antigen has protein kinase activity towards its own IgG antibody, which is a fortuitous substrate.

The research reported in this communication has been conducted on the hypothesis that there are several physiological substrates in the cell that react with the 60,000 dalton sarc-specific protein kinase during transformation and that the pleiotypic response of the cell to viral transformation can be explained in terms of the action of this enzyme.

The elaboration of a plasminogen activator(s) is especially characteristic of a transformed cell. Since the more commonly studied cellular plasminogen activator is a so-called "serine" protease, it reacts with and is covalently labeled by ^{3}H-labeled DFP (10). In this communication we have made a search for a putative precursor in normal cells that is converted to an active plasminogen activator during transformation. The chemical tool for this investigation has been DFP. We have taken this direct chemical approach based on a metabolic property of the transformed cell as a means of following cell surface changes that are specifically related to the transformation process.

We have been able to identify a 100,000 dalton protein of either growing or resting chick embryo fibroblasts that is labeled with DFP and that is lost when cells are infected with a non-defective transforming virus. The retention of this protein in cells infected with the transformation-defective counterpart is evidence that the disappearance of this protein is transformation-specific.

A plasminogen activator of 37,000 daltons has been identified in the plasma membranes of transformed cells. Plasminogen activators of several sizes are found in the harvest fluids of transformed cells but not of normal cells. One species of approximately 50,000 daltons is readily labeled by relatively low concentrations (10 μM) of ^{3}H-DFP. We are currently isolating this protein and the 100,000 dalton protein of normal cells to establish their structural relationship, if any. By this procedure we would like to pinpoint one membrane protein of normal cells as a target of action of the sarcoma-specific protein kinase.

ACKNOWLEDGMENT

This work was supported by grant number BC-206B from the American Cancer Society. We wish to thank Mrs. Nancy Armstrong for technical assistance.

REFERENCES

1. Hynes, R.O., Cell Surface proteins and Malignant Transformation, Biochim. Biophys. Acta 458, 73 (1976).

2. Kamine, J. & Buchanan, J.M., Cell Free Synthesis of Two Proteins Unique to RNA of Transforming Virions of Rous Sarcoma Virus, Proc. Natl. Acad. Sci., USA 74, 2011 (1977).

3. Kamine, J., Burr, J.G. & Buchanan, J.M., Multiple Forms of Sarc Proteins from Rous Sarcoma Virus RNA, Proc. Natl. Acad. Sci., USA 75, 366 (1978).

4. Beemon, K. & Hunter, T., In Vitro Translation Yields a Possible Rous Sarcoma Virus SRC Gene Product, Proc. Natl. Acad. Sci., USA 74, 3302 (1977).

5. Purchio, A.F., Erikson, E. & Erikson, R.L., Translation of 35S and Subgenomic Regions of Avian Sarcoma Virus RNA, Proc. Natl. Acad. Sci., USA 74, 4661 (1977).

6. Brugge, J.S. & Erikson, R.L., Identification of a Transformation-Specific Antigen Induced by an Avian Sarcoma Virus, Nature 269, 346 (1977).

7. Collett, M.S. & Erikson, R.L., Protein Kinase Activity Associated with the Avian Sarcoma Virus Gene Product, Proc. Natl. Acad. Sci., USA 75, 2021 (1978).

8. Christman, J.K. & Acs, G., Purification and Characterization of a Cellular Fibrinolytic Factor Associated with Oncogenic Transformation: The Plasminogen Activator from SV-40-Transformed Hamster Cells, Biochim. Biophys. Acta 340, 339 (1974).

9. Rifkin, D., Loeb, J., Moore, G., & Reich, E., Properties of Plasminogen Activators Formed by Neoplastic Human Cell Cultures, J. Exp. Med. 139, 1317 (1974).

10. Unkeless, J., Danø, K., Kellerman, G.M. & Reich, E., Fibrinolysis Associated with Oncogenic Transformation, J. Biol. Chem. 249, 4295 (1974).

11. Quigley, J.P., Association of a Protease (Plasminogen Activator) with a Specific Membrane Fraction Isolated from Transformed Cells, J. Cell Biol. 71, 472 (1976).

12. Chen, L.B. & Buchanan, J.M., Plasminogen-Independent Fibrinolysis by Proteases Produced by Transformed Chick Embryo Fibroblasts, Proc. Natl. Acad. Sci., USA 72, 1132 (1975).

13. Haverkate, F. & Traas, D.W., Dose-Response Curves in the Fibrin Plate Assay: Fibrinolytic Activity of Proteases, Thromb. Diath. Haemorrh. 32, 356 (1974).

14. Laemmli, U.K., Cleavage of Structural Proteins During the Assembly of the Head of Bacteriophage T4, Nature 227, 680 (1970).

15. Laskey, R.A. & Mills, A.D., Quantitative Film Detection of ^{3}H and ^{14}C in Polyacrylamide Gels by Fluorography, Eur. J. Biochem. 56, 335 (1975).

16. Perdue, J.F., personal communication.

17. Cohen, J.A. & Warringa, M.G.P.J., Purification and Properties of Dialkylfluorophosphatase, Biochim. Biophys. Acta 26, 29 (1957).

18. Duesberg, P.H. & Vogt, P.K., RNA Species Obtained from Clonal Lines of Avian Sarcoma and from Avian Leukosis Virus, Virology 54, 207 (1973).

19. Coffin, J.M., Genes Responsible for Transformation by Avian RNA Tumor Viruses, Cancer Res. 36, 4282 (1976).

20. Bernstein, A., MacCormick, R. & Martin, G.S., Transformation-Defective Mutants of Avian Sarcoma Viruses: The Genetic Relationships between Conditional and Non-Conditional Mutants, Virology 70, 206 (1976).

21. Wang, L-H., Duesberg, D., Beemon, K. & Vogt, P.K., Mapping RNase T1-Resistant Oligonucleotides of Avian Tumor Virus RNAs: Sarcoma-Specific Oligonucleotides are Near the Poly (A) End and Oligonucleotides Common to Sarcoma and Transformation-Defective Viruses are at the Poly (A) End, J. Virol. 16, 1051 (1975).

22. Joho, R.H., Billeter, M.A. & Weissman, C., Mapping of Biological Functions on RNA of Avian Tumor Viruses: Location of Regions Required for Transformation and Determination of Host Range, Proc. Natl. Acad. Sci., USA 72, 4772 (1975).

23. Junghans, R.P., Hu, S., Knight, C.A. & Davidson, N., Heteroduplex Analysis of Avian RNA Tumor Viruses, Proc. Natl. Acad. Sci., USA 74, 477 (1977).

ASPECTS ON BIOCHEMISTRY AND PATHOPHYSIOLOGY OF α_1-ANTITRYPSIN

Carl-Bertil Laurell
Department of Clinical Chemistry, University of Lund,
Malmö General Hospital, S-214 01 Malmö, Sweden

Fourteen years ago I had the privilege to give the first report on inherited α-1-antitrypsin deficiency at this Protein Foundation (ref. 1). This deficiency state was detectable by paper electrophoresis and was shown to be related to the early development of pulmonary emphysema. This relationship has since attracted considerable interest because emphysema is a common debilitating disease of unknown origin. The primary problem was to settle whether low α-1-AT levels in plasma in deficiency states was a secondary phenomenon to a metabolic disorder or whether the low level was secondary to a structural plasma protein abnormality. The technique of crossed immunoelectrophoresis in agarose gels was developed to study electrophoretic heterogeneity of α-1-AT in native plasma. The first patterns obtained by crossed immunoelectrophoresis were however confusing because electrophoretic heterogeneity of α-1-AT both in healthy subjects and in deficiency cases were obtained. The major α-1-AT fraction in plasma from deficiency cases seemed to migrate like the minor fraction observed in normal plasma. This could be in conformity with both hypotheses.

Genetic variants

Detection of a series of inherited, electrophoretic α-1-AT variants soon followed and supported the occurrence of structural variants for α-1-AT similar to that of hemoglobin. Characteristic phenotypic patterns were recognized for various genotypes with the aid of acid starch gel electrophoresis (ref. 2) which gave higher resolution than did agarose gel electrophoresis. The electrophoretic five band patterns of α-1-AT resolved by acid starch gel electrophoresis initiated a phenotyping system known now as the protease inhibitor (Pi) system (ref. 3). α-1-AT has been identified as the major protease inhibitor of plasma (ref. 4). The charge heterogeneity of α-1-AT has been an obstacle both in developing methods for its isolation and also for the structural studies of α-1-AT. This protein contains a single peptide chain (ref. 5). More than 25 alleles for α-1-AT have now been recognized (ref. 6). It is reasonable to assume missense mutations with single amino acid substitutions for most of them but only two substitutions have so far been pinpointed. Sequence studies have concentrated on phenotypes with decreased levels of α-1-AT in plasma. In classical PiZ deficiency a GLU-LYS substitution has been found (ref. 7.8) while in PiS deficiency the substitution is GLU-VAL (ref. 9). These substitutions concern two different glutamyl residues in the same cyanogen-bromide fragment. It is a challenge to explain on which metabolic level the missense mutations produce decreased plasma levels of α-1-AT.

The inheritence of α-1-AT is co-dominant with expression of both alleles so that plasma of all heterozygotes contain a mixture of two molecular species (ref. 3). An exception to this rule is the rare Pi null allele which probably represents a deletion or a nonsense mutation. No α-1-AT is found in plasma of the Pi null homozygote - the complete α-1-AT deficiency (ref. 10.11).

Microheterogeneity

In each Pi-homozygote five major molecular α-1-AT species (ref. 2.4.6.7.8 according to Fagerhol) are regularly found in plasma. This heterogeneity is assumed to originate when oligosaccharide chains are linked to the protein backbone by hepatocyte rough endoplasmic reticulum or when the core oligosaccharides are completed in the smooth endoplasmic reticulum prior to secretion. One charge unit difference is found by isoelectric focusing between each major fraction which can be eliminated after sialidase treatment. This indicates a difference in the number of sialic acids (ref. 11). The major fractions 4 and 6 focusing at pH 4.52 and 4.59 have 8 and 7 sialic acids respectively. Two types of glycopeptides have been isolated. In both the non-reducing terminal is -D-galactose-sialic acid. The average number of oligosaccharide chains is four according to Chan et al. (13). It is still unproven whether all five major fractions contain four chains and if the terminal sugars vary. These problems have physiological importance because missing sialidation for the ultimate galactose of the sugar chains would result in a markedly shortened biological half life if more than one galactose is available for reaction with the galactose receptors of the hepatocytes (ref. 14). Therefore the number, the branching and the terminal sugar of each oligosaccharide chains of the five fractions are of prime importance to define. All genetic variants so far found give the same electrophoretic five band pattern which indicates that the missense mutations do not alter any of the sequence Asn-X-Ser which are important for attachment of oligosaccharide chains. The quantitative distribution of the α-1-AT molecules between the five fractions shows a metabolic variation. Normally the concentration order is $6>4>7\geqslant 8>2$. Pregnancy and administration of estrogens induce increased α-1-AT synthesis, doubling the plasma level in pregnancy and change this sequence to $4>6>7>8>2$ indicating a slightly higher mean sialylation. Alteration of the microheterogeneity pattern suggests that estrogens induce higher activity of one or more of the glycosylating enzymes lining the endoplasmic reticulum of the hepatocytes. A higher degree of branching would produce the observed band pattern if sialic acid regularly terminates the chains.

The single cysteinyl

Another α-1-AT characteristic of metabolic interest is its single cysteinyl. This occurs in plasma partly in reactive form and partly as a mixed disulfide, where the most frequent partners are cysteine, probably γ-glutamylcysteine and IgA through its penultimate cysteinyl in the heavy chain. It is remarkable that only about half the cysteinyls normally occur in oxidized state at physiological pH in spite the reduced form has a greater tendency than most other plasma proteins to form SS-bridges with thiol compounds. Therefore this property may be used for thiol-disulfide interchange chromatography to isolate α-1-AT from the bulk of the plasma proteins which contain no reactive thiol group (ref. 15). The SH-SS interchange reaction is independent of variation in charge of the subfractions and therefore this method allows harvest of α-1-AT with all native microheterogeneity retained in contrast to methods utilizing ionic exchange chromatography.

The relative stability of the thiol group of α-1-AT in reduced state suggests that it is protected in a crevice. This is supported by the finding that SS-linked dimers do not occur in α-1-AT. Nor are any complexes formed with albumin, the most abundant thiol protein in plasma which has its reactive thiol located in a pouch on the surface. However, the terminal cysteinyls of light Ig κ-chains and the penultimate cysteinyl of the heavy IgA-chains, which are more readily exposed, form SS-linked complexes with α-1-AT. Normally about 4 % of the IgA circulate as α-1-AT-IgA complexes (ref. 16).

The exchange rate of cysteine between α-1-AT and free cystine in plasma has been measured in the dog by injection of 131-I-α-1-AT-35-S-cysteine. The half life of this Cys was only 1 hour contrasted to 4 days for 131-I-α-1-AT. The disappearance from plasma of injected cysteine was still faster (Fig. 1). Our results indicate a rapid interchange reaction between cysteine in plasma, cysteine of Cys-α-1-AT and the intracellular cysteine pool. The average concentration of cysteine and cystine in plasma have been reported to be 20 and 40 μmole/l respectively (ref. 17). This represents a small pool compared with the total amount of reactive thiol groups of plasma proteins (200-300 μmole/l) in human. Therefore α-1-AT and albumin may possibly serve as a buffer preventing fast changes of the cystein:cystine ratio of plasma. Causes of microheterogeneity of α-1-AT are summarized on fig. 2.

This reaction between the thiol groups of various compounds contributes to the heterogeneity of α-1-AT as observed by electrofocusing. The pattern may be simplified by treating the sample with excess cysteine, transferring the mixed disulfides of α-1-AT into α-1-AT-Cys (ref. 18).

Interaction with proteases

On reaction of α-1-AT with most serine proteases relatively stable complexes are formed. However measurable amounts of complexes between α-1-AT and any of these proteases have not been identified in plasma from healthy subjects. But they may occur in very low concentrations in plasma during disease. Such complexes containing granulocytic serine proteases have been identified in lymph and local tissue fluids from abscesses (ref. 19). Pancreatic elastase has been found linked to α-1-AT in the exudate from pancreas after acute lesions but no apparent changes of the protease inhibitors of plasma have been recognized. These observations supported rapid elimination of protease inhibitor complexes when they were formed (ref. 20.21).

On addition of serine proteases to α-1-AT *in vitro* complexes are formed on a mole to mole ratio. In presence of slight excess of α-1-AT the reaction is complete within about a minute for pancreatic chymotrypsin and takes several minutes for cathodal trypsin and is not finished within half an hour for *e.g.* plasminogen. Other serine proteases show a reaction rate between these extremes. The species differences are very marked (ref. 22). An asymmetric cleavage of the chain of α-1-AT is generally accepted (ref. 23.24). Trypsin cleaves off a peptide of 6-8.000 daltons. This may be released or may be loosely bound to the complex and has not been isolated. As a second step, acylation of serine at the active center of the protease with α-1-AT is thought to occur (ref. 23). The reaction of α-1-AT with pancreatic elastase gives rise to multiple products in presence of excess α-1-AT. Three bonds on α-1-AT may be attacked "one such attack cleaves the inhibitor into two inactive fragments, and the other two yield complexes with a lower molecular weight than the sum of the weights of the reactants" (ref. 25). Inhibitory inactive α-1-AT molecules with physical properties very similar to native α-1-AT were found. Their turn over rates are unknown.

The initial trypsin-α-1-AT complex has relatively low stability when formed *in*

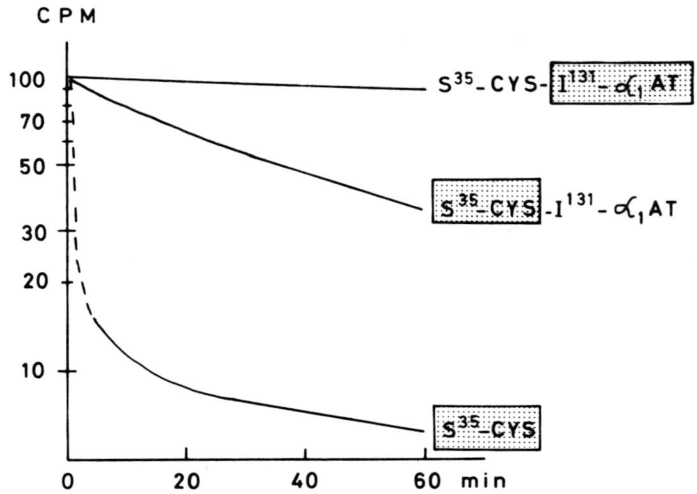

Fig. 1 Comparison between disappearance of S^{35} and I^{131} on injection of S^{35}-Cys-I^{131}-α-1-AT and of S^{35}-cystine.

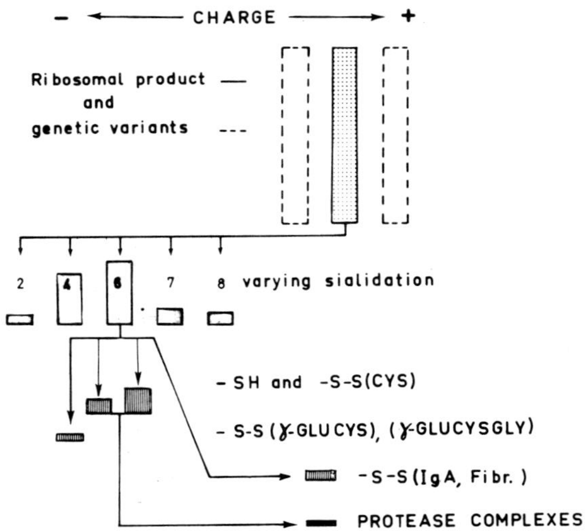

Fig. 2 Various causes of microheterogeneity of α-1-AT.

vitro with a slightest excess of the protease and decays by autodigestion if excess of protective α-1-AT is not present (ref. 23.26.27.28). The variation in cleavage points between the various serine proteases and the lability of the complexes has hampered both structural and metabolic studies. The biologic fate of freshly prepared human trypsin-α-1-AT-complexes and granulocyte elastase-α-1-AT have been studied in dog (ref. 29) and human (ref. 30). In both species a transfer of trypsin occurs from the α-1-AT-complex to α-macroglobulin. The dog trypsin-α-1-AT complex is more labile than the human and transfer to α-macroglobulin is faster in the dog. Superficially nothing seems to happen if large amounts of trypsin-α-1-AT complexes are injected into the dog but a gradual saturation of α-macroglobulin develops (Fig. 2). After about 2 hours all α-macroglobulin molecules are saturated and at that moment the dog goes into shock because any molecules of trypsin released from the α-1-AT-complex and not bound by α-macroglobulin will cause a catastrophic release of vasoactive kinins. The sensibility of the dog to elastase- and chymotrypin-α-AT complexes are less than for trypsin because the enzyme release from these complexes is slower. A firmer linkage of chymotrypsin and elastase than of trypsin has been confirmed on the injection of free enzymes into the dog. Greater amounts of chymotrypsin than trypsin are tolerated before death. The relative binding rates of the enzymes to the inhibitors are reflected by the partition of the enzyme between the various inhibitors immediately after the injection (ref. 29).

From the experimental studies it is evident that the serine proteases released locally into the intercellular fluids are linked to α-macroglobulin or to α-1-AT. The complexes are partly absorbed by the local lymph glands. Complexes between enzyme and α-macroglobulin entering the blood will be cleared by the reticuloendothelial system with a half life of minutes. Complexes between α-1-AT and serine proteases are less efficiently absorbed by RES but when entering blood through the lymphatics an immediate dilution occurs and excess α-macroglobulin guarantees rapid elimination (ref. 31). This explains why such small amounts of complexes between serine proteases and α-1-AT are found in plasma in conditions characterized by increased protease release.

Metabolism

The hepatocytes are the only body cells with high α-1-AT synthesis. Secreted protein approaches equilibration in distribution between plasma and extracellular fluids within two days. The size of 55.000 daltons for α-1-AT gives a ratio of about 60 % outside and 40 % within the vascular tree (ref. 32). *In vivo* studies of α-1-AT biosynthesis have not been reported, but catabolic rates have been estimated in PiM, PiZ and Pi null subjects for the α-1-AT variants PiS, Z and M^{Malton} all of which are characterized by decreased plasma levels (Table 1) (ref. 33.34). When compartment equilibrium has been reached after injection of labeled α-1-AT calculation of the fractional catabolic rate have given constant values for all Pi proteins studied. This indicates that major subfractions of α-1-AT with variable content of sialic acid have roughly identical fractional catabolic rates. The FCR of α-1-AT rapidly increases with increasing degree of desialidation (ref. 33.34) similar to many other proteins (ref. 14). This constant FCR supports that subfractions with lowest sialic acid content have no terminal galactose. It is thus reasonable to assume that the branching of the oligosaccharides varies in the subfractions and that some chains end with sugars other than sialic acid or galactose. Therefore the efficiency of the sialylation of the galactose residue by the Golgi apparatus seems thus not to be the primary cause of the microheterogeneity of α-1-AT.

The fractional catabolic rate calculated from the final disappearance slopes indicates there is a slightly faster or normal catabolism for the allele products

TABLE 1 α_1-Antitrypsin concentration in homozygous α_1-antitrypsin deficiency

Phenotype	Plasma conc. g/l	% of normal
Pi MM	1.4	100
PiSS	0.85	60
PiZZ	0.2	15
$Pi(M^{Malton})$ ·2	0.2	15
Pi (null) ·2	<0.002	-

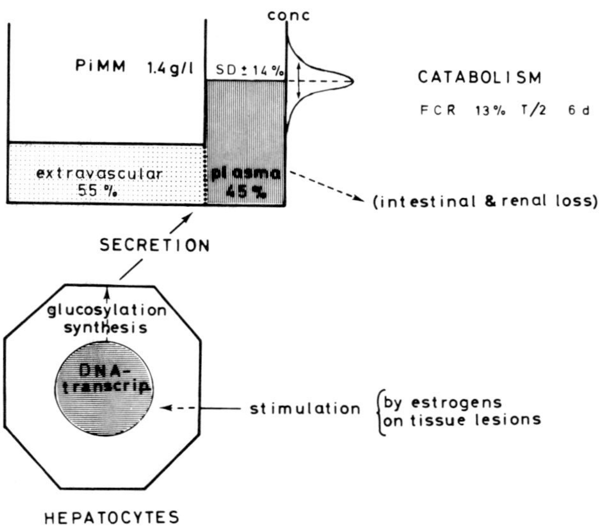

Fig. 3 Metabolic main routes of α-1-AT.

in subjects with missense mutations (Table 2) but these differences are much too small to explain the decreased plasma content of α-1-AT in the various types of α-1-AT-deficiency. Similar catabolic rates of PiM protein has been found in PiM and in Pi null subjects (ref. 35) which clearly shows that the catabolic machinary is not dependent on the biosynthetic rate of α-1-AT or plasma level of α-1-AT. Thus variation in plasma level is governed by altered rates in biosynthesis and secretion of α-1-AT. Decreased plasma levels during disease occur because of increased catabolism has only been observed after severe renal and intestinal losses of plasma (ref. 36). The plasma level of α-1-AT markedly increases on inflammation and after increased influence of estrogens but not after androgens or anabolic steroids. This reaction pattern of α-1-AT on steroid administration is unusual but resembles that found for ceruloplasmin and transcortin.

It may be stated from comparison of plasma α-1-AT variations in PiM and PiZ subjects during inflammatory response, estrogen administration or in pregnancy, that the α-1-AT increases in these conditions are proportional to the basic concentration level (ref. 37). This implies a much smaller absolute rise in PiZ subjects than in PiM subjects. Estrogens and other steroids usually effect the protein synthesis by influencing DNA transcriptional rate. The collected observations suggest that the missense mutations followed by decreased concentration of α-1-AT in plasma markedly modulate the biosynthetic rate before, or at the DNA transcriptional level. It remains to explain why a few, single sequence changes in the genetic code of α-1-AT have such an influence on the transcriptional rate, that the α-1-AT secretion falls to a small fraction. This is a basic problem and makes it particularly interesting to study the α-1-AT structure of various mutants which produce reduced plasma levels. Metabolic main routes of α-1-AT are summarized on fig. 3.

Biological function

α-1-AT belongs to the group of acute phase reactants that increase during inflammatory response. α-1-AT starts to increase in plasma on the second day after a tissue injury and reaches a peak two or three days later. The granulocytes invade the injured area within the first hours after tissue lesions while macrophages accumulate after a delay of one or two days. These time courses suggest that the α-1-AT increase will result in an increased local capacity to neutralize the protease release during the macrophage phase more efficiently than during the earlier granulocytic phase. But the increased local fluid exchange early during the inflammatory response also implies an enhanced local access to α-1-AT. The general effect of α-1-AT complexing with the proteases is neutralization and retardation of spread of active enzymes from the inflamed area. Eriksson´s clinical studies of patients with various degrees of α-1-AT deficiency have given the first insights into the biological importance of α-1-AT (ref. 38). α-1-AT levels in plasma below half normal predisposes individuals to premature ageing of the elastin fibers in lung tissue with impaired lung recoil as an early manifestation (ref. 38). Lower the extracellular α-1-AT level, higher the risk for loss of lung tissue elasticity and development of a wasting lung. This ageing process is greatly accelerated on exposure to polluted air with an early appearance of pulmonary insufficiency.

The early functional lung lesions in subjects with severe α-1-AT-deficiency suggest a primary injury of the elastin fibres. How are the elastic fibres damaged? Granulocytes contain about 1 % elastase and release part of it during phagocytosis (ref. 39.40). Therefore local elastin destruction might occur secondary to enhanced phagocytosis by localized granulocytic accumulation. Pulmonary emphysema has been induced on inhalation of human leucocyte elastase(ref. 41). How is elastase normally inhibited in the body? α-1-AT is more efficient as an inhibitor of elastase than any other protease inhibitor in the body fluids because its avid reaction, firm linkage and high extracellular concentration (ref. 42). These collected facts have focused the interest on occurrence of elastase rich cells in the lung tissues.

The primary suspect for the elastin destruction was the elastase rich neutrophils but lately interest has switched to the alveolar macrophage. Both types of cells invade the lungs in large amounts on smoking. The alveolar macrophages are said to increase 10-20 times with heavy smoking while granulocyte invasion is less regular and more dependent on infections. The granulocytes primarily invade the bronchial tree, pass out into the lumen, through the mucosa and are swept unward by ciliary activity, while the macrophages invade and proliferate in the alveolar zone. They have also the capacity to migrate backwards into the supporting tissue which has not been observed normally for granulocytes. Macrophages perform their phagocytosing activity in the alveolar zone. It has recently been shown by Larsson (43) that smoking PiZ subjects have on the average 20 years shorter survival than non smoking PiZ subjects. PiMZ subjects with 45 to 70 % of the normal α-1-AT concentration in tissue fluids seem to be only little more affected by smoking than normal PiM subjects (ref. 44). From these longitudinal studies of PiZ and observations on PiSZ subjects it is probable that the critical level of α-1-AT required for adequate protection of lung tissue needs to be at least 30-45 % of the normal concentration if the subject is exposed to polluted air. The critical border for subjects not exposed to air pollution lies at about half that level where some do some do not develop overt signs of emphysema.

Clinical findings in α-1-AT deficiency of various phenotypes suggest that the major biological function of α-1-AT is to balance and localize the effect of elastase released from the macrophages and granulocytes during their cleaning up activities of lung tissue (ref. 45). It is of interest that no premature ageing has been observed of other elastin rich tissues in α-1-AT deficiency. Thus there seems to be no premature ageing of skin or of the vessels which ought to be the case if α-1-AT deficiency is followed by a general early elastin wasting. Furthermore, the lungs usually retain a good function after an acute lobar pneumoniae which is characterized by an enormous granulocytic invasion during the acute phase but emphysema does usually not develop in the reconvalescence. Local tissue destruction with abscess formation may be caused by granulocytes that phagocytize foreign material indigestible to them. The tubercle bacillus is such a microorganism which resists the granulocytes and which has a tendency to cause formation of local caverns in the affected tissue because of tissue disintergration.

The quietly wasting lung is the only common characteristic of all types of severe α-1-AT deficiencies which is why we have good reason to believe that a major biological function of α-1-AT is self protection against the effect of proteases released by the phagocytes while fullfilling their sanitary functions. To neutralize the secreted macrophage elastase appears to be an essential function of α-1-AT.

A relatively benign glomerular lesion has been recognized in α-1-AT deficiency. Its origin is obscure but the macrophages and granulocytes while cleaning glomerular membranes of protein complexes may produce this lesion because of the protease release (ref. 46).

The most pronounced and regular α-1-AT increase that occurs is related to pregnancy and estrogen administration. Whether this is of biological importance or not is unknown. We have observed no complications during pregnancy in PiZ subjects even though estrogen induction of α-1-AT-synthesis in such subjects does not raise the plasma level above 1/3 of the average non pregnant level while most normal pregnant women double their plasma level. The abortion frequency in PiZ subjects is unknown. No pregnant Pi null subject has so far been studied. The increasing difference in α-1-AT levels developing between PiM and PiZ subjects during pregnancy suggests that pregnant PiZ subjects need special attention since α-1-AT may have an additional protective function during pregnancy. The PiZ subjects ought to be prone to manifest deficiency symptoms.

The course of acute pancreatitis in PiM, -MZ and -Z subjects suggests that α-1-AT is of little importance for self protection during the acute local spread of proteolytic enzymes in this condition when compared with the protective importance of α-macroglobulin (ref. 47).

Hepatological disorders in PiZ subjects such as neonatal icterus, juvenile cirrhosis, periportal cirrhosis and the increased frequency of primary hepatoma are strictly linked to the Z-type and are not found in any other Pi type with low plasma α-1-AT such as PiM^{Malton}, PiM^{Duarte} or Pi null. The cellular hepatic weakness in PiZ subjects seems to be in some way linked to the GLU-LYS amino acid substitution. The leading clue has been characteristic inclusion bodies first recognized by Sharp in the hepatocytes of PiZ subjects (ref. 48). They accumulate in the endoplasmic reticulum and increase in number and size with increasing age and are also found but in less number in PiMZ heterozygotes. These inclusion bodies contain the complete peptide chain of α-1-AT but the glycosylation process is probably not finished (ref. 49.50). The cause of this molecular aggregation is still unknown.

The hypothesis that the inclusion bodies represent aggregated pro-α-1-AT with a peptide attached to the N-terminal end may be rejected. It has recently been shown in our laboratory that α-1-AT from inclusion bodies have the same amino acid composition and N-terminal amino acid sequence up to 10 residues as the secreted plasma α-1-AT (J.-O. Jeppsson & S. Eriksson, to be published). The intracellular aggregates may produce a metabolic disturbance which in turn increases the turn over of the hepatocytes with a resultant predisposition to hepatic disorders like juvenile hepatitis, cirrhosis and primary cancer of the liver (ref. 51).

In conclusion it may be stated that the structure of genetic α-1-AT variants followed by depressed α-1-AT plasma levels are of special interest for general studies concerning the relationship between metabolism and structure of extracellular proteins. No influence has been found between α-1-AT plasma levels and the biosynthetic rate or the fractional catabolic rate. Little effect of single amino acid substitutions on the rate of α-1-AT catabolism has been found.

Strong enhancement of α-1-AT biosynthesis is induced by inflammation and estrogens yet the hepatocytes have no "estrogen receptors". It remains to determine how estrogens modulate the DNA transcription rate or stabilize a selective group of hepatic cell ribosomes and how this is related to single amino acid substitutions within the α-1-AT-molecule.

Further studies on the interaction of α-1-AT with the various serine-proteases are necessary for understanding better the function of α-1-AT. Rate of reaction, stability of complexes, the fate of cleavage products and complexes have to be estimated for several serine-proteases. From clinical studies it may be concluded that the major function of α-1-AT is to neutralize the activity of proteases released in the intercellular spaces - especially macrophage elastase released during phagocytosis. The α-1-AT complexes formed are not detected in blood because of complex absorption in RES,protease transfer to α-macroglobulin and dilution on return to blood through lymphatics. The blood concentration of α-1-AT can therefore only be used as "whitewashed" reflection of the antiprotease capacity in the extracellular space.

Clinical α-1-AT deficiency states are easily detected (ref. 52), and individual preventive steps of importance are within reach.

Acknowledgement

This investigation was supported by a grant from the Swedish Medical Research Council (Project no. B79-13X- 00581-15B).

TABLE 2 Distribution and catabolism of α_1-antitrypsins of various Pi-types

Recipient Pi-type	Nr exp	Administered Pi-protein	Extravasc. to plasma ratio (E/P ratio)	Fractional catabolic rate (FCR)d^{-1}	Final T/2 d^{-1}	Ref
M	4	M	1.41	0.28	6.7	32
M	7	M	1.07	0.33	4.6	34
M	1	S	1.36	0.36	5.5	33
M	2	Z	1.42	0.40	5.0	32
M	2	M^{Malton}	1.56	0.34	6.2	33
null	1	M	-	-	6	35
MZ	2	M	-	-	5.5	35

REFERENCES

(1) C.-B. Laurell, Genetic variants of α-1-antitrypsin, Vox Sang 10, 363 (1965).

(2) M. Fagerhol and M. Braend, Serum prealbumin: Polymorphism in man, Science 149, 986 (1965).

(3) M. Fagerhol and C.-B. Laurell, The polymorphism of "pre-albumins" and α-1-antitrypsin in human sera, Clin. Chim. Acta 16, 199 (1967).

(4) H.E. Schultze, K. Heide and H. Haupt, α-1-Antitrypsin aus Humanserum, Klin. Wschr. 40, 427 (1962).

(5) I.P. Crawford, Purification and properties of normal human α-1-antitrypsin, Arch. Biochem. Biophys. 156, 215 (1973).

(6) D. Cox and L. Celhoffer, Inherited variants of α-1-antitrypsin: A new allele Pi-N, Can. J. Genet. Cytol. 16, 297 (1974).

(7) J.-O. Jeppsson, Amino acid substitution - Glu Lys in α-1-antitrypsin PiZ, FEBS Letters 65, 195 (1976).

(8) A. Yoshida, J. Lieberman, L. Gaidulis and C. Ewing, Molecular abnormality of human α-1-antitrypsin variant (Pi-ZZ) associated with plasma activity deficiency, Proc. Nat. Acad. Sciences of USA, 73, 1324 (1976).

(9) M.C. Owen and R.W. Carrell, Alpha-1 antitrypsin: Molecular abnormality of S variant, Brit. Med. J., I, 130 (1976).

(10) R.C. Talamo, C.E. Langley, C.E. Reed and S. Makino, Alpha-1-antitrypsin deficiency: A variant with no detectable alpha-1-antitrypsin, Science 181, 80 (1970).

(11) J.P. Martin, D. Vandeville and C. Ropartz, α-1-antitrypsin deficiency: PiO, Lancet II, 845 (1973)

(12) J.-O. Jeppsson, C.-B. Laurell and M. Fagerhol, Properties of isolated human α-1-antitrypsins of Pi types M, S and Z, Eur. J. Biochem. 83, 143 (1978).

(13) S.K. Chan, D.C. Rees, S.-C. Li and Y.T. Li, Linear structure of the oligosaccharide chains in α -1 protease inhibitor isolated from human plasma, J. Biol. Chem. 251, 471 (1976

(14) A.G. Morell, G. Gregoriados, H. Scheinberg, J. Hickman and G. Ashwell, The role of sialic acid in determining the survival of glycoproteins in the circulation, J. Biol. Chem. 246, 1461 (1971).

(15) C.-B. Laurell, J. Pierce, U. Persson and E. Thulin, Purification of α-1-antitrypsin from plasma through thiol-disulfide interchange, Eur. J. Biochem. 57, 107 (1975).

(16) C.-B. Laurell, A. Grubb and E. Thulin, J. chain and α-1-antitrypsin-IgA complexes in sera with poly- and mono-clonal IgA, La Ricerca Clin. Lab. 6 (Suppl. no. 3) 57, (1976).

(17) W.D. Block, M. Markovs and B. Steele, Methionine, cysteine, cystine and taurine interrelationships in human plasma, Am. J. Clin. Nutr. 22, 33 (1969).

(18) J.A. Pierce, J.-O. Jeppsson and C.-B. Laurell, α-1-Antitrypsin phenotypes determined by isoelectric focusing of the cysteine-antitrypsin mixed disulfide in serum, Anal. Biochem. 74, 227 (1976).

(19) K. Ohlsson, Collagenase and elastase released during peritonitis are complexed by plasma protease inhibitors, Surgery 79, 652, (1976).

(20) K. Ohlsson and A. Eddeland, Release of proteolytic enzymes in bile-induced pancreatitis in dogs, Gastroenterology 69, 668 (1975).

(21) K. Ohlsson and C.-B. Laurell, Catabolic rate of α-1-antitrypsin of Pi types S, and M-Malton and of asialylated M-protein in man, Clin. Science & Mol. Med. 51, 87 (1976).

(22) M. Anbry and J. Bieth, Kinetics of the inactivation of human bovine trypsins and chymotrypsins by α-1-proteinase inhibitor and of their reactivation by α-2-macroglobulin, Clin. Chim. Acta 78, 371 (1977).

(23) J.M. Moroi and M. Yamasaki, Mechanism of interaction of bovine trypsin with human α-1-antitrypsin, Biochem. Biophys. Acta 359, 130,(1974).

(24) D. Johnson and J. Travis, Human α-1-protease inhibitor mechanism of action: Evidence for activation by limited proteolysis, Biochem. Biophys. Res. Commun, 72, 33 (1976).

(25) Theresa Lo, A. Cohen and H. James, The interaction of α-1-antitrypsin with soluble and Sepharose bound elastase, Biochim. Biophys. Acta 453, 344 (1976).

(26) K. Oda, M. Laskowski, Sr., L.F. Kress and D. Kowalski, Human plasma α_1-proteinase inhibitor: temporary inhibition and multiple molecular forms of the complex with porcine trypsin. Biochem. Biophys. Res. Commun, 76, 1062 (1977).

(27) J. Bloom and M. Hunter, Interaction of α-1-antitrypsin with trypsin and chymotrypsin, J. Biol. Chem. 253, 547 (1978).

(28) A. Cohen, D. Geczy and H. James, Interaction of human α-1-antitrypsin with porcine trypsin. Biochemistry 17, 392 (1978).

(29) K. Ohlsson, Interaction in vitro and in vivo between dog trypsin and dog plasma protease inhibitors, Scand. J.Clin. Lab. Invest. 28, 219 (1971).

(30) K. Ohlsson and C.-B. Laurell, The disappearance of enzyme-inhibitor complexes from the circulation of man, Clin. Science and Mol. Med. 51, 87 (1976).

(31) K. Ohlsson, Interaction between α-1-antitrypsin and α-2-macroglobulin in the elimination of proteolytic enzymes (1976) Protides of the biological fluids, Brügge 1975, Pergamon Press Ltd. , New York.

(32) C.-B. Laurell, B. Nosslin and J.-O. Jeppsson, Catabolic rate of α-1-antitrypsin of Pi-type M and Z in man. Clin. Science & Mol. Med. 52, 457 (1977).

(33) J.-O. Jeppsson, C.-B. Laurell, B. Nosslin and D.W. Cox, Catabolic rate of α-1-antitrypsin of Pi types S, and M-Malton and of asialylated M-protein in man. Clin. Science & Mol. Med. 55, 103 (1978).

(34) E.A. Jones, J. Vergalla, C.J. Steer, P.R. Bradley-Moore and J.M. Vierling, Metabolism of intact and desialylated α-1-antitrypsin. Clin. Science & Mol. Med. 55, 139 (1978).

(35) S. Makino and C.E. Reed, Distribution and elimination of exogenous α-1-antitrypsin, J. Lab.Clin. Med. 75, 742 (1970)

(36) J.J. Bernier, Ch. Desmazures, Ch. Florent, Ch. L´Hirondel and Ch. Aymes, Diagnosis of protein-losing enteropathy by gastrointestinal clearance of α-1-antitrypsin, Lancet 763, (1978).

(37) C.-B. Laurell, Variation of the α-1-antitrypsin level of plasma. (1972) Pulmonary Emphysema and Proteolysis, Academic Press, Inc., New York.

(38) S. Eriksson, Studies in α-1-antitrypsin deficiency, Acta Med. Scand. 177, Suppl. 432 (1965).

(39) A. Janoff and J. Scherer, IX Mediators of inflammation in leukocyte lysosomes Elastinolytic activity in granules of human polymorphnuclear leukocytes, J. Exp. Med. 128, 1137 (1968).

(40) K. Ohlsson and I. Olsson, The neutral proteases of human granulocytes, Eur. J. Biochem. 42, 519 (1974).

(41) R.M. Senior, H. Tegner, C. Kuhn, K. Ohlsson, B.C. Starcher and J.A. Pierce, The induction of emphysema with human leukocyte elastase, Am. Rev. Resp. Dis., 116, 469 (1977).

(42) K. Ohlsson and I. Olsson, Neutral proteases of human granulocytes III Interaction between human granulocyte elastase and plasma protease inhibitors, Scand. J. Clin. Lab. Invest. 34, 349 (1974).

(43) Ch. Larsson, Natural history and life expectancy in severe α-1-antitrypsin deficiency, PiZ, Acta Med. Scand. In press (1978).

(44) Ch. Larsson, S. Eriksson and H. Dirksen, Smoking and intermediate α-1-antitrypsin deficiency and lung function of middle-aged men, Brit. Med. J., 2, 922 (1977).

(45) W.L. Coudon and J.O. Harris, Human alveolar macrophage proteolytic enzyme activities in chronic obstructive pulmonary disease. Lack of correlation with functional abnormalities. Chest 73, 364 (1978).

(46) M. Davies, A.J. Barrett, A.J. Tracis, E. Sanders and G.A. Coles, The degradation of human glomerular basement membrane with purified lysosomal proteinases: Evidence for the pathogenic role of the polymorphnuclear leucocyte in glomerulonephritis, Clin. Science & Mol. Med. 54, 233 (1978).

(47) A. Borgström and K. Ohlsson, Immunoreactive trypsin in serum and peritoneal fluid in acute pancreatitis, Hoppe-Seyler Z. Physiol. Chem. In press (1978).

(48) H.L. Sharp, Alpha-1-antitrypsin deficiency, Hosp. Pract. 6, 83 (1971).

(49) J.-O. Jeppsson, C. Larsson and S. Eriksson, Characterization of α-1-antitrypsin in the inclusion bodies from the liver in α-1-antitrypsin deficiency, New Eng. J. Med. 293, 576 (1975).

(50) A. Herz, E. Katona, E. Cutz, J. Wilson and M. Barton, α_1-Antitrypsin: The presence of excess mannose in the Z variant isolated from liver, Science 201, 1229 (1978).

(51) S. Eriksson and I. Hägerstrand, Cirrhosis and malignant hepatoma in α-1-antitrypsin deficiency, Acta Med. Scand. 195, 451 (1974).

(52) T. Sveger, Liver disease in α_1-antitrypsin deficiency detected by screening of 200 000 infants, New Eng. J. Med. 294, 1316 (1976).

HUMAN ALPHA-1-PROTEINASE INHIBITOR AND HUMAN ALPHA-1-ANTICHYMOTRYPSIN: PROPERTIES AND MECHANISM STUDIES

James Travis, Nancy Matheson, David Johnson, and Keith Beatty
Dept. of Biochemistry, University of Georgia, Athens, Georgia 30602

ABSTRACT

Human α-1-Proteinase Inhibitor (α-1-PI) and human α-1-Antichymotrypsin (α-1-Achy) are plasma glycoproteins which have the specific function of inhibiting serine proteinases from a number of sources. In particular, α-1-PI has the strongest binding constant for leukocyte elastase while α-1-Achy interacts most strongly with leukocyte cathepsin G. Oxidizing agents inactivate α-1-PI by probable interaction with the reactive site methionine residue in this protein. This reaction may be paralleled in vivo by cigarette smoke or other noxious gases, resulting in uncontrolled proteolysis of lung tissue and the development of pulmonary emphysema.

INTRODUCTION

Although proteinase inhibitors have been known to exist in plasma for seventy-five years (1), no significant interest in the role of this class of proteins in maintaining homeostasis was shown until 1963 when Laurell and Eriksson (2) established a relationship between α-1-PI deficiency and the development of pulmonary emphysema. At the present time seven proteinase inhibitors have been isolated from human plasma (Table 1) and others, including a collagenase inhibitor (3), and a specific inhibitor of thiol proteinases (4), have been detected.

The specific function of many of the plasma proteinase inhibitors such as the inter-α-trypsin inhibitor (5) and α-1-Achy (6) have not yet been clarified. However, deficiencies in the concentration of other inhibitors in plasma due to genetic variation have given us valuable information on their probable role in controlling proteolytic activity associated with normal metabolic processes. Thus, beside α-1-PI, we now know that antithrombin III normally controls the activity of Factor X_a and Factor II_a (7) while a deficiency results in thrombotic episodes; similarly, C_1 esterase inhibitor regulates the activity of the complement cascade and in the deficiency state leads to the development of hereditary angioneurotic edema (8). No deficiency state has been reported for α-2-macroglobulin but it has recently been suggested that a genetic alteration in this protein may be present in individuals with cystic fibrosis (9). Finally, it seems certain that the α-2-plasmin inhibitor must control the fibrinolytic system since it is a fast reacting and specific inhibitor of plasmin (10).

TABLE 1: PROTEINASE INHIBITORS OF HUMAN PLASMA

NAME	CONCENTRATION (moles/100 ml)	MOL. WT.	CHO (%)	$E_{280\ NM}$
α-1-PROTEINASE INHIBITOR	25.0	52,000	12.5	5.2
α-1-ANTICHYMOTRYPSIN	7.7	68,000	24.6	6.2
INTER-α-TRYPSIN INHIBITOR	3.1	160,000	8.4	7.1
ANTITHROMBIN III	4.4	65,000	13.4	-
C_1 ESTERASE INHIBITOR	2.3	104,000	34.7	5.0
α-2-MACROGLOBULIN	6.8	725,000	7.7	8.1
α-2-PLASMIN INHIBITOR	0.9	67,000	11.7	7.0

In this laboratory we have been examining the mechanism by which plasma proteinase inhibitors protect tissues from proteolytic damage, especially that due to proteinases released from granulocytes during phagocytosis or cell death. Two of these enzymes, neutrophil elastase and neutrophil cathepsin G are capable of degrading structural proteins, including elastin (11), collagen (12), and proteoglycan (13). The data presented here summarizes our earlier observations with regard to the function of α-1-PI in controlling these proteolytic activities, as well as some recent results obtained during a study of the mechanism by which this inhibitor functions. In the course of this investigation we became interested in the role played by α-1-Achy in regulating the activity of chymotrypsin like enzymes, such as cathepsin G. In this report we also summarize some of the properties of the inhibitor, as purified in our laboratory.

THE REACTIVE CENTER OF HUMAN ALPHA-]-PROTEINASE INHIBITOR

One of the most intriguing properties of most of the plasma proteinase inhibitors involves the extreme stability of complexes formed with proteolytic enzymes. In particular, we now know that α-1-PI (14), α-1-Achy (15), C_1 esterase inhibitor (16), α-2-plasmin inhibitor (10), and anthithrombin III (17) interact with serine proteinases to form complexes which are not dissociated by denaturing in boiling sodium dodecyl sulfate. Only α-2-macroglobulin, the function of which is described elsewhere in this volume, and inter-α-trypsin inhibitor appear to form complexes with proteinases in a different manner.

The elucidation of the mechanism by which α-1-PI inhibits proteinases has been facilitated by the fact that complexes with this inhibitor can be dissociated by the addition of nucleophilic reagents (18). This effect has proven extremely useful, especially since α-1-PI obtained from dissociated complexes (referred to as α-1-PI*) has a lower molecular weight than that of native α-1-PI. Using α-1-PI*) obtained from complexes with trypsin, chymotrypsin, elastase, and thrombin, we have found that a new amino terminal sequence was now present in this modified protein and that, as a consequence of dissociation, bond cleavage must have occurred at what may be presumed to be the reactive center of this inhibitor. Significantly, the new sequence obtained was the same no matter which enzyme-inhibitor complex was dissociated indicative of a single, unique site apparently recognized by all of the proteinases tested. The unique structure in the vicinity of this section of the molecule was further confirmed by results which showed that both papain and cathepsin B, two thiol proteinases which are not inactivated by α-1-PI, directly convert this inhibitor to α-1-PI* by cleavage at the reactive center (19).

Recently (20), we isolated and determined the structure of a peptide fragment from papain digests of denatured α-1-PI. The sequence of this peptide was found to overlap with the amino terminal sequence of α-1-PI*. Part of the structure of this peptide is given below as well as a delineation of the residues in terms of their subsite importance in binding to proteinases.

...-GLU-ALA-ILE-PRO-MET-SER-ILE-PRO-PRO-GLU-...

P_5 P_4 P_3 P_2 P_1 ↑ P_1' P_2' P_3' P_4' P_5'

←-----α-1-PI*--------...

Two significant features of this structure should be noted. First, residues P_1' - P_4' are completely homologous with the reactive center residues of several proteinase inhibitors from plant sources. Second, and almost certainly of more importance, the P_1 residue which forms a critical role in proteinase interaction is methionine. This amino acid residue is not normally cleaved by trypsin, elastase, or papain but has been shown to be a substrate for chymotrypsin action. It should be noted that acid denatured α-1-PI is not cleaved at the MET-SER linkage by any of these proteinases indicative of a specific reactive conformation in the native protein.

OXIDATIVE INACTIVATION OF HUMAN ALPHA-1-PROTEINASE INHIBITOR

The development of pulmonary emphysema in individuals with either normal or heterozygous levels of α-1-PI cannot be easily explained on the basis of uncontrolled proteolysis of lung tissue unless a biological reaction occurs whereby the inhibitor is inactivated. The presence of methionine at the reactive site of α-1-PI suggested to us that, possibly, oxidative agents might convert this residue to methionine sulfoxide, thereby impairing the inhibitor. We, therefore, tested the effect of both a chemical and biochemical oxidant on the inhibitory activity of α-1-PI towards serine proteinases.

In the chemical oxidation experiments, N-chlorosuccinimide was tested (21) and the results shown in Figure 1 were obtained. Both a rapid loss of immediate inhibitory activity towards leukocyte elastase and a concomitant oxidation of two of the eight methionine residues of α-1-PI was obtained (the latter even at N-chlorosuccinimide:α-1-PI molar ratios of 40:1. Inhibitory activity towards trypsin and porcine pancreatic elastase was also destroyed but, curiously, only a 25% loss in chymotrypsin inhibition was detected. When oxidized α-1-PI was incubated for extended periods with these same serine proteinases most of the inhibitory activity was still observable, except for porcine elastase. These results suggest a difference in the association rate of native α-1-PI and oxidized α-1-PI with these enzymes and is confirmed by the kinetic analyses given in Table 2.

The biochemical oxidation of α-1-PI was performed using human leukocyte myeloperoxidase, a major constituent of neutrophil granules. As shown in Figure 2 this enzyme rapidly destroyed the inhibitory activity of α-1-PI towards pancreatic elastase at an inhibitor:enzyme molar ratio of 50:1. We have also found, by amino acid analysis, that between two and three residues of methionine are oxidized by this treatment. With either chemical or biochemical oxidation we found no losses in histidine or tryptophan, two amino acids which may be susceptible to oxidizing agents.

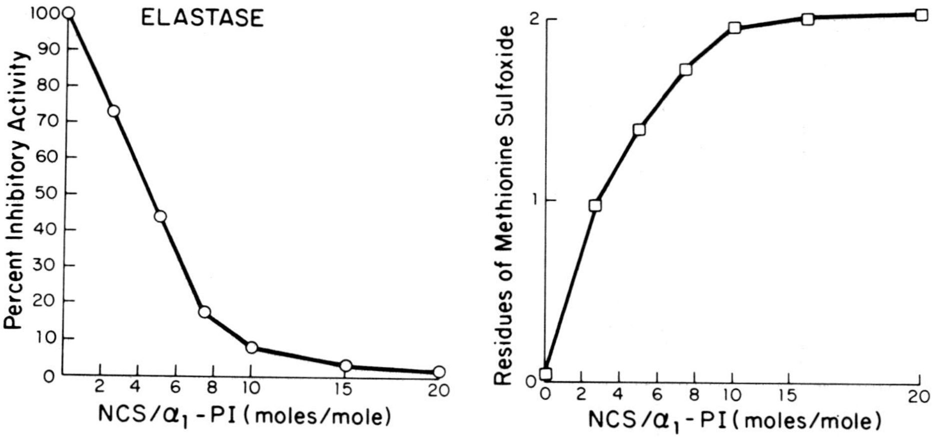

Fig. 1. Inactivation of Human α-1-Proteinase Inhibitor by N-chlorosuccinimide. A. Effect of Oxidation on Inhibitory Activity towards Leukocyte Elastase. B. Residues of Methionine Oxidized per Mole of α-1-PI Treated.

TABLE 2: ASSOCIATION CONSTANTS OF SERINE PROTEINASES WITH PLASMA PROTEINASE INHIBITORS

ENZYME	INHIBITOR		
	α-1-PI_{native}	α-1-$PI_{oxidized}$	α-1-Achy
Human Chymotrypsin	5.4×10^6	1.0×10^6	3.5×10^4
Leukocyte Elastase	6.5×10^7	3.0×10^4	-
Leukocyte Cathepsin G	4.1×10^5	6.4×10^2	6.0×10^7
Porcine Elastase	1.0×10^5	zero	-
Porcine Trypsin	4.2×10^4	5.0×10^3	-

These results indicate that myeloperoxidase may play an important role in phagocytic processes by oxidizing α-1-PI in order to maintain the enzymatic activity of leukocyte elastase. This could, however, prove to be deleterious to surrounding tissue during the leakage of leukocyte lysosomal enzymes from phagocytizing or dying cells since limited protection of oxidized α-1-PI would be

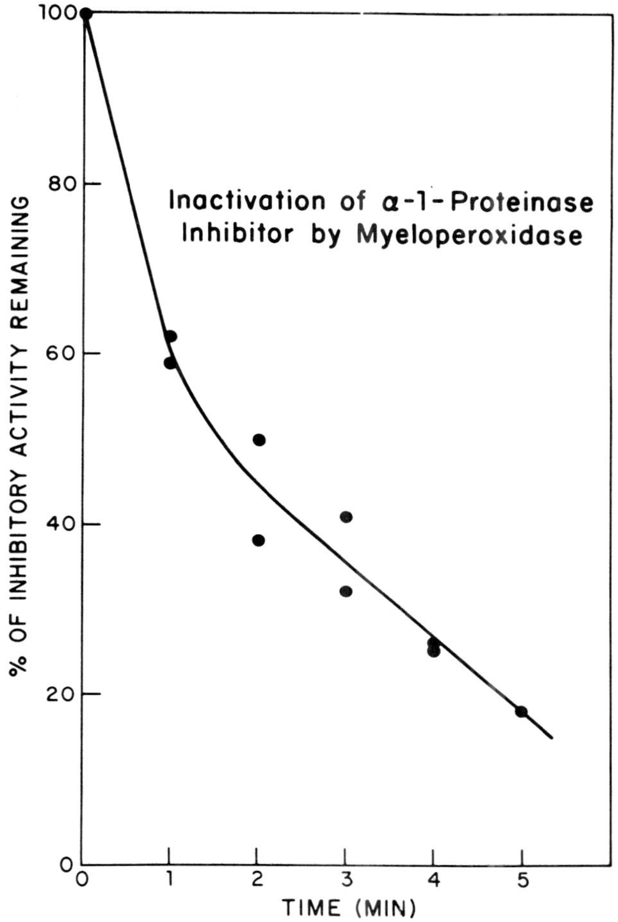

Fig. 2. Inactivation of Human α-1-Proteinase Inhibitor by Human Neutrophil Myeloperoxidase. (E:I molar ratio = 50:1).

afforded. Significantly, α-1-Achy, used as a control, was not inactivated by chemical oxidants and would still be capable of inhibiting cathepsin G.

Although we have not yet proven that the reactive site methionyl residue is oxidized under the experimental conditions described above, the effect of the oxidants utilized and the loss of methionine residues in the protein logically suggest that this is, indeed, what is occurring. It should be mentioned that cigarette smoke bubbled through solutions of α-1-PI saturated with oxygen also inactivates the protein with a loss of methionine residues. Thus, it is possible that potential oxidants present in cigarette smoke, polluted air, etc. may be able to inactivate the protective α-1-PI present in or near lung tissue. If such an effect does occur it would explain at a biochemical level exactly how tissue damage associated with the development of pulmonary emphysema can occur in individuals with apparently normal levels of α-1-PI.

A summary of the possible methods by which proteolysis of tissue could occur through α-1-PI deficiency is given in Figure 3. Four pathways are suggested which include (1) a normal phagocyte mediated process which could effectively titrate all of the α-1-PI used to defend against proteolysis; (2) a reductive pathway by which potential reducing agents such as HCN or H_2S present in inhaled gases could penetrate tissues and activate thiol proteinases, indirectly causing the enzymatic conversion of α-1-PI to α-1-PI*; (3) an oxidative pathway, described in detail in this contribution, by which both chemical and biochemical oxidants could inactivate α-1-PI directly; (4) a genetic deficiency pathway in which the classical emphysema picture described by Laurell and Eriksson (ref. 2) might occur. All of these pathways would, ultimately, cause an imbalance in the levels of protective inhibitors in the tissue resulting in uncontrolled proteolysis and subsequent tissue damage.

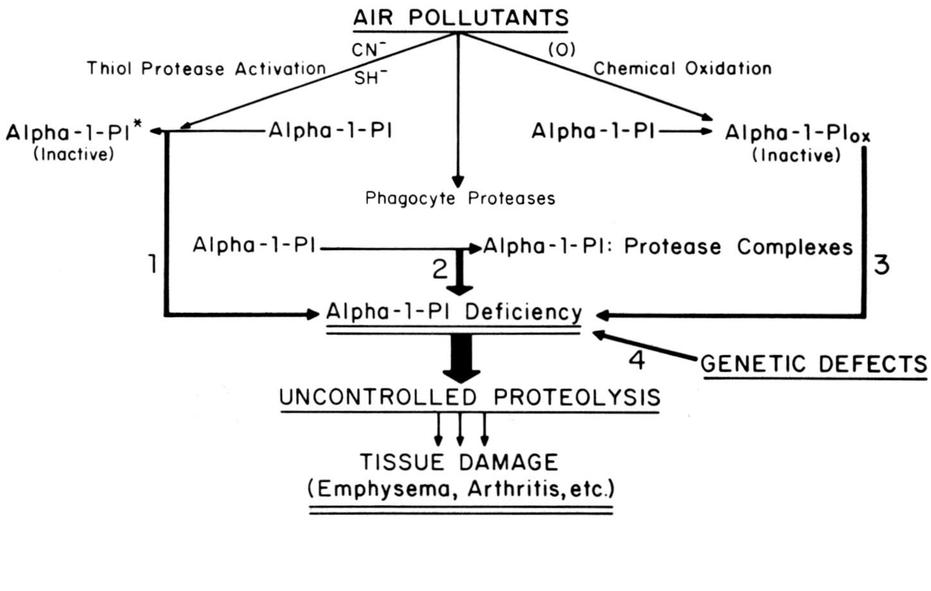

Fig. 3. Potential Pathways Leading to Uncontrolled Proteolysis and Tissue Damage.

PROPERTIES OF HUMAN ALPHA-1-ANTICHYMOTRYPSIN

Human α-1-Achy was originally isolated by Schultze and co-workers (22) using a relatively complex purification procedure. The isolated protein, while homogeneous, had low inhibitory activity and seemed to us to be unsuitable for mechanism studies. We have, therefore, developed a simple three step procedure for the isolation of this protein which involves (1) ammonium sulfate fractionation between 0.50 sat. and 0.80 sat.; (2) adsorption on and elution from Cibacron Blue sepharose at pH 7.0; (3) chromatography on SP-sephadex at pH 5.5 (23) (Figure 4). The resulting protein is homogeneous by all criteria and has the properties listed in Table 3 in comparison to those of human α-1-PI.

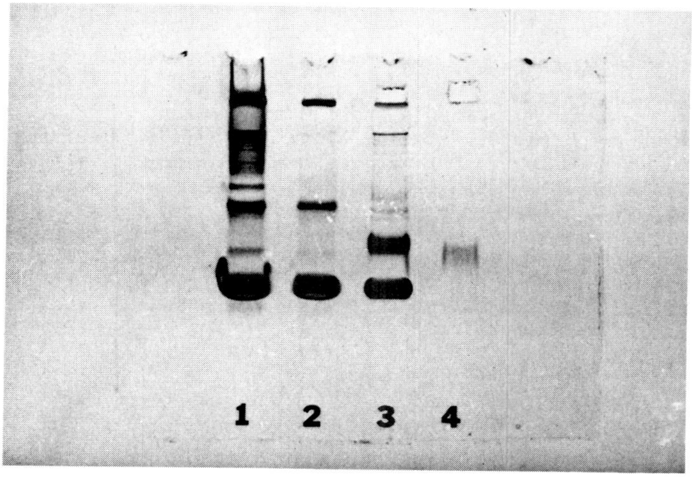

Fig. 4. Gel Electrophoresis of Human α-1-Antichymotrypsin Containing Fractions during the Purification from Plasma. (1) Whole Plasma; (2) $(NH_4)_2SO_4$ Fraction; (3) Cibacron Blue sepharose chromatography; (4) SP-sephadex chromatography.

TABLE 3: COMPARATIVE PROPERTIES OF ALPHA-1-ACHY AND ALPHA-1-PI

PROPERTY	ALPHA-1-ACHY	ALPHA-1-PI
MOLECULAR WEIGHT	68,000	52,000
EXTINCTION COEFFICIENT ($E^{1\%}_{280\ nm}$)	6.2	5.2
CARBOHYDRATE CONTENT (%)	24.4	12.6
PLASMA CONCENTRATION (mg%)	40	130
AMINO TERMINUS	Arginine	Glutamic Acid
CARBOXY TERMINUS	Glycine	Lysine
REACTIVE CENTER	Unknown	Methionyl-Serine
EFFECT OF OXIDANTS	No Effect	Inactivated

As previously shown (Table 2), the inhibitor has a higher association constant for cathepsin G than α-1-PI. Furthermore, when mixtures of α-1-PI and α-1-Achy are combined with chymotrypsin-like enzymes, the leukocyte proteinase cathepsin G complexes entirely with α-1-Achy while pancreatic chymotrypsin binds exclusively to α-1-PI (15). These results, therefore, suggest that α-1-Achy specifically functions as an inhibitor of chymotrypsin-like proteinases elicited by phagocytic cells, including neutrophils, basophils, and mast cells. In fact, this inhibitor probably has little or no function in the control of proteolysis by pancreatic chymotrypsin.

Acknowledgements:

We wish to thank Dr. J. Bieth for helpful discussions during the course of this work. Supported by grants from NIH and The Council for Tobacco Research-U.S.A.

REFERENCES

1. L. Camus and E. Gley, Action du serum sanguin sur quelques ferment digestif, C.R. Soc. Biol. 49, 8 (1897).

2. C.B. Laurell and S. Eriksson, The electrophoretic α_1-globulin pattern of serum in α-1-antitrypsin deficiency, Scand. J. Clin. Lab. Invest. 15, 132 (1963).

3. D.E. Wooley, D.R. Roberts, and J.M. Everson, Inhibition of Human collagenase activity by a small molecular weight serum protein, Biochem. Biophys. Res. Commun. 66, 747 (1975).

4. M. Sasaki, K. Minakata, H. Yamamoto, M. Niwa, T. Kato, and N. Ito, A new serum component which specifically inhibits thiol proteinases, Biochem. Biophys. Res. Commun. 76, 917 (1977).

5. K. Heide, N. Heimburger, and H. Haupt, An inter-α-trypsin inhibitor of human serum, Clin. Chim. Acta, 11, 82 (1965).

6. N. Heimburger and H. Haupt, Characterisierung von α_1X-glycoprotein als chymotrypsin-inhibitor des humanplasmas, Clin. Chim. Acta, 12, 116 (1965).

7. P.C. Harpel and R.D. Rosenberg, α-2-macroglobulin and antithrombin-heparin cofactor: modulators of hemostatic and inflammatory reactions, Progress in Hemostasis and Thrombosis, 3, 145 (1976).

8. V.H. Donaldson and R.R. Evans, Biochemical abnormality in hereditary angioneurotic edema: absence of serum inhibitor of C_1 esterase, Amer. J. Med. 35, 37 (1963).

9. E. Shapira, C.L. Martin and H. Nadler, Comparison between purified α-2-macroglobulin preparation from normal controls and patients with cystic fibrosis, J. Biol. Chem. 252, 7923 (1977).

10. M. Moroi and N. Aoki, Isolation and Characterization of α-2-plasmin inhibitor from human plasma, J. Biol. Chem. 251, 5956 (1976).

11. P.M. Starkey and A.J. Barrett, Human lysosomal elastase: catalytic and immunological properties, Biochem. J. 155, 265 (1976)

12. P.M. Starkey and A.J. Barrett, Human cathepsin G: catalytic and immunological properties, Biochem. J. 155, 273 (1976).

13. P.J. Roughley and A.J. Barrett, The degradation of cartilage proteoglycans by tissue proteinases, Biochem. J. 167, 629 (1977).

14. R. Baugh and J. Travis, Human leukocyte granule elastase: rapid purification and characterization, Biochemistry 15, 836 (1976).

15. J. Travis, J. Bowen, and R. Baugh, Human α-1-antichymotrypsin: interaction with chymotrypsin-like proteinases, Biochemistry (in press, 1978).

16. P.C. Harpel and N.R. Cooper, Studies on human plasma C_1' inactivator-enzyme interactions. 1. Mechanism of interaction with C_{1s}, plasmin, and trypsin, J. Clin. Invest. 55, 593 (1975).

17. R. Rosenberg and P.S. Damus, The purification and mechanism of action of human antithrombin-heparin cofactor, J. Biol. Chem. 248, 6490 (1973).

18. D. Johnson and J. Travis, Human α-1-proteinase inhibitor mechanism of action: evidence for activation by limited proteolysis, Biochem. Biophys. Res. Commun. 72, 33 (1976).

19. D. Johnson and J. Travis, Inactivation of human α-1-proteinase inhibitor by thiol proteinases, Biochem. J. 163, 639 (1977).

20. D. Johnson and J. Travis, Structural Evidence for methionine at the reactive center of human α-1-proteinase inhibitor, J. Biol. Chem. 253, 7142 (1978).

21. Y. Schechter, Y. Burstein, and A. Patchornik, Selective oxidation of methionine residues in proteins, Biochemistry, 14, 4497 (1975).

22. H.E. Schultze, K. Heide, and H. Haupt, Uber ein noch nicht beschreibenes α-1-glycoprotein des menschlichen serums, Naturwissenschaften 49, 133 (1962).

23. J. Travis, D. Garner, and J. Bowen, Human α-1-antichymotrypsin: purification and properties, Biochemistry (in press, 1978).

MECHANISM OF ANTITHROMBIN ACTION AND THE STRUCTURAL BASIS OF HEPARIN'S ANTICOAGULANT FUNCTION

Robert D. Rosenberg
Sidney Farber Cancer Institute, Beth Israel Hospital, and Harvard Medical School, Boston, Mass. 02115. Supported by NIH-HLB 19131. RDR is an Established Investigator of the American Heart Association.

INTRODUCTION

Early in this century, several investigators recognized that thrombin gradually lost activity when added to defibinated plasma or serum (1). On this basis, they suspected that a specific inactivator of this enzyme, antithrombin, must be present under normal physiological conditions. In 1916, McLean isolated heparin from the liver as well as the heart and demonstrated its potent anticoagulant action (2). Subsequently, Brinkhous and his coworkers showed that heparin was effective as an anticoagulant only in the presence of a plasma component which they termed heparin-cofactor (3). In the 1950's, work from several laboratories suggested that plasma antithrombin and plasma heparin cofactor activities were manifestations of the same molecular entity (4,5,6). Furthermore, it was hypothesized that heparin must act by accelerating the rate at which antithrombin neutralizes thrombin. In 1968, this thesis was substantiated by Abildgaard who obtained small amounts of a purified human plasma protein that functioned as an antithrombin and a heparin cofactor (7). We have subsequently confirmed these observations, provided methods for the isolation of large quantities of this substance and examined the heparin-antithrombin interaction in considerable detail (8).

MECHANISM OF INHIBITOR ACTION

Human antithrombin was purified by a series of chromatographic and isoelectric focusing steps to obtain a final product that is homogeneous by disc gel electrophoresis (8). To demonstrate that this single protein possesses both antithrombin and heparin cofactor activity, we studied the inactivation of purified human thrombin in the presence and absence of heparin, Fig. 1. If thrombin is added to buffer with or without heparin, no loss in enzymatic activity is noted. If thrombin is incubated for varying periods of time with antithrombin, a slow, progressive decline in the enzyme's activity is observed. If thrombin is incubated with a mixture of heparin and antithrombin, its enzymatic activity is inhibited virtually instantaneously. The equivalence point of the reaction in the presence and absence of mucopolysaccharide occurs at a 1:1 molar ratio of enzyme to inhibitor. Thus, heparin acts by accelerating the rate at which antithrombin neutralizes thrombin without altering the stoichiometry of this interaction (8).

To prove that this protease inhibitor is responsible for most of the antithrombin and heparin cofactor activities normally present in the blood, we immunoprecipitated this component from defibrinated plasmas with a specific γ-globulin fraction directed against the protein and measured these residual activities in

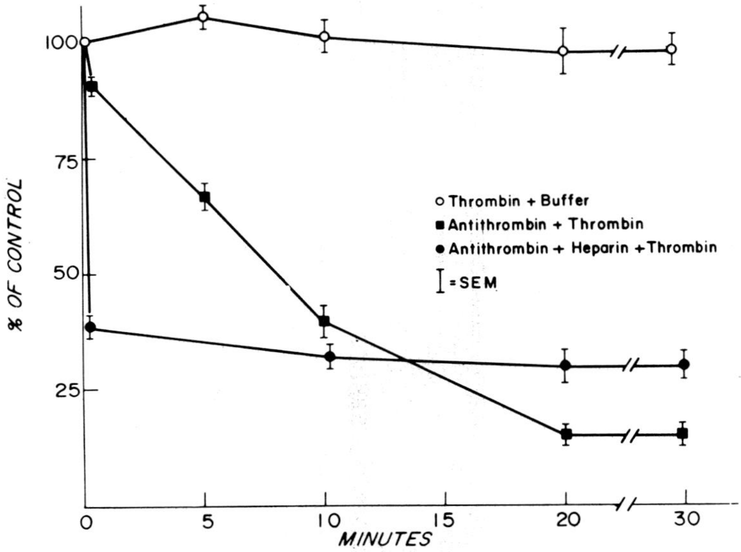

Fig. 1 Inhibition of thrombin by antithrombin in the presence and absence of heparin. Thrombin activity is expressed as percentage of the control value.

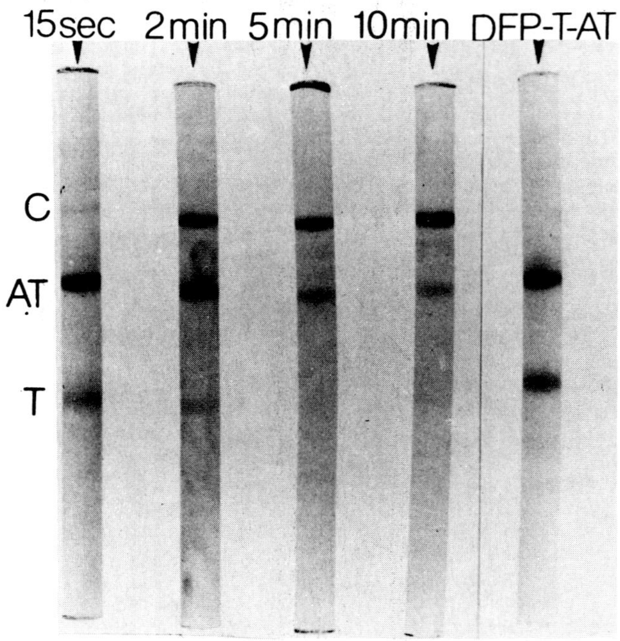

Fig. 2 Electrophoretic analysis of interactions between thrombin and antithrombin and between diisopropylfluorophosphate (DFP)-treated thrombin and antithrombin. Electrophoresis was performed in sodium dodecyl sulfate gels. C represents the complex formed by thrombin and antithrombin, AT represents antithrombin, and T represents thrombin.

the resultant supernatants. The data revealed that antithrombin and heparin cofactor activities declined in parallel fashion as the concentration of γ-globulin was increased and that less than 10% of either activity remained at the highest level of immunoglobulin utilized (8).

We have directly monitored the physical formation of a remarkably stable thrombin-antithrombin complex by sodium dodecyl sulfate gel electrophoresis. As expected from estimates of reaction stoichiometry, the complex has a molecular weight approximately equal to the sum of the molecular weights of thrombin and antithrombin. In the absence of heparin, complex formation occurs at a relatively slow rate, consonant with the gradual inhibition of enzymatic activity. In the presence of heparin, complex formation is virtually instantaneous (8), Figs. 2,3.

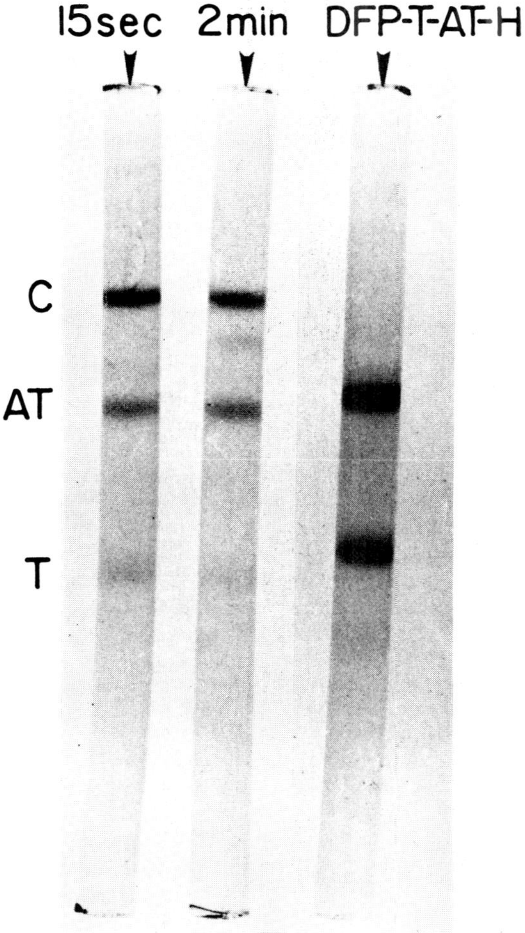

Fig. 3 Electrophoretic analysis of interactions between thrombin, antithrombin, and heparin and between diisopropylfluorophosphate (DFP)-treated thrombin, antithrombin and heparin: Electrophoresis was performed in sodium dodecylsulfate gels. C represents complex, AT denotes antithrombin, and T represents thrombin.

The formation of this enzyme-inhibitor complex, both in the presence and absence of heparin, is critically dependent upon the active serine center of thrombin. If this residue is blocked by the addition of diisopropylfluorophosphate, interaction between thrombin and antithrombin is totally inhibited, Fig. 2 and Fig. 3. As noted by other observers, thrombin's capacity to transform fibrinogen to fibrin depends on its ability to specifically cleave arginine-glycine bonds. Therefore, we expected that the reactive site of the inhibitor that binds the active serine center of the enzyme would contain an arginine residue. Indeed, our modification of this group on antithrombin with 2,3 - butanedione or 1,2 - cyclohexanedione virtually eliminates the ability of this protein to inhibit thrombin in the presence or absence of heparin (8). Given the highly acidic nature of heparin, one would expect that positive groups on antithrombin such as ε-amino lysyl residues form the binding site for this negatively charged anticoagulant. We have shown that the chemical alteration of these residues with *o*-methylisourea prevents the binding of heparin to this protein and suppresses the acceleration of inhibitor action by this anticoagulant. However the slow, progressive inactivation of thrombin by antithrombin is not appreciably affected (8).

Thus, antithrombin neutralizates the activity of thrombin by the formation of a 1:1 stoichiometric complex through an interaction between the reactive site (arginine) on the inhibitor and the active center (serine) on the enzyme. Heparin functions as an anticoagulant by binding to antithrombin and dramatically increasing the rate at which the enzyme-inhibitor complex is formed.

The hemostatic mechanism is composed of a series of linked proteolytic reactions. At each stage of this cascade, a parent zymogen is converted to a serine protease which catalyzes a subsequent zymogen-serine protease transition. Thus, of the eleven proteins that are part of the coagulation system, six are ultimately activated to serine proteases (prothrombin, factors VII, IX, X, XI, and XII); three are cofactors for these conversions (factors V, VIII, and high molecular weight kininogen); one is transformed into a transamidinating enzyme with an-SH group at its active center (factor XIII); and one is the final substrate for these multiple interactions (fibrinogen).

The nature of the antithrombin-heparin mechanism of action led us to predict that all serine proteases within the coagulation system would be neutralized by antithrombin and that the mucopolysaccharide would accelerate each of these interactions (8,9,10). We were particularly encouraged in this belief by the data of other investigators, obtained by coagulation assay, that antithrombin also neutralized the activity of factor Xa (11,12,13). To test this hypothesis, we analyzed the interaction of this protein with virtually all of the serine proteases of the hemostatic system: factor IXa (14), factor IXa (10), and factor XIIa (15).

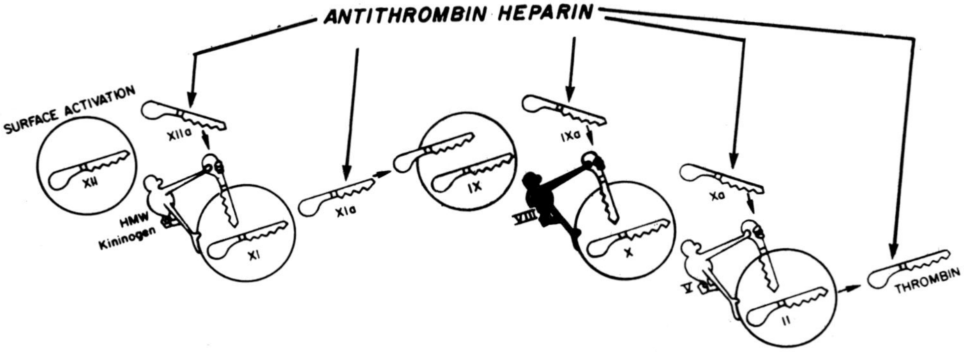

Fig. 4 The sites of action of antithrombin and heparin within the coagulation cascade.

In each of these cases, a slow but progressive inhibition of enzymatic activity occurred in the presence of antithrombin. This process of inactivation is due to the formation of a 1:1 stoichiometric complex of enzyme and inhibitor. In each instance, the addition of heparin dramatically accelerated the rate of neutralization without altering the stoichiometry or nature of complex formation (8,9,14, 15,16), Fig. 4. These unsuspected observations have been confirmed by work from other laboratories (17,18,19). The only exception to this generalized view of heparin's action may be in the inhibition of factor VIIa by antithrombin. There has been a preliminary report that heparin's effect on this interaction is minimal (20). However, the maintenance of an enzymatically active form of factor VII requires a stable interaction of the proenzyme with tissue factor-phospholipid complexes. This renders interpretation of these findings difficult, since the tissue factor-phospholipid surface is highly negatively charged and would repel the similarly charged heparin-inhibitor complex. Other steps of the coagulation system that do not involve serine proteases are only minimally affected by heparin. These include the binding of cofactors such as factor V and the polymerization or crosslinking of fibrin. Thus, antithrombin functions as a classical protease inhibitor within the hemostatic mechanism except that the ligand heparin can accelerate its action in a unique fashion.

HEPARIN

This mucopolysaccharide is initially synthesized as an alternating copolymer of N-acetylglucosamine and glucuronic acid (21). In subsequent postsynthetic steps, glucosamine residues are variably N-deacetylated and N-sulfated, glucuronic acid residues are variably epimerized to form iduronic acid, and glucosamine as well as iduronic acid residues are variably ester sulfated (22). The final structure of the mucopolysaccharide is depicted in Fig. 5. It is important to note that this represents only one of many possible arrangements of hexosamine and uronic acid residues.

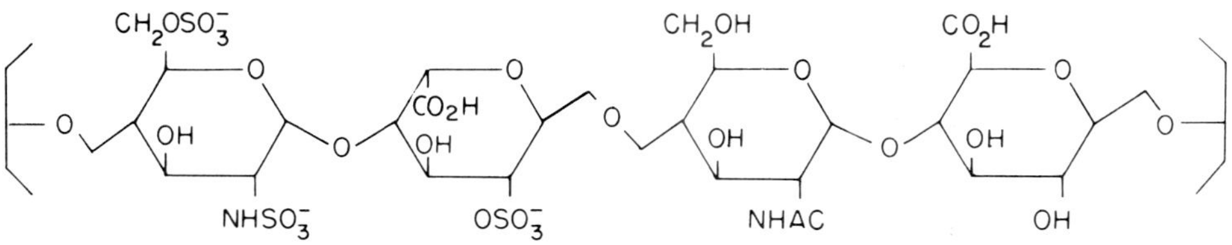

Hexosamine Iduronic acid Hexosamine Glucuronic acid

Fig. 5 One of the many possible arrangements of hexosamine and uronic acid residues present within the heparin polymer.

Considerable effort has been expended in defining the linear sequence and three-dimensional configuration of heparin (23,24,25). However, the precise relationship between its structure and anticoagulant properties remained elusive until very recently. Heparin preparations have exhibited considerable polydispersity in molecular size (26), variations in the ratio of glucuronic acid to iduronic acid (27), alterations in the amount of ester and N-sulfation and differing extents of N-acetylation (28). Changes in each of these parameters correlate only to a limited degree with anticoagulant potency. Thus, it has been tacitly assumed that this mucopolysaccharide may exhibit *numerous alternative structures equally capable of activating antithrombin*. Given these observations, it is surprising that chemically related mucopolysaccharides such as heparan sulfate and dermatan sulfate have minimal anticoagulant activity.

We thought it unlikely that heparin would exhibit the unique specificity described in this review if it possessed such an ill-defined molecular structure. Therefore, we considered the possibility that these products might be grossly impure and that only a small fraction of the molecules were responsible for its distinctive biologic properties. In this case, attempts to relate the structure of the bulk material to its anticoagulant functions would prove meaningless.

FRACTIONATION OF HEPARIN SPECIES

Numerous investigators have subjected heparin to gel filtration, ion exchange chromatography or electrophoresis without observing any substantial increase in its anticoagulant activity per mg of mucopolysaccharide. Therefore, we attempted to employ a more biologic approach in fractionating preparations of this complex sugar. To this end, we added a large molar excess of antithrombin to heparin.

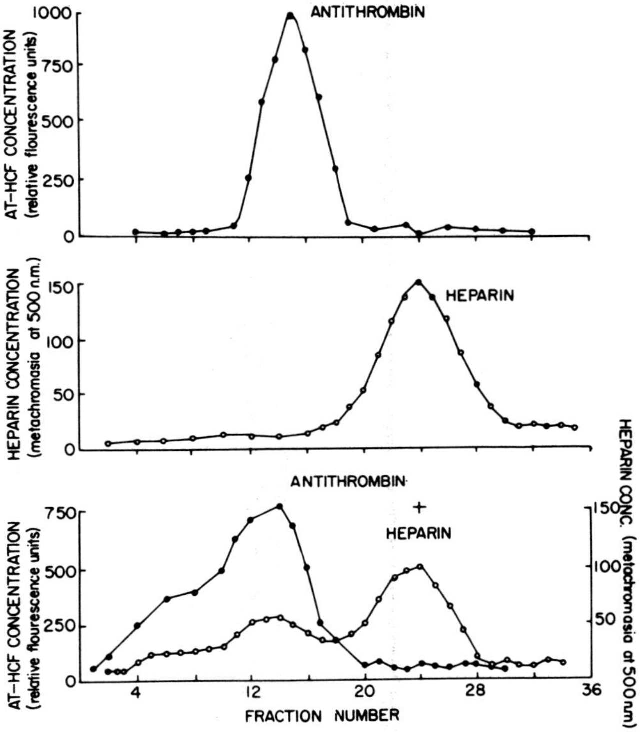

Fig. 6 Sucrose density gradient centrifugation of antithrombin and heparin.

Subsequently, sucrose density gradient centrifugation was utilized to separate mucopolysaccharide that bound to antithrombin from that unable to complex with the inhibitor (29). Our data indicated that preparations of heparin consisted of two distinct populations of the mucopolysaccharide which differed greatly in their ability to bind to and activate antithrombin. The first form constituted approximately two-thirds of the chemical mass of the unfractionated heparin and was unable to complex with the inhibitor under the conditions of these experiments. This fraction was responsible for less than 15% of the total anticoagulant activity of the starting material. The second form comprised one-third of the remaining chemical mass of unfractionated heparin and was capable of binding tightly to antithrombin. This material possessed more than 85% of the total anticoagulant activity of the starting material (29), Fig. 6. The heparin utilized in these studies was indistinguishable from other preparations of the mucopolysaccharide. Indeed, we have recently analyzed heparin isolated from a variety of sources including the human lung and have obtained data identical to that provided above (30). The existence of active and relatively inactive species of mucopolysaccharide has been confirmed by Lindahl and his coworkers (31).

We have subsequently demonstrated that the *active heparin* species that are capable of binding to antithrombin are *quite heterogeneous* and have provided a new highly discriminating methodology for the affinity fractionation of low molecular weight forms of this mucopolysaccharide (6000-8000 daltons) (32). The low molecular weight species isolated from commercial preparations of heparin were separated by a technique based upon their affinity for antithrombin. Cycle I of this process was initiated by adding the protease inhibitor to the heparin pool at a molar ratio of 0.08. The resultant mixture was filtered through columns of Sephadex G-100 equilibrated with 0.15 M NaCl in 0.01 M Tris-HCl, pH 7.5. The column effluents were monitored for protein by absorbance at 280 nm and for mucopolysaccharide by the carbazole reaction. These measurements revealed two discrete peaks. The first peak contained protein as well as mucopolysaccharide and represented a stable heparin-antithrombin complex. Mucopolysaccharide present in this region of the chromatogram is designed highly active heparin. The second peak consisted only of free mucopolysaccharide. Its elution position was identical to that observed when the low molecular weight heparin fraction was gel filtered as described above but in the absence of antithrombin. Mucopolysaccharide located in this area of the chromatogram consisted of active and relatively inactive heparin species. The highly active heparin-antithrombin complex was concentrated and filtered through columns of Sephadex G-100 equilibrated with 3.0 M NaCl in 0.01 M Tris-HCl, pH 7.5. The increase in ionic strength of the solvent disrupted the complex such that discrete peaks of protein as well as mucopolysaccharide were generated. Cycle II of the fractionation was initiated by mixing antithrombin with the pool of active and relatively inactive heparin species at a molar ratio of 1.5. The resultant solution was processed as described above to separate the active from the relatively inactive material. Further addition of antithrombin to this latter species did not result in the formation of a protein mucopolysaccharide complex as judged by gel filtration. The relative abundance of the highly active, active, and relatively inactive forms of heparin were 7.9, 25.1, and 67.0%, respectively. Their specific anticoagulant activities were 360, 267, and 4 units/mg.,respectively (32).

Additional experiments were conducted to determine the homogeneity of highly active and active heparin species. When the molar ratio of antithrombin to mucopolysaccharide was increased to 0.15 during cycle I of affinity fractionation, the specific anticoagulant activity of the heparin that bound to antithrombin was significantly decreased compared to the highly active material. On the other hand, when the molar ratio of antithrombin to mucopolysaccharide was decreased to 0.04 during cycle I of the isolation technique, the resultant heparin bound to antithrombin was found to have a specific anticoagulant activity equivalent to that of highly active material. These critical experiments suggest that highly active heparin is homogeneous with respect to its ability to bind to and activate antithrombin. A similar analysis of the active material indicated that this fraction is composed of several heparin species with different affinities for antithrombin and differing anticoagulant potencies (32).

FUNCTIONAL PROPERTIES OF HEPARIN SPECIES

We initially examined the binding of highly active as well as relatively inactive heparin species to antithrombin (33). Chromatographic isolation of the radiolabeled highly active heparin-antithrombin interaction product permitted us to show that the protease inhibitor possesses only one binding site for the low molecular weight species and therefore can complex with only one molecule of this mucopolysaccharide. The formation of the highly active heparin-antithrombin complex is accompanied by an increase in the intrinsic fluorescence of the protease inhibitor at 330 nm (33). Einarsson and Andersson have made similar observations with poorly characterized active heparin products of unknown binding stoichiometry (34). In a recent communication, we have demonstrated that the progressive enhancement in the intrinsic fluorescence of antithrombin at increasing concentrations of highly active heparin can be fitted to a mass action equation with a K_{DISS} of 1.8×10^{-7} M and a binding stoichometry of 1:1 (33). The excellent agreement between our experimental observations and this simple single site model indicates that the mucopolysaccharide behaves as a nearly ideal ligand despite its extraordinary charge density. Data obtained for relatively inactive heparin could also be fitted to the same single site binding model except that K_{DISS} averaged 1.0×10^{-4} M (33).

As expected, variations in protein concentration from 5×10^{-8} M to 4×10^{-7} M did not alter the binding isotherm for the highly active heparin-antithrombin interaction. However, changes in the level of inhibitor from 2×10^{-8} M to 5×10^{-6}M markedly displaced the binding isotherm for the relatively inactive heparin-antithrombin interaction. These results point to the unexpected conclusion that highly active heparin is quite homogeneous whereas only a small subpopulation within the relatively inactive mucopolysaccharide is able to bind tightly to antithrombin (33). A computer fit of the experimental data indicates that this anomalous shift in the binding isotherm of relatively inactive heparin is best explained by the contamination of this material with 1-2% of active mucopolysaccharide (33).

We have also analyzed the ability of the two heparin species to accelerate thrombin-antithrombin interactions (33). Prior to examining these properties in a quantitative manner it was necessary to probe the kinetic relationships between mucopolysaccharide and protease inhibitor. Various investigators have suspected that heparin might function as a catalyst during the neutralization of thrombin by antithrombin (35,36,37,38,39). To examine this possibility, we have utilized concentrations of reactants sufficiently reduced to permit monitoring of enzyme inactivation by manual assay techniques. When highly active heparin was admixed with antithrombin and thrombin at final concentrations of 5×10^{-9} M, 1×10^{-8} M, and 1×10^{-8} M, respectively, complete inhibition of enzyme took place over 150 sec. Minimal amounts of thrombin are inhibited at the same point in time when mucopolysaccharide is absent. Given the 1:1 molar binding stoichiometry of highly active heparin and antithrombin, we calculate that the mucopolysaccharide must be reutilized eighteen to twenty times during the course of this reaction (33).

It is apparent that highly active heparin might function as a catalyst if the mucopolysaccharide were released from antithrombin during formation of the enzyme-inhibitor complex and were able to bind anew to free protease inhibitor. We have validated this hypothesis by demonstrating that three critical aspects of the mechanism are correct. Firstly, we have shown that the binding of thrombin to the highly active heparin-antithrombin complex results in the discharge of mucopolysaccharide from the protease inhibitor on a 1:1 molar basis. Secondly, we have provided evidence that release of mucopolysaccharide is linked to its inability to bind tightly to the thrombin-antithrombin complex as compared to free inhibitor. Thirdly, we have shown that highly active heparin discharged from the protease inhibitor during enzyme inactivation retains its ability to bind to antithrombin.

In most instances, the rate of enzyme neutralization is limited by the recycling of mucopolysaccharide. The inactivation of thrombin is exceedingly rapid once the heparin-antithrombin complex has formed (33). Thus, the amount of highly active heparin-antithrombin complex formed at time zero should determine the initial rate of the thrombin-antithrombin interaction (33). In Fig. 7, we provide a plot of the initial velocity of this reaction versus the concentration of highly active heparin present in the incubation mixture. An increasing rate of thrombin inhibition is noted as the concentration of highly active heparin is raised from 1×10^{-9} M to 2×10^{-7}. Also depicted is the binding of this mucopolysaccharide fraction to antithrombin as monitored by fluorescence spectroscopy. A close correspondence is evident between the initial velocity plot as a function of highly active heparin concentration and the amount of mucopolysaccharide bound to antithrombin. We have provided a rigorous mathematical proof that *superimposition* of these two sets of data strongly suggests a *primary role* for the *Heparin-Antithrombin* interaction product in the enzymatic neutralization process (33).

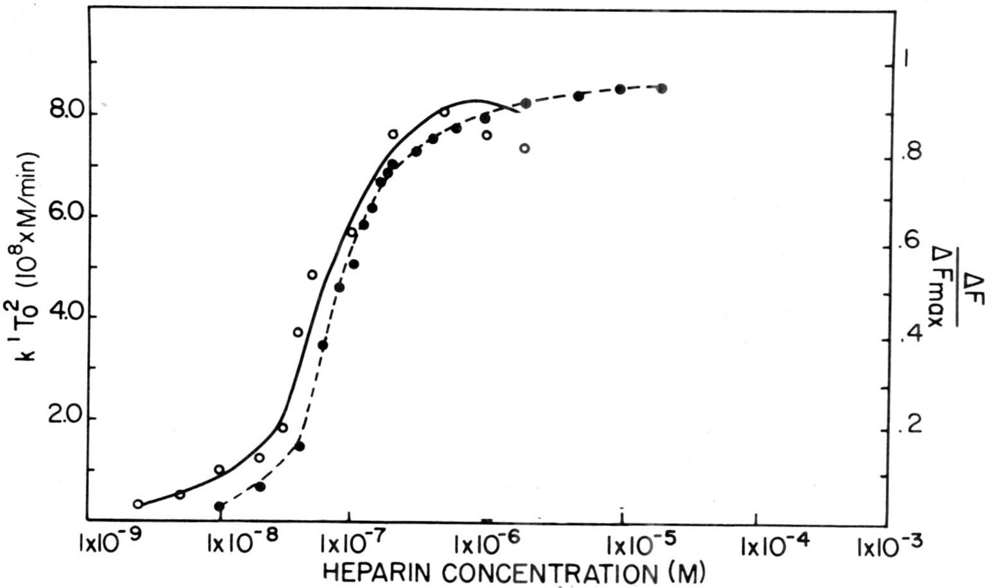

Fig. 7 The extent of binding of heparin to antithrombin and its ability to accelerate the thrombin-antithrombin interaction. The fluorescence binding curve was obtained with the same fraction of highly active heparin (•--•) utilized in the kinetic analysis. The binding data is plotted as the fluorescence charge at 330 nm for a given concentration of mucopolysaccharides normalized to the projected maximal increase in this parameter ($\Delta F/\Delta F_{MAX}$). The kinetics of the thrombin-antithrombin interaction were examined in the presence of varying concentrations of highly active (o——o) heparin. The initial velocity of this process is plotted as $K^1 To^2$ where To represents the nominal starting concentration of thrombin and K^1 is the negative value of the bimolecular rate constant multiplied by:

$$\frac{[\text{Heparin-Antithrombin}]}{[\text{Antithrombin}]} \times \left(1 - \frac{[\text{Heparin-Thrombin}]}{[\text{Thrombin}]}\right)$$

Further inspection of the data reveals that a pseudoplateau in the initial velocity of the thrombin-antithrombin interaction occurs between highly active heparin concentrations of 2×10^{-7} M and 5×10^{-6} M. The region of relatively constant initial velocity coincides with the saturation of the inhibitor by mucopolysaccharide as judged by the fluorescence binding curve. The bimolecular rate constant for the thrombin-antithrombin interaction at these saturating levels of highly active heparin is $1.0 \times 10^9\ M^{-1}min^{-1}$. This represents a 2300 fold increase over the bimolecular rate constant obtained in the absence of mucopolysaccharide. At higher concentrations of highly active heparin, a *decrease* in the initial velocity of this inhibitory process is apparent when compared to pseudoplateau values obtained at lower levels of mucopolysaccharide (not shown). This phenomenon is independent of the heparin-antithrombin interaction (33). Our data suggests that the decreased rates of inhibition must be due to the interaction of mucopolysaccharide with thrombin. Thus, a thrombin-mucopolysaccharide complex is inhibited only slowly by the antithrombin-heparin interaction product (33).

The relatively inactive heparin was examined in similar fashion to determine its effect upon the thrombin-antithrombin interaction. Several hundred fold higher concentrations of this molecular species are required to achieve a similar increase in the rate of thrombin interaction as compared to the highly active fraction (33). Furthermore, when sufficiently high levels of this mucopolysaccharide are employed the maximal rate of enzyme inactivation is approximately 10% of that achieved with the highly active heparin. This kinetic data is in complete accord with the presence of a small amount of active heparin (1-2%) contaminating the relatively inactive fraction (33).

STRUCTURAL ANALYSIS OF HEPARIN SPECIES

Highly active and relatively inactive heparin species were also analyzed with respect to uronic acid composition and sulfate group placements, Table 1 (32). Based upon molecular weight analysis, monosaccharide composition, and sulfate group distribution, we estimate that the highly active form has 1.1 additional residues of glucuronic acid per molecule and 1.5 fewer residues of N-sulfated glucosamine per molecule when compared to the relatively inactive species. High resolution nuclear magnetic resonance measurements suggest that the latter reduction in N-sulfated glucosamine is secondary to a concomitant increased in N-acetyl glucosamine. We suspected that the additional glucuronic acid and N-acetyl glucosamine residues might be located at adjacent sites on the highly active heparin polymer (32).

TABLE 1 Chemical and Functional Characteristics

Heparin	Glucuronic* acid %	Sulfate/ disaccharide	N-sulfate/ disaccharide	O-sulfate/ disaccharide
Highly active	30.7	2.26	0.70	1.56
Relatively inactive	19.3	2.37	0.95	1.42

*The iduronic acid value can be calculated by substracting the glucuronic acid value from 100%.

Nitrous acid degradation of mucopolysaccharide at pH 1.5 converts N-sulfated glucosamine residues to 2,5 anhydromannose moieties with resultant cleavage of the respective glycosidic bonds. This treatment has no effect upon N-acetyl glucosamine groups. Therefore, heparin polymers exposed to the above chemical agent would be transformed into disaccharides except where N-acetyl substituents are present on the mucopolysaccharide chain. If our supposition concerning the position of the additional glucuronic acid and N-acetyl glucosamine moieties is correct, these residues should be captured as a tetrasaccharide after nitrous acid degradation of highly active heparin.

To test this hypothesis, we individually subjected the two heparin species to nitrous acid cleavage at pH 1.5, radiolabeled the newly formed reducing ends with sodium [H^3] borohydride, separated the various components by paper chromatography and quantitated the respective peaks by scintillation counting (32). Our analyses indicated that larger amounts of a specific oligosaccharide, 1β, are found within the tetrasaccharide zone of highly active heparin as compared to a similar structure, isolated from mucopolysaccharide, Fig. 8. Indeed, 1.1 1β oligosaccharide sequences per molecule, 1β*a*, are present within highly active heparin whereas only 0.3 1β structures per molecule, 1β*i*, are found in the relatively inactive mucopolysaccharide.

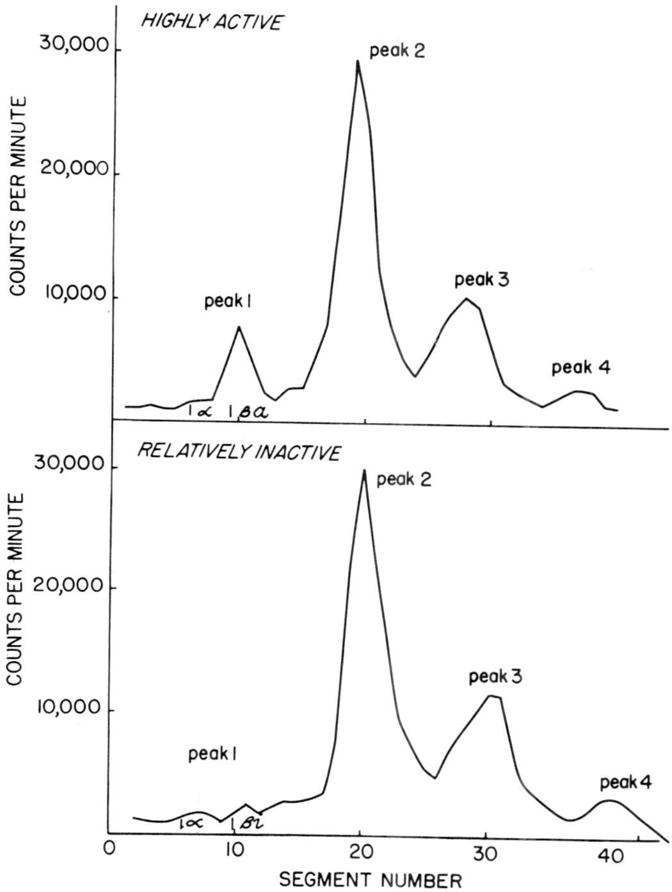

Fig. 8 Nitrous acid degradation patterns for highly active (upper) and relatively inactive (lower) heparin species. The 1β*a* and 1β*i* tetrasaccharides are indicated in the upper and lower panel, respectively.

Detailed chemical studies demonstrated that both oligosaccharides possess two uronic acid moieties per reducing end group, contain equimolar amounts of iduronic acid as well as glucuronic acid, and terminate in [^{3}H] anhydromannitol at the reducing end position. In addition, a complete destruction of all uronic acid residues resulted when 1β*a* was treated at pH 3.9 and 5° with 0.1 M sodium periodate for 48 hr (40). Furthermore, the internal glucosamine residue of 1β*a* and 1β*i* appears to be N-acetylated since the two components are completely resistant to cleavage with nitrous acid at pH 4.2 (40). Given the known alternating glucosamine-uronic acid structure of heparin, these experiments indicate that both 1β*a* and 1β*i* are tetrasaccharides with a monosaccharide sequence of uronic acid → N-acetyl glucosamine → uronic acid → [H^3] anhydromannitol. The relative abundance of 1β*a* and 1β*i* within the two mucopolysaccharide fractions are consistent with the differences in uronic acid composition and N-acetyl glucosamine content of the parent polymers cited above (40).

Of course, 1β*a* and 1β*i* may be subtly different in structure. For this reason, we examined these tetrasaccharides by high voltage electrophoresis at pH 3.6 and pH 5.3 while utilizing monosulfated disaccharide, disulfated disaccharide, and tetrasulfated tetrasaccharide markers. Both 1β*a* and 1β*i* migrated slightly faster than the monosulfated disaccharide marker at pH 3.6 (40). These findings suggested that each component contains two sulfated monosaccharide moieties. The patterns also indicated that 1β*i* is considerably more heterogeneous than 1β*a*.

To elucidate the possible structural differences in 1β*a* and 1β*i*, we determined the type and degree of sulfation of the uronic acid residue present at the non-reducing end of these species (40). This was accomplished by employing exoglycosidases to remove single uronic acid residues from the non-reducing ends of these oligosaccharides. The reaction mixtures were subsequently filtered on columns of P2 - polyacrylamide to determine the extent of enzymatic cleavage. In this system, tetrasaccharides, disulfated disaccharides as well as sulfated monosaccharides elute at fixed positions relative to radiolabeled glucose utilized as a column marker (40).

The 1β*a* migrated within the tetrasaccharide zone prior to treatment with enzyme. The uronic acid composition of this species was 51% iduronic acid and 49% glucuronic acid. The ratio of uronic acid to anhydromannitol was 2.1. After enzymatic degradation with β-glucuronidase, virtually 100% of this component continued to migrate within the tetrasaccharide region. The uronic acid composition of this species, and the ratio of uronic acid to anhydromannitol was unchanged. When the same component was exposed to a crude enzyme mixture containing α-iduronidase and iduronate sulfatase, ~95% of the material shifted its elution position into a region of the chromatogram located between the tetrasaccharide and disaccharide zones. Analysis of the uronic acid composition of this material revealed that it contained 100% glucuronic acid. Furthermore, the newly generated species exhibited a ratio of uronic acid to anhydromannitol of 1.1. The residue liberated from 1β*a* migrated within the sulfated monosaccharide region. This group was identified as iduronic acid after conversion to iditol and subsequent paper chromatography with appropriate standards. To determine whether the iduronic acid moiety present at the non-reducing end of 1β*a* possesses an ester sulfate substituent, we subjected this component to degradation with partially purified α-iduronidase. This treatment shifted the elution position of 95% of the tetrasaccharide mass into the trisaccharide zone. Thus, virtually all 1β*a* exhibits a non-sulfated iduronic acid residue at the non-reducing end position. The 1β*i* was examined in a similar fashion. This material migrated within the tetrasaccharide zone prior to treatment with β-glucuronidase. Its uronic acid content was 51% iduronic acid and 49% glucuronic acid. The ratio of uronic acid to anhydromannitol was 2.1. After degradation with β-glucuronidase, the elution position of 29% of 1β*i* mass shifted into the trisaccharide zone. Species which remained within the tetrasaccharide region exhibited no alteration in uronic acid composition or in the ratio of uronic acid to anhydromannitol. Material that migrated within the trisaccharide zone showed an iduronic acid content of >95% and a ratio of uronic acid to anhydromannitol of 1.1. Thus, 29% of 1β*i* contains a glucuronic acid residue at the non-reducing end. To demonstrate that the remaining 71% possesses an iduronic acid residue at the non-reducing position, we degraded material that was resistant to β-glucuronidase with a crude enzyme mixture of α-iduronidase and iduronate sulfatase. As expected, the elution position of 87% of this tetrasaccharide shifted to the trisaccharide zone. The material that migrated as a trisaccharide contained only glucuronic acid and the ratio of uronic acid to anhydromannitol was quantitated as 1.1. To determine whether the iduronic acid liberated from 1β*i* possessed an ester sulfate substituent when present on the parent molecule, we treated species resistant to β-glucuronidase with partially purified α-iduronidase. Approximately 88% of 1β*i* was uneffected by exposure to this enzyme. Thus, only 12% of this component contains a non-sulfated iduronic acid at the non-reducing position (40).

We have also utilized an alternate method to directly quantitate the degree of sulfation of the iduronic acid located at the non-reducing end of 1β*a* and 1β*i* tetrasaccharides that were resistant to treatment with β-glucuronidase (40). This approach is based upon the observations of Shively and Conrad that carboxy-reduction of iduronsyl-2-sulfate-anhydromannitol-6-sulfate will permit scissioning of the glycosidic bond of this disaccharide with dilute HCl without producing complete desulfation of the liberated monosaccharides (41,42). These authors have identified the resultant cleavage fragments by paper chromatography and rigorously confirmed the assigned structures by mass spectroscopy (41,42). Initially, we repeated the work of these investigators on this model disaccharide. This allowed us to establish the relative mobilities of various well characterized fragments in our chromatographic system. Furthermore, results obtained with this model disaccharide could be employed as a control when estimating the extent to which sulfate substituents initially present on the idose residue are retained by this hexose moiety upon release by dilute acid hydrolysis. Subsequently, we have conducted identical studies employing 1β*a* and 1β*i* tetrasaccharides that were resistant to degradation with β-glucuronidase. Complete hydrolysis of the idose-N-acetylglucosamine bond was achieved with both components. In the case of 1β*a* we calculated that 5.5% of iduronic acid residues present at the non-reducing position are sulfated. With respect to 1β*i*, we estimate that 89% of the iduronic acid residues located at the non-reducing end of the tetrasaccharide must bear ester sulfate substituents (40).

Thus, highly active heparin possesses 1.1 1β*a* tetrasaccharide per molecule. Careful examination of this nitrous acid fragment by chemical as well as enzymatic degradation techniques has revealed that 95% of the non-reducing end group consists of non-sulfated iduronic acid while 5.0% may bear an ester sulfate substituent. This minor degree of heterogeneity may be due to trace contamination of our sample with oligosaccharides such as 1α tetrasaccharide that migrate close to 1β*a* and contain sulfated iduronic acid as the predominant uronic acid residue (2). If the above data is employed in conjunction with the uronic acid composition, electrophoretic mobility, periodate sensitivity, and high pH nitrous acid resistance of this 1β*a* tetrasaccharide, it is possible to propose a structure for this component. On the basis of the available evidence, we conclude that 1β*a* should be represented by the following monosaccharide sequence at the polymer level:

L-IDURONIC ACID → N-ACETYLATED-D-GLUCOSAMINE 6 SULFATE → D-GLUCURONIC ACID → N-SULFATED-D-GLUCOSAMINE 6 SULFATE

The relatively inactive mucopolysaccharide possesses 0.3 1β*i* fragments per molecule. Treatment of this component with purified β-glucuronidase indicates that only 71% of this component exhibits an iduronic acid at the non-reducing position. Furthermore, chemical as well as enzymatic degradation techniques demonstrate that 88% of 1β*i* resistant to degradation with β-glucuronidase contain an ester sulfate substituent on the iduronic acid residue. Thus, only 2.6% of the molecules present within the relatively inactive mucopolysaccharide can possess the unique 1β*a* tetrasaccharide sequence found within each molecule of highly active heparin, Table 2. It should be noted that the preparations of relatively inactive mucopolysaccharide utilized in this study are not completely depleted of active species. Indeed, we estimate that these products contain 2-3% of heparin components which exhibit anticoagulant activity (32,33). The observed correlation between the relative abundance of the unique tetrasaccharide structure and the anticoagulant potency of these preparations strongly suggests that this critical sequence must represent a binding site on porcine heparin which is recognized by antithrombin. Our conclusion concerning the importance of this sequence is considerably strengthened by the invariant nature of this structure within the highly active heparin as well as the presence of two relatively rare non-sulfated uronic acid moieties in close proximity. It is of particular interest that a non-sulfated iduronic acid residue has been found within the critical tetrasaccharide since this moiety can assume unique conformations in the heparin polymer (43). Of course, it remains to be seen whether minor variations within the critical tetrasaccharide sequence such as the replacement of the N-acetyl glucosamine 6-sulfate residue by an N-sulfated glucosamine 6-sulfate group will alter the functional properties of highly active heparin. In addition, it may be necessary to position elements such as trisulfated iduronsyl-glucosamine disaccharides on either side of the critical tetrasaccharide sequence to attain a complete protease inhibitor binding site on the mucopolysaccharide. These structural features constitute 60-70% of the chemical mass of the heparin molecule.

TABLE 2 Summary of Data on 1β*a* and 1β*i* Tetrasaccharides

Heparin	1β*a* or 1β*i* Content	Uronic Acid Residue at the Non-Reducing End, %			1β*a* Content	Anticoagulant Activity Normalized to the Highly Active Fraction
		Glucuronic Acid	Sulfated Iduronic Acid	Non-Sulfated Iduronic Acid		
Highly Active	1.1	0	0.05	0.95	1.05[b]	1.0
Relatively Inactive	0.3	0.29	0.625	0.085[a]	0.026[b]	0.03

a) This value represents 12% of the 71% of 1β*i* tetrasaccharide possessing iduronic acid at the non-reducing end.

b) This value represents column 1 multiplied by column 4.

Despite these uncertainties, we believe that our data provides the first example of a well defined structure-function relationship for a mucopolysaccharide. Thus, our findings suggest that this class of biologic macromolecules may prove to be quite similar in this regard to proteins and nucleic acids.

REFERENCES

(1) C. Contejean, Recherches sur les injections intraveineuses de peptone et leur influence sur la coagulabilité du sang chez le chien, Arch. Phyisol Norm Pathol. 7, 45-53 (1895).

(2) J. McLean, The thromboplastic action of cephalin, Am. J. Physiol. 41, 250-257. (1916).

(3) K.M. Brinkhous, H.P. Smith, E.D. Warner, The inhibition of blood clotting: an unidentified substance which acts in conjunction with heparin to prevent the conversion of prothrombin into thrombin, Am. J. Physiol. 125, 683-687 (1939).

(4) Morowitz, P. (1968) The Chemistry of Blood Coagulation, Springfield, Ill., Charles C. Thomas Publisher.

(5) D.F. Waugh, M.A. Fitzgerald, Quantitative aspects of antithrombin and heparin in plasma, Am. J. Physiol. 184, 627-639 (1956).

(6) F.C. Monkhouse, E.S. France, W.H. Seegers, Studies on the antithrombin and heparin cofactor activities of a fraction adsorbed from plasma by aluminum hydroxide, Circ. Res. 3, 397-402 (1955).

(7) U. Abildgaard, Highly purified antithrombin III with heparin cofactor activity prepared by disc electrophoresis, Scand. J. Clin. Lab. Invest. 21, 89-91 (1968).

(8) R.D. Rosenberg, P.S. Damus, The purification and mechanism of action of human antithrombin-heparin cofactor, J. Biol. Chem. 248, 6490-6505 (1973).

(9) P.S. Damus, M. Hicks, R.D. Rosenberg, A generalized view of heparin's anticoagulant action, Nature (Lond) 246, 355-357 (1973).

(10) R.D. Rosenberg, Heparin action, Circulation 49, 603-605 (1973).

(11) W.H. Seegers, E.R. Cole, C.R. Harmison, et al. Neutralization of autoprothrombin C activity with antithrombin, Can. J. Biochem. 42, 359-364 (1964).

(12) R. Briggs, K.W.E. Denson, N. Akman, et al. Antithrombin III, antifactor Xa and heparin, Br. J. Haematol. 19, 283-305 (1970).

(13) E.T. Yin, S. Wessler, P.J. Stoll, Identity of plasma-activated factor X inhibitor with antithrombin III and heparin co-factor, J. Biol. Chem. 246, 3712-3719 (1971).

(14) J.S. Rosenberg, P. McKenna, R.D. Rosenberg, The inhibition of human factor IXa by human antithrombin-heparin co-factor, J. Biol. Chem. 250, 8883-8888 (1975).

(15) N. Stead, A. Kaplan, R.D. Rosenberg, Inhibition of Factor XIIa with antithrombin, Clin. Res. 24, 321A (1976)

(16) N. Stead, A. Kaplan, R.D. Rosenberg, Inhibition of activator factor XII by antithrombin-heparin co-factor, J. Biol. Chem. 251, 6481-6488 (1976).

(17) K. Kurachi, K. Fujikawa, G. Schmier, E.W. Davie, Inhibition of bovine factor IXa and factor Xβ by antithrombin III, Biochem. 373-377 (1976).

(18) J. Chen, C. Burrowes, F. Habal, H. Movat, The inhibition of activated factor XII (Hageman factor) by antithrombin III: the effect of other plasma proteinase inhibitor, Biochem. Biophys. Res. Commun. 74, 150-158 (1977).

(19) K. Fujikawa, K. Kurachi, E.W. Davie, Characterization of bovine factor XIIa, Biochemistry, 16, 4182-4188 (1977).

(20) H.C. Godal, M. Ryah, K. Laake, Progressive inactivation of purified Factor VII by heparin and antithrombin III, Thromb. Res. 5, 773-776 (1974).

(21) Stoolmiller, A.C., Dorfman, N. (1969) Comprehensive Chemistry, XVII, 241 Academic Press, New York.

(22) Fransson, L.A. (1970) The Chemistry and Molecular Biology of the Intercellular Matrix, II, 823 Grune and Stratton, New York.

(23) M.E. Silva, C.P. Dietrich, Structure of heparin, J. Biol. Chem. 250, 6841-6846 (1975).

(24) R.L. Taylor, J.T. Shively, H.E. Conrad, J.A. Cifonelli, Uronic acid composition of heparins and heparan sulfates, Biochemistry 3633-3636 (1973).

(25) J.A. Nieduszynski, E.D.T. Atkins, Conformation of the mucopolysaccharides-X-ray Fibre diffraction of heparin, Biochemistry 135, 729-733 (1973).

(26) T.C. Laurent, Studies on fractionated heparin, Arch. Biochem. Biophys. 92, 224-231 (1961).

(27) P. Hovingh, A. Linker, The enzymatic degradation of heparin and heparitin sulfate, J. Biol. Chem. 245, 6170-6175 (1970).

(28) I.H. Danishefsky, A. Steiner, A. Friedlander, Investigations on the chemistry of heparin, J. Biol. Chem. 244, 1741-1745 (1969).

(29) L.H. Lam, J.E. Silbert, R.D. Rosenberg, Separation of active and inactive forms of heparin, Biochem. Biophys. Res. Commun. 69, 570-577 (1976).

(30) D.D. Metcalfe, R.A. Lewis, J.E. Silbert, R.D. Rosenberg, S.I. Wasserman, K.F. Austen, Isolation, identification, and characterization of heparin from human lung, Fed. Proc. 37, 1776 (1978).

(31) M. Höök, J. Bjork, J. Hopwood, U. Lindahl, Anticoagulant activity of heparin: separation of high-activity and low-activity heparin species by affinity chromatography on immobilized antithrombin, FEBS Letters 66, 90-93 (1976)

(32) R.D. Rosenberg, G. Armand, L.H. Lam, Structure-function relationships of heparin species, Pro. Nat. Acad. Sci. (U.S.) 75, 3065-3069 (1978).

(33) R. Jordan, D. Beeler, R.D. Rosenberg, Fractionation of low molecular weight heparin species and their interaction with antithrombin, J. Biol. Chem. (in press) (1979).
(34) R. Einarsson, L-O Andersson, Binding of heparin to human antithrombin III as studied by measurements of tryptophan fluorescence, Biochem. Bio. Phys. Acta 490, 104-111 (1977).
(35) W.B. Person, A criterion for reliability of formation constants of weak complexes, J.Amer.Chem. Soc. 87, 167-170 (1965).
(36) F. Markwardt, P. Walzmann, P., Untersuchungen iiben cen mechanismus der antithrombiirkung des heparins, Hoppe-Seylers Z-Physiol Chemie 317, 64-77 (1960).
(37) H.H. Hanstell, M. Kligerman, The nature of heparin antithrombin action, Thromb. Diath. et Haemorrh 18, 167-178 (1967).
(38) Gitel, S.N. (1975) Heparin: Structure, Function and Clinical Implications (Bradshaw, R.A. and Wessler, S., eds) 243-247, Plenum Press, New York.
(39) I. Björk, B. Nordenman, Acceleration of the reaction between thrombin and antithrombin III by non-stoichiometric amounts of heparin, Eur. J. Biochem. 68, 507-511 (1976).
(40) R.D. Rosenberg, L.H. Lam, A correlation between the structure and function of heparin, Pro. Nat. Acad. Sci. (U.S.) (in press).
(41) J.E. Shively, H.E. Conrad, Formation of Anhydrosugars in the chemical depolymerization of heparin, Biochemistry 15, 3932-3942 (1976).
(42) J.E. Shively, H.E. Conrad, Nearest neighbor analysis of heparin:Identification and quantitation of the products formed by selective depolymerization procedures, Biochemistry 15, 3942-3950 (1976).
(43) L-Å. Fransson, T.N. Huckerby I.A. Nieduszynski, α-L-Iduronate ring conformations in heparin and heparin derivatives, Biochem. J. 175, 299-309 (1978).

SERUM C$\bar{1}$ INHIBITOR (C$\bar{1}$-INH)

Virginia H. Donaldson, M.D.
Departments of Pediatrics and Medicine,
University of Cincinnati College of Medicine
Children's Hospital Research Foundation
Cincinnati, Ohio 45229

The complement system consists of seventeen or more separable proteins found in fresh normal human serum, that can participate in immune lysis of sensitized cells and in the release of biologically active fragments which can in turn cause non-cytolytic inflammation. Immunologically-induced function of the classical pathway (Figure 1) of complement involves 11 of its components and occurs through the activation of the first component, C1. When the C1q subunit of the C1 macromolecule binds to the Fc portions of certain immunoglobulins, the C1r and C1s subunits are then converted to active enzymes, C1$\bar{r}$ and C1$\bar{s}$ (C1 esterase) which can hydrolyze certain synthetic amino acid esters (1-6). C1$\bar{s}$ and activated macromolecular C$\bar{1}$ can hydrolyze the fourth (C4) and second (C2) components of complement. Once this has occurred, an active C$\overline{42}$ complex forms which can enzymatically cleave and activate the third (C3) component of complement, releasing a biologically active fragment, C3a, which can release histamine from mast cells. If C$\bar{1}$ attacks C4 and C2 in the fluid phase they may be rendered hemolytically inactive, a functional C$\overline{42}$ complex will not form, and the C3 may not become active (1,4,7). Once C3 is activated upon a sensitized cell, however, it can split C5 and the late acting components of complement then generate a lytic lesion in the membrane of the cell, leading to its destruction. It is teleologically reasonable that a series of enzymatic events such as these, which can have broad and serious biological consequences, should be carefully regulated to prevent spontaneous activation and anomalous complement action which might lead to the release of cytotoxic and noncytotoxic mediators in the body (Table I). An inhibitor (C$\bar{1}$-INH) directed against the action of activated C1 (C$\bar{1}$ or C1-esterase) is critical to this regulatory process.

TABLE I: BIOLOGICALLY ACTIVE FRAGMENTS RELEASED DURING COMPLEMENT ACTION

Interacting Components	Fragment	Pathophysiologic Change
C1 - C4 - C2 (+ plasmin)	Kinin	Increased vascular permeability
C3 Activation: C$\overline{42}$ or C3$\overline{bB}$	C3a Anaphylatoxin	Histamine release; Increased vascular permeability
C5 Activation: C$\overline{3b}$	C5a Anaphylatoxin	"
C3 fragment	Chemotaxin	Cellular infiltration
C5, C6, C7	C$\overline{567}$ Chemotaxin	"

Figure 1

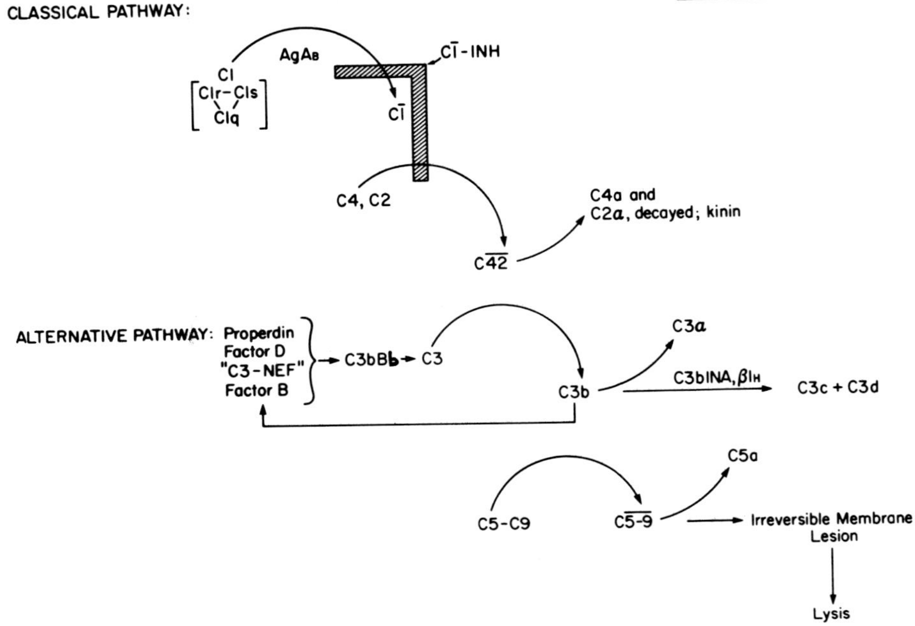

Almost coincident with the discovery of the enzymatic nature of C1 (1), Ratnoff and Lepow (4) noted that normal human serum inhibited the enzymatic activity of partially purified preparations of C1̄. The inhibitory property was due to a heat and acid labile protein which was isolated in an alpha-2 globulin fraction of serum by Pensky and his associates (8). This inhibitor of C1-esterase, or C1̄ inhibitor (C1̄-INH), has been designated C1-inactivator (C1-INA) by an international committee (9), but since the latter term implies that the inhibitor blocks the action of C1̄ by an enzymatic mechanism, the term C1̄-INH is more appropriate.

C1̄-INH interacts with the activated first component of complement (C1̄) in a stoichiometric manner (Figure 1) (10). In solution, C1̄-INH blocks the esterolytic activity of C1̄ (10). Further, it blocks the action of activated C1, which is bound to a sensitized cell, so as to prevent its interaction with the fourth (C4) and the second (C2) components of complement (11, 12). C1̄-INH can also impair the enzymatic action of preparations of the C1̄r subcomponent of C1 in the activation of C1s preparations (13). Once the stepwise interactions of components of complement upon the surface of a sensitized cell that lead to complement mediated immune lysis have proceeded beyond the point of action of C2, C1̄-INH can no longer function, for it does not inhibit membrane attack by the late-acting (C3-C9) components (11).

Each of these properties of C1̄-INH has been used in measuring its concentration in body fluids. Levy and Lepow (10) defined the stoichiometric, irreversible interaction of the inhibitor with C1̄ in solution and designated one unit of C1̄-INH in this assay as that amount which inhibited 10 units of C1 esterase activity. In this esterolytic assay, a tyrosine ester (N-acetyl-L-tyrosine ethyl ester or ALTEE) was used as substrate, since it is not known to be susceptible to hydrolysis by enzymes other than C1̄ which may be found in human serum, but the esterolytic action of C1̄ can also be measured against arginine and lysine esters (4, 15). Gigli and her colleagues (14) have devised a much more sensitive hemolytic assay in which sensitized erythrocytes (EA) are complexed to C1. Next, the ability of serum to impair the interaction of this EAC1̄ with C4 and C2 and later acting components (C3 - C9) which lyse the cell (C3 - C9) is measured.

Inhibition of Other Plasma Enzymes by C1̄-INH:

The broad spectrum of inhibitory functions of C1̄-INH first became clear when Kagan and Becker found that partially purified preparations of C1̄-INH could impair the esterolytic activity and permeability increasing activity of preparations of two chromatographically separable permeability-enhancing globulins from human plasma (16-18). One of these globulins appeared to be a permeability factor described by Miles and his colleagues, known as PF/DIL (19) because the permeability-increasing activity of this substance evolved when diluted plasma or serum was incubated in a glass tube. Ratnoff and Miles (19) found that the activation of PF/DIL required the presence of Hageman factor (20), thus indicating a link between intrinsically initiated blood coagulation and the aspect of inflammatory responses due to increased vascular permeability. Johnston and his associates have reported experiments suggesting that PF/DIL may be a property of surface-activated Hageman factor (21). Ratnoff and his colleagues found that C1̄-INH inhibited the formation of PF/DIL much more effectively than the action of pre-formed PF/DIL in an assay measuring increased vascular permeability (13), rather than esterase activity measured by others (16, 22). The other globulin separated by Kagan and Becker was believed to be plasma kallikrein, which is a proteolytic enzyme which releases vasoactive polypeptide kinins, such as bradykinin, from plasma globulins called kininogens. The inhibition of plasma kallikrein by C1̄-INH was confirmed later by others (13,23). A plasma prekallikrein has been shown to function in the clotting of blood plasma following the activation of Hageman factor by an appropriate surface (24). The clotting factor function of this prekallikrein has been called Fletcher factor after the surname of the first propositus reported to have an inherited deficiency of this clotting activity (25).

Fibrinolytic activity can evolve in human plasma when it is exposed to substances which activate Hageman factor (26), streptokinase, a substance produced by certain beta hemolytic streptococci (27), urokinase, a substance found in normal human urine (28) and certain organic solvents (29). In each instance, the activity results from the conversion of plasminogen in plasma to plasmin, which is a proteolytic enzyme able to digest fibrin, fibrinogen and a number of other proteins and synthetic substrates (30). Using more highly purified preparations of C1̄-INH than previously available, Ratnoff and his associates (13) found that physiologic concentrations of C1̄-INH delayed the lysis of fibrin clots by plasma in which fibrinolytic activity was generated by exposure to kaolin, which activates Hageman factor and Hageman factor dependent reactions in plasma. C1̄-INH also inhibited fibrinolysis by spontaneously activated human plasmin preparations, and blocked the digestion of casein by human plasmin. C1̄-INH did not block the generation of fibrinolytic activity in plasma euglobulins exposed to kaolin even in high concentrations, even though physiologic concentrations blocked already active plasmin (13). Similarly, C1̄-INH failed to inhibit the action of urokinase, an activator of plasminogen from normal urine, upon a synthetic lysine ester which it is known to hydrolyze (13).

Gigli and her colleagues examined the nature of the interaction between C1̄-INH and plasma kallikrein. She found that an apparent stoichiometric reaction took place between these proteins that resulted in inhibition of kallikrein activity as measured by esterolysis and by the generation of kinin-releasing activity (23). Their studies added a dimension for future investigation. Serum containing an inherited variant of the normal C1̄-INH molecule (from a patient with hereditary angioneurotic edema) which did not block the hemolytic activity of C1 could inhibit the esterolytic activity of plasma kallikrein (23), as if certain genetically determined structural alterations of this C1̄-INH did not deplete it of all of its functions.

The inhibitory effect of C$\bar{1}$-INH upon the generation of permeability-enhancing activity in plasma pointed to its role in regulation of surface dependent reactions in which Hageman factor initiates a number of plasma enzyme reactions. Consonant with this possibility, Forbes, et al., and Harpel (31, 32) demonstrated a direct inhibitory effect of C$\bar{1}$-INH upon the clot-promoting activity of preparations of activated Hageman factor, and activated plasma thromboplastin antecedent (P.T.A., factor XI). Certain non-functional C$\bar{1}$-INH proteins may react with P.T.A., for when a preparation of C$\bar{1}$ was added to plasmas from persons with hereditary angioneurotic edema containing non-functional inhibitors, the P.T.A.-inhibitory activity of certain plasmas was partially quenched by this maneuver (33). Schreiber and his associates further demonstrated that C$\bar{1}$-INH blocked the capacity of certain fragments of Hageman factor isolated chromatographically to release kinin in plasma through the activation of prekallikrein, to convert plasminogen to plasmin by a plasma fraction, and to convert P.T.A. to an active clot-promoting substance (34). In the latter experiment, a large Hageman factor molecule (80,000 mol. wt.) was used (34). C$\bar{1}$-INH did not block the later steps in clotting involving thrombin or activated Stuart factor (factor Xa) (31).

The biological impact of the functional potential of C$\bar{1}$-INH is impressive, but its most significant action is probably in its regulation of C$\bar{1}$ action, for there are other plasma proteins in plasma which can inhibit the action of plasmin, P.T.A., possibly Hageman factor, and kallikrein (35, 36). To our knowledge, there are no other inhibitors of C$\bar{1}$. Therefore, in the face of its deficiency, the complement system is most susceptible to uncontrolled activation. Hageman factor-dependent reactions which lead to plasma coagulation, release of vasoactive polypeptide kinins , to the generation of fibrinolytic activity and even to the activation of C1, through the action of plasmin are illustrated in Figure 2. Although there may be some other controls upon the action of Hageman factor in the ultimate conversion of plasminogen to plasmin by direct (37) or indirect (38) means, only C$\bar{1}$-INH can regulate the action of activated C1 (C$\bar{1}$).

Figure 2

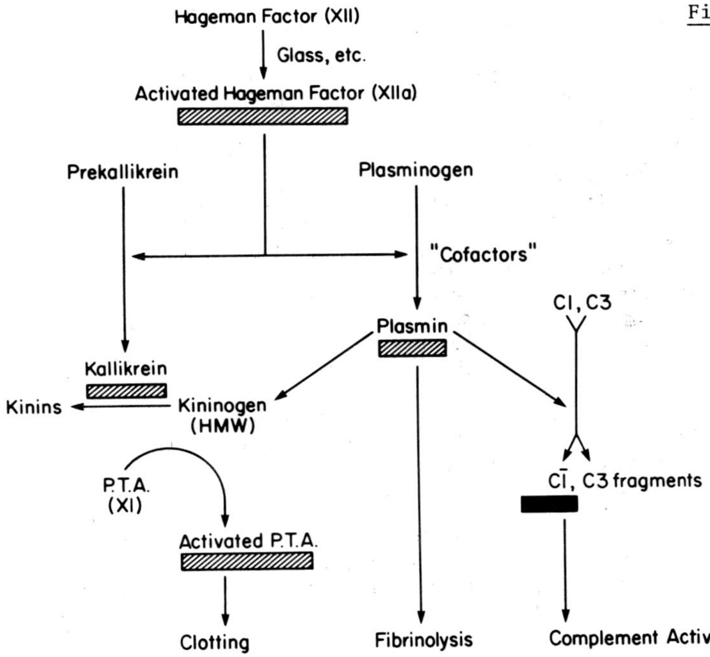

Chemical Properties of C1̄-INH and its Mechanisms of Inhibitory Actions:

C1̄-INH is an alpha-2 globulin with a high content of amino sugars, (8, 39, 40) which becomes inactive when exposed to hydrogen ion concentrations of pH 5.2 or less and to temperatures above 40°C (8). It is present in serum of normal humans in concentrations of 18-22 mg./dl, and is detectable in serum from a number of other species (10, 41). Its function is also destroyed upon exposure to ether(42), certain aliphatic alcohols (8), and other organic solvents including chloroform and a mixture of chloroform and methanol (43). Its stability characteristics and its unusually high concentration of amino sugars resembled the properties of an alpha-2 neuraminoglycoprotein which had been isolated from human serum by Schultze, et al. (40), and C1̄-INH was, in fact, found to be immunologically identical to this protein (39). The fact that the alpha-2 neuraminoglycoprotein lacked the capacity to inhibit preparations of partially purified C1 esterase was doubtless due to the fact that it had been isolated from serum at an acid pH known to destroy the function of C1̄-INH (39).

C1̄-INH, as isolated by Pensky, et al. (8), behaved as a 4.5 S protein in analytical ultracentrifugation, and, therefore, appeared to have a molecular weight of approximately 106,000, but it behaves as a 7 S protein during gel filtration (44). This apparent discrepancy in molecular weight may relate to the fact that glycoproteins can exhibit anomalous gel filtration behavior (44). A minor component in Pensky's preparation could not be further characterized (8). Preparations of C1̄-INH examined by Harpel and his associates contained 2 components when examined in polyacrylamide analytical disc gel electrophoresis, one with a molecular weight of about 105,000 and the other of which weighed about 96,000 (45). The heavier band predominated, but both contained high concentrations of PAS reactive material (carbohydrates), and both reacted with a monospecific antibody to the inhibitor giving reactions of complete immunological identity with one another. Thus, both appeared to represent C1̄-INH glycoprotein. Both forms appeared to consist of a single polypeptide chain (45). When examined in sodium dodecyl sulfate-containing polyacrylamide gels, preparations of purified C1̄s subunit of C1 (C1 esterase) appeared to form a stoichiometric complex with each of the C1̄-INH bands. The site on the C1s̄ molecule which combined with each species of C1̄-INH was on the light chain of the enzyme (45). Alper and Rosen have suggested that C1̄-INH consists of 3 repeating subunits (46).

In recent experiments Ziccardi and Cooper (47) have determined that when C1 in normal human serum is activated either with aggregated IgG, immune complexes, or a lipopolysaccharide (Salmonella Minnesota), the concentration of C1r antigenic determinants in that serum was decreased. A similar loss in C1s antigen concentration was found using certain antisera which seemed to recognize antigenic determinants of C1s close to the region of its interaction with C1̄-INH. No loss in C1r or C1s antigens was observed when serum deficient in C1̄-INH from persons who had hereditary angioneurotic edema (H.A.N.E.) was activated by these means supporting their view that the loss in antigen concentration was due to the interaction of each subunit with C1̄-INH in a manner in which the inhibitor covers certain antigenic determinant of each (47). Moreover, when C1̄-INH was restored to H.A.N.E. sera by addition of a purified preparation of the inhibitor, the concentrations of C1r and C1s antigens were then reduced upon activation of the serum, moreover, after the addition of purified C1̄-INH to purified C1r, the intensity of the precipitin reaction between purified C1r and anti-C1r was reduced (47). Thus, C1̄-INH seems to mask antigenic determinants of C1r and C1s.

Ziccardi and Cooper additionally provided important information concerning the probable mechanism of interaction of C1̄r and C1̄s with C1̄-INH when C1 was activated by an immune mechanism. Serum which had been activated with aggregated IgG contained soluble complexes of C1r, C1s and C1̄-INH as if the C1̄r and C1̄s each were bound to the inhibitor and dissociate from the C1q subunit when C1 was activated. Indeed, Laurell and her colleagues also found soluble complexes of C1r and C1s in certain pathological sera (48). Some of these complexes also contained C1̄-INH.

Harpel and Cooper have also elucidated the mechanisms through which $C\bar{1}$-INH interacts with proteolytic enzymes (45). When $C\bar{1}$-INH interacts with plasmin, it may either inhibit the enzyme, or it may be inactivated by the enzyme (44), depending upon the ratios of molar concentrations of $C\bar{1}$-INH to plasmin. When plasmin was incubated with equimolar amounts of $C\bar{1}$-INH, complexes evolved in which the inhibitor interacted with a region of the light chain of plasmin, as it did in the case of $C\bar{1}s$ (45). In contrast to the preferential binding of $C\bar{1}s$ to the cathodal (band I) species of $C\bar{1}$-INH separated by polyacrylamide disc gel electrophoresis (45), plasmin appeared to interact preferentially with band II of the inhibitor (45). With increasing molar ratios of concentrations of plasmin to $C\bar{1}$-INH, however, the enzyme appeared to cleave band I and then bind to a cleavage product (45). It could not be shown that the band II $C\bar{1}$-INH found in all purified preparations was actually generated by plasmin, nor could the appearance of this band in purified preparations of inhibitor be prevented by drawing blood from which the inhibitor was to be isolated directly into protease inhibitors (Polybrene and soy bean trypsin inhibitor) (45). Two functionally distinguishable products of band I cleavage by plasmin seemed to form, for some of the derivative material did not bind to plasmin when generated in mixtures containing high molar ratios of plasmin to $C\bar{1}$-INH (45). Thus, one derivative plasmin cleavage product of $C\bar{1}$-INH was functional while the other was not. The non-functional plasmin derivative also failed to bind to or inhibit preparations of $C\bar{1}s$ (45). These interactions are diagrammatically represented in figures 3 and 4. The requirement for enzymatic hydrolysis of $C\bar{1}$-INH by plasmin in inhibition of plasmin in a plasmin $C\bar{1}$-INH complex is quite distinct from the interaction of $C\bar{1}s$ with $C\bar{1}$-INH, for in this reaction the inhibitor is not measurably cleaved by $C1\bar{s}$ as if it were not a substrate of the enzyme.

Figure 3

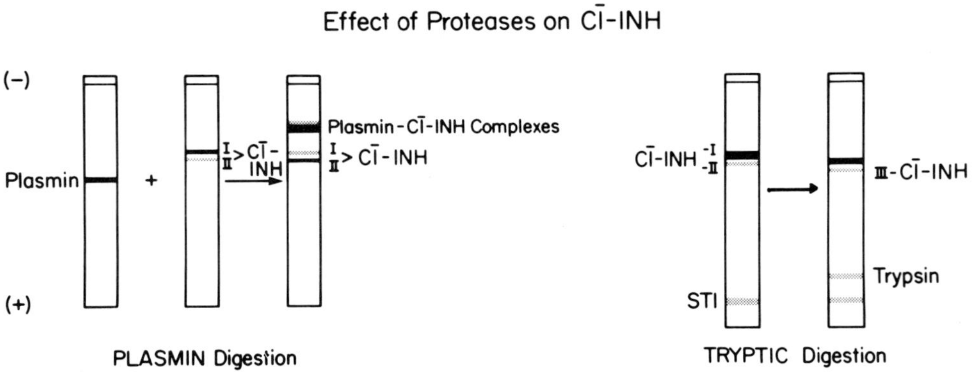

from Harpel and Cooper

Figure 3: Diagrams of the electrophoretic mobilities of plasmin and C$\bar{1}$-INH (left) and trypsin and C$\bar{1}$-INH in SDS polyacrylamide gels (5%). Plasmin forms an inhibited complex with C$\bar{1}$-INH, and digests the cathodal component of C$\bar{1}$-INH (third gel, left). Trypsin did not form inhibited complexes, but digested C$\bar{1}$-INH to inactive derivatives. (From Harpel and Cooper, reference No. 45.)

Figure 4

Changes in C$\bar{1}$-INH upon interacting with C1$\bar{s}$, Trypsin and Plasmin

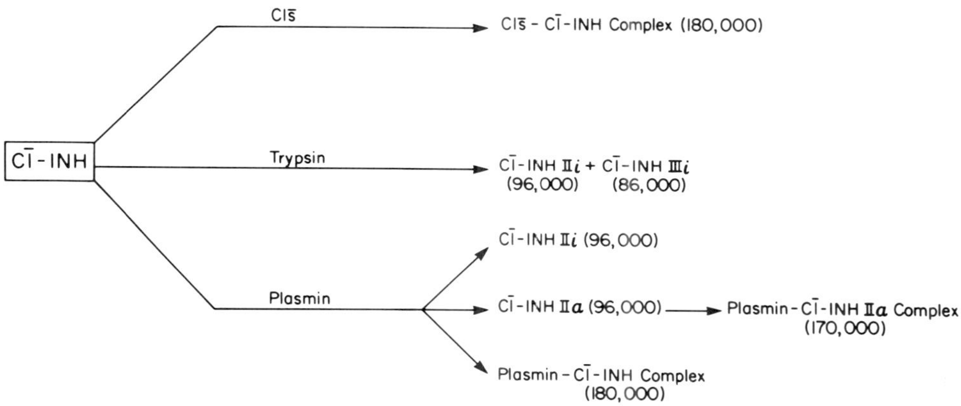

Figure 4: The molecular changes of C$\bar{1}$-INH upon interacting with C1$\bar{s}$, trypsin and plasmin. Trypsin generated C$\bar{1}$-INH II i and III i are active fragments. Plasmin-generated C$\bar{1}$-INH IIa is an inhibitory cleavage product of band II and C$\bar{1}$-INH IIi is an inactive cleavage product generated from band II by plasmin. The molecular weights of the C$\bar{1}$-INH derivatives and the complexes which they form are in parentheses (45).

Trypsin also depleted the cathodal band I of C$\bar{1}$-INH in a cleavage reaction generating inhibitor protein that had an electrophoretic mobility like that of band II inhibitor protein and it could also extensively degrade the inhibitor molecule (45). At molar ratios of trypsin to C$\bar{1}$-INH as low as 0.025 the ability of the digested inhibitor to interact with C1$\bar{s}$ was partially lost and it was totally destroyed at a ratio of 0.1 (45). At molar ratios of 1.0 or more, the band I C$\bar{1}$-INH was completely destroyed by trypsin and a product with a molecular weight of about 86,000 designated band III evolved that had an electrophoretic mobility in polyacrylamide disc gels more anodal than either band I or band II of the "native" C$\bar{1}$-INH (45). Band III was probably a tryptic derivative of band II inhibitor (45) (figures 3, 4). In these cleavage reactions by trypsin and plasmin the carbohydrate part of the inhibitor was retained in bands II and III (45). Trypsin generated band II lacked inhibitory properties, for it would not interact with trypsin or with C$\bar{1}$s, whereas plasmin generated band II did (45); it failed to block the enzymatic reaction between C1$\bar{s}$ and C4 or C2 in which the hemolytic properties of these two components are normally destroyed.

C$\bar{1}$-INH function is labile at acid pH (8). Harpel and Cooper found that loss of inhibitory activity at acid pH was not associated with detectable degradation of the inhibitor molecule (45). Even so, the acidified inhibitor failed to form demonstrable complexes with plasmin or with C1$\bar{s}$. Both plasmin and trypsin, however, degraded the acid-denatured C$\bar{1}$-INH, producing low molecular weight fragments.

Genetic Regulation of Biosynthesis of C$\bar{1}$-INH:

The complex mechanisms of gene action designating biosynthesis of C$\bar{1}$-INH have come to light largely through studies of serums from individuals with hereditary angioneurotic edema (H.A.N.E.), in whom the deficiency of serum inhibition of activated C1 is inherited as an autosomal dominant trait (49). Similarly, the tendency of H.A.N.E. patients to have circumscribed bouts of subepithelial swelling, often severe and sometimes fatal, is inherited in the manner of an autosomal dominant trait (49). The genetic mechanisms are more complex, however, for in about 85% of kindred with H.A.N.E. affected persons are deficient in the antigenic as well as functional properties of C$\bar{1}$-INH, and therefore appear to fail to synthesize this protein. In the remaining kindred, affected members have a serum protein with normal antigenic determinants which fails to block the action of C$\bar{1}$ (50, 51). Even these abnormal inhibitor proteins are heterogeneous (51), as defined below (Table II). The inheritance pattern of each form of C$\bar{1}$-INH deficiency is consistent with the expression of an autosomal dominant trait, and to my knowledge no affected kindred demonstrates more than one form of C$\bar{1}$-INH deficiency. Thus, the non-functional proteins must reflect genetically determined errors in biosynthesis of this protein, rather than the presence of inhibitor bound to another plasma enzyme, and therefore non-reactive with C$\bar{1}$, as one group of investigators has proposed (52). A 2-component non-functional C$\bar{1}$-INH protein in one kindred with H.A.N.E. which we reported earlier (50) may have represented the products of proteolytic degradation by plasmin of the abnormal inhibitor in stored serum. But the components of this protein were immunologically identical with one another, whereas a reaction of partial identity was seen between fragments of a purified preparation of C$\bar{1}$-INH which had been digested by plasmin when the digests were examined immunoelectrophoretically (44, 50). Subsequent examination of sera from the same kindred using a different immunoelectrophoretic technique revealed a single band of C$\bar{1}$-INH antigens.

Table II

NON-FUNCTIONAL ALLOTYPES OF C$\bar{1}$-INH IN HANE:

Electrophoretic Mobility	-	Normal Fast Very Fast 2-components
Concentration	-	100% 400% <30%
Function	-	Blocks neither esterolysis or C4 inactivation by C$\bar{1}$ Blocks esterolysis but not C4 inactivation by C$\bar{1}$

The inheritance of deficient C$\bar{1}$-INH function in HANE presents a unique problem in understanding genetic mechanisms of inheritance of autosomal dominant traits. All affected kindred with HANE demonstrate autosomal dominant inheritance of the deficiency whether it is associated with an apparent failure to synthesize

C$\bar{1}$-INH protein (CRM$^-$) or with normal amounts of immunoreactive C$\bar{1}$-INH protein which lacks normal function (CRM$^+$). Moreover, the marked heterogeneity of gene products displayed among CRM$^+$ kindred is difficult to explain in terms of simple autosomal dominance. For example, in several kindred, the concentrations of serum C$\bar{1}$-INH protein which lacks function was about four times that in normal serum (51, 53); in addition, there were two bands of immunoreactive C$\bar{1}$-INH protein detected by immunoelectrophoresis, one of which was of the mobility of albumin and appeared to represent a non-covalently linked complex of inhibitor and albumin, while the other band had normal electrophoretic mobility (51, 53). Other variant forms of non-functional C$\bar{1}$-INH behaved as if they were slightly more positively charged than the normal inhibitor in immunoelectrophoretic analysis, and still others were even more positively charged (51). Additional variability in the binding affinity for C1$\bar{s}$ was found among CRM$^+$ sera. For example, in 3 unrelated kindred the defective C$\bar{1}$-INH of intermediately increased positive charge impaired the esterolytic activity of preparations of C$\bar{1}$, but failed to prevent the destruction of the hemolytic activity of the C4 endogenous to that serum or of added exogenous crude C4 by the active C1 in the individual CRM$^+$ sera (51). These findings are summarized in Table II. Harpel and his colleagues found that non-functional C$\bar{1}$-INH proteins isolated from serums from 2 members of a kindred with this form of H.A.N.E. had a slightly higher molecular weight than normal inhibitor proteins (54). This C$\bar{1}$-INH appeared to differ from the normal in its primary structure and had a lower concentration of phenylalanine than the normal, despite its normal electrophoretic mobility in alkaline acrylamide gels (54).

Despite all of these variations in the expression of the apparent action of an autosomal dominant gene, the severity of the attacks of edema which the propositi sustain are unrelated to the type of defect, as far as has been demonstrated to date. The means through which the abnormal gene dominates and "blocks" the expression of the normal gene in this and other autosomal dominant traits is obscure. All affected individuals with whom we have been acquainted are heterozygous, for only one parent has the disease. Virtually none demonstrate half normal serum levels of functional or antigenic properties of C$\bar{1}$-INH protein, however. The CRM$^-$ patients in whom we have evaluated the range of concentration of C$\bar{1}$-INH antigen concentrations has varied from 5 to 30% of that in normal sera (14, 51).

These inhibitor proteins in serum from CRM$^-$ patients are of normal electrophoretic mobility and bind to C1$\bar{s}$ preparations (51). We did not find a rapid rate of clearance of radioactively labelled purified inhibitor protein from the vascular compartment of CRM$^-$ patients in remission as compared to the rate of clearance of normal individuals (51); others have reported similar data (55). We determined an intravascular half-life of about 4 days, once equilibration between intra and extravascular spaces has occurred (51), while Brackertz et al. estimated that the half life was 63 to 72 hours (55).

C$\bar{1}$-INH is normally synthesized by the liver (56). In some CRM$^-$ individuals whose liver tissue could be examined pathologically, the cytoplasm of the hepatic parenchymal cells failed to fluoresce following exposure to a fluorescent antibody to the normal C$\bar{1}$-INH which did produce a fluorescent pattern of these cells from normal individuals (56). Therefore, there appeared to be a failure to synthesize any C$\bar{1}$-INH protein in persons with this type of deficiency. It is possible, however, that an inhibitor protein is synthesized which is structurally distorted to such a degree as to be unable to react with any available antisera.

The Repair of the Biochemical in H.A.N.E. Associated with Long-term Remission Induced with a Synthetic Androgen:

In 1960, Spaulding reported that several individuals with H.A.N.E. who were treated with testosterone sustained long-term remissions, indicating that the testosterone in some way exerted a significant preventive effect (57). Davis, et al. observed sustained remissions in patients given testosterone preparations for a period of years (58). More recent observations suggest that the effectiveness of androgenic compounds was due to the synthesis of $C\bar{1}$-INH, for Rosse and his colleagues reported increased levels of the inhibitor in serums from H.A.N.E. patients taking synthetic androgens (59, 60). We have failed to find increased levels of $C\bar{1}$-INH in the serum of several patients taking testosterone including one subject who has had a sustained remission of 11 years duration during testosterone therapy; a different procedure (that of Laurell) was used to measure the inhibitor.

In 1976 Gelfand and his colleagues clearly demonstrated that a synthetic attenuated androgen (Danazol), which impedes the pituitary gonadal axis, not only prevented affected individuals from having attacks of H.A.N.E. but induced the appearance of functional and antigenic $C\bar{1}$-INH in plasma or serum from these individuals (61). Thus, these synthetic androgens had either invoked the biosynthesis of normal inhibitor proteins, presumably by allowing the normal gene designating its synthesis to function, or the androgens induced the release of the protein into the circulation from some extravascular depot. The latter possibility is unlikely for in CRM$^-$ HANE, $C\bar{1}$-INH protein was not demonstrated in immunofluorescent studies of the liver (56). It is possible that the attenuated androgen, which has significant anabolic effects, in some way induces the function of the silent gene by derepression, but direct evidence favoring this is limited to the observed effect of this compound upon the biochemical defect in H.A.N.E. When normal individuals were given Danazol, the serum concentration of $C\bar{1}$-INH also increased significantly (61).

When CRM$^+$ patients with H.A.N.E. were given Danazol, they developed serum inhibitory activity which was associated with the appearance of a component of inhibitor protein in serum which had normal electrophoretic mobility, again suggesting that a normal biosynthetic mechanism had been released from some form of inhibition (62). The nonfunctional protein of the abnormal electrophoretic mobility persists in such sera, so that during remissions induced with Danazol these individuals develop 2 species of $C\bar{1}$-INH protein, one of which is normal and the other which is abnormal.

The serum concentrations of C4 in H.A.N.E. are reduced below the normal level, and may be undetectable during episodes of edema (63). This deficiency of C4 occurs because of the activation of C1 in serum in which $C\bar{1}$-INH is absent or markedly reduced (63). The $C\bar{1}$ in turn <u>inactivates</u> the C4. When the deficiency of $C\bar{1}$-INH is repaired in patients with H.A.N.E. during Danazol induced remissions, the other alterations in complement are also repaired and serum levels of C4 return to normal (61). In our own studies, the serum concentrations of C4 were within the normal range when the $C\bar{1}$-INH concentration reached about half of that in normal serum (64) as if this amount may provide satisfactory regulation of complement action. These therapeutic experiments have provided in vivo confirmation of the role of $C\bar{1}$-INH in modulating the action of complement.

Acquired Deficiency of $C\bar{1}$-INH:

Several reports have described individuals who have had a deficiency of $C\bar{1}$-INH in association with dysproteinemias or lymphoproliferative syndromes (64-68). In the individual whose case we reported (65), a 7S monoclonal cryoglobulin was demonstrated to interact with, and activate the first component of complement, thus allowing it to bind subsequently to the inhibitor in the serum. This individual had a low serum level of $C\bar{1}$-INH, but the protein was not absent from his serum. He was subject to cold urticaria, but did not have the remarkably bland swellings typical of H.A.N.E. Other patients have developed angioneurotic edema in association with virtual absence of the inhibitor from their serum (65, 66).

Concluding Remarks:

The $C\bar{1}$-INH is named for its ability to block the action of the activated form of the first component of complement ($C\bar{1}$) but resembles the other protease inhibitors found in normal human plasma in that it can inhibit other plasma enzymes as well. If an individual is markedly deficient in serum C$\bar{1}$-INH, either because of an acquired disease or of an inherited trait, that individual is likely to have a clinical disorder, angioneurotic edema. Since individuals with normal levels of this serum inhibitor may also develop angioneurotic edema, other factors are important to the development of this symptom. Deficiencies of other plasma inhibitors may predispose an individual to certain disorders; persons deficient in antithrombin III may develop thromboembolism (69), and alpha-1-antitrypsin deficiency may predispose an individual to pulmonary disease and cirrhosis of the liver (70-72), Thus, each of these broadly acting plasma inhibitors appears to be more critical to certain areas of plasma enzyme functions than others and each is essential to normal health. The unregulated plasma enzyme system is potentially dangerous to the health of that individual.

References:

1. Lepow, I.H., Ratnoff, O.D., Rosen, F.S., Pillimer, L. Observations on a pro-esterase associated with partially purified first component of complement (C1). Proc. Soc. Exp. Biol. & Med. 92: 32, (1956).

2. Lepow, I.H., Naff, G.B., Todd, E.W., Pensky, J., Hinz, C.F. Chromatographic resolution of the first component of human complement into three activities. J. Exp. Med. 117: 983, (1963).

3. Naff, G. B., Pensky, J., Lepow, I.H. The macromolecular nature of the first component of human complement. J. Exp. Med. 119: 593, (1964).

4. Ratnoff, O.D. and Lepow, I.H. Some properties of an esterase derived from preparations of the first component of complement. J. Exp. Med. 106: 327, (1957).

5. Laurell, A.-B., Martensson, J. Interactions between C1q, C1r, and C1s from human serum. Acta. Path. Microbiol. Scand. Sec. B 82: 585, (1974).

6. Muller-Eberhard, H.-J. "Complement" in Ann. Rev. Biochemistry 44: 697, (1975).

7. Donaldson, V.H., Rosen, F.S., Bing, D.H. Role of the second component of complement (C2) and plasmin in kinin release in hereditary angioneurotic edema (HANE) Plasma. Trans. Assoc. Amer. Phys. 90: 174, (1977).

8. Pensky, J., Levy, L.R., Lepow, I.H. Partial purification of a serum inhibitor of C'1-esterase. J. Biol. Chem. 236: 1674, (1961).

9. Bulletin of World Health Org. 39: 935, (1968).

10. Levy, L. R.,& Lepow, I.H. Assay and properties of serum inhibitor of C'1-esterase. Proc. Soc. Exp. Biol. Med. 101: 608, (1959).

11. Lepow, I.H., Leon, M.A. Interaction of serum inhibitor of C'1-esterase with intermediate complexes of the immune haemolytic system. I Specificity of inhibition of C'1 activity associated with intermediate complexes. Immunology 5: 222, (1962).

12. Leon, M.A., Lepow, I.H. Interaction of a serum inhibitor of C'1 esterase with intermediate complexes of the immune haemolytic systems. II Kinetics and mechanism of the interaction. Immunology 5: 235, (1962).

13. Ratnoff, O.D., Pensky, J., Ogston, D., Naff, G.B. The inhibition of plasmin, plasma kallikrein, plasma permeability factor, and the Clr subcomponent of the first component of complement by serum C'1-esterase inhibitor. J. Exp. Med. 129: 315, (1969).

14. Gigli, I., Ruddy, S., Austen, K.F. The stoichiometric measurement of the serum inhibitor of the first component of complement by the inhibition of immune hemolysis. J. Immunol. 100: 1154, (1968).

15. Harpel, P.C. A sensitive colorometric method for the measurement of serum C$\bar{1}$ Inactivator using the substrate N-α-acetyl-L-Lysine methyl ester. J. Immunol. 104: 1024, (1970).

16. Kagan, L.J., Becker, E.L. Inhibition of permeability globulins by C'1 esterase inhibitor. Fed. Proc. 20: 613, (1963).

17. Kagan, L.J. Some biochemical and physical properties of the human permeability globulins. Brit. J. Exp. Path. 45: 604, (1964).

18. Kagan, L.J., Leddy, J.P., Becker, E.L. The presence of two permeability globulins in human serum. J. Clin. Invest. 42: 1353, (1963).

19. Miles, A.A., Wilhelm, D.L. Enzyme-like globulins from serum reproducing the vascular phenomena of inflammation. I. An activable permeability factor and its inhibitor in guinea pig serum. Brit. J. Exp. Path. 36: 71, (1955).

20. Ratnoff, O.D., and Miles, A.A. The induction of permeability increasing activity in human plasma by activated Hageman factor. Brit. J. Exp. Path. 45: 328, (1964).

21. Johnston, A.R., Cochrane, C.G., Revak, S.D. The relationship between PF/DIL and activated human Hageman factor. J. Immunol. 113: 103, (1974).

22. Landerman, N.S., Webster, M.E., Becker, E.L. Ratcliffe, H.S. Hereditary angioneurotic edema. II Deficiency of inhibitor for serum globulin permeability factor and/or plasma kallikrein. J. Allergy 33: 330,(1962).

23. Gigli, I., Mason, J.W., Colman, R.W., Austen, K.F. Interaction of plasma kallikrein with the C$\bar{1}$ inhibitor. J. Immunol. 104: 579, (1970).

24. Wuepper, K.D. Prekallikrein deficiency in man. J. Exp. Med. 138: 1345,(1973).

25. Hathaway, W.E., Belhasen, L.P., Hathaway, J.S. Evidence for a new plasma thromboplastin factor. I. Case report, coagulation studies and physicochemical properties. Blood 26: 521, (1965).

26. Niewiarowski, S., Prou-Wartelle, O. Role du facteur Hageman dans la fibrinolyse. Thromb. et Diath. Haemorr. 3: 593, (1959).

27. Tillett, W.S., Garner, R.L. The fibrinolytic activity of hemolytic streptococci. J. Exp. Med. 58: 545, (1933).

28. Williams, J.R.B. The fibrinolytic activity of urine. Brit. J. Exp. Path. 32: 530, (1951).

29. Denys, J., de Marbaix, J. Sur les peptonization provoquées par le chloroforme et quelques autres substances. Cellule 5: 197, (1889).

30. Donaldson, V.H. The effect of plasmin in vitro on clotting factors in plasma. J. Lab. Clin. Med. 56: 644, (1960).

31. Forbes, C.D., Pensky, J., Ratnoff, O.D., Inhibition of activated Hageman factor and activated plasma thromboplastin antecedent by purified serum C$\bar{1}$ inactivator. J. Lab. Clin. Med. 76: 809, (1970).

32. Harpel, P.C. Separation of plasma thromboplastin antecedent from kallikrein by the plasma α_2-macroglobulin kallikrein inhibitor. J. Clin. Invest. 50: 2084, (1971).

33. Ratnoff, O.D., Pensky, J., Donaldson, V.H., Amir, J. The inhibitory properties of plasma against activated plasma thromboplastin antecedent (factor Xla) in hereditary angioneurotic edema. J. Lab. Clin. Med. 80: 803, (1972).

34. Schreiber, A.D., Kaplan, A.P., Austen, K.F. Inhibition by C$\bar{1}$-INH of Hageman factor fragment activation of coagulation fibrinolysis and kinin generation. J. Clin. Invest. 52: 1402, (1973).

35. Schreiber, A.D., Kaplan, A.P., Austen, K.F. Plasma inhibitors of the components of the fibrinolytic pathway in man. J. Clin. Invest. 52: 1394, (1973).

36. Harpel, P.C., Rosenberg, R.D. α_2 Macroglobulin and antithrombin-heparin cofactor: Modulator of hemostatic and inflammatory reactions, in "Progress in Hemostasis and Thrombosis", T.H. Spaet, editor, III: 145, (1976).

37. Goldsmith, G.H., Jr., Saito, H., Ratnoff, O.D. The activation of plasminogen by Hageman factor (Factor XII) and Hageman factor fragments. J. Clin. Invest. 62: 54, (1978).

38. Ogston, D., Ogston, C.M., Ratnoff, O.D., Forbes, C.D. Studies on a complex mechanism for the activation of a plasminogen by kaolin and by chloroform: The participation of Hageman factor and additive co-factors. J. Clin. Invest. 48: 1786, (1969).

39. Pensky, J., Schwick, H.G. Human serum inhibitor of C1 esterase: identity with alpha-2 neuraminoglycoprotein. Science 163: 698, (1969).

40. Schultze, H.E., Heide, K., Haupt, H. Uber ein bisher unbekanntes saures alpha 2 glykoprotein. Naturwissenschaften 49: 133, (1962).

41. Donaldson, V.H., Pensky, J. Some observations on the phylogeny of serum inhibitor of C1 esterase. J. Immunol. 104: 1388, (1970).

42. Donaldson, V.H. Studies on the activation of a serum esterase with ether and its relationship to C'1-esterase. J. Clin. Invest. 40: 673, (1961).

43. Donaldson, V.H. Unpublished observations, (1961).

44. Harpel, P.C. C$\bar{1}$ Inactivator inhibition by plasmin. J. Clin. Invest. 49: 568 (1970).

45. Harpel, P.C., Cooper, N.R. Studies on human plasma C$\bar{1}$ inactivator-enzyme reactions. I. Mechanisms of interaction with C1$\bar{s}$, plasmin and trypsin. J. Clin. Invest. 55: 593, (1975).

46. Alper, C.A. and Rosen, F.S. Genetics of the complement system, in "Advances in Human Genetics". Editors H. Harris and K. Hirschhorn. Plenum Press, N.Y. 7: 141, (1976).

47. Ziccardi, R.J. Cooper, N.R. Modulation of the antigenicity of C1r̄ and C1s̄ by C1̄ inactivator. J. Immunol. in press.

48. Laurell, A.-B., Martensson, U., Sjoholm, A.G. C1 subcomponent complexes in normal and pathological sera studied by crossed immunoelectrophoresis. Acta. Path. Microbiol. Scand. Sect. C. 84: 455, (1976).

49. Donaldson, V.H., and Evans, R.R. A biochemical abnormality in hereditary angioneurotic edema: Absence of serum inhibitor of C'1-esterase. Am. J. Med. 35: 37, (1963).

50. Rosen, F.S., Charache, P., Donaldson, V.H., Pensky, J. Hereditary angioneurotic edema: Two genetic variants. Science. 148: 957, (1965).

51. Rosen, F.S., Alper, C.A., Pensky, J., Klemperer, M.R., Donaldson, V.H. Genetically determined heterogeneity of the C1 esterase inhibitor in patients with hereditary angioneurotic edema. J. Clin. Invest. 50: 2143, (1971).

52. van Royen, E.A., Lohman, S., Voss, M., Pondman, K.W. C1̄ Inactivator and cold promoted activation of factor VII. J. Lab. Clin. Med. 92: 152, (1978).

53. Laurell, A.-B., Martensson, U. C1 inactivator protein complexed with albumin in plasma from a patient with hereditary angioneurotic edema. Eur. J. Immunol. 1: 146, (1971).

54. Harpel, P.C., Hugli, T.E., Cooper, N.R. Studies on human plasma C1̄-Inactivator-enzyme interactions. II. Structural studies of an abnormal C1̄ inactivator from a kindred with hereditary angioneurotic edema. J.Clin. Invest. 55: 605, (1975).

55. Brackertz, D., Isler, E., Kueppers, F. Half life of C1̄-INH in hereditary angioneurotic oedema, Clin. Allergy 1: 89, (1975).

56. Johnson, A.M., Alper, C.A., Rosen, F.S., Craig, J.M. C1̄ inhibitor: Evidences for decreased hepatic synthesis in hereditary angioneurotic edema. Science. 173: 553, (1971).

57. Spaulding, W.B. Methyltestosterone therapy for hereditary episodic edema (hereditary angioneurotic edema). Ann. Int. Med. 53: 739, (1960).

58. Davis, P.J., Davis, F.B., Charache P. Long term therapy of hereditary angioedema (HAE). Preventive management with fluoxymesterone and oxymetholone in severely affected males and females. Hopkins Med. J. 135: 391, (1974).

59. Rosse, W., Logue, G.L., Silberman, H.R. The effect of synthetic androgens on the clinical course and C1̄ esterase inhibitor (C1̄-INH) levels in hereditary angioneurotic edema. (HANE). Clin. Res. 24: 42A, (1976).

60. Rosse, W.F., Logue, G.L., Silberman, H.R., Frank, M.M. The effect of synthetic androgens in hereditary angioneurotic edema: Alteration of C1 inhibitor and C4 levels. Trans Assoc. Amer. Phys. 89: 122, (1976).

61. Gelfand, J.A., Sherins, R.J., Alling, D.W., Frank, M.M. Treatment of hereditary angioneurotic edema with Danazol. Reversal of clinical and biochemical abnormalities. New Eng. J. Med. 295: 1444, (1976).

62. Gadek, J.E., Hosea, S.W., Gelfand, J.A., Frank, M.M. C1 Inhibitor phenotypes in hereditary angioneurotic edema: Genetic implications of Danazol therapy. Clin. Res. 25: 357A, (1977).

63. Donaldson, V.H., Rosen, F.S. Action of complement in hereditary angioneurotic edema. The role of C'1 esterase. J. Clin. Invest. 43: 2204, (1964).

64. Pitts, J., Donaldson, V.H., Wyatt, R., Forristal, J. Remissions in hereditary angioneurotic edema (H.A.N.E.) induced with an attenuated androgen (Danazol): Correllation between concentrations of C$\bar{1}$-inhibitor (C$\bar{1}$-INH)and the fourth (C4) and second (C2) components of complement. J. Lab. Clin. Med. 92: 501, (1978).

65. Costanzi, J.J., Coltman, C.A., Donaldson, V.H. Activation of complement by a monoclonal cryoglobulin associated with cold urticaria, J.Lab. Clin.Med. 74: 902, (1969).

66. Caldwell, J.R., Ruddy, S., Schur, P.H., Austen, K.F. Acquired C$\bar{1}$ inhibitor deficiency in lymphosarcoma. Clin. Immunol. and Immunopath. 1: 39, (1972).

67. Oberling, F., Hauptmann, G., Lang, J.M., Bergerat, J.P., Mayer, G., Batzenschlager, A., Hammann, B., Gillet, B. Acquired C1-esterase inhibitor deficiencies during lymphoid syndromes. Nouv. Presse Med. 4: 2705, (1975).

68. Schreiber, A.D., Zweiman, B., Atkins, P., Goldwein, F., Dietra, G., Atkinson, B., Abdou, N.I. Acquired angioedema with lymphoproliferative disorder: Association of C1 inhibitor deficiency with cellular abnormality. Blood. 48: 567, (1976).

69. Marciniak, E., Farley, C.H., DeSimone, P.A. Familial thrombosis due to antithrombin III deficiency. Blood. 43: 219, (1974).

70. Laurell, C.-B., Eriksson, S. The electrophonetic α_1 globulin pattern of serum in α_1 antitrypsin deficiency. Scand. J. Clin. Lab. Invest. 15: 132, (1963).

71. Eriksson, S. Studies in α_1 antitrypsin deficiency. Acta. Med. Scand.(Suppl.) 432: 1, (1965).

72. Sharp, H.L. Alpha$_1$ antitrypsin deficiency. Hospital Practice. 6: 83, (1971).

α_2-MACROGLOBULIN

Peter C. Harpel
Cornell University Medical College
New York, New York 10021

Twenty four years ago, Schultze and colleagues (1) isolated a high molecular weight globulin from serum which subsequently was found to differ from IgM (2,3). This protein was named α_2-macroglobulin (α_2M) to reflect two of its major physical properties - an electrophoretic mobility as an α_2-globulin and its large molecular weight. Several years following these biochemical studies of α_2M, the enzyme-binding properties of this glycoprotein were discovered (4,5). The α_2M was found to possess a unique characteristic in comparison with other plasma protease inhibitors in that the enzyme in the α_2M-enzyme complex still retained an active catalytic site, although its substrate specificity had been altered. Thus, the protease was apparently sterically hindered from degrading high molecular weight substrates but it retained its ability to hydrolyze low molecular weight substrates.

The α_2M has been shown to form a complex with and to inhibit to a varying degree a remarkably diverse group of protein cleaving enzymes derived not only from the circulating blood, but from cells, bacteria and from snake venoms (6,7). The potential physiologic importance of the α_2M and its unusual physical-chemical properties have stimulated a number of laboratories to investigate various properties of the α_2M and several reports serve to summarize these studies (7-10). In the present chapter I will review recent work from our laboratory as well as others which clarifies our concepts regarding the nature of the α_2M subunit structure as well as of the molecular events that occur when the α_2M interacts with its enzymes. A new observation, that the α_2M subunit chain fragments into two polypeptide chains when heated under denaturing and reducing conditions, will be considered. Finally, the relationship of α_2M to cell surfaces including the lymphocyte, platelet, and human vascular endothelium will be reviewed.

Subunit Structure of α_2-Macroglobulin: Modification by Proteolytic Enzymes

The α_2M is a high molecular weight protein composed of multiple subunits. The native molecule has an apparent molecular weight of 725,000 (10). Under acid conditions, or following incubation with a denaturing agent such as urea or dodecyl sulfate, α_2M dissociates into two major components with a sedimentation constant of 11 (11,12). Thus the α_2M molecule possesses a dimeric structure consisting of two half-molecules joined by noncovalent forces. Cleavage of disulfide bonds in the α_2M molecule with β-mercaptoethanol or dithiothreitol produces α_2M subunits with an estimated molecular weight of 185,000 when analyzed by dodecyl sulfate polyacrylamide gel electrophoresis (13). This is in close agreement with a subunit chain molecular weight of 196,000 as determined by density-gradient equilibrium ultracentrifugation of reduced α_2M (11,12). These data indicate that each α_2M half-molecule consists of two subunit chains held together by disulfide bridges.

Studies in my laboratory have demonstrated that the interaction between α_2M and the proteolytic enzymes with which it forms a high molecular weight complex is accompanied by proteolytic modification of the subunit structure of α_2M (13). When trypsin was incubated with α_2M and the resulting enzyme-α_2M complex analyzed by dodecyl sulfate polyacrylamide gel electrophoresis, cleavage of the 185,000 molecular weight subunit chain was observed. The molecular weight of the cleavage product, 85,000, indicated that the α_2M subunit had been hydrolyzed near or at its center. The trypsin-induced proteolytic derivative was only identified by dodecyl sulfate gel electrophoretic analysis following treatment of the α_2M, trypsin incubation mixture with dithiothreitol thereby establishing that the 85,000 molecular weight proteolytic derivative was bound to the parent molecule by disulfide bridges.

Additional experiments have permitted the conclusion that once trypsin is bound to the α_2M molecule, no further cleavage of the subunit chain occurs (13). Increasing amounts of trypsin were incubated with a constant quantity of α_2M. The reaction was terminated after 1 and 61 minutes by the addition of a solution containing 1% dodecyl sulfate, 8 M urea, and 14 mM dithiothreitol. Dodecyl sulfate gel electrophoretic analysis of these mixtures showed that the loss of 185,000 molecular weight subunit chain and the reciprocal production of the 85,000 molecular weight proteolytic derivative were proportional to the concentration of trypsin in the α_2M, trypsin mixture. There was no increase in the amount of the 85,000 molecular weight derivative chain at 61 minutes as compared to the 1 minute sample. Since the concentration of the proteolytic derivative did not increase during the hour of incubation, the enzyme must have been fully inhibited by the α_2M following the initial proteolytic cleavage of the α_2M.

Both the catalytic site of trypsin and the native form of α_2M were found to be necessary for the cleavage of the subunit chain of α_2M to the lower molecular weight derivative. The appearance of this product was prevented when trypsin was preincubated with a trypsin inhibitor such as soybean or pancreatic trypsin inhibitor as well as by DFP, which blocks serine in the active site of trypsin. The functional state of α_2M also influenced the pattern of interaction between trypsin and α_2M. Acidification of α_2M (pH 2.0 for 30 minutes at 37°C), followed by neutralization, destroyed the activity of α_2M in inhibiting trypsin. This treatment did not change the subunit structure as analyzed by dodecyl sulfate gel electrophoresis. When trypsin was incubated with acid-treated α_2M in molar ratios of trypsin:α_2M as low as 0.002, the α_2M was found to be cleaved into many polypeptide chains with molecular weights lower than that of the 85,000 molecular weight derivative. These results indicated that functionally intact α_2M restricted the catalytic attack of trypsin to a limited and specific region of the molecule.

Proteases other than trypsin were found to cleave the α_2M in a manner similar to that documented for trypsin. When α_2M was incubated with either thrombin, plasmin, plasma kallikrein or chymotrypsin and each mixture analyzed by dodecyl sulfate gel electrophoresis, after reduction with a thiol, the 85,000 molecular weight derivative polypeptide chain was observed. Chymotrypsin produced, in addition, two other fragments of 90,000 and 75,000 molecular weight. Barrett, Starkey, and Munn (14) have subsequently demonstrated that a 85,000 molecular weight product was produced when α_2M interacted with cathepsins B and D, thermolysin, and rabbit fibroblast collagenase.

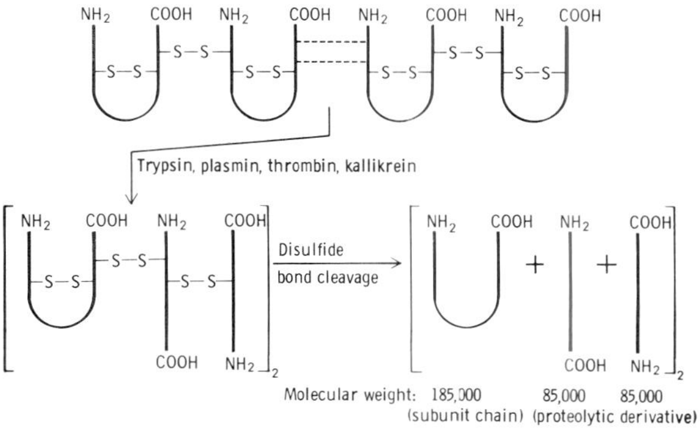

Fig. 1.

A model of the subunit structure of α_2-macroglobulin indicating the cleavages induced in the molecule by interaction with proteases. Reprinted with permission from Ref. 13.

From these considerations, a model for the covalent structure of α_2M has been proposed (Fig. 1). As illustrated in Fig. 1, the α_2M consists of two half-molecules held together by electrostatic and hydrophobic forces (indicated by dashed lines). Since the molecular weight of the α_2M is 725,000, the molecule consists of four chains, 185,000 molecular weight each. As discussed previously, each half-molecule possesses two polypeptide chains linked by disulfide bridges. In Fig. 1 the placement of the NH_2- and C terminal ends of the subunit chains is arbitrary and the minimum number of inter- and intrachain disulfide bridges is indicated. The subunit chains are cleaved at their center by proteolytic enzymes as indicated. Since the product 85,000 molecular weight chain which result from the α_2M-protease interaction is observed only after reduction, it follows that this cleaved chain is apparently linked to the parent α_2M molecule by disulfide bridges.

Binding of Plasmin to α_2-Macroglobulin Subunits

The studies that have been reviewed focus on the changes which occur in the covalent structure of α_2M when this molecule interacts with proteases. A question which is under study in our laboratory regards the mechanism of the binding of the protease to the α_2M and the relationship of the protease molecule to the subunit chains of α_2M. The α_2M, plasmin interaction has proven to be a fruitful model with which to study these molecular reactions. Earlier reports in the literature have suggested that plasmin could dissociate from its plasma inhibitors when substrate was present (15,16). More recent studies have suggested that binding of a proteinase to α_2M is irreversible (17,18). In fact, radiolabeled plasmin remains bound to α_2M even in the presence of a dodecyl sulfate-urea solution (19,20).

The reaction between plasmin and α_2M was studied utilizing ^{125}I-plasmin, prepared by activating radiolabeled plasminogen with urokinase. Following incubation of the enzyme with α_2M in the approximate molar ratio of 1, the mixture was reduced with dithiothreitol in the presence of dodecyl sulfate, and then applied to dodecyl sulfate polyacrylamide gels (21). After staining of the gels with Coomassie brilliant blue, the gels were scanned in a densitometer. The gels containing the

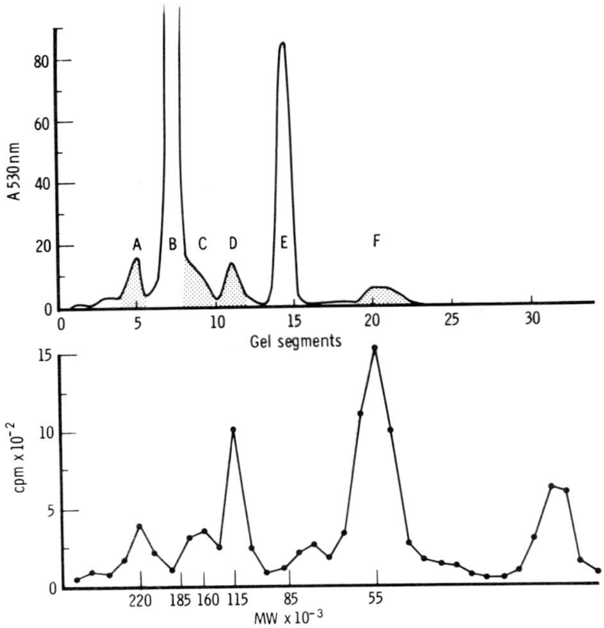

Fig. 2.

Analysis of the ^{125}I-plasmin, α_2-macroglobulin interaction by dodecyl sulfate polyacrylamide (5%) gel electrophoresis. α_2M was incubated with radiolabeled plasmin. After treatment with 2% dodecyl sulfate and 14 mM dithiothreitol at 37°C for 45 minutes, the sample was analyzed by gel electrophoresis. The stained gel was scanned in a densitometer (top panel), then sliced into segments and counted in a gamma counter (bottom panel). Shaded areas in the peaks (top panel) indicate the corresponding radioactive bands. The molecular weight of the major peaks is indicated on the abscissa. Reprinted with permission from Ref. 21.

radiolabeled plasmin were sliced into 2 mm segments and counted in a gamma counter. As shown in Fig. 2 (top panel), six Coomassie blue staining peaks, labeled A-F, were observed. The protein peaks which possessed radioactivity (A,C,D,F) are indicated in shaded areas in the top panel. The radioactivity of the sliced gels is shown in the lower panel of Fig. 2. In gels which are not shown, radiolabeled plasmin, following reduction with dithiothreitol, displayed two peaks of radioactivity consistent with its heavy chain (Mr = 55,000) and its light chain (Mr = 26,000), that contains the enzyme's catalytic site. The peak of these two chains are in gel segments 20 and 31 in the gel shown. After incubation with α_2M, a significant portion of the plasmin-associated radioactivity appears in the dodecyl sulfate gel with apparent molecular weight significantly greater than either unreduced plasmin (Mr = 75,000) or of the heavy chain of the enzyme. It is apparent that complexes have formed between α_2M polypeptide chains and plasmin chains which resist disruption by dithiothreitol and dodecyl sulfate. This suggests that the bonds which have formed are covalent.

Examination of the molecular weights of these products suggests that the light chain of plasmin has formed a complex with a 1:1 molar stoichiometry with both the 185,000 molecular weight subunit chain of α_2M (band A) as well as the 85,000 molecular weight proteolytic derivative (band D). The molecular weight of the radioactive complex band C (160,000) suggests that either a complete plasmin molecule containing both chains has formed a complex with the proteolytic derivative, or that the light chain, 185,000 molecular weight subunit complex has undergone proteolytic degradation. Further studies are in progress to clarify these reactions. In addition to these studies with plasmin, unpublished observations from our laboratory indicate that β trypsin remains in a complex with both the subunit chain as well as the proteolytic derivative of α_2M in a manner analogous to that demonstrated for plasmin. These findings do not support the entrappment theory presented by Barrett and Starkey (6) to explain the α_2M, protease reaction. This theory suggests that following cleavage of a peptide bond in the α_2M molecule by a protease, the enzyme is entrapped in the enveloping inhibitor molecule. The demonstration of a complex between the plasmin light chain and the α_2M subunit chain indicates that covalent bond formation accompanies the reaction and thus explains the irreversibility of the binding between proteases and the α_2M.

Formation of a "Macroprotease": Studies of the Effect of Acid on the α_2-Macroglobulin-Trypsin Complex

The interesting effect of acid treatment on the properties of α_2M has been outlined in this report. Dr. Hayes and I (22) have investigated the effect of a low pH on the α_2M-trypsin complex to determine if conditions could be found which might result in the release of bound trypsin from the α_2M, an unlikely possibility given the electrophoretic studies described above. Alternatively, we wished to explore whether acid treatment might unmask trypsin's proteolytic activity while the protease was still bound to the α_2M. In order to assay for alterations in the α_2M-trypsin complex as a result of acid treatment, several different properties of trypsin, α_2M, and the α_2M-trypsin complex were determined. The proteolytic activity of trypsin was measured using the particulate protein substrate Remazolbrilliant Blue Hide (RBB-Hide) according to the method of Rinderknecht et al. (23). Trypsin, when incubated at pH 3.9 and 37°C for one hour, lost very little RBB-Hide activity. α_2M completely lost its ability to protect trypsin against the action of soybean trypsin inhibitor within five minutes at pH 3.9 and 37°C. Finally, the α_2M-trypsin complex incubated at pH 8.0 and 37°C demonstrated no proteolytic activity towards RBB-Hide.

Based on these properties, experiments were designed to test for changes in the nature of the α_2M-trypsin complex as a result of alterations in pH and temperature. In Table 1, the results of an experiment testing the effect of acid treatment is presented. The complex was prepared by mixing a 1.5 molar excess of α_2M with trypsin at 4°C, incubating the solution for 3 minutes at 37°C, then cooling the mixture in an ice bath. The buffer used was 0.1 M Tris-HCl, pH 8.3 (25°C) containing 1.25 mM $CaCl_2$. Portions of the α_2M-trypsin complex were adjusted to pH 3.9 with 1.275 M acetic acid. The control complex was diluted with a volume of cold buffer similar to that of the acetic acid added. An amount of trypsin equal to that present in the complex was acid treated or kept at basic pH in an identical manner to that of the α_2M-trypsin complex. The samples were then incubated at 37° for 60 minutes and the activities measured in the absence and presence of soybean trypsin inhibitor.

As demonstrated in Table 1 the α_2M-trypsin complex maintained at basic pH had no proteolytic activity when assayed using the model protein substrate. In contrast, significant RBB-Hide hydrolyzing activity is expressed as a result of the acid treatment at 37°. Furthermore, the newly exposed RBB-Hide activity is completely abolished by soybean inhibitor. These results indicate that acid treatment of the α_2M-trypsin complex has modified the complex in such a way that the properties of trypsin seem to be intermediate between those of the untreated complex and that of free trypsin. These findings are compatible with two alternatives: 1) either acid treatment results in release of free trypsin, or 2) the newly expressed activities and susceptibility to soybean trypsin inhibitor are a result of the exposure of trypsin's catalytic site while the enzyme is still bound to α_2M.

TABLE 1 Effect of Acid Treatment on Activities of the α_2M-Trypsin Complex

	RBB-Hide Activity -SBI	+SBI
Trypsin	100%	0
α_2M-Trypsin	0	0
Acidified α_2M-Trypsin	35%	0

To test for these possibilities, gel filtration of the acid treated complex was carried out on a calibrated Sephadex G-100 superfine column. The acid treated complex was eluted in the void volume as a single peak of ultraviolet absorbing material. Since the amount of trypsin used to prepare the α_2M trypsin complex could not be detected by light absorption, an activity profile was performed using the small molecular weight trypsin substrate, BAPNA (α-N-benzoyl-D, L-arginine ρ-nitroaniline). In the absence of soybean inhibitor, the area corresponding to the elution volume of trypsin represented only 5% of the total ρ-nitroaniline production whereas the main peak contained 90% of the total. In the presence of soybean inhibitor, the small amount of free trypsin was totally inhibited while there was 68% inhibition of the main peak.

These results indicate that the α_2M-trypsin complex, when incubated in an acid milieu is modified so that an entity is produced which must be regarded as a macroprotease. Dr. Hayes and I have defined a macroprotease as a modified inhibitor-protease complex capable of hydrolyzing protein substrates to which it was refractory prior to an alteration in its physical structure. In studies not detailed in this chapter, the stability of the α_2M-bound trypsin, following acid treatment, was greater than that of free trypsin. The tryptic activity of the acid modified complex was relatively unaffected by both prolonged incubation at basic pH and elevated temperature whereas the activity of free trypsin decayed rapidly under these conditions. These considerations raise the possibility that such α_2M-enzyme complexes may be modified in vivo by an acid environment at sites of inflammation or within cells so that the proteolytic activity of the bound protease is expressed in the organism.

Fragmentation of α_2-Macroglobulin

The following studies detail a phenomenon that has recently been observed in our laboratory (22) and that contributes to our knowledge regarding the covalent structure of α_2M. As reviewed in this report, when α_2M is incubated in the presence of dodecyl sulfate and a disulfide bond cleaving agent at neutral pH for 45 minutes at 37°C, one major polypeptide chain (Mr = 185,000) is identified when analyzed by dodecyl sulfate polyacrylamide gel electrophoresis. We have observed that a variety of experimental conditions induce a time dependent decrease in the 185,000 molecular weight subunit chain of α_2M in association with the progressive generation of two new polypeptide chains, termed bands II and III, whose apparent molecular weights are 125,000 and 62,000 respectively. This fragmentation of the α_2M subunit chain is illustrated in Fig. 3.

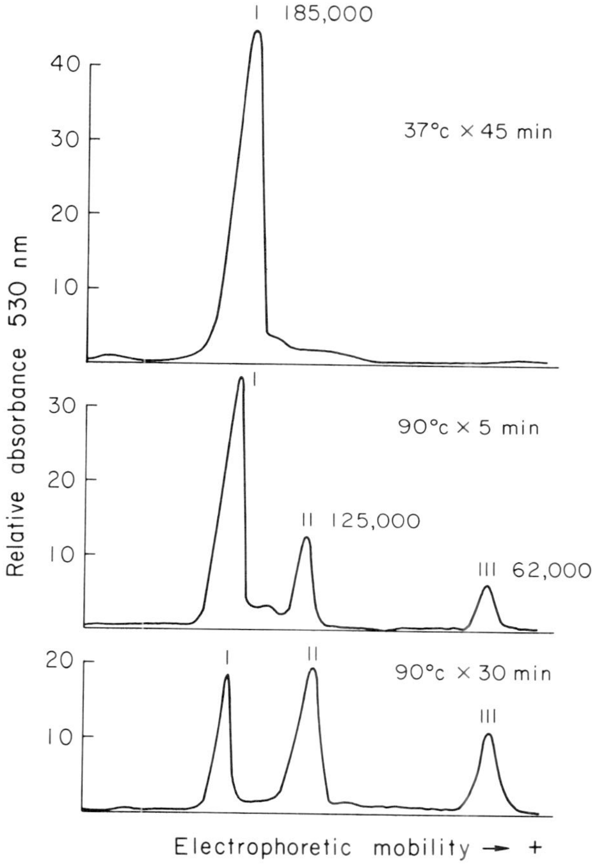

Fig. 3.

Fragmentation of the subunit chain of α_2M as illustrated by densitometric scans of dodecyl sulfate polyarcylamide (5%) gels. α_2M was incubated with dodecyl sulfate and dithiothreitol at 37°C for 45 minutes (top panel), 90°C for 5 minutes (middle panel), or for 30 minutes (bottom panel). The apparent molecular weights of the three peaks (bands I, II, and III) are indicated. The electrophoresis is from left to right. Reprinted with permission from Ref. 21.

In this experiment α_2M was mixed with 1% dodecyl sulfate, 14 mM dithiothreitol in 0.02 M sodium phosphate buffer at pH 7.0. Portions of this mixture were incubated at 37°C for 45 minutes, or at 90°C for 5 or 30 minutes. These solutions were then analyzed by dodecyl sulfate gel electrophoresis and the stained gels were scanned in a densitometer. The α_2M treated at 90° fragmented into band II and III material. The amount of bands II and III generated increased between 5 and 30 minutes of heating in a boiling water bath. Comparison of the area of each peak in Fig. 3 demonstrated that the band III polypeptide chain represented approximately 50% of the area of peak II indicating that band I fragments directly into the two new products whose combined molecular weight (187,000) is equivalent to that of the parent subunit chain. Reduction of disulfide chains was a requirement for the generation of bands II and III, since in the absence of dithiothreitol, these bands were not observed.

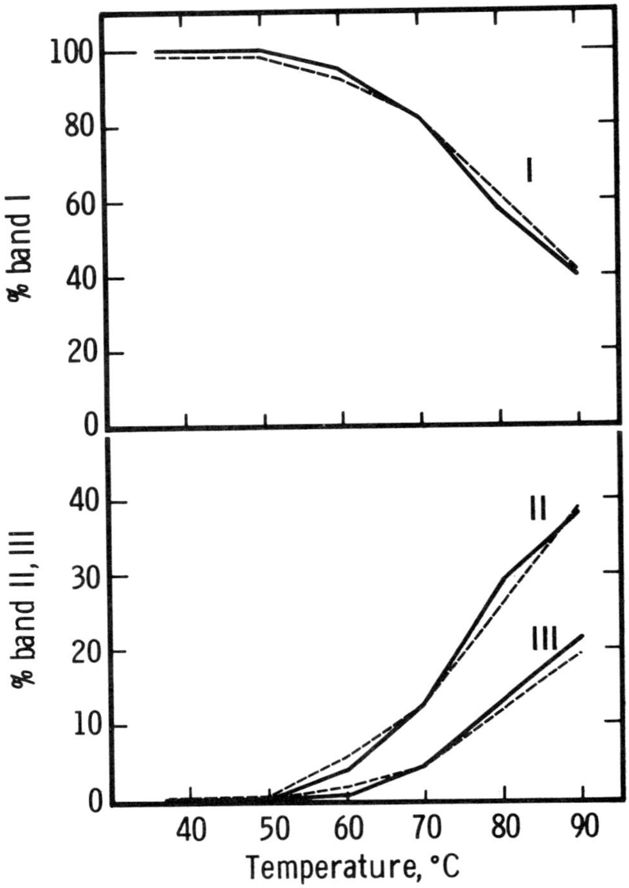

Fig. 4.

Effect of temperature on α_2M subunit structure. A mixture of radiolabeled and native α_2M was incubated with dodecyl sulfate and dithiothreitol at pH 7.0 for 30 minutes at the temperatures indicated. After dodecyl sulfate gel electrophoresis, the stained gels were scanned at 550 nm and the area of each peak expressed as a percent of the sum of peaks I, II and III. The gels were cut and the radioactivity quantitated in a γ counter. The radioactivity of each peak was expressed as the sum of all three peaks. The solid lines represent the scanned peaks and the dashed lines, the radioactive peaks.

Prolonged heating, in excess of the 30 minute period indicated in Fig. 3, caused a progressive loss in both band I and II material indicating that additional fragmentation had occurred. Band II and III material was also generated at room temperature by prolonged incubation of α_2M under denaturing and reducing conditions. A variety of experimental conditions were designed to establish those parameters which effected the fragmentation of the subunit chain. The effect of alteration of temperature is illustrated in Fig. 4.

A mixture of native and ^{125}I-labeled α_2M was incubated at pH 7.0 with dodecyl sulfate and dithiothreitol for 30 minutes at six different temperatures (37, 50, 60, 70, 80, 90°C). After dodecyl sulfate gel electrophoresis, the stained gels were scanned and the areas under the three major peaks determined by densitometry. The gels were then sliced into 2 mm segments and the radioactivity counted in a gamma counter. Band II and III were first identified as the temperature of the mixture was raised to 60°C. Thereafter there was a decrease in band I material and a progressive increase in the product bands II and III. The radioactivity which accompanied the stained bands exactly paralleled the densitometric data and confirmed the validity of the scanning results.

In addition to the effect of heat on accelerating the production of bands II and III, alteration in the pH of the incubation mixture above pH 8.0, enhanced the fragmentation of the band I subunit chain. Changes in ionic strength over a five fold range, dodecyl sulfate concentration or in α_2M concentration failed to influence the heat-induced generation of bands II and III. The α_2M fragments could also be generated in the absence of dodecyl sulfate. Radioiodinated α_2M was incubated at 90°C in 6 M quanidine-HCl at pH 9.0, with 0.05% β-mercaptoethanol and applied to a Sephadex CL-6B column equilibrated with the same buffer. The elution profile demonstrated three radioactive peaks which when analyzed by dodecyl sulfate gel electrophoresis were identified as corresponding to bands I, II and III.

Examination of the ^{125}I-labelled tryptic peptide digests obtained from bands I, II and III respectively, by the method of Elder et al. (24), have clarified the relationship of these three polypeptide chains. The findings, to be reported in detail elsewhere, demonstrate that bands II and III have peptide maps which are entirely unrelated. A mixture of the tryptic digest of bands II plus III produces a peptide map indistinguishable from the map of band I. These experiments support the data obtained in gel scanning experiments and indicate that bands II and III are the result of asymmetric fragmentation of the α_2M subunit chain.

Of great interest was the relationship of bands II and III to the 85,000 molecular weight proteolytic derivative that results when α_2M reacts with proteases. To assess the effect of the trypsin, α_2M interaction on the subsequent generation of bands II and III, increasing concentrations of trypsin were incubated with a mixture of native and radiolabelled α_2M (Fig. 5). The mixtures were then heated at 90°C for 30 minutes with dodecyl sulfate and dithiothreitol and applied to dodecyl sulfate gels. The gels were sliced into segments and counted in a gamma counter. In the control mixture consisting of α_2M and buffer (Fig. 5, top panel) radiolabeled bands I, II, and III can be appreciated. Increasing amounts of trypsin (middle and lower panel) induced a progressive increase in the 85,000 molecular weight proteolytic derivative (labeled PD in the Fig.) that was accompanied by a parallel decrease in material at the band I, II and III position. These results are consistent with the thesis that as the band I, 185,000 molecular weight subunit chain of α_2M is cleaved by trypsin there is less band I material for heat-accelerated fragmentation into the bands II and III. In Fig. 5, radioactive material possessing an electrophoretic mobility slower than that of band I, can be identified in the trypsin, α_2M incubation mixtures. These higher molecular weight components were found to represent complexes between trypsin and the 185,000 molecular weight chain of α_2M.

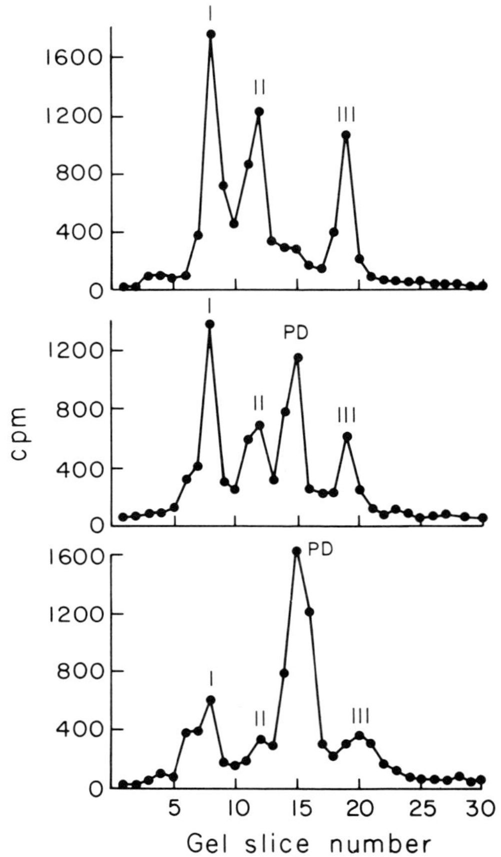

Fig. 5.

Effect of the trypsin, α_2M interaction on the generation of α_2M fragments II and III. A mixture of ^{125}I-α_2M and native α_2M was incubated with buffer (top panel), or with bovine trypsin in the trypsin/α_2M molar ratio of 0.5 (middle panel) or 1.0 (lower panel) at 37°C for 5 min. The samples were then treated with 2% dodecyl sulfate and 14 mM dithiothreitol at 90°C for 30 minutes and analyzed by dodecyl sulfate polyacrylamide gel (5%) electrophoresis. The gels were sliced in 2.0 mm segments and counted in a gamma counter. Reprinted with permission from Ref. 21.

These results indicate that bands II and III do not represent true subunits of α_2M since they clearly did not exist prior to incubation of α_2M with trypsin. How then, is the cleavage of the α_2M subunit chain accomplished? It is unlikely that enzyme catalyzed proteolysis of the denatured α_2M by an accompanying protease as has been described for both hexokinase and thyroglobulin (25-27) is responsible for our observations. Several arguments against such a mechanism are provided by our studies. Heating at 90°C for 5 minutes in the presence of dodecyl sulfate and the potent reducing agent, dithiothreitol, should have inactivated any contaminating proteases (25). Bands II and III, however, were found to increase in concentration between 5 and 30 minutes of incubation at 90°C (Fig. 3). In addition, in studies not detailed here, a number of protease inhibitors including DFP, benzamidine, pepstatin, iodoacetamide, or 0-phenanthroline failed to inhibit the heat-induced fragmentation of α_2M.

Our results are consistent with the thesis that a bond exists in the α_2M which is uniquely susceptible to thermal induced hydrolysis, and that following the action of trypsin in cleaving the 185,000 molecular weight subunit chain, the putative covalent bond is no longer susceptible to hydrolysis. Thus, the α_2M may be relatively unique in its susceptibility to heat-induced fragmentation since Deutsch has shown that the covalent structure of eight proteins was not altered by treatment in dodecyl sulfate and a reducing agent for 30 minutes (28).

α_2-Macroglobulin, Lymphocytes, and Platelets

The relationship of α_2M to cell surface represents a new and fascinating area in α_2M research. McCormick et al. (29) first identified α_2M as a surface antigen of both human and murine B lymphocytes. Many of the lymphocytes, presumably of the B type, from patients with chronic lymphocytic leukemia have α_2M on their surface (30). The presence of α_2M on the lymphocyte surface may not be related to adsorption from the plasma. Gelder et al. (31) have reported that α_2M is resynthesized on the lymphocyte surface after proteolytic digestion of the membrane proteins. Tunstall and James (32) have presented preliminary studies which also suggest that α_2M is synthesized by the circulating lymphocyte.

Nachman and I (33) have demonstrated that membrane and granule fractions derived from human platelets contain immunologically identifiable α_2M as well as α_1-antitrypsin. For the purpose of this review, I will consider only the data that pertains to the α_2M. The platelets were washed extensively prior to homogenization, and the final wash which was concentrated 100-fold by ultrafiltration contained no α_2M as assayed by immunodiffusion analysis. The platelet subcellular fractions were obtained as has been detailed in the presence of proteolytic enzyme inhibitors, and solubilized in Lubrol PX solution. The soluble membrane or granule preparations were further fractionated by ammonium sulfate. Four different subfractions were obtained from each (0 to 30, 30 to 50, 50 to 80, and greater than 80% saturation with ammonium sulfate). By immunodiffusion analysis, α_2M was identified in both the membrane and granule fractions in the 30 to 50% ammonium sulfate precipitate. The α_2M was not detected in other fractions or in the platelet cytosol.

The platelet-derived α_2M showed a reaction of immunologic identity when compared to α_2M purified from plasma. Furthermore, the α_2M from both the membrane and granule fraction possessed a similar subunit polypeptide chain structure to purified α_2M as determined by dodecyl sulfate gel electrophoresis. The 185,000 molecular weight chain was intact in the platelet α_2M and no 85,000 molecular weight derivative was observed indicating that the platelet α_2M had not previously interacted with a protease. Confirmation that the platelet α_2M was functionally active was obtained by determining the binding of ^{125}I-trypsin to the α_2M containing fractions using sucrose density gradient ultracentrifugation. The radiolabeled trypsin formed a complex with the α_2M obtained from both platelet membrane and granule fractions.

Quantitation of the amount of α_2M in the platelet by electroimmunoassay indicated that the amount of this protein is quite small compared to the amount present in platelet-poor plasma. The platelets in one ml of blood contain approximately 1/2500 of the α_2M present in one ml of platelet-poor plasma. The function of the α_2M in platelets is unknown. The possibility exists that the α_2M may modulate the activity of several different proteases in environments where platelets are highly concentrated, such as in platelet hemostatic plugs and in thrombi.

α_2-Macroglobulin on Human Vascular Endothelium

Becker and I have demonstrated by the indirect immunofluorescent technique that α_2M antigen is located on the endothelial surface of human blood vessels and lymphatics (34). In these studies tissues were obtained at autopsy or immediately after surgical removal. Frozen sections were cut from the tissues which had been embedded in gelatin prior to freezing. The tissue sections on glass slides were washed extensively following which a drop of rabbit anti-human α_2M, normal rabbit serum or rabbit anti-human α_2M previously absorbed with purified α_2M was applied. Rabbit antisera to other human proteins were also tested. After incubation in a moist chamber at 37°C for 30 minutes, the antisera was washed in three changes of buffer and a drop of fluoresceinated goat anti-rabbit IgG was applied. After a second incubation and washing, the slides were examined by immunofluorescence microscopy. The tissues examined by this technique included medium sized branches of the external mammary artery, mesenteric artery, liver with an intrahepatic vein and a lymphatic vessel adjacent to the mesenteric artery.

A thin, continuous band of yellow-green immunofluorescence was observed on the luminal surface of endothelial cells when sections of human blood vessels and lymphatics were treated as detailed. The α_2M appeared to localize to the glycocalyx of the endothelial cells since there appeared to be very little staining of the cytoplasm. No immunofluorescence was associated with the basement membrane beneath endothelial cells, elastic lamina and myointimal and medial smooth muscle cells of arteries, smooth muscle cells of veins, and connective tissue surrounding blood and lymphatic vessels.

Sections of human liver, when treated with rabbit anti-human α_2M, followed by the fluoresceinated goat anti-rabbit IgG, demonstrated immunofluorescence in hepatic parenchymal cells as well as the surfaces of endothelial cells lining arteries, veins and the sinusoids. In sections of human kidney, the endothelial surface of the blood vessels contained the α_2M antigen whereas the renal tubular epithelium was not stained.

Specificity of the staining was confirmed by prior absorption at equivalence of anti-α_2M serum with purified α_2M. In addition, pooled normal rabbit serum failed to stain the vessel wall when followed by the fluoresceinated antibody. Of especial significance was the plasma proteins which were not identified on the blood vessel wall. Neither antiserum directed against antithrombin III nor against α_1-antitrypsin reacted with any components of the tissue sections examined. Since the plasma concentration of α_1-antitrypsin is approximately 45 µM as compared with 3.5 µM for α_2M, the lack of α_1-antitrypsin on the vessel wall argues strongly for the specificity of the endothelial surface, α_2M interaction. In other words, it is likely that the α_2M is associated with the endothelial surface in a specific manner and not as a result of passive absorption that might have occurred during tissue processing. Other proteins that were not found on the vessel wall include IgG, IgA, IgM, C3 or fibrinogen.

The location of α_2M on the luminal surface of endothelial cells in sections of normal human arteries, veins and lymphatics suggests that this protein may play an important role in the physiology of the blood vessel wall. Since the α_2M is capable of modulating the activity of many different proteases, it is tempting to speculate that the α_2M protects the endothelium against potentially injurious plasma and cellular enzymes which are activated adjacent to the vessel wall during inflammatory and hemostatic events. Alternatively, the α_2M may be binding directly to endothelial cell surface oriented proteases. Finally, it is also possible that α_2M, enzyme complexes formed *in vivo* may bind to receptors on the endothelial cell surface, as has been detailed for the binding of such complexes to macrophages (35).

Biologic Role of α_2-Macroglobulin

In this chapter we have reviewed some recent advances regarding the structure of α_2M and the manner in which it reacts with proteases. The role of this interesting protein in human physiology remains poorly defined. This is due in part to the fact that no inherited deficiency of α_2M in humans has yet been described. In contrast, clues as to the function of α_1-antitrypsin, $C\bar{1}$ inactivator and antithrombin-heparin cofactor have been provided by the study of individuals with inherited deficiencies of these proteins (c.f. reviews by Drs. Laurell, Donaldson and Rosenberg in this symposium).

It seems reasonable to postulate that a major role of the α_2M is to protect the organism from protease mediated injury. Once a complex has been formed between the enzyme and α_2M in the plasma, the complex appears to be removed rapidly from the circulation (7), probably by tissue macrophages (35,36). The α_2M-enzyme complex may itself possess important biological activity. Several investigations have established that the enzyme bound to the α_2M possesses a portion of the biological activity of the free protease. Thus, α_2M purified from plasma degrades fibrinogen in a manner similar to plasmin (37). Rinderknecht and Geokas (38) have provided experimental data that α_2M purified from serum and presumably being complexed with thrombin was able to clot a fibrinogen solution. Largman and coworkers (*Nature* 269, 168, 1977) have also demonstrated that the α_2M-trypsin complex can convert proinsulin to active desalanyl insulin. These considerations suggest that the binding of an enzyme to α_2M provides an additional mechanism whereby certain proteases can express their activity in a highly restricted manner *in vivo*.

Acknowledgement

The investigations by the author which are cited in this chapter were supported in part by U.S. Public Health Service grant HL-18828 (Specialized Center of Research in Thrombosis) and by a grant from the Cystic Fibrosis Foundation. The author extends special thanks to Ms. Susan Anderson for her expert secretarial assistance.

REFERENCES

1. H.E. Schultze, I. Göllner, K. Heide, et al, Zur kenntnis der α-globuline des menschlichen normalserums, *Z. Naturforsch* Teil B 10, 463 (1955).

2. H.J. Müller-Eberhard, H.G. Kunkel, E.C. Franklin, Two types of γ-globulins differing in carbohydrate content, *Proc. Soc. Exp. Biol. Med.* 93, 146 (1956).

3. G. Wallenius, R.T. Trautman, H.G. Kunkel, E.C. Franklin, Ultracentrifugal studies of major non-lipid electrophoretic components of normal human serum, *J. Biol. Chem.* 225, 253 (1957).

4. B.J. Haverback, B. Dyce, H.F. Bundy, et al, Protein binding of pancreatic proteolytic enzymes, *J. Clin. Invest.* 41, 972 (1962).

5. J.W. Mehl, W. O'Connell, J. DeGroot, Macroglobulin from human plasma which forms an enzymatically active compound with trypsin, *Science* 145, 821 (1964).

6. A.J. Barrett, P.M. Starkey, The interaction of α_2-macroglobulin with proteinases, Biochem. J. 133, 709 (1973).

7. P.C. Harpel, R.D. Rosenberg, α_2-macroglobulin and antithrombin-heparin cofactor modulators of hemostatic and inflammatory reactions, In Progress in Hemostasis and Thrombosis. T.H. Spaet, editor, Grune & Stratton, Inc., New York 3, 145 (1976).

8. P.C. Harpel, Human α_2-macroglobulin, In Methods in Enzymology, Proteolytic Enzymes. L. Lorand, editor, Academic Press, New York 45, 639 (1976).

9. P.M. Starkey, A.J. Barrett, α_2-macroglobulin, a physiologic regulator of proteinase activity, In Proteinases in Mammalian Cells and Tissues. A.J. Barrett, editor, Elsevier North-Holland, Amsterdam 663 (1977).

10. P.K. Hall, R.C. Roberts, Physical and chemical properties of human plasma α_2-macroglobulin, Biochem. J. (London) 171, 27 (1978).

11. C. Gentou, Structure quaternaire des α_2-macroglobulines humaines normales, C.R. Acad. Sci. 266, 2358 (1968).

12. J.M. Jones, J.M. Creeth, R.A. Kekwick, Thiol reduction of human α_2-macroglobuli The subunit structure, Biochem. J. (London) 127, 187 (1972).

13. P.C. Harpel, Studies on human plasma α_2-macroglobulin-enzyme interactions. Evidence for proteolytic modification of the subunit chain structure, J. Exp. Med. 138, 508 (1973).

14. A.J. Barrett, P.M. Starkey, E.A. Munn, The unique nature of the interaction of α_2-macroglobulin with proteinases, In Bayer Symposium V Proteinase Inhibitor H. Fritz, H. Tschesche, L.J. Greene, editors, Springer-Verlag, Berlin 72 (1974

15. P.S. Norman, B.M. Hill, Studies of the plasmin system. III. Physical propertie of two plasmin inhibitors in plasma, J. Exp. Med. 108, 639 (1958).

16. C.M. Ambrus, G. Markus, Plasmin-antiplasmin complex as a reservoir of fibrinolytic enzyme, Amer. J. Physiol. 199, 491 (1960).

17. R. Saunders, B.J. Dyce, W.E. Vannier, B.J. Haverback, The separation of alpha 2-macroglobulin into five components with differing electrophoretic and enzyme-binding properties, J. Clin. Invest. 50, 2376 (1971).

18. S. Abe, Y. Nagai, Interaction between tadpole collagenase and human α_2 macroglobulin, Biochim. Biophys. Acta 278, 125 (1972).

19. P.C. Harpel, Relative affinity of plasmin for the α_2-macroglobulin, $C\bar{1}$ inactivat and α_1-antitrypsin inhibitors, Fed. Proc. 34, 344 (1974).

20. M. Steinbuch, R. Audran, P. Lambin, J.M. Fine, Subunit structure of human alpha 2-macroglobulin. Its relationship with its biological activity, In Protides of the Biological Fluids. H. Peeters, editor, Elsevier, Amsterdam, 133 (1975).

21. P.C. Harpel, M.B. Hayes, Studies on the subunit structure of α_2-macroglobulin, In The Physiological Inhibitors of Blood Coagulation and Fibrinolysis. D. Colle B. Wiman, M. Verstraete, editors, Elsevier (1979).

22. M.B. Hayes, P.C. Harpel, The effect of acid on the α_2-macroglobulin-trypsin complex, In The Physiological Inhibitors of Blood Coagulation and Fibrinolysis. D. Collen, B. Wiman, M. Verstraete, editors, in press, Elsevier/North Holland Press, Amsterdam (1979).

23. H. Rinderknecht, M.C. Geokas, P. Silverman, B.J. Haverback, Determination of trypsin and chymotrypsin with remazolbrilliant blue-hide, Clin. Chim. Acta 28, 239 (1970).

24. J.H. Elder, R.A. Pickett, J. Hampton, R.A. Lerner, Radioiodination of proteins in single polyacrylamide gel slices. Tryptic peptide analysis of all the major members of complex multicomponent systems using microgram quantities of total protein, J. Biol. Chem. 252, 6510 (1977).

25. J.R. Pringle, The molecular weight of the undegraded polypeptide chain of yeast hexokinase, Biochem. Biophys. Res. Commun. 39, 46 (1970).

26. R. Pitt-Rivers, Molecular Mechanisms and Regulation of Thyroid Hormone Biosynthesis, Academia Nazionale dei Lincei, Roma 1, 47 (1975).

27. M. Rolland, S. Lissitzky, Endogenous proteolytic activity and constituent polypeptide chains of sheep and pig 19S thyroglobulin, Biochim. Biophys. Acta 427, 696 (1976).

28. D.G. Deutsch, Effect of prolonged 100°C heat treatment in sodium dodecyl sulfate upon peptide bond cleavage, Anal. Biochem. 71, 300 (1976).

29. J.N. McCormick, D. Nelson, A.M. Tunstall, K. James, Association of α_2-macroglobulins with lymphoid cells, Nature New Biology 246, 78 (1973).

30. K. James, A.M. Tunstall, A.C. Parker et al, The association of alpha 2-macroglobulin with lymphocyte membranes in chronic lymphocytic leukaemia and other disorders, Clin. Exp. Immunol. 19, 237 (1975).

31. F. Gelder, P. Hurtubise, J. Scillian et al, The association of α_2-macroglobulin with the Fc receptor on B lymphocytes, Clin. Res. 23, 291A (1975).

32. A.M. Tunstall, K. James, Preliminary studies on the synthesis of alpha 2-macroglobulin by human lymphocytes in vitro, Clin. Exp. Immunol. 17, 697 (1974).

33. R.L. Nachman, P.C. Harpel, Platelet α_2-macroglobulin and α_1-antitrypsin, J. Biol. Chem. 251, 4514 (1976).

34. C. Becker, P.C. Harpel, α_2-Macroglobulin on human vascular endothelium, J. Exp. Med. 144, 1 (1976).

35. M.T. Debanne, R. Bell, J. Dolovich, Characteristics of the macrophage uptake of proteinase-α-macroglobulin complexes, Biochim. Biophys. Acta 428, 466 (1976).

36. K. Ohlsson, Elimination of ^{125}I-trypsin α-macroglobulin complexes from blood by reticuloendothelial cells in dog, Acta Physiol. Scand. 81, 269 (1971).

37. P.C. Harpel, M.W. Mosesson, Degradation of human fibrinogen by plasma α_2-macroglobulin-enzyme complexes, J. Clin. Invest. 52, 2175 (1973).

38. H. Rinderknecht, M.C. Geokas, On the physiological role of α_2-macroglobulin, Biochim. Biophys. Acta 295, 233 (1973).

INDEX